T0140373

Current Clinical Neurology

Series Editor

Daniel Tarsy, MD
Department of Neurology
Beth Israel Deaconness Hospital
Boston, MA
USA

More information about this series at http://www.springer.com/series/7630

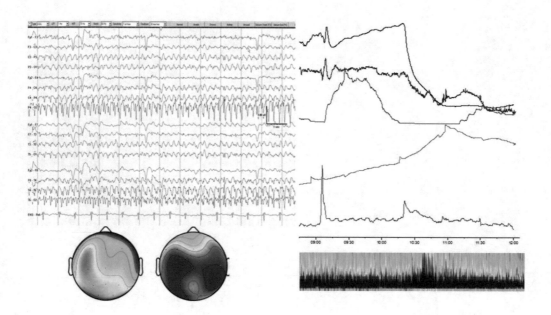

Panayiotis N. Varelas • Jan Claassen

Editors

Seizures in Critical Care

A Guide to Diagnosis and Therapeutics

Third Edition

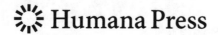 Humana Press

Editors
Panayiotis N. Varelas, MD, PhD, FNCS
Departments of Neurology and Neurosurgery
Henry Ford Hospital
Detroit, MI, USA

Department of Neurology
Wayne State University
Detroit, MI, USA

Jan Claassen, MD, Ph.D, FNCS
Neurocritical Care
Columbia University College of Physicians
   & Surgeons
New York, NY, USA

Division of Critical Care and Hospitalist
   Neurology
Department of Neurology
Columbia

University Medical Center
New York Presbyterian Hospital
New York, NY, USA

Current Clinical Neurology
ISBN 978-3-319-84187-8   ISBN 978-3-319-49557-6 (eBook)
DOI 10.1007/978-3-319-49557-6

Printed on acid-free paper

This Humana Press imprint is published by Springer Nature
The registered company is Springer International Publishing AG
The registered company address is: Gewerbestrasse 11, 6330 Cham, Switzerland

Series Editor Introduction

The first two editions of *Seizures in Critical Care: A Guide to Diagnosis and Therapeutics* were published in 2005 and 2010. Both of these volumes provided much needed support for medical, neurological, and neurosurgical intensive care specialists who deal with critically ill patients who suffer seizures in the ICU setting. At one time seizures, especially of the nonconvulsive type, were quite often poorly recognized in unresponsive ICU patients. This situation has certainly been remedied over the past couple of decades, due in large part to the wealth of information summarized in these volumes. As stated in my introductions to the first two volumes, seizures in ICU patients are typically secondary phenomena indicative of underlying medical and neurological complications in individuals with serious medical and surgical illness. Rapid identification of the cause of these seizures, analysis of various contributing factors, and providing appropriate and rapid management and treatment are crucial to the survival of these patients. Dr. Varelas, together with his co-editor Dr. Jan Claasen, has now recruited a larger number of new experts in various aspects of the field in order to provide additional information concerning basic pathophysiology as learned both from animal models and from new clinical technologies such as quantitative EEG and multimodal monitoring which have improved the care of these patients. New clinical chapters in this third edition include an overview of the management of critical care seizures which is then followed by a series of chapters on the many clinical situations in which seizures occur in the ICU. Many of these appeared in the earlier volumes but have been updated with several of these written by newly recruited authors. These issues are all addressed in great depth and with much sophistication by the very impressive array of contributors to this volume.

Boston, MA, USA   Daniel Tarsy, MD

Contents

Contributors

Nicholas S. Abend Department of Neurology and Pediatrics, Children's Hospital of Philadelphia and Perelman School of Medicine, University of Pennsylvania, Philadelphia, PA, USA

Edilberto Amorim Department of Neurology, Harvard Medical School, Massachusetts General Hospital, Boston, MA, USA

Andrew Beaumont Department of Neurosurgery, Aspirus Spine and Neuroscience Institute, Aspirus Wausau Hospital, Wausau, WI, USA

Siddharth Biswal Department of Neurology, Harvard Medical School, Massachusetts General Hospital, Boston, MA, USA

Thomas P. Bleck Department of Neurological Sciences, Neurosurgery, Anesthesiology, and Medicine, Rush Medical College, Chicago, IL, USA

James W.Y. Chen Department of Neurology, VA Greater Los Angeles Health Care System, Los Angeles, CA, USA

Jan Claassen Neurocritical Care, Columbia University College of Physicians and Surgeons, New York, NY, USA

Division of Critical Care and Hospitalist Neurology, Department of Neurology, Columbia University Medical Center, New York Presbyterian Hospital, New York, NY, USA

Jens P. Dreier Center for Stroke Research Berlin, Charité University Medicine Berlin, Berlin, Germany

Department of Neurology, Charité University Medicine Berlin, Berlin, Germany

Department of Experimental Neurology, Charité University Medicine Berlin, Berlin, Germany

Iván Sánchez Fernández Division of Epilepsy and Clinical Neurophysiology, Department of Neurology, Boston Children's Hospital, Harvard Medical School, Boston, MA, USA

Department of Child Neurology, Hospital Sant Joan de Déu, University of Barcelona, Barcelona, Spain

Brandon Foreman University of Cincinnati Medical Center, Cincinnati, OH, USA

Department of Neurology and Rehabilitation Medicine, University of Cincinnati, Cincinnati, OH, USA

Hans-Peter Frey Division of Critical Care and Hospitalist Neurology, Department of Neurology, Columbia University Medical Center, New York Presbyterian Hospital, New York, NY, USA

Daniel Friedman Comprehensive Epilepsy Center, Department of Neurology, New York University, New York, NY, USA

Nicolas Gaspard Service de Neurologie–Centre de Référence pour le Traitement de l'Epilepsie Réfractaire, Université Libre de Bruxelles–Hôpital Erasme, Bruxelles, Belgium

Department of Neurology, Comprehensive Epilepsy Center, Yale University School of Medicine, New Haven, CT, USA

Romergryko Geocadin Department of Neurology, Johns Hopkins University School of Medicine, Baltimore, MD, USA

Department of Anesthesiology and Critical Care Medicine, Johns Hopkins University School of Medicine, Baltimore, MD, USA

Lotfi Hacein-Bey Sutter Imaging Division, Interventional and Diagnostic Neuroradiology, Sacramento, CA, USA

Radiology Department, UC Davis School of Medicine, Sacramento, CA, USA

Jed A. Hartings Department of Neurosurgery, University of Cincinnati College of Medicine, Cincinnati, OH, USA

Mayfield Clinic, Cincinnati, OH, USA

Uwe Heinemann Neuroscience Research Center, Charité University Medicine Berlin, Berlin, Germany

Lawrence J. Hirsch Comprehensive Epilepsy Center, Department of Neurology, Yale University, New Haven, CT, USA

Sara Hocker Division of Critical Care Neurology, Mayo Clinic, Rochester, MN, USA

Aatif M. Husain Department of Neurology, Duke University Medical Center, Durham, NC, USA

Neurodiagnostic Center, Department of Veterans Affairs Medical Center, Durham, NC, USA

Inna Keselman Department of Neurology, David Geffen School of Medicine at UCLA, Los Angeles, CA, USA

Department of Neurology, VA Greater Los Angeles Health Care System, Los Angeles, CA, USA

Jennifer A. Kim Department of Neurology, Harvard Medical School, Massachusetts General Hospital, Boston, MA, USA

Matthew A. Koenig Neuroscience Institute, The Queens Medical Center, Honolulu, HI, USA

Lauren Koffman Department of Neurology, Johns Hopkins University School of Medicine, Baltimore, MD, USA

Department of Anesthesiology and Critical Care Medicine, Johns Hopkins University School of Medicine, Baltimore, MD, USA

Georgia Korbakis Department of Neurosurgery, UCLA David Geffen School of Medicine, Los Angeles, CA, USA

Tobias Loddenkemper Division of Epilepsy and Clinical Neurophysiology, Department of Neurology, Boston Children's Hospital, Harvard Medical School, Boston, MA, USA

Andreas Luft Department of Vascular Neurology and Rehabilitation, University Hospital of Zurich, Zurich, Switzerland

Julian Macedo University of Cincinnati Medical Center, Cincinnati, OH, USA

Ali Mahta Division of Neurological Intensive Care, Department of Neurology, Columbia University College of Physicians and Surgeon, New York, NY, USA

Sebastian Major Center for Stroke Research Berlin, Charité University Medicine Berlin, Berlin, Germany

Department of Neurology, Charité University Medicine Berlin, Berlin, Germany

Department of Experimental Neurology, Charité University Medicine Berlin, Berlin, Germany

Maggie L. McNulty Department of Neurological Sciences, Rush Medical College, Rush University Medical Center, Chicago, IL, USA

Chandan Mehta Departments of Neurology and Neurosurgery, K-11, Henry Ford Hospital, Detroit, MI, USA

Nicholas A. Morris Division of Critical Care and Hospitalist Neurology, Department of Neurology, Columbia University Medical Center, New York Presbyterian Hospital, New York, NY, USA

Lidia M.V.R. Moura Department of Neurology, Harvard Medical School, Massachusetts General Hospital, Boston, MA, USA

Deena M. Nasr Department of Neurology, Mayo Clinic, Rochester, MN, USA

Barnett R. Nathan Division of Neurocritical Care, Department of Neurology, University of Virginia, Charlottesville, VA, USA

Jerome Niquet Department of Neurology, David Geffen School of Medicine at UCLA, Los Angeles, CA, USA

Department of Neurology, VA Greater Los Angeles Health Care System, Los Angeles, CA, USA

Gamaleldin Osman Comprehensive Epilepsy Center, Department of Neurology, Yale University, New Haven, CT, USA

Department of Neurology and Psychiatry, Ain Shams University, Cairo, Egypt

Mohammed Rehman Departments of Neurology and Neurosurgery, K-11, Henry Ford Hospital, Detroit, MI, USA

Gajanan S. Revankar Center for Stroke Research Berlin, Charité University Medicine Berlin, Berlin, Germany

Denise H. Rhoney Division of Practice Advancement and Clinical Education, UNC Eshelman School of Pharmacy, Chapel Hill, NC, USA

David Roh Division of Critical Care and Hospitalist Neurology, Department of Neurology, Columbia University Medical Center, New York Presbyterian Hospital, New York, NY, USA

Karl Schoknecht Center for Stroke Research Berlin, Charité University Medicine Berlin, Berlin, Germany

Department of Neurology, Charité University Medicine Berlin, Berlin, Germany

Neuroscience Research Center, Charité University Medicine, Berlin, Germany

Andrew C. Schomer Division of Neurocritical Care, Department of Neurology, University of Virginia, Charlottesville, VA, USA

Claudine Sculier Service de Neurologie–Centre de Référence pour le Traitement de l'Epilepsie Réfractaire, Université Libre de Bruxelles–Hôpital Erasme, Bruxelles, Belgium

Greene Shepherd Division of Practice Advancement and Clinical Education, UNC Eshelman School of Pharmacy, Asheville, NC, USA

Marianna V. Spanaki Henry Ford Hospital, Detroit, MI, USA

Wayne State University, Detroit, MI, USA

Jose Ignacio Suarez Baylor College of Medicine, Houston, TX, USA

Christa B. Swisher Department of Neurology, Duke University Medical Center, Durham, NC, USA

Michel T. Torbey Neurology and Neurosurgery Department, Cerebrovascular and Neurocritical Care Division, The Ohio State University College of Medicine, Columbus, OH, USA

Panayiotis N. Varelas Departments of Neurology and Neurosurgery, Henry Ford Hospital, Detroit, MI, USA

Department of Neurology, Wayne State University, Detroit, MI, USA

Paul M. Vespa Department of Neurosurgery, UCLA David Geffen School of Medicine, Los Angeles, CA, USA

Claude G. Wasterlain Department of Neurology, VA Greater Los Angeles Health Care System, Los Angeles, CA, USA

M. Brandon Westover Department of Neurology, Harvard Medical School, Massachusetts General Hospital, Boston, MA, USA

Eelco F.M. Wijdicks Division of Critical Care Neurology, Mayo Clinic, Rochester, MN, USA

Craig Williamson Department of Neurology and Neurological Surgery, University of Michigan, University Hospital, Ann Arbor, MI, USA

Maren K.L. Winkler Center for Stroke Research Berlin, Charité University Medicine Berlin, Berlin, Germany

Jens Witsch Division of Critical Care and Hospitalist Neurology, Department of Neurology, Columbia University Medical Center, New York Presbyterian Hospital, New York, NY, USA

Johannes Woitzik Department of Neurosurgery, Charité University Medicine Berlin, Berlin, Germany

Sahar Zafar Department of Neurology, Harvard Medical School, Massachusetts General Hospital, Boston, MA, USA

Wendy Ziai Neurosciences Critical Care Division, Departments of Neurology, Neurosurgery, and Anesthesiology – Critical Care Medicine, Johns Hopkins Hospital, Baltimore, MD, USA

Part I

General Section

Status Epilepticus - Lessons and Challenges from Animal Models

Inna Keselman, Claude G. Wasterlain, Jerome Niquet, and James W.Y. Chen

Introduction

The first reference to status epilepticus (SE) dates back to 700–600 BC in Babylonian cuneiform tablets, yet our understanding of this condition remains limited. SE is not simply a long seizure; mechanistically, it is a different entity. Our clinical experience suggests that an underlying etiology, systemic factors, and genetic background influence the generation and progression of SE as well as its sequelae. Understanding the underlying pathophysiology of SE is key to developing effective treatment and a topic of rigorous scientific research.

In this chapter, we will review different forms of SE and delineate available treatments. We will describe common animal models of SE used to study basic physiology in order to develop novel treatments, as well as discuss challenges that the scientific community faces when trying to translate animal data into clinical practice.

History and Definition of SE

The first known description of SE was in the XXV-XXVI tablets of the Sakikku cuneiform from the Neo-Babylonian era, estimated to have been carved between 718 and 612 BC, as "if the possessing demon possesses him many times during the middle watch of the night, and at the time of his possession his hands and feet are cold, he is much darkened,

keeps opening and shutting his mouth…he will die". This vivid description has captured two important aspects of SE: repeated seizures and high mortality rate. In addition, it attributed the cause of SE to demonic possession, a concept, which is still accepted today by certain people and cultures around the world.

There were a couple of notable descriptions of SE before the nineteenth century. In 1824 Calmeil coined the term *Etat de mal* in his thesis, describing patients in Paris asylum, where they resided due to the condition reminiscent of refractory epilepsy and SE. It was not until 1876 that Bourneville used a clinical presentation to define SE as "more or less incessant seizures." He also described the characteristic features of SE which included coma, hemiplegia, rise in body temperature, heart rate, and respiratory rate changes.

The English term status epilepticus came from of *Etat de mal* when Bazire translated the medical works of Trousseau, who in 1868 saliently stated that "in the status epilepticus, something specific happens (in the brain) which requires an explanation." This is an important conceptual departure from a view that SE is just a prolonged seizure or multiple seizures. In 1904, Clark and Prout described the natural course of SE in 38 patients without pharmacotherapy and recognized three distinct conditions: an early pseudostatus phase (described as aborted, imperfect, or incomplete), convulsive SE, and stuporous SE [1]. Henri Gastaut expressed the complexity of clinical definition of SE as "there are as many types of status as there are types of epileptic seizures."

In 1962, he held the Xth Marseilles Colloquium, the first major conference devoted to SE. There the modern clinical definition of SE was adopted as "a term used whenever a seizure persists for a sufficient length of time or is repeated frequently enough to produce a fixed or enduring epileptic condition." Gastaut suggested that a sufficient length of time to be about 30–60 min. However, because that time period was not demarcated, it was difficult to apply this new definition in a clinical setting. Moreover, this lack of a well-defined time parameter led to several decades of academic debates

I. Keselman • J. Niquet
Department of Neurology, David Geffen School of Medicine at UCLA, Los Angeles, CA, USA

Department of Neurology, VA Greater Los Angeles Health Care System, 11301 Wilshire Blvd, Los Angeles, CA 90073, USA
e-mail: ikeselman@mednet.ucla.edu; jniquet@ucla.edu

C.G. Wasterlain • J.W.Y. Chen (✉)
Department of Neurology, VA Greater Los Angeles Health Care System, 11301 Wilshire Blvd, Los Angeles, CA 90073, USA
e-mail: wasterla@ucla.edu; jwychen@ucla.edu

P.N. Varelas, J. Claassen (eds.), *Seizures in Critical Care*, Current Clinical Neurology, DOI 10.1007/978-3-319-49557-6_1

about it. In addition, there was overwhelming evidence that argued for treatment of SE as soon after its onset as possible in order to prevent neuronal injuries rather than wait for 60 min.

Evidence from animal studies argues that repetitive seizures transform into a state of self-sustaining and pharmacoresistance develops within 15–30 min. The development of neuronal injury also occurs in a similar timeframe. Mostly driven by the clinical necessity for early treatment to prevent neuronal death and complications from SE, the time definition of status epilepticus has been progressively shrinking from 30 min in the guidelines of the Epilepsy Foundation of America's Working Group on Status Epilepticus to 20 min in the Veterans Affairs Status Epilepticus Cooperation Study and again to 5 min in the Santa Monica Meeting [1].

However, shortening the time definition of SE to 5 min to satisfy this clinical need would lead to inclusion of cases other than an established SE (please see below for definition) and as such complicate outcome data obtained from that heterogeneous population. It is appropriate to separate out the early phase of convulsive SE, before it is fully established, as impending SE.

Impending convulsive SE [1] is a different clinical and physiological entity from prolonged seizures and is defined as "continuous or intermittent seizures lasting more than 5 minutes, without full recovery of consciousness between seizures." Five minutes was chosen here because it is almost 20 standard deviations (SD) removed from the mean duration of a single convulsive seizure. This calculation is based on work by Theodore and colleagues [2] who found the mean duration of a convulsive seizure to be 62.2 s, based on clinical presentation, and 69.9 ± 12 s based on electrographic findings, thus making 5 min (300 s) 19 SD away from the mean electrographic and 20 SD away from the mean clinical duration of convulsive seizures [2]. The transformation from impending SE to established SE is likely to be a continuum and can be modeled by a single exponential curve with a time constant of 30 min [1]. It suggests that at 30 min, about two-thirds of continuously seizing cases have completed the transformation into an established SE. There are overwhelming animal and human data to support using 30 min as a practical cutoff time point. Once the SE is established, it can easily become refractory SE (RSE) or superrefractory SE (SRSE), which are defined based on the lack of therapeutic response. RSE [2] is defined as SE that has not responded to first-line therapy [a benzodiazepine (BDZ)] and second-line therapy [an antiepileptic drug (AED)] and requires the application of general anesthetics. Superrefractory SE is defined as SE that has continued or recurred despite 24 h of general anesthesia (or coma-inducing anticonvulsants) [3].

Most recently, the new definition of SE has been proposed by the International League Against Epilepsy (ILAE) to be: "SE is a condition resulting either from the failure of the mechanisms responsible for seizure termination or from the initiation of mechanisms, which lead to abnormally prolonged seizures (after time point t1). It is a condition, which can have long-term consequences (after time point t2), including neuronal death, neuronal injury, and alteration of neuronal networks, depending on the type and duration of seizure" [4]. This is a conceptual definition with two variables t1 and t2, which are SE type dependent.

Epidemiology

There have been three population-based prospective studies to investigate the incidence of SE, based on the 30 min definition of SE. The first study done in Richmond, VA, USA [5], demonstrated an overall incidence of 41/100,000 individuals per year, with the rate being 27/100,000 per year for young adults (aged 16–59 years) and 86/100,000 per year in the elderly (aged 60 years and above). Two studies have shown the incidence of SE to be three times higher in African-Americans than Caucasians [6–8]. Mortality was higher in the elderly, 38% versus 14% for younger adults. The incidence from two prospective studies in Europe was 17.1/100,000 per year in Germany and 10.3/100,000 per year in the French-speaking part of Switzerland [1].

Etiology

Any normal brain can generate seizures if sufficiently perturbed, such as from electrolyte or glucose derangements, head injury, intracranial hemorrhages, etc. When the perturbed conditions are not rectified, these seizures can become incessant and transform into SE. SE can occur in a patient who did not have a prior history of seizures. The common etiologies for SE include low antiepileptic drug (AED) blood levels in patients with chronic epilepsy (often occurs when a medication is abruptly discontinued), anoxia/hypoxia, metabolic derangements, intoxication, trauma, stroke, and alcohol/drug withdrawal [1].

Animal Models of SE

The observation that SE is not a simple summation of seizures was made in the nineteenth century; but it is not until we were able to use animal models that we understood the physiology behind this clinical observation [1]. Animals became an important tool to study basic mechanisms of SE (and disease in general) because of obvious ethical constraints. There are many animal models of seizures and epilepsy, but only a few are available for SE. These have been used because they have demonstrated similarities to human

SE (both convulsive and non-convulsive types), clinically, electrographically, and histopathologically as well as in their response to known treatment. SE-induced epileptogenesis occurs in the vast majority of animals in several models of SE [9–11]. In humans presenting with SE, the incidence of chronic epilepsy is high, but harder to interpret [12]. Epileptic patients and animals which develop chronic epilepsy after a bout of SE exhibit chronic cellular hyperexcitability, neuronal degeneration, mossy fiber sprouting, and synaptic reorganization in the dentate gyrus of the hippocampus [13]. Due to the space constraints, we provide a brief description of the most commonly used models and will focus on those used in our own laboratory; for more details, please refer to *Models of Seizures and Epilepsy* [13].

The following are commonly used models of SE.

Electrical Stimulation Models

The first model of self-sustaining SE (SSSE) derived from the serendipitous observation that, when rats were paralyzed, ventilated with oxygen, and kept in good metabolic balance, repetitive application of electroconvulsive shocks (ECS) once a minute for over 25 min resulted in seizures which continued after stimulation stopped (Fig. 1.1-I). Duration and severity of these self-sustaining seizures depended on the duration of stimulation [14, 15]. After repeated ECS for 25 min, self-sustaining seizures lasted for a few minutes. After 50 min they lasted for up to an hour, and rats stimulated for 100 min remained in self-sustaining SE for hours and expired, in spite of the fact that their oxygenation, acid-base balance, and other metabolic parameters remained stable.

Following the discovery of the kindling phenomenon, Taber et al. [16] and de Campos and Cavalheiro [17] modified the method of stimulation to obtain SE. McIntyre et al. [18, 19] showed that continuous stimulation for 60 min of basolateral amygdala of kindled animals induced SE, demonstrating that the kindled state predisposes to the development of SE. Both high-[20] and low-frequency [21] stimulation of limbic structures can induce SSSE. Inoue et al. [22, 23] produced SE in naïve rats by electrical stimulation of prepiriform cortex. Handforth and Ackerman [24, 25] used continuous high-frequency stimulation of the hippocampus or amygdala and analyzed the functional anatomy of SE with [^{14}C]-deoxyglucose. They delineated several types of SE, ranging from a very restricted limbic pattern around the site of stimulation with mild behavioral manifestations to bilateral involvement of limbic and extralimbic structures accompanied by widespread clonic seizures. Lothman and colleagues [26] showed that stimulation of dorsal hippocampus for 60 min with high-frequency trains with very short inter-train intervals, a protocol which they called "continuous hippocampal stimulation" (CHS), resulted in

the development, in many animals, of SE characterized by non-convulsive or mild convulsive seizures which lasted for hours after the end of CHS. Metabolic activity was increased in many brain structures and decreased in others [27]; these seizures lead to loss of GABAergic hippocampal inhibition, to hippocampal interictal spiking, and to delayed (1 month after CHS) spontaneous seizures [28].

Vicedomini and Nadler [29] showed that intermittent stimulation of excitatory pathways could generate SE in many regions. SE developed in each animal that showed at least ten consecutive afterdischarges. We used a protocol derived from those of Vicedomini and Nadler [29] and Sloviter [30]. We stimulated the perforant path in awake rats with 10 s, with 20 Hz trains (1 ms square wave, 20 V) delivered every minute, and with 2 Hz continuous stimulation and recorded from dentate gyrus [31] (Fig. 1.1-II). Nissinen et al. [32] developed a similar model based on amygdala stimulation. Other variations of the perforant path model have been used [33]. The perforant path stimulation model provides a tool to study epileptic pathways, histopathological changes, sequelae of SE, systemic factors, as well as genetic background influencing the physiology of SE and to test the effects of AEDs. The EEG and clinical evolution of SE (Fig. 1.1 -I) is similar to that described for clinical SE [34, 35], starting with individual seizures which merge into nearly continuous polyspikes, which later are interrupted by slow waves, which increase in duration and interrupt seizure activity while polyspikes decrease in amplitude. Eventually, after many hours, this evolves into a burst-suppression pattern of progressively decreasing power.

Chemical Models of SE: Pilocarpine and Lithium–Pilocarpine

Pilocarpine is an agonist at muscarinic receptors. Its induction of SE has been shown to occur primarily through activation of muscarinic 1 receptors (M1R), but its actions on muscarinic 2 receptors (M2R) may also contribute to the SE propagation and sequelae development by affecting systemic factors, such as inflammation [36]. Lithium is administered prior to pilocarpine in order to decrease animal mortality, but pilocarpine may be used alone.

Many different protocols of pilocarpine administration exist [37]. Pilocarpine is injected either systemically (i.e., intraperitoneal route) or directly into the brain (intracerebroventricular or intrahippocampal route), while electrical activity is being monitored in the cortex and hippocampus. The amount of injected chemical can be variable, depending on intended outcome. Male rats or mice are most often used in these experiments, but females have shown similar responses. Just as with electrical stimulation models, and similar to human patients, induction of SE with pilocarpine

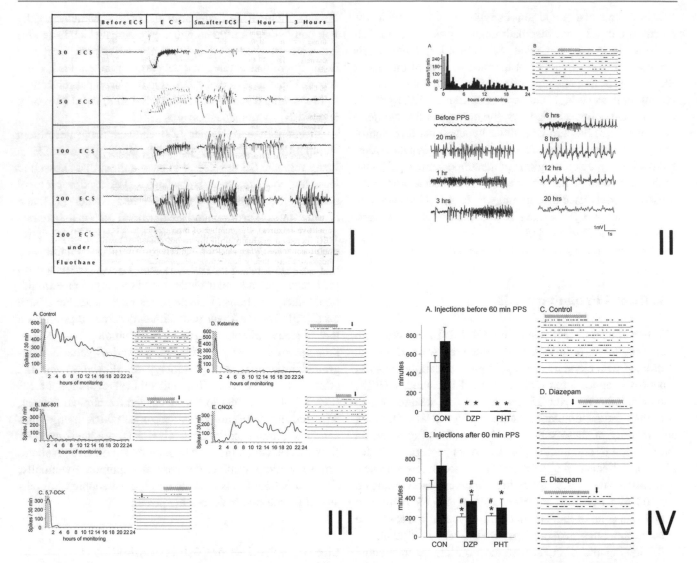

Fig. 1.1 (**I**) Initial observation that repeated electroconvulsive shocks induce self-sustaining SE in rats. Representative electrographic recordings from skull screw electrodes in paralyzed and O_2-ventilated rats maintained in good acid-base balance. Animals shocked repeatedly for 25 min (50 ECS) or longer showed self-sustaining seizure activity after the end of electrical stimulation. Increasing the duration of stimulation resulted in longer lasting self-sustaining SE *(Reproduced from* [14], @ *Elsevier 1972 and 15 @ Epilepsia)*. (**II**) EEG during SE induced by 30 min of intermittent perforant path stimulation (PPS). (**a**) Representative course of spikes. (**b**) 24 h distribution of seizures (*black bars*). The period of stimulation is indicated by the *gray bar* on the top. *Each line* represents 2 h of monitoring. (**c**) Evolution of EEG activity in the dentate gyrus during SE. Software- recognized seizures are underlined *(Reproduced with changes from* [31]*, © Elsevier, 1998)*. (**III**) The effects of NMDA (**a–d**) and AMPA/kainate (**e**) receptor blockers on SE induced by PPS. Each graph shows frequency of spikes plotted against time during SE. PPS is indicated by the *gray bar*. Representative time course of seizures detected by the software is shown in the graphs immediately to the right. Each line represents 2 h of monitoring, and each seizure is indicated by a *black bar*. *Arrows* indicate drug administration. Notice that in this model, NMDA receptor blockers MK-801 (0.5 mg/kg i.p.), 2,5-DCK (10 nmol into the

stimulated hilus), and ketamine (10 mg/kg i.p.) are administered 10 min after the end of PPS aborted SE soon after injection. CNQX (10 nmol into the hilus) injected after PPS induced only transient suppression of seizures, which reappeared 2–4 h after CNQX injection *(Reproduced with changes from* [72]*, © Elsevier 1999)*. (**IV**) Time-dependent development of pharmacoresistance in SE induced by 60 min PPS. (**a**) Pretreatment with diazepam (DZP) or phenytoin (PHT) prevented the development of SE. (**b**) *Top*: When injected 10 min after PPS, neither of them aborted SSSE, although they shortened its duration. *$p < 0.05$ vs. control. #$p < 0.05$ vs. DZP and PHT, respectively, in **a** (pretreatment). *Open bars* show cumulative seizure time, and *black bars* show the duration of SE. (**c–e**) Representative time course of seizures in a control animal (**c**), an animal pretreated with diazepam (**d**), or an animal Fig. 1.1 (continued) injected with diazepam 10 min after PPS (**e**). *Each line* represents 2 h of EEG monitoring. Each software-recognized seizure is shown by a *small black bar*. PPS is indicated by *gray bars* on the top. Injection of diazepam is indicated by an *arrow* in **d** and **e**. Notice that, in the control animal, SE lasted for 17 h. In diazepam-pretreated rats, seizures occurred during PPS, but only a few seizures were observed within the first 20 min after PPS. In the diazepam-posttreated animal, SE continued for 8 h. *(Reproduced with changes from* 44*, © Elsevier 1998)* leads to increased synaptic activity in limbic areas. Acutely, following injections of pilocarpine, normal hippocampal and cortical rhythms are transformed to spiking and then electrographic seizures, which within an hour after injection become sustained, similar to human SE. This electrical activity is correlated with behavior, which consists of facial automatisms, akinesia, ataxia, and eventually motor seizures and SE. Pathologic changes seen following induction of SE are similar to those seen in human brains and are an important paradigm in our effort to understand the pathologic process of epileptogenesis.

Turski et al. [9] developed the pilocarpine model of SE. Honchar and Olney [11] showed that lithium pretreatment reduces the dose of pilocarpine needed and the mortality from SE. Buterbaugh [38] and Morrisett et al. [39] showed that, in these chemical models, seizures become independent from the initial trigger, and self-sustaining, as they do in electrical stimulation models. Morissett et al. [39] administered atropine sulfate, which removed the cholinergic stimulus. This was effective in blocking status epilepticus when given before the onset of behavioral seizures, but failed to stop SE after onset of overt seizures, demonstrating that different mechanisms are responsible for initiation and maintenance of SE and that self-sustaining SE can be triggered by chemical as well as electrical stimulation. These results were extended to juvenile animals by Suchomelova et al. [40]. The pilocarpine model can also be used to test potential AEDs for their effects on SE, as well as on the induction and evolution to chronic epilepsy.

Studies of the Transition from Single Seizures to SE: GABA$_A$R

GABAergic agents lose their therapeutic effectiveness as status epilepticus (SE) proceeds, and brief convulsant stimuli result in a diminished inhibitory tone of hippocampal circuits [41], as indicated by loss of paired-pulse inhibition in vivo. To examine the effects of SE on GABA$_A$ synapses, whole-cell patch-clamp recordings of GABA$_A$ miniature inhibitory postsynaptic currents (mIPSCs) were obtained from dentate gyrus granule cell in hippocampal slices from 4- to 8-week-old Wistar rats after 1 h of lithium–pilocarpine SE and compared to controls [42]. Figure 1.2a shows that mIPSCs recorded from granule cells in slices prepared 1 h into SE showed a decreased peak amplitude to $61.8 \pm 11.9\%$ of controls (-31.5 ± 6.1 picoAmpere (pA) for SE vs. -51.0 ± 17.0 pA for controls; $p < 0.001$) and an increase of decay time to $127.9 \pm 27.6\%$ of controls (7.75 ± 1.67 ms for SE vs. 6.06 ± 1.17 ms for controls; $p < 0.001$). Unlike mIPSCs, tonic currents (Fig. 1.2b) increased in amplitude to a mean of -130.0 (±73.6) pA in SE vs. $-44.8(\pm19.2)$ pA in controls ($p < 0.05$). Tonic currents are thought to be mediated by extrasynaptic receptors containing δ subunits, which are known to display low levels of desensitization and internalization.

Their persistence during SE might suggest that drugs with strong affinity for extrasynaptic receptors, such as neurosteroids, may be effective. Mathematical modeling of GABA$_A$ synapses using mean–variance fluctuation analysis and seven-state GABA$_A$ receptor models suggested that SE reduced postsynaptic receptor number by 47% [from 38 ± 15 (control) to 20 ± 6 (SE) receptors per synapse; $p < 0.001$] (Fig. 1.2a). This may underestimate the acute changes, since slices collected from animals in SE were examined after 1–2 seizure-free hours in vitro.

Immunocytochemistry was performed in rats perfused after 60 min of seizures induced by lithium–pilocarpine (Fig. 1.2c, d). These anatomical studies indicate that the decrease in number of synaptic receptors observed physiologically reflects, at least in part, receptor internalization. They show colocalization of the β2/3 subunits with the presynaptic marker synaptophysin on the surface of soma and proximal dendrites of dentate granule cells and CA3a pyramids in controls, with internalization of those subunits in SE (Fig. 1.2d). In the lithium–pilocarpine model at 60 min, $12 \pm 17\%$ of β2/3 subunits are internalized in control CA3 compared to $54 \pm 15\%$ in slices from rats in SE ($p < 0.001$). Numbers in CA1 were similar. We also found that the γ2 subunits are internalized during SE [42].

In conclusion, a decrease in synaptic GABA$_A$ currents and an increase in extrasynaptic tonic currents are observed with SE. Internalization/desensitization of postsynaptic GABAA receptors (possibly from increased GABA exposure) can explain the decreased amplitude of synaptic mIPSCs, although an increase in intracellular chloride concentration may also play a role. These changes at GABAergic synapses may represent important events in the transition from single seizures to self-sustaining SE (Fig. 1.1). Since internalized receptors are not functional, this internalization may reduce the response of inhibitory synapses to additional seizures and may in part explain the failure of inhibitory GABAergic mechanisms which characterizes the initiation phase of self-sustaining SE. The reduced synaptic receptor numbers also may explain the diminished effect of benzodiazepines and other GABAergic drugs as SE proceeds [43, 44] (Fig. 1.3, Table 1.1).

Studies of the Transition from Single Seizures to SE: NMDAR

The self-perpetuating nature of SE suggests that synaptic potentiation may account for some of the maintenance mechanisms of SE. Indeed, we found that SE is accompanied by increased long-term potentiation (LTP) in the perforant path-dentate gyrus pathway [45]. Several mechanisms may underlie facilitation of LTP during SE. SE-induced loss of GABA inhibition, which occurs at a very early stage of stimulation, may contribute to facilitation of LTP. However, direct changes affecting excitatory NMDA receptors seem to

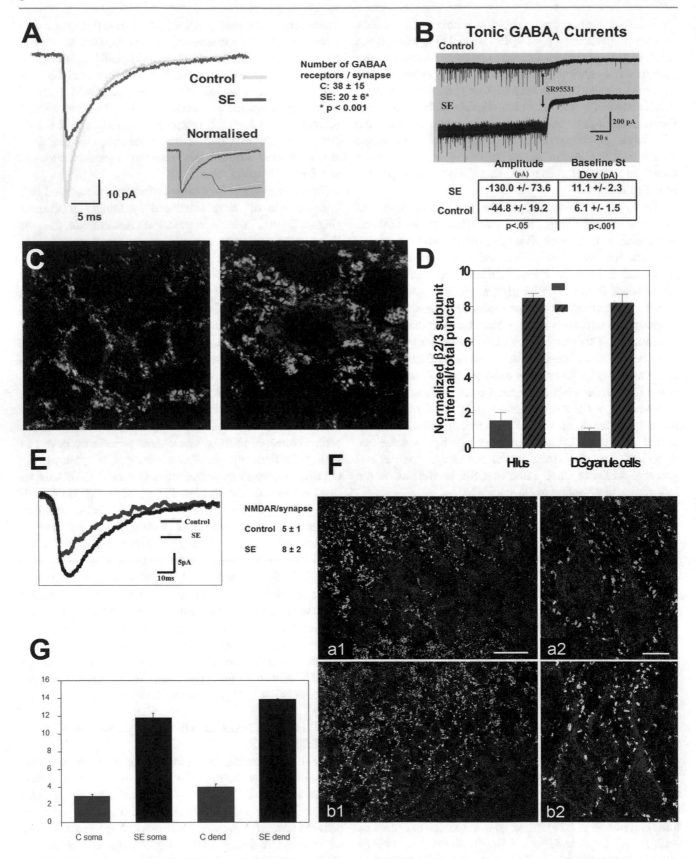

Fig. 1.2 (a) γ-Aminobutyric acid (GABA)$_A$ miniature inhibitory postsynaptic currents (IPSCs) recorded from the soma of granule cells in hippocampal slices prepared from rats in lithium–pilocarpine-induced SE for 1 h show reduced amplitude but little change in kinetics. Our model predicts that this reflects reduced number of GABA$_A$ receptors from 38 ± 15 in controls to 20 ± 6 per synapse in slices from animals in SE. (b) In slices from rats in SE, tonic currents generated by extrasynaptic GABA$_A$ receptors are increased, reflecting (at least in part)

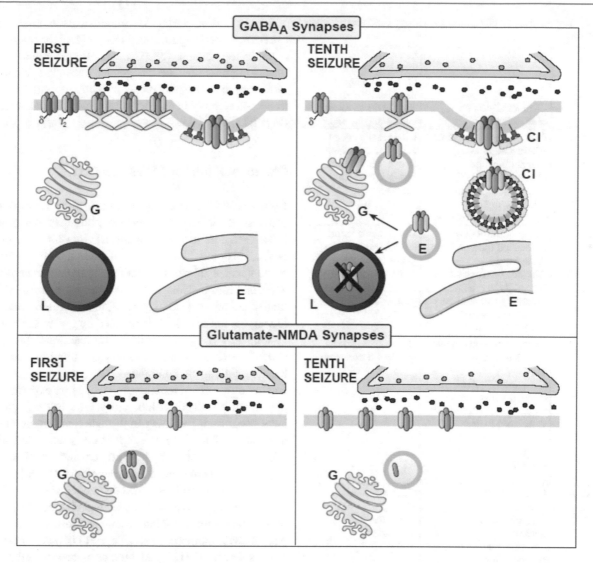

Fig. 1.3 Model summarizing our hypothesis on the role of receptor trafficking in the transition from single seizures to SE. After repeated seizures, the synaptic membrane surrounding GABA_A receptors forms clathrin-coated pits (Cl), which internalize as clathrin-coated vesicles, inactivating the receptors since they are no longer within reach of the neurotransmitter GABA. These vesicles evolve into endosomes, which can deliver the receptors to lysosomes (L) where they are destroyed, or to the Golgi apparatus (G) from where they are recycled to the membrane. By contrast, in NMDA synapses, after repeated seizures, receptor subunits are mobilized to the synaptic membrane and assemble into additional receptors. As a result of this trafficking, the number of functional NMDA receptors per synapse increases while the number of functional GABA_A receptors decreases [37, 41]. Reproduced from Chen and Wasterlain ([1] @ Elsevier 2006)

Fig. 1.2 (continued) increased extracellular GABA concentration during SE. (**c**) Subcellular distribution of β2–3 subunits of GABA_A receptors after 1 h of SE. In control granule cells (*left*) the β2–3 subunits of GABA_A receptors (*red*) localize to the vicinity of the presynaptic marker synaptophysin (*green*), whereas after an hour of SE induced by lithium and pilocarpine (*right*), many have moved to the cell interior. (**d**) The graph shows an increase in β2–3 subunits internalization following SE in the hilus and in the Fig. 1.2 (continued) dentate gyrus granule cell layer. (**e**) NMDA miniature excitatory postsynaptic currents (NMDA-mEPSCs) mean traces from a typical granule cell from a control (*red*) and a SE animal (*black*), demonstrating larger amplitude and area-under-the curve (AUC) in the latter, indicating an increased response of the postsynaptic membrane to a quantum of glutamate released from a single vesicle, and suggesting an increase in NMDAR from 5 ± 1 NMDAR/synapse in controls to 8 ± 2 NMDAR/synapse in slices from rats in SE. (**f**) Subcellular distribution of NMDA NR1 subunit-like immunoreactivity (LI) after 1 h of SE. Hippocampal sections through CA3 of control (a1) and SE (b1) brains stained with antibodies against the NR1 subunit-LI (*red*) and against the presynaptic marker synaptophysin-LI (*green*), with overlaps appearing *yellow*. Hippocampal sections of CA3 at higher magnification are shown in a2 and b2. Note increased NR1 subunit-LI colocalization with synaptophysin-LI in pyramidal cells for SE rat (bar—40 μm *left panel*; 10 μm *right panel*). (**g**) The number of colocalizations between NR1 subunits and synaptophysin increases with SE at both the soma and proximal dendrites of CA3 pyramidal cells (error bars as ± SEM). *Modified from Naylor et al.* ([42]: *A-D. presented at a Meeting of Society of Neuroscience 2005) and 47: E-G, @ Elsevier 2013)*

Table 1.1 Time-dependent changes in physiology of SE and treatment implications

Time	Changes/effects on excitability	Classes of medications working at this level and likely becoming inefficient due to status-induced changes in underlying physiology
Milliseconds–seconds	Protein phosphorylation Alternation in ion channel function Changes in neuromodulators and neurotransmitters Receptor desensitization	Drugs that work on GABA transmission Drugs that work on Na+, K+, Ca++ ion channels
Seconds–minutes	Receptor trafficking (relocation from and into the synapse) Alterations in excitability secondary to changes in excitatory and inhibitory receptors at synapse BBB dysfunction	Drugs that work on GABA transmission Drugs that work on carbonic anhydrase and synaptic vesicle protein 2A
Minutes–hours	Changes in neuropeptide modulators of excitability Often maladaptive changes with overall increase in excitatory (substance P) and decrease in inhibitory (substance Y) peptides causing overall increase in excitability	Downstream effects are overall excitation
Hours–days/weeks	Long-term effects in gene expression (i.e., inflammatory genes) BBB dysfunction persists Inflammation	Gene modification therapy Anti-inflammatory medications

also be involved. We compared 4–8-week-old rats in self-sustaining SE for 1 h to controls [46]. Physiological measurements included NMDA miniature excitatory postsynaptic currents (mEPSCs) recorded from granule cells in the hippocampal slice with visualized whole-cell patch (Fig. 1.2e). The mEPSCs showed an increase in peak amplitude from -16.2 ± 0.4 pA for controls to -19.5 ± 2.4 for SE ($p < 0.001$). No significant changes in event decay time were noted. A slight increase in mEPSC frequency was noted for SE cells (1.15 ± 0.51 Hz vs. 0.73 ± 0.37 Hz; $0.05 < p < 0.01$). Mean–variance analysis of the mEPSCs showed an increase from 5.2 ± 1.2 receptors per synapse in controls to 7.8 ± 2 receptors during SE (50% increase; $p < 0.001$). Immunocytochemical analysis with antibodies to the NR1 subunit of NMDA receptors showed a movement of NR1 subunits from cytoplasmic sites to the neuronal surface and an increase in colocalization with the presynaptic marker synaptophysin, suggesting a mobilization of "spare" subunits to the synapse (Fig. 1.2f, g).

In conclusion, during SE, endocytosis/internalization of GABAA postsynaptic receptors is accompanied by an increase in excitatory NMDA synaptic receptors. Receptor trafficking may regulate the balance between excitatory and inhibitory postsynaptic receptor numbers and may be an important element in the transition to and maintenance of SE (Fig. 1.3, Table 1.1).

Chemical Models of SE: Kainic Acid

Kainic acid is a naturally occurring algal neurotoxin that activates excitatory kainate-type glutamate receptors and causes seizures in marine mammals and birds up the food chain. This model has been used since the observation was made that the injection of kainate generates repetitive seizures and causes damage in hippocampal neurons [13]. This model and others lead to generation of chronic seizures following the initial SE. SE is induced by giving kainate either systemically (i.e., intravenously, intraperitoneally) or intracranially (i.e., intraventricularly, intrahippocampally). Kainic acid can be administered as a large single dose or smaller doses given repetitively [13]. Most experiments are performed on standard laboratory rats, but other animals have been used, including both male and female mice and dogs. Recordings from the hippocampal and cortical leads will show spikes and repetitive clinical and subclinical (electrographic) seizures and SE. These animals usually go on to develop chronic epilepsy with spontaneous convulsive and non-convulsive seizures. Pathological changes seen following kainate administration resemble those seen in human patients with temporal lobe epilepsy (TLE) and mesial temporal sclerosis (MTS) and include neuronal cell loss and gliosis. As with prior models, these animals can be used to test potential AED treatment in SE, as well as effects on behavior and on induction and course of chronic epilepsy.

Chemical Models of SE: Nerve Agents

Soman, or GD, is an organophosphate (pinacolyl methylphosphonofluoridate) that inactivates acetylcholinesterase, thus causing increased acetylcholine concentration in the central and peripheral nervous system synapses; this leads to induction of SE as well as to salivary hypersecretion, neuromuscular junction block, depressed respiration, and death. SE induces neuroinflammation leading to neuronal cell death and gliosis in the piriform cortex, hippocampus, amygdala, and thalamus [47]. Rat models have been mostly used, and in most animals, epileptiform activity continues for 4 h and in some survivors lasts up to 24 h.

Similar to the pilocarpine model of SE, the soman model can be used to study the role of the cholinergic system in SE.

Unlike the pilocarpine model, however, organophosphate administration leads to alteration in nicotinic receptor signaling in addition to the muscarinic receptors. Moreover, GABAergic and glutamatergic systems have been shown to play an important role in this model, once again supporting the complex physiology of SE [48, 49].

Sarin, or GB, is an organophosphate developed in Germany in 1938. It is a clear and odorless liquid which constitutes a weapon of mass destruction, according to the Centers of Disease Control and Prevention [50]. When administered at high doses, sarin causes seizures and respiratory suppression in humans [51]. It was used by terrorists in Japan in 1994 and 1995 in a subway attack. The epidemiological consequences of the 1994 exposure were analyzed and revealed hundreds of affected people including seven deaths [52].

In addition to commonly used models of pilocarpine, kainate, and soman/sarin, many of the chemical convulsants are able to induce SE when used in high-enough doses. Among other well-studied models are cobalt–homocysteine [53], flurothyl [54], bicuculline [55], and pentylenetetrazol [56].

In Vitro Models Used to Study Basic Physiology of SE

Here we will describe a few commonly used techniques used to study molecular, cellular, and network changes, resulting from SE; a more detailed review of basic science techniques is beyond the scope of this chapter.

Brain Slices

A special preparation of brain tissue, termed brain slices [57], is used to study basic physiology of SE and neural tissue in general. Slice preparation allows investigators to answer questions, which would otherwise be difficult to address in vivo. This preparation gives access to deep brain structures and allows one to study tissue properties in the context of preserved local networks. Depending on a study question, a researcher can slice a whole brain or a structure of interest, i.e., hippocampus.

Slice preparations are used to look at acute or chronic changes: acute, by inducing epileptiform discharges directly in the slice, and chronic by using brains from animal models of SE described in prior sections. Slices, once prepared, are then manipulated using electrical or pharmacological methods. Composition of the perfusion solution is usually altered in order to address specific questions.

The following models are used to study physiology of SE [58]:

4-Aminopyridine Model

4-Aminopyridine (4-AP) is a potassium channel blocker that mainly acts on presynaptic sites to decrease repolarization of cell membranes. Administration of 4-AP reproducibly induced epileptiform discharges in in vitro preparations and has been reported to be a proconvulsant in humans. Its effect at the network circuitry has been attributed to enhancement of the glutaminergic tone and neutralization of the GABAergic inhibition [59].

In hippocampal slices, stimulating electrode is usually positioned in the dentate gyrus, and extracellular recordings are made via a recording electrode in CA3, while the slice is continuously perfused with artificial cerebrospinal fluid (aCSF) containing 4-AP. Bipolar stimulating electrode is used to induce spontaneous epileptiform bursting, which starts within 5 min following application of 4-AP and disappear following its removal. In a recent paper, Salami et al. studied effects of 4-AP on high-frequency oscillations (HFOs) showing correlation between presence of HFOs and seizure progression to SE [60].

Low Magnesium Model

This model is used in entorhinal–hippocampal slices while testing effects of drugs on epileptic discharges by measuring extracellular field potential recordings in areas of interest, i.e., the entorhinal cortex or CA1. In these slices, epileptiform activity evolves over time and becomes resistant to BDZ. Similarly to 4-AP model, effects of potential antiepileptic on extracellular field recordings and single-cell physiology can be studied in real time; Heinemann et al. used this model to study effects of SE on energy metabolism and cell survival and showed that calcium played an important role in coupling mitochondrial ATP production to ionic homeostasis [61].

High Potassium Model

Solution containing high potassium evokes epileptiform discharges [62]. Different concentrations of potassium are needed to evoke this activity in different areas, and its effects are studied by using extracellular field recording and whole-cell techniques. Furthermore, lowering extracellular calcium concentration or blocking synaptic transmission in addition to high potassium leads to induction of long-lasting ictal patterns [63, 64].

Organotypic Slice Culture Model

Obtained from neonatal rodents, this preparation allows for slices to be kept in culture for weeks, while cells continue to differentiate eventually producing tissue organization similar to that in situ [65, 66]. However, the circuitry is modified by mossy fiber sprouting and other factors. Just as other slice models, this one can be used to study physiology of SE using EP and intracellular techniques described above. This model is unique in that it allows slices to be kept for longer periods of time thus allowing one to study long-term changes in physiology in the absence of acute trauma and chronic drug effects including effects of reactive oxygen species [67].

Brain slice preparation is an important technique, which enables one to access and study status-induced changes in network physiology and individual cell types. It also allows one to easily test potential lifesaving medications. However, one has to be aware of its limitations while interpreting experimental results. One of the biggest limitations is an ability to examine only a microcircuit within a given slice, because connections to other parts of the brain are cut.

In summary, slice preparation allowed the scientific community to easily access and examine otherwise hard to reach brain areas. However, one should be aware of the limitations of slice preparation in interpreting experimental results. Correlation with other in vitro or in vivo techniques is often required to validate study results.

Other Techniques

A variety of in vitro techniques are used in combination with in vivo models to address specific questions in status epilepticus physiology, as well as to run necessary controls (i.e., animals injected with saline instead of kainate). This is an important point to mention, because most experiments done on human tissue, which are usually performed in the context of epilepsy surgery, lack them.

Intrinsic Optical Imaging

Intrinsic optical imaging technique performed on the intact cortex or a brain slice allows study of SE-induced dynamic changes in network anatomy and physiology, i.e., induction of neuronal hypersynchrony, by visualization fluctuations in light reflection that correlate to changes in neuronal activity [68].

Dissociated Cultures

In addition, brains or hippocampi can be dissociated into individual cells in order to study specific cellular effects. For example, hippocampal calcium levels have been shown to be elevated in animals that develop chronic seizures following episode of SE. For example, SE-induced changes in ion metabolism can be addressed by using hippocampal neuronal cultures. Phillips et al. have used this technique to study effects of hyperthermia on calcium entry and showed that temperature changes specifically effected NMDA and ryanodine receptors, but not voltage-gated calcium channels [69].

However, it is important to point out that in vitro preparations lack the behavioral manifestations of clinical seizures or SE to confirm the validity of the models. When interpreting data obtained using these experimental techniques, one should be cognitive of the uncertainties inherent in these models.

Combination of various techniques allows scientists to address a problem at multiple levels, i.e., looking at synaptic changes at subcellular level, studying whole-cell effects, and examining alterations of neuronal network properties. In addition, imaging techniques that were developed initially for humans, i.e., magnetic resonance imaging (MRI), computed tomography (CT), and PET, are also adopted for animals. This type of approach might bring a more comprehensive understanding of the basic mechanisms of SE.

Pathophysiological Changes During SE

Experimental evidence from animal models points to SE being a complex self-sustaining phenomenon associated with changes in molecular, cellular, and network physiology (Table 1.1).

It is now evident that basic physiology gets altered in as quickly as milliseconds after onset of SE and continues to change for hours, weeks, and months after its termination. Within seconds of initial SE, changes in protein phosphorylation and ion channel function are seen. Within minutes, alterations in synaptic function become apparent, which are followed by, at least in part, maladaptive changes in excitatory/inhibitory balance. Within hours, increases in gene expression and new synthesis of neuropeptides occur, leading to increase in proconvulsant neuropeptides (i.e., substance P) and decrease in inhibitory neuropeptides (i.e., neuropeptide Y) [70] which bring further imbalance toward excitability. On this time scale, changes in the blood–brain barrier (BBB) are seen as well. These persist for weeks after SE is terminated. The above changes are then followed by long-term changes in gene expression, which among other things lead to extensive changes in neuronal firing and induction of neuroinflammation and result in extensive cell death as seen on pathological specimens collected from patients who die as a consequence of SE [1]. This process is also important for epileptogenesis since animal models of SE also develop chronic epilepsy.

Due to differences in etiology and genetic factors, these changes and their progression rate most likely vary from individual to individual, and one could expect that antiseizure measures, medications, or otherwise will have different effects in different patients. Thus, it is not surprising that treatment of SE is different than that of a single seizure or chronic epilepsy and changes in time as SE progresses and transforms from impending to established to refractory/superrefractory or subtle form [71].

Lessons from Animal Models of SE

SE Is Maintained by an Underlying Change in Limbic Circuit Excitability That Does Not Depend on Continuous Seizure Activity

Perihilar injection of the α-amino-3-hydroxy-5-methyl-4-isoxazolepropionic acid receptor (AMPA)/kainate receptor blocker 6-cyano-7-nitroquinoxaline-2,3-dione (CNQX), 10 min after 30 min performant path stimulation (PPS), strongly suppressed electrographic and behavioral seizures (Fig. 1.1-III-E). However, 4–5 h after injection of CNQX, electrographic spikes and seizures reappeared, and soon after that, behavioral convulsions recurred. Despite the effective seizure and spike suppression for hours, total time spent in seizures over 24 h (253 + 60 min vs. 352 + 80 min in controls) and the time of occurrence of the last seizure (627 + 40 min vs. 644 + 95 in controls) did not significantly differ from controls [72]. The change in excitability triggered by SE had outlasted the drug and did not depend on continuous seizure activity in recurrent limbic circuits. The anatomical substrate of that change resides in limbic circuits. The limbic circuit that maintains SSSE, however, is very similar (but not identical) in many models and types of SE: once it gets going, it is self-sustaining, stereotyped, and no longer depends on the original stimulus.

The Initiation and Maintenance Phases of SE Are Pharmacologically Distinct

Pharmacologically, a large number of agents are able to induce SSSE (Table 1.2), suggesting that the circuit that maintains self-sustaining seizures has many potential points of entry. However, pharmacological responsiveness during initiation of SSSE and during established SSSE are strikingly different. Minute amounts of many agents, which enhance inhibitory transmission or reduce excitatory transmission, easily block the development of SSSE (Table 1.2), suggesting that brain circuits are biased against it and that all systems must "go" in order for the phenomenon to develop.

Table 1.2 Agents important in different stages of SE

Initiators	Blockers of initiation phase	Blockers of maintenance phase
• Low Na_o^+, High K_o^+ • $GABA_A$ antagonists • Glutamate agonists: NMDA, AMPA, kainate, low Mg_o^{++}, low Ca_o^{++}, stimulation of glutamatergic pathways • Cholinergic muscarinic agonists, stimulation of muscarinic pathways • Tachykinins (SP, NKB) • Galanin antagonists • Opiate δ agonists • Opiate κ antagonists	• Na^+ channel blockers • $GABA_A$ agonists • NMDA antagonists, high Mg_o^{++} • AMPA/kainate antagonists • Cholinergic muscarinic antagonists • SP, neurokinin B antagonists • Galanin • Somatostatin • NPY • Opiate δ antagonists • Dynorphin (κ agonist)	• NMDA antagonists • Tachykinin antagonists • Galanin • Dynorphin

However, once seizures are self-sustaining, few agents are effective in terminating them, and they usually work only in large concentration. The most efficacious agents are blockers of NMDA synapses or presynaptic inhibitors of glutamate release (Table 1.2).

Initiation Is Accompanied by a Loss of GABA Inhibition

Prolonged loss of paired-pulse inhibition occurs after brief (<5 min) perforant path stimulation in vivo, with the paired-pulse population spike amplitude ratio (P2/P1) increasing from the baseline, consistent with the involvement of $GABA_A$ synaptic receptors, and confirming the results of Lothman, Kapur, and others [26, 42–44]. Intracellular recordings showing SE-associated loss of mIPSCs (Fig. 1.2a) and immunohistochemical evidence of $GABA_AR$ internalization (Fig. 1.2c, d) confirm the loss of GABA inhibition during SE.

Maintenance of SSSE Depends on the Activation of NMDA Receptors

Intraperitoneal administration of the NMDA receptor blocker MK801 (0.5 mg/kg) after 60 min of performant path stimulation effectively aborted SE [72]. Other NMDA receptor blockers, 5,7-dichlorokinurenic acid (10 nmoles injected into the hilus), and ketamine (10 mg/kg i.p.) stopped both behavioral and electrographic seizures within 10 min after drug injection (Fig. 1.1-III-B, C, D). However, in more severe models of SE, NMDAR blockers used alone are less successful and need to be combined to $GABA_AR$ agonists to terminate SE [73].

Time-Dependent Development of Pharmacoresistance

Pretreatment with diazepam (0.5–10 mg/kg), or phenytoin (50 mg/kg), before beginning stimulation, effectively prevented the development of SSSE (Fig. 1.1-IV). When administered 10 min after the end of 30 min PPS, diazepam in the same doses induced strong muscle relaxation and ataxia. However, electrographic seizures continued. Phenytoin (50 mg/kg) effectively aborted SSSE when injected 10 min after 30 min PPS, but failed when injected 10 min after 60 min PPS [44]. In other words, the same dose which was very effective as pretreatment failed after SSSE was established. The reduction through endocytosis of the number of $GABA_A$ receptors available at the synapse (Fig. 1.2a, c, d) may explain the loss of benzodiazepine potency: the clathrin-binding site, which is the mediator of endocytosis, is located on the benzodiazepine-binding γ2 subunit of $GABA_A$ receptors. SE can also decrease $GABA_A$ receptor effectiveness due to desensitization, and to chloride shift into neurons, making the opening of chloride channels less effective [43, 74].

Maladaptive Seizure-Induced Receptor Trafficking Plays a Role in the Development of Pharmacoresistance

Once SE gets going, standard anticonvulsants loose much of their effectiveness, as discussed above. A prominent component of that change is a decrease in the number of synaptic $GABA_A$ receptors (Fig. 1.2a), due mainly to $GABA_A$ receptor internalization into endosomes (Fig. 1.2c), where the receptor no longer behaves as a functional ion channel, greatly reducing the response to benzodiazepines [42, 75].

Potentiation of NMDA Synaptic Responses May Play a Role in Maintaining SE

This is due principally to receptor trafficking which increases the number of active NMDA receptors at the synapse (Fig. 1.2e, f, g), with consequences for maintenance of seizure activity and for development of excitotoxic neuronal injury [46, 76].

Therapeutic Implications of Seizure-Associated Receptor Trafficking

The Case for Polytherapy

Standard treatment (benzodiazepine monotherapy) is aimed at enhancing the function of the remaining synaptic $GABA_A R$. [1, 77]. Benzodiazepines allosterically stimulate chloride flux through γ2-containing synaptic $GABA_A R$, and this can restore inhibition as long as a sufficient number of receptors remain on the postsynaptic membrane. If treatment is late, and a high proportion of $GABA_A R$ are internalized, benzodiazepines may not be able to fully restore GABA-mediated fast inhibition. However, even if GABAergic inhibition is successfully restored, this only addresses half the problem. The increase in functional NMDAR and the resulting runaway excitation and potential excitotoxicity remain untreated. Treating both changes induced by seizure-induced receptor trafficking would require using two drugs when treating early and three drugs when treating late. This may be why, in some models of SE, NMDA antagonists have been reported to remain effective late in the course of SE [72]: they correct maladaptive changes, which are usually untreated. Optimal treatment to reverse the results of seizure-induced receptor trafficking would include a $GABA_A R$ agonist (e.g., a benzodiazepine), an NMDAR antagonist, and if treating late, an antiepileptic drug (AED) to restore inhibition by stimulating a non-benzodiazepine site.

If Treatment Is Delayed, Triple Therapy May Be Needed

The increasing internalization of $GABA_A R$ with time (or more likely with seizure burden, which during SE increases with time) makes it unlikely that a high number of synaptic $GABA_A R$ will remain available in synapses for ligand binding. Even maximal stimulation with benzodiazepines may not be able to fully restore GABAergic inhibition. In addition to midazolam and ketamine, a third drug (e.g., an AED) is then needed to enhance inhibition at a non-benzodiazepine site. The choice of the best drug which works synergistically with midazolam and ketamine is critical and is the focus of our current research [73].

Timing of Polytherapy Is Critical

Standard treatment of SE and CSE uses sequential polytherapy, since each drug that fails to stop seizures is rapidly followed by another drug or treatment. Typically, a benzodiazepine (midazolam, lorazepam, or diazepam) is followed by another AED (e.g., fosphenytoin), then by a "newer" AED (e.g., valproate, levetiracetam, or lacosamide), then by general anesthesia, and, after several anesthetics fail, by ketamine or other less commonly used drugs. However sequential polytherapy takes time, since one has to wait for a drug to fail before starting the next one. During that time, receptor changes which are not treated by the initial drug (e.g., NMDAR changes if the first drug is a benzodiazepine) are likely to get worse and may be intractable by the time a drug which targets them (e.g., ketamine) is used many hours or even days later. We should consider giving drug combinations early (simultaneous polytherapy) in order to reverse the effects of receptor trafficking before they become irreversible.

The Earlier the Better

Early treatment is essential, the progressive nature of receptor changes, and the fact that they probably occur quite early [41, 42] suggests that time is of the essence. One should treat as early in the course of SE as possible. The success of prehospital treatment [78] and the impressive clinical benefit of early intramuscular drug delivery [78] support the applicability of that principle to clinical SE.

In summary, recent progress in our understanding of the pathophysiology of SE and CSE requires a drastic reevaluation of the way we treat those syndromes. The unquestionable benefits of monotherapy for chronic epilepsy may not apply to SE/CSE, an acute, life- and brain-threatening condition. Polytherapy with drug cocktails addressing the seizure-induced maladaptive changes that occur needs to be evaluated and may provide at least a partial solution to the problem of overcoming pharmacoresistance during SE.

Issues Commonly Encountered in Translational Research

The scientific community learned a tremendous amount about SE from the animal models. But despite this progress, our knowledge of human condition and its treatments remains to be improved. Animal models use a homogenous population of healthy animals and induce SE with one particular method, electrical stimulation of a specific brain region or drug, acting on a particular neurotransmitter system. In contrast, human SE develops on an individual genetic background and has a variable etiology such as stroke, TBI, inflammation, infection, or metabolic derangement. This interplay between the etiology of SE itself and the individual's genetic background may explain some of the difficulty in treating SE that we encounter in clinical practice. But despite these limitations, experimental evidence collected from the aforementioned animal models helps us understand the underlying pathophysiology and guides us toward development of better, more effective antiepileptic treatments. Animal models remain a necessary tool in our fight against disease in general and SE in particular.

Conclusions

SE is a medical emergency with high morbidity and mortality, especially in the elderly. The scientific community learned a tremendous amount about SE from animal models, but translation from bench to bedside has been extremely slow. Unfortunately, economic disincentives to large-scale clinical trials in a field with limited potential sales have restricted the role of industry, but strong recent interest in SE and its treatment may offer hope for the future. Our knowledge of this grave human condition and its treatment needs to be improved. A transformation from discrete seizure to SE, which is not fully understood, makes the brain proconvulsant and hyperexcitable and leads to development of pharmacoresistance to most, if not all, pharmacological agents. Established SE requires ICU level of care with availability of ventilation support. Continuous EEG monitoring is helpful in guiding the treatment and providing prognostic predictions. It should be used if available. A well-organized team approach among the members of the ICU, neurology, EEG/epilepsy specialists, and the clinical neuropharmacist is crucial to managing SE successfully. Good clinical evidence for treating refractory SE is sparse, and it will take many years before evidence-based standardized guideline could be established. In this conundrum gap, as we learn more and more about pathophysiology of SE, it will become even more important for practicing physicians to utilize their clinical judgment that adheres to the principles established from basic researches, such as awareness of the fast development of pharmacoresistance or including antiepileptic agents with anti-glutamate receptor properties in treating refractory cases. By doing so, we might have the best chance of optimizing neuroprotection in treating SE.

Acknowledgments We would like to extend special thank you to Roland McFarland, Dorota Kaminska, Ph.D., and Lyn Clarito, Pharm.D for their helpful comments on this manuscript. This work was supported by Merit Review Award # I01 BX000273-07 from the United States Department of Veterans Affairs, by NINDS (grant UO1 NS074926; CW), and by the James and Debbie Cho Foundation.

References

1. Chen JW, Wasterlain CG. Status epilepticus: pathophysiology and management in adults. Lancet Neurol. 2006;5(3):246–56.
2. Shorvon S. Super-refractory status epilepticus: an approach to therapy in this difficult clinical situation. Epilepsia. 2011;52(Suppl 8):53–6.
3. Alvarez V, Drislane FW. Is favorable outcome possible after prolonged refractory status epilepticus? J Clin Neurophysiol. 2016;33(1):32–41.
4. Trinka E, Cock H, Hesdorffer D, et al. A definition and classification of status epilepticus--report of the ILAE task force on classification of status epilepticus. Epilepsia. 2015;56(10):1515–23.
5. DeLorenzo RJ, Hauser WA, Towne AR, et al. A prospective, population-based epidemiologic study of status epilepticus in Richmond, Virginia. Neurology. 1996;46(4):1029–35.
6. Rosenow F, Hamer HM, Knake S. The epidemiology of convulsive and nonconvulsive status epilepticus. Epilepsia. 2007;48(Suppl 8): 82–4.
7. Wu YW, Shek DW, Garcia PA, et al. Incidence and mortality of generalized convulsive status epilepticus in California. Neurology. 2002;58(7):1070–6.
8. DeLorenzo RJ. Epidemiology and clinical presentation of status epilepticus. Adv Neurol. 2006;97:199–215.
9. Turski WA, Cavalheiro EA, Schwarz M, et al. Limbic seizures produced by pilocarpine in rats: behavioural, electroencephalographic and neuropathological study. Behav Brain Res. 1983;9(3):315–35.
10. Ben-Ari Y, Tremblay E, Ottersen OP, et al. Evidence suggesting secondary epileptogenic lesion after kainic acid: pre treatment with diazepam reduces distant but not local brain damage. Brain Res. 1979;165(2):362–5.
11. Honchar MP, Olney JW, Sherman WR. Systemic cholinergic agents induce seizures and brain damage in lithium-treated rats. Science. 1983;220(4594):323–5.
12. Punia V, Garcia CG, Hantus S. Incidence of recurrent seizures following hospital discharge in patients with LPDs (PLEDs) and nonconvulsive seizures recorded on continuous EEG in the critical care setting. Epilepsy Behav. 2015;49:250–4.
13. Pitkänen A, Schwartzkroin PA, Moshé SL. Models of seizures and epilepsy. Amsterdam; Boston: Elsevier Academic Press; 2006.
14. Wasterlain CG. Breakdown of brain polysomes in status epilepticus. Brain Res. 1972;39(1):278–84.
15. Wasterlain CG. Mortality and morbidity from serial seizures. An experimental study. Epilepsia. 1974;15(2):155–76.
16. Taber KH, McNamera JJ, Zornetzer SF. Status epilepticus: a new rodent model. Electroencephalogr Clin Neurophysiol. 1977;43(5): 707–24.
17. de Campos CJ, Cavalheiro EA. Modification of the "kindling" method for obtaining experimental status epilepticus in rats. Arq Neuropsiquiatr. 1980;38(1):81–8.
18. McIntyre DC, Nathanson D, Edson N. A new model of partial status epilepticus based on kindling. Brain Res. 1982;250(1):53–63.
19. McIntyre DC, Stokes KA, Edson N. Status epilepticus following stimulation of a kindled hippocampal focus in intact and commissurotomized rats. Exp Neurol. 1986;94(3):554–70.

20. Milgram NW, Green I, Liberman M, et al. Establishment of status epilepticus by limbic system stimulation in previously unstimulated rats. Exp Neurol. 1985;88(2):253–64.

21. Cain DP, McKitrick DJ, Boon F. Rapid and reliable induction of partial status epilepticus in naive rats by low-frequency (3-Hz) stimulation of the amygdala. Epilepsy Res. 1992;12(1):51–5.

22. Inoue K, Morimoto K, Sato K, et al. Mechanisms in the development of limbic status epilepticus and hippocampal neuron loss: an experimental study in a model of status epilepticus induced by kindling-like electrical stimulation of the deep prepyriform cortex in rats. Acta Med Okayama. 1992;46(2):129–39.

23. Inoue K, Morimoto K, Sato K, et al. A model of status epilepticus induced by intermittent electrical stimulation of the deep prepyriform cortex in rats. Jpn J Psychiatry Neurol. 1992;46(2):361–7.

24. Handforth A, Ackermann RF. Hierarchy of seizure states in the electrogenic limbic status epilepticus model: behavioral and electrographic observations of initial states and temporal progression. Epilepsia. 1992;33(4):589–600.

25. Handforth A, Ackermann RF. Mapping of limbic seizure progressions utilizing the electrogenic status epilepticus model and the 14C-2-deoxyglucose method. Brain Res Brain Res Rev. 1995;20(1):1–23.

26. Lothman EW, Bertram EH, Bekenstein JW, et al. Self-sustaining limbic status epilepticus induced by 'continuous' hippocampal stimulation: electrographic and behavioral characteristics. Epilepsy Res. 1989;3(2):107–19.

27. VanLandingham KE, Lothman EW. Self-sustaining limbic status epilepticus. I. Acute and chronic cerebral metabolic studies: limbic hypermetabolism and neocortical hypometabolism. Neurology. 1991;41(12):1942–9.

28. Lothman EW, Bertram EH, Kapur J, et al. Recurrent spontaneous hippocampal seizures in the rat as a chronic sequela to limbic status epilepticus. Epilepsy Res. 1990;6(2):110–8.

29. Vicedomini JP, Nadler JV. A model of status epilepticus based on electrical stimulation of hippocampal afferent pathways. Exp Neurol. 1987;96(3):681–91.

30. Sloviter RS. Decreased hippocampal inhibition and a selective loss of interneurons in experimental epilepsy. Science. 1987;235(4784):73–6.

31. Mazarati AM, Wasterlain CG, Sankar R, et al. Self-sustaining status epilepticus after brief electrical stimulation of the perforant path. Brain Res. 1998;801(1–2):251–3.

32. Nissinen J, Halonen T, Koivisto E, et al. A new model of chronic temporal lobe epilepsy induced by electrical stimulation of the amygdala in rat. Epilepsy Res. 2000;38(2–3):177–205.

33. van Vliet EA, Aronica E, Tolner EA, et al. Progression of temporal lobe epilepsy in the rat is associated with immunocytochemical changes in inhibitory interneurons in specific regions of the hippocampal formation. Exp Neurol. 2004;187(2):367–79.

34. Wang NC, Good LB, Marsh ST, et al. EEG stages predict treatment response in experimental status epilepticus. Epilepsia. 2009;50(4):949–52.

35. Treiman DM, Walton NY, Kendrick C. A progressive sequence of electroencephalographic changes during generalized convulsive status epilepticus. Epilepsy Res. 1990;5(1):49–60.

36. Sales ME. Muscarinic receptors as targets for anti-inflammatory therapy. Curr Opin Investig Drugs. 2010;11(11):1239–45.

37. Curia G, Longo D, Biagini G, et al. The pilocarpine model of temporal lobe epilepsy. J Neurosci Methods. 2008;172(2):143–57.

38. Buterbaugh GG, Michelson HB, Keyser DO. Status epilepticus facilitated by pilocarpine in amygdala-kindled rats. Exp Neurol. 1986;94(1):91–102.

39. Morrisett RA, Jope RS, Snead OC, 3rd. Effects of drugs on the initiation and maintenance of status epilepticus induced by administration of pilocarpine to lithium-pretreated rats. Exp Neurol 1987;97(1):193–200.

40. Suchomelova L, Baldwin RA, Kubova H, et al. Treatment of experimental status epilepticus in immature rats: dissociation between anticonvulsant and antiepileptogenic effects. Pediatr Res. 2006;59(2):237–43.

41. Naylor DE, Wasterlain CG. GABA synapses and the rapid loss of inhibition to dentate gyrus granule cells after brief perforant-path stimulation. Epilepsia. 2005;46(Suppl 5):142–7.

42. Naylor DE, Liu H, Wasterlain CG. Trafficking of GABA(A) receptors, loss of inhibition, and a mechanism for pharmacoresistance in status epilepticus. J Neurosci. 2005;25(34):7724–33.

43. Kapur J, Macdonald RL. Rapid seizure-induced reduction of benzodiazepine and Zn2+ sensitivity of hippocampal dentate granule cell GABAA receptors. J Neurosci. 1997;17(19):7532–40.

44. Mazarati AM, Baldwin RA, Sankar R, et al. Time-dependent decrease in the effectiveness of antiepileptic drugs during the course of self-sustaining status epilepticus. Brain Res. 1998;814(1–2):179–85.

45. 22nd IEC Proceedings. Epilepsia 1997;**38**:1–284.

46. Naylor DE, Liu H, Niquet J, et al. Rapid surface accumulation of NMDA receptors increases glutamatergic excitation during status epilepticus. Neurobiol Dis. 2013;54:225–38.

47. Johnson EA, Kan RK. The acute phase response and soman-induced status epilepticus: temporal, regional and cellular changes in rat brain cytokine concentrations. J Neuroinflammation. 2010;7:40.

48. Miller SL, Aroniadou-Anderjaska V, Figueiredo TH, et al. A rat model of nerve agent exposure applicable to the pediatric population: The anticonvulsant efficacies of atropine and GluK1 antagonists. Toxicol Appl Pharmacol. 2015;284(2):204–16.

49. McDonough Jr JH, Shih TM. Pharmacological modulation of soman-induced seizures. Neurosci Biobehav Rev. 1993;17(2):203–15.

50. CDC, http://www.bt.cdc.gov/agent/sarin/basics/facts.asp.

51. Smythies J, Golomb B. Nerve gas antidotes. J R Soc Med. 2004;97(1):32.

52. Nakajima T, Ohta S, Morita H, et al. Epidemiological study of sarin poisoning in Matsumoto City, Japan. J Epidemiol. 1998;8(1):33–41.

53. Walton NY, Treiman DM. Experimental secondarily generalized convulsive status epilepticus induced by D,L-homocysteine thiolactone. Epilepsy Res. 1988;2(2):79–86.

54. Wasterlain CG. Developmental brain damage after chemically induced epileptic seizures. Eur Neurol. 1975;13(6):495–8.

55. Soderfeldt B, Kalimo H, Olsson Y, et al. Bicuculline-induced epileptic brain injury. Transient and persistent cell changes in rat cerebral cortex in the early recovery period. Acta Neuropathol. 1983;62(1–2):87–95.

56. el Hamdi G, de Vasconcelos AP, Vert P, et al. An experimental model of generalized seizures for the measurement of local cerebral glucose utilization in the immature rat. I. Behavioral characterization and determination of lumped constant. Brain Res Dev Brain Res. 1992;69(2):233–42.

57. Bernard C. Chapter 6—Hippocampal slices: designing and interpreting studies in epilepsy research A2. In: Pitkänen A, Schwartzkroin PA, Moshé SL, editors. Models of Seizures and Epilepsy. Burlington: Academic Press; 2006. p. 59–72.

58. Reddy DS, Kuruba R. Experimental models of status epilepticus and neuronal injury for evaluation of therapeutic interventions. Int J Mol Sci. 2013;14(9):18284–318.

59. Avoli M, Barbarosie M, Lucke A, et al. Synchronous GABA-mediated potentials and epileptiform discharges in the rat limbic system in vitro. J Neurosci. 1996;16(12):3912–24.

60. Salami P, Levesque M, Avoli M. High frequency oscillations can pinpoint seizures progressing to status epilepticus. Exp Neurol. 2016;280:24–9.

61. Heinemann U, Buchheim K, Gabriel S, et al. Coupling of electrical and metabolic activity during epileptiform discharges. Epilepsia. 2002;43(Suppl 5):168–73.

62. Traynelis SF, Dingledine R. Potassium-induced spontaneous electrographic seizures in the rat hippocampal slice. J Neurophysiol. 1988;59(1):259–76.

63. Feng Z, Durand DM. Effects of potassium concentration on firing patterns of low-calcium epileptiform activity in anesthetized rat hippocampus: inducing of persistent spike activity. Epilepsia. 2006;47(4):727–36.

64. Xiong ZQ, Stringer JL. Prolonged bursts occur in normal calcium in hippocampal slices after raising excitability and blocking synaptic transmission. J Neurophysiol. 2001;86(5):2625–8.

65. Stoppini L, Buchs PA, Muller D. A simple method for organotypic cultures of nervous tissue. J Neurosci Methods. 1991;37(2): 173–82.

66. Heinemann UWE, Kann O, Schuchmann S. Chapter 4—An overview of in vitro seizure models in acute and organotypic slices A2. In: Pitkänen A, Schwartzkroin PA, Moshé SL, editors. Models of Seizures and Epilepsy. Burlington: Academic Press; 2006. p. 35–44.

67. Kovacs R, Schuchmann S, Gabriel S, et al. Free radical-mediated cell damage after experimental status epilepticus in hippocampal slice cultures. J Neurophysiol. 2002;88(6):2909–18.

68. Zepeda A, Arias C, Sengpiel F. Optical imaging of intrinsic signals: recent developments in the methodology and its applications. J Neurosci Methods. 2004;136(1):1–21.

69. Phillips KF, Deshpande LS, DeLorenzo RJ. Hypothermia reduces calcium entry via the N-methyl-D-aspartate and ryanodine receptors in cultured hippocampal neurons. Eur J Pharmacol. 2013; 698(1–3):186–92.

70. Wasterlain C, Treiman D, et al. Status epilepticus: Mechanisms of brain damage and treatment. New York: Raven Press; 1983. p. 15–35.

71. Fernandez-Torre JL, Kaplan PW, Hernandez-Hernandez MA. New understanding of nonconvulsive status epilepticus in adults: treatments and challenges. Expert Rev Neurother. 2015;15(12):1455–73.

72. Mazarati AM, Wasterlain CG. N-methyl-D-asparate receptor antagonists abolish the maintenance phase of self-sustaining status epilepticus in rat. Neurosci Lett. 1999;265(3):187–90.

73. Wasterlain CG, Baldwin R, Naylor DE, et al. Rational polytherapy in the treatment of acute seizures and status epilepticus. Epilepsia. 2011;52(Suppl 8):70–1.

74. Staley KJ, Soldo BL, Proctor WR. Ionic mechanisms of neuronal excitation by inhibitory GABAA receptors. Science. 1995; 269(5226):977–81.

75. Goodkin HP, Yeh JL, Kapur J. Status epilepticus increases the intracellular accumulation of GABAA receptors. J Neurosci. 2005;25(23):5511–20.

76. Bertram EH, Lothman EW. NMDA receptor antagonists and limbic status epilepticus: a comparison with standard anticonvulsants. Epilepsy Res. 1990;5(3):177–84.

77. Glauser T, Shinnar S, Gloss D, et al. Evidence-Based Guideline: Treatment of Convulsive Status Epilepticus in Children and Adults: Report of the Guideline Committee of the American Epilepsy Society. Epilepsy Curr. 2016;16(1):48–61.

78. Silbergleit R, Durkalski V, Lowenstein D, et al. Intramuscular versus intravenous therapy for prehospital status epilepticus. N Engl J Med. 2012;366(7):591–600.

Iván Sánchez Fernández and Tobias Loddenkemper

Introduction

Electrographic seizures in the intensive care unit (ICU) are frequent and often subclinical. In a series of 570 patients (495 adults and 75 patients younger than 18 years of age) who underwent continuous EEG monitoring (cEEG), seizures were detected in 110 (19%), and seizures were exclusively nonconvulsive (subclinical) in 101 (92%) [1]. In a series of 550 pediatric patients (ages 1 month to 21 years) who underwent cEEG in the ICU, 162 (30%) had electrographic seizures, and 61 of 162 (38%) had electrographic status epilepticus (SE) [2].

Electrographic seizures and electrographic SE are increasingly recognized, and they are associated with worse outcomes in neonates [3–6], children [2, 4, 5, 7–9], and adults [10–12]. However, it is currently unknown whether they impact outcome or are a biomarker of a more severe underlying etiology, hence the lack of clear guidelines on how aggressively to treat them. This chapter aims to address this gap in knowledge by summarizing currently available literature on how electrographic seizures and electrographic SE influence outcome in different populations of critically ill patients.

I. Sánchez Fernández
Division of Epilepsy and Clinical Neurophysiology, Department of Neurology, Boston Children's Hospital, Harvard Medical School, 300 Longwood Ave, Boston, MA 02115, USA

Department of Child Neurology, Hospital Sant Joan de Déu, University of Barcelona, Barcelona, Spain
e-mail: ivan.fernandez@childrens.harvard.edu

T. Loddenkemper (✉)
Division of Epilepsy and Clinical Neurophysiology, Department of Neurology, Boston Children's Hospital, Harvard Medical School, 300 Longwood Ave, Boston, MA 02115, USA
e-mail: Tobias.Loddenkemper@childrens.harvard.edu

Continuous Electroencephalogram Monitoring

The burden of electrographic seizures in the ICU is increasingly recognized as cEEG becomes more available. cEEG monitoring is growing exponentially at a pace of approximately 30% per year both in adults [13] and children [14]. In a large series of 5949 adults (>17 years of age) with mechanical ventilation in the USA, cEEG use increased by 263%, and the number of hospitals reporting cEEG use nearly doubled from 135 to 244 over the 4-year study period between 2005 and 2009 [13]. cEEG use increased by an average of 33% per year—much more than the average 8% increase per year in routine EEG use during the same period [13]. A survey of pediatric neurologists from 50 US and 11 Canadian leading hospitals showed that cEEG use also increased by approximately 30% from August 2010 to August 2011 [14]. During that 1-year period, the number of patients with cEEG monitoring per month and per site increased from a median [and 25th and 75th percentiles (p_{25}–p_{75})] of 6 (5–15) to 10 (6.3–15) in the USA and from 2 (1–2.5) to 3 (2–4.5) in Canada [14]. ICUs are the main drivers of this increase in cEEG monitoring. A survey of 137 intensivists and neurophysiologists from 97 adult ICUs in the USA reported a 43% increase in the number of cEEG per month during a 1-year period [15]. Further, in an ideal situation with unlimited resources, respondents would monitor between 10 and 30% more patients (depending on specific cEEG indications), and 18% would increase cEEG duration [15].

However, resources are limited and relatively minor changes in cEEG monitoring strategies can lead to major differences in the rate of seizure detection and in costs [16], specifically by identifying patients at greatest risk. Using readily available variables, a proposed model can guide the use of limited resources to those patients who will benefit more from EEG monitoring [17]. In a cost-effectiveness analysis of electrographic seizures in the pediatric ICU, cEEG monitoring for 1 h, 24 h, and 48 h would identify 55%,

© Springer International Publishing AG 2017
P.N. Varelas, J. Claassen (eds.), *Seizures in Critical Care*, Current Clinical Neurology, DOI 10.1007/978-3-319-49557-6_2

85%, and 89% of children experiencing electrographic seizures, respectively [18]. The preferred strategy (specifically, higher cost-effectiveness for detection of a patient with seizures) would be cEEG monitoring for 1 h if the decision-maker was willing to pay <$1666, for 24 h if willingness to pay was $1666–$22,648, and for 48 h if willingness to pay was >$22,648 [18]. Seizure detection is used as a surrogate end point for the real outcome of interest: outcome improvement. Several studies show that electrographic seizures and electrographic SE are independently associated with worse outcomes in neonates [3–6], children [2, 4, 5, 7–9], and adults [12, 19], but there is no conclusive evidence that early detection and treatment of electrographic seizures improves outcome [16]. However, a study showed that even minor improvements in outcome may make up for the tentative economic burden of cEEG monitoring [20]. If cEEG yielded an increase in quality-adjusted life years (QALYs) of as little as 3%, cEEG monitoring for 24 h would be more cost-effective than not performing an EEG or performing a one-hour EEG [20]. For QALY increases of 3–6%, both 24 h and 48 h monitoring (depending on willingness to pay per QUALY) would be cost-effective compared to not performing an EEG or a one-hour EEG [20]. For QUALY increases of more than seven percent cEEG monitoring for 48 h would be the more cost-effectiveness strategy [20]. Unfortunately, these cost-effectiveness data cannot be translated into objective clinical decision-making because there is no data on how much—if at all—detection and treatment of electrographic seizures influences outcome. Hence, there is an urgent need for high-quality and quantitative estimates of the influence of electrographic seizures on outcome.

Terminology

For the purposes of this review, we define electrographic seizures as abnormal, paroxysmal electroencephalographic events that differ from the background activity and evolve in frequency, morphology, and spatial distribution on EEG [21]. We classified seizures into electroclinical seizures when there is a clinical correlate and electrographic-only seizures when they are asymptomatic or have very subtle clinical features detected only during video-EEG review [21]. For the purposes of this overview, we refer to electrographic SE as uninterrupted electrographic seizures lasting at least 30 min or repeated electrographic seizures totaling more than 30 min in any 1 h period [2, 6, 9, 22, 23], although lower time thresholds like 5 min are gaining popularity following the literature on convulsive SE [24].

We only considered outcomes that were objectively defined in the primary studies such as in-hospital death, death at 30 days after an index event (such as stroke or sepsis), or functional outcomes defined with a widely used scale such as the Glasgow Outcome Scale. The literature is skewed toward short-term outcomes, and this review reflects the available data. We focused our review on outcome data from adult studies.

Literature Search Methods

We performed a PubMed search up to September 2015 using different combinations of the following terms: "seizures," "nonconvulsive seizures," "electrographic seizures," "epilepsy," "critical," "intensive care unit," "sepsis," "septic shock," "traumatic brain injury," "subarachnoid hemorrhage," "stroke," "brain infarct," "intracranial bleeding," "cardiac surgery," "cardiac arrest," and "brain tumor." The initial searches returned 4627 articles. Additional 589 papers were identified from relevant articles from a manual search of cited references. After screening and exclusion of abstracts (and when relevant, full-text manuscripts), 76 articles were included in this literature review (Fig. 2.1).

Electrographic Seizures in the Intensive Care Unit

Electrographic seizures and electrographic SE are frequent and are often associated with poor outcome in critically ill patients [11]. In a study of 201 adults in a medical ICU without known acute neurologic injury, 21 patients (10%) had electrographic seizures, 34 (17%) had periodic epileptiform discharges, 10 (5%) had both, and 45 (22%) had either electrographic seizures or periodic epileptiform discharges [12]. Electrographic seizures were electrographic-only (not clinically detectable) in most patients (67%) [12]. After controlling for age, coma, renal failure, hepatic failure, and circulatory shock, the presence of electrographic seizures or periodic epileptiform discharges was associated with death or severe disability, with an odds ratio of 19.1 (95% CI, 6.3–74.6) [12]. In a large series of 5949 adult (>17 years) patients who underwent mechanical ventilation (as a proxy for ICU stay) and in whom a routine EEG or a cEEG was performed, the use of EEG was independently associated with lower in-hospital mortality (OR = 0.63, 95% CI, 0.51–0.76) with no significant difference in cost or length of stay [13].

However, electrographic seizures are not always an independent predictor of poor outcome. In a series of 247 adult (>17 years) patients presenting to the emergency department with seizures who either died in the emergency department or were admitted to the ICU, ten patients died in hospital, and nine were discharged to hospice for a total of 19 (7.7%) patients with a poor prognosis [25]. The causes of death (septic shock in three patients, cocaine-associated intracranial hemorrhage in two, cardiac death in two, ruptured

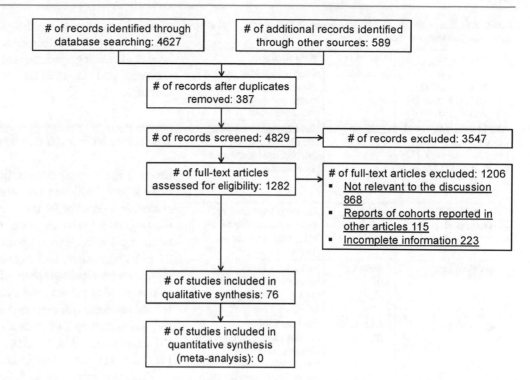

Fig. 2.1 PRISMA flowchart of the literature search methods and results

cerebral aneurysm in one, acute ischemic stroke in one, and ethylene glycol ingestion in one) suggest that the primary etiology and not the seizures was largely responsible for mortality [25]. Independent risk factors for poor outcome were early intubation (OR 6.44, 95% CI, 1.88–26.6) and acute intracranial disease (OR 5.78, 95% CI, 1.97–18.6) [25]. In contrast, presence of SE was not associated with a poor outcome in this series [25].

Whether electrographic seizures worsen outcome independent of the underlying etiology or whether they are just a biomarker of a more severe underlying lesion is a matter of ongoing discussions and study, and there are significant hurdles to appropriately answer this question best. First, the frequency of electrographic seizures reported in the literature is inherently biased due to confounding by indication as most patients only undergo cEEG when clinically indicated. A survey of 330 neurologists showed that the most common indications for performing cEEG monitoring in critically ill patients were altered mental status with or without seizures, subtle eye movements, acute brain lesion, and paralyzed patient in the ICU [26], but indications vary between and within centers. Second, patients might be misclassified as not having electrographic-only seizures because they occur prior to initiation of monitoring or after cEEG is discontinued. cEEG is most commonly used for at least 24 h if there are no electrographic seizures and, when detected, maintained for at least 24 h after the last seizure [26]. However, in certain populations such as patients with non-traumatic subarachnoid hemorrhage, the first seizure can occur later than 48 h [27] and might be missed when monitoring routinely for

24–48 h. Last, the impact of seizures on outcome might be etiology specific; electrographic seizures might cause marked outcome worsening in subarachnoid hemorrhage but not in brain tumors. Studies that analyze heterogeneous and broad etiologic categories jointly might bury associations in individual subgroups. In the following sections, we summarize the impact of electrographic seizures on outcome in different subgroups of critically ill patients (Tables 2.1 and 2.2).

Outcome in Sepsis

EEG background abnormalities and electrographic seizures are common in patients with sepsis [28]. In a series of 71 adults with septic shock, 43 patients underwent EEG for clinical signs of coma, delirium, or seizure, and 13 (30.2%) had electrographic seizures [29]. Based on the limited literature available, sepsis is a risk factor for electrographic seizures, and when patients present with seizures and sepsis, outcomes are poor. In a series of 201 patients admitted to the ICU for acute neurologic injury, sepsis on admission was the only independent predictor of electrographic seizures, and electrographic seizures were independent predictors of death or severe disability at hospital discharge with an OR of 19.1 (95% CI, 6.3–74.6) [12]. In another series, 100 of 154 adults in a surgical ICU developed sepsis, and among these patients 24 (15.6%) had electrographic seizures and 8 of 24 (33.3%) patients had electrographic SE [30]. Electrographic seizures (including electrographic SE) were independently associated with poor outcome (death, vegetative state, or severe

Table 2.1 Summary of studies that suggest that electrographic seizures independently worsen outcome

Author and year	Population	Main finding
Glass et al. [3], Lambrechtsen et al. [4], McBride et al. [5], Pisani et al. [6]	Neonates	Electrographic seizures and electrographic SE are independent predictors of poor outcomes
Abend et al. [2], Lambrechtsen et al. [4], McBride et al. [5], Gwer et al. [7], Payne et al. [8], Topjian et al. [9]	Children	Electrographic seizures and electrographic SE are independent predictors of poor outcomes
Oddo et al. [12], Foreman et al. [11], Claassen et al. [10]	Adults	Electrographic seizures and electrographic SE are independent predictors of poor outcomes
Vespa et al. [36]	Adults with TBI	Increase in brain extracellular glutamate during electrographic seizures
Vespa et al. [37]	Adults with TBI	Patients with electrographic seizures had higher elevations of intracranial pressure and lactate/pyruvate ratio than matched controls
Ko et al. [79]	Single adult post-cardiac arrest	Electrographic seizures were time-locked with reductions in brain tissue oxygen tension, increases in cerebral blood flow, and increases in brain temperature

SE Status epilepticus, *TBI* Traumatic brain injury

disability) at hospital discharge, with an OR of 10.4 (95% CI, 1–53.7) [30]. Further data are needed to evaluate the impact of electrographic seizures during sepsis on long-term outcome and to elucidate whether treatment modifies outcome.

Outcome in Traumatic Brain Injury

Electrographic seizures are frequent following traumatic brain injury (TBI) and are often associated with poor outcomes. In a series of 94 adults with moderate to severe TBI, electrographic seizures occurred in 21 (22.3%) patients including 6 with electrographic SE [31]. In this study, 11 of 21 (52.4%) patients had electrographic-only seizures [31]. Patients with electrographic seizures had similar outcomes as compared to patients without electrographic seizures, but the six patients with electrographic SE died (100% mortality), compared to 24% mortality in the non-seizure group [31], suggesting that the presence of SE (and not only the presence of seizures) was associated with worse outcomes.

Electrographic seizures following TBI are also frequent in children, especially during the first 2 years of life [32, 33]. In a series of 144 children with TBI and cEEG, 43 (29.9%) patients had electrographic seizures, 17 of whom had electrographic-only seizures [33]. The presence or absence of electrographic seizures or status epilepticus did not correlate with discharge outcome, classified in only three broad categories: death, discharge to rehabilitation facility, and discharge to home [33]. In a series of 87 children with TBI and

Table 2.2 Summary of the association of seizures with worse outcomes in different conditions

	Experimental models	Clinical studies: short-term outcomes	Clinical studies: long-term outcomes	Comments
Sepsis	?	+	?	Unclear whether electrographic seizures impact outcomes or just reflect a more severe underlying lesion
Traumatic brain injury	+	+	−	Unclear whether electrographic seizures impact outcomes or just reflect a more severe underlying lesion
Subarachnoid hemorrhage	+	+	+	The inflammatory cascade of blood products in the brain causes worse outcomes through electrographic seizures
Stroke (ischemic or hemorrhagic)	?	−	−	Electrographic seizures are not independent predictors of outcome in most studies
Cardiac surgery	?	+	+	Heterogeneous group with multiple potential confounders
Cardiac arrest	+	+	+	Electrographic seizures cause additional damage in the human brain
Tumor	−	−	−	Electrographic seizures more frequent in slow-growing tumors

+ Data supporting a positive association, − Data supporting lack of an association, ? Unknown/limited evidence cEEG admitted to the ICU, 37 (42.5%) patients had electrographic seizures, 14 of whom had electrographic-only seizures [32]. Outcomes at hospital discharge—measured more precisely with the King's Outcome Scale for Childhood Head Injury—were worse in patients with clinical and subclinical SE, electrographic-only seizures, and electrographic SE [32].

Worse outcomes might simply reflect a more severe underlying etiology. However, some studies suggest that electrographic seizures contribute to poor outcomes. In a series of 140 patients with moderate to severe TBI and cEEG, 32 (22.9%) patients had electrographic seizures [34]. A subgroup of patients had volumetric MRI at baseline (within 2 weeks of TBI) and 6 months after TBI [34]. Among these, six had electrographic seizures and were compared with a control group of ten patients matched by Glasgow Coma Scale, CT lesion, and occurrence of surgery [34]. Patients with electrographic seizures had greater hippocampal atrophy on follow-up as compared to those without seizures (21% vs 12%, $p = 0.017$) [34]. Further, hippocampi ipsilateral to the electrographic seizure focus demonstrated a greater degree of atrophy as compared with contralateral hippocampi (28% vs 13%, $p = 0.007$) [34]. These data suggest that post-TBI electrographic seizures cause long-term anatomic damage [34].

The underlying mechanism by which post-TBI electrographic seizures cause worse outcomes may be related to the dysregulation between excitation and inhibition. In a mouse model of TBI, glutamate signaling was elevated and GABAergic interneurons were reduced following controlled cortical impact—an experimental equivalent to moderate to severe TBI [35]. In parallel, spontaneous excitatory postsynaptic current increased, and inhibitory postsynaptic current decreased after controlled cortical impact [35]. Similar dysregulation is described in humans. In a series of 17 adults with severe TBI, a microdialysis probe measured extracellular glutamate during the first week post-TBI [36]. Transient elevations in extracellular glutamate occurred during periods of decreased cerebral perfusion pressures of less than 70 mmHg, but also during seizures with normal cerebral blood perfusion [36]. Dysregulation of brain metabolism may elevate intracranial pressure and may lead to worse outcomes. A study in adults with moderate to severe non-penetrating traumatic brain injury evaluated cEEG and cerebral microdialysis for 7 days after the traumatic brain injury [37]. Matched for age, CT lesion, and initial Glasgow Coma Scale, ten patients with electrographic-only seizures (seven with electrographic SE) were compared with ten patients without electrographic seizures [37]. Patients with post-traumatic electrographic-only seizures experienced a higher mean intracranial pressure, a greater percentage of time of elevated intracranial pressure, and a more prolonged elevation of intracranial pressure beyond post-injury hour 100 as compared with patients with no post-traumatic electrographic seizures [37]. Similarly, the lactate/pyruvate ratio was elevated for a longer period of time and more often in patients with post-traumatic electrographic-only seizures [37]. In ten patients with electrographic-only seizures, a within-subject design compared the time periods 12 h before seizure and 12 h after seizure onset within the same patients [37]. Seizures led to episodic increases in intracranial pressure, in lactate/pyruvate ratio, and in mean glutamate level [37]. These findings have been confirmed on a series of 34 patients with severe traumatic brain injury in whom brain microdialysis showed that the lactate/pyruvate ratio increased during seizures and pseudoperiodic discharges, but not during non-epileptic epochs [38]. These results suggest that intracranial pressure and lactate/pyruvate ratio go up in response to electrographic-only seizures, and not vice versa. Electrographic-only seizures may therefore not only represent a simple biomarker of brain damage, but may contribute to further brain damage, at least in the context of traumatic brain injury.

Prior studies suggest that seizures contribute to worse outcomes by causing additional damage. Therefore, prophylactic AED use to reduce seizure burden, and to improve outcomes, has been contemplated. However, a Cochrane review of randomized clinical trials found that AED prophylaxis in TBI reduced the risk of early seizures (within 1 week of TBI) but not late seizures or mortality [39]. In summary, post-TBI electrographic seizures lead to further brain damage, but to date there is lack of evidence that electrographic seizure control after TBI improves outcomes.

Outcome in Subarachnoid Hemorrhage

Electrographic seizures are particularly frequent and appear relatively late in patients with subarachnoid hemorrhage. Electrographic seizures occurred in 8 of 69 (11.6%) patients with non-traumatic high-grade subarachnoid hemorrhage [27]. In this study, the initial 17 patients underwent cEEG for clinical suspicion of electrographic seizures, which occurred in 3 (17.7%) patients [27]. The following 52 patients underwent cEEG as part of a protocol for subarachnoid hemorrhage, regardless of clinical suspicion, and electrographic seizures occurred in 5 (9.6%) patients [27]. Among the 35 patients monitored per protocol and without a clinical suspicion of seizures, electrographic seizures occurred in 3 (8.6%) patients [27]. While high clinical grade of the subarachnoid hemorrhage was associated with poor outcome, the presence of electrographic seizures was not [27]. In a series of 402 patients with subarachnoid hemorrhage, seizure burden was independently associated with outcome so that every hour of seizure on cEEG was associated with an OR of 1.1 (95% CI, 1.01–1.21) to 3-month disability and mortality [40].

In contrast, other studies showed an association between electrographic seizures and poor outcome. In a series of 479 adult patients with subarachnoid hemorrhage, 53 (11%) had electrographic seizures [10]. Patients with electrographic seizures had increased clinical and laboratory inflammatory biomarkers, and the degree of inflammation was an independent predictor of electrographic seizures [10]. On univariate analysis, both inflammatory burden during the first 4 days and the presence of electrographic seizures were associated with poor outcome [10]. But after correction for other potential confounders, only electrographic seizures remained a predictor of poor outcome [10]. Further, mediation analysis showed that the effect of inflammation on outcome was mediated through the presence of electrographic seizures [10]. In summary, this study suggests that blood products in the brain may trigger an inflammatory cascade which causes electrographic seizures and, eventually, poor outcomes [10].

The concept that inflammatory cascades cause or contribute to seizures, and these impact outcome, is clinically relevant because it implies that anti-inflammatory products may reduce seizures. In fact, targeted anti-inflammatory treatments have controlled seizures or brain damage in animal models. In a rat model of inflammation—induced either by intestinal inflammation which increases tumor necrosis factor alpha (TNFα) or by direct infusion of TNFα—neuronal excitability increased with severity of inflammation. Central antagonism of TNFα prevented increase in seizure susceptibility [41]. Further, in a rat model of subarachnoid hemorrhage, the administration of IL-1RA—an interleukin-1 (IL-1) antagonist—reduced blood-brain barrier breakdown and the extent of brain injury [42].

Despite promising animal models, anti-inflammatory therapy for seizure prevention in subarachnoid hemorrhage is not ready for clinical use. A more realistic goal in subarachnoid hemorrhage may be outcome prediction based on cEEG results. In a series of 116 patients on cEEG following subarachnoid hemorrhage and with 3 months functional follow-up (measured with the modified Rankin Scale), the absence of sleep architecture (OR, 4.3) and the presence of periodic lateralized discharges (OR, 18.8) independently predicted poor outcome [43]. Additionally, outcome was poor in all patients with lack of EEG reactivity or state changes within the first 24 h, generalized periodic epileptiform discharges, or bilateral independent periodic lateralized epileptiform discharges and in 92% of patients with nonconvulsive SE [43].

cEEG may not only predict, but it may also modify outcome in patients with subarachnoid hemorrhage by early detection of delayed cerebral ischemia. In a series of 34 patients with subarachnoid hemorrhage, 9 (26.5%) patients developed delayed cerebral ischemia [44]. Visual analysis of cEEG demonstrated new onset slowing or focal attenuation in seven of nine patients with delayed cerebral ischemia (77.8%) [44]. Further, decreases in alpha power to delta power ratio identified patients with delayed cerebral ischemia with a very high sensitivity and a reasonable specificity: a cutoff of six consecutive recordings with more than 10% decrease in alpha power to delta power ratio from baseline yielded a sensitivity of 100% and a specificity of 76%; a cutoff of any single measurement with more than 50% decrease in the ratio yielded a sensitivity of 89% and a specificity of 84% [44]. In summary, cEEG detects electrographic seizures and/or delayed cerebral ischemia in patients with subarachnoid hemorrhage and in the appropriate clinical setting may improve outcomes.

Outcome in Stroke

Seizures occur frequently after stroke, particularly when it involves a hemorrhagic component or conversion from ischemic to hemorrhagic. In a study of 6044 patients with stroke, 190 (3.1%) patients experienced clinical seizures within the first 24 h, and these were more frequent in hemorrhagic than in ischemic stroke [45]. On univariate analysis, patients with seizures had a higher 30-day mortality rate than patients without seizures (32.1% vs 13.3%) [45]. Clinical seizures might represent only "the tip of the iceberg" as electrographic-only seizures might be overlooked without cEEG monitoring. In a series of 109 patients with stroke, electrographic seizures within 72 h occurred in 21 (19.3%) patients: 18 of 63 (28.6%) patients with intracranial hemorrhage, and in 3 of 46 (6.5%) patients with ischemic stroke [46]. On univariate analysis, posthemorrhagic seizures worsened the NIH Stroke Scale and increased midline shift [46]. However, on multivariate analysis, seizures did not independently predict outcome [45, 46]. Similarly, clinical seizures within 30 days of non-traumatic supratentorial hemorrhage occurred in 57 of 761 (7.5%) patients, but seizures were not independent predictors of in-hospital mortality [47]. In concordance with these results, electrographic seizures occurred in 32 of 102 (31%) adults with non-traumatic intracerebral hemorrhage who underwent cEEG monitoring [48]. In this series, 20 (20%) patients died in the hospital, and 5 patients had poor neurological outcome including coma, persistent vegetative state, or minimally conscious state [48]. Independent factors associated with poor outcome (defined as death, vegetative or minimally conscious state) at hospital discharge were coma at the time of hospital admission (OR 9, 95% CI, 2.4–34.3), intracranial hemorrhage volume of 60 ml or more (OR 4.4, 95% CI, 1.2–15.7), presence of periodic epileptiform discharges (OR 7.6, 95% CI, 2.1–27.3), periodic lateralized epileptiform discharges (PLEDs) (OR 11.9, 95% CI, 2.9–49.2), and focal stimulus-induced rhythmic, periodic, or ictal discharges (SIRPIDs) [48]. In this series, lower systolic blood pressure on admission was protective (OR 0.9, 95% CI, 0.9–1 per mmHg), but the presence of electrographic seizures did not influence outcome [48]. In summary, after nontraumatic intracranial hemorrhage, clinical seizures occur in approximately 3–8% of patients, but many seizures are subclinical, and EEG detects electrographic seizures in approximately 20–30% of patients. However, based on available data, seizures were not independent predictors of outcome.

Further, seizures were also not clearly associated with acute deterioration following stroke. In a series of 266 patients with non-traumatic intracranial hemorrhage, early neurological deterioration occurred in 61 (22.9%) patients and was associated with an eightfold increase in poor outcome; however, seizures were not a predictor of early neurological deterioration [49].

Considering more detailed outcome features, late seizures are weakly associated with subsequent development of epilepsy. In a series of 1897 patients with stroke, seizures occurred in 168 (8.9%) patients: 28 of 265 (10.6%) patients with hemorrhagic stroke and 140 of 1632 (8.6%) patients with ischemic stroke [50]. Recurrent seizures occurred in 47 of 1897 (2.5%) patients with late first seizure onset as sole risk factor for epilepsy following ischemic stroke. In this series, the authors did not find risk factors following hemorrhagic stroke [50]. Mechanistically, early seizures may frequently reflect brain irritation by blood products, while late seizures may often be related to gliosis and scarring [51]. In a series of 110 patients who underwent clot evacuation after intracerebral hemorrhage, the frequency of seizures was particularly high, occurring in 41%: early-onset seizures (within 2 weeks) in 31% and late-onset seizures in 10% [52]. Independent predictors of early-onset seizures were volume of hemorrhage, presence of subarachnoid hemorrhage, and subdural hemorrhage, and independent predictors of late-onset seizures were subdural hemorrhage and increased admission international normalized ratio (INR) [52]. These results suggest that the severity of the bleeding is related to seizure development. Therefore, these authors recommended prophylactic antiepileptic therapy for patients with severe intracranial hemorrhage [52]. However, the value of AEDs in intracranial hemorrhage remains unclear. In a study where 5 of 295 (1.7%) patients with intracranial hemorrhage had seizures, the use of AEDs was an independent risk factor for poor outcome after 90 days [53]. The deleterious effects of stroke and SE appear to act synergistically, so that mortality is three times higher when there is SE on an ischemic stroke compared to when there is only an ischemic stroke [54]. In summary, poststroke seizures are not independent predictors of outcome [50, 51], and their treatment does not necessarily improve prognosis [53]. However, the presence of SE may worsen prognosis, especially in ischemic stroke [54].

Outcome After Cardiac Surgery

Seizures after cardiac surgery are relatively frequent, especially in neonates, and are associated with worse short-term outcome in most studies. In a series of 2578 patients who underwent cardiac surgery, clinical seizures occurred in 31 (1.2%) cases [55]. Compared to patients without seizures, patients with seizures experienced an almost fivefold increase (29% vs 6%) in in-hospital mortality, a higher incidence of all major postoperative complications, and a lower one-year survival rate (53% vs 84%) [55]. In contrast, a study of 101 adult patients (>18 years) who underwent sub-hairline cEEG after cardiac surgery found that 3 (3%) had electrographic seizures—two electroclinical and one electrographic-only—but the presence of electrographic seizures did not affect morbidity or mortality [56]. Of note, lack of correlation between electrographic seizures and outcome in this particular study may have been related to a limited EEG montage utilizing a four-channel subhairline EEG applied in the frontal and temporal regions with a typical sensitivity of 68% (95% CI, 45–86%) and a specificity of 98% (95% CI, 89–100%) for detecting seizures as compared to a regular 10–20 electrode placement [56, 57]. Further, only three patients had seizures, limiting statistical analyses in the series [56].

In newborns, electrographic seizures following cardiac surgery are particularly frequent and associated with worse short-term outcomes. Thirteen of 161 (8%) neonates undergoing cardiac surgery had seizures, and these were electrographic-only seizures in most patients (11; 85%) [58]. Acute mortality was higher among neonates with seizures (38% vs 3%) [58]. In contrast, the effect of electrographic seizures on more subtle outcomes, such as neurodevelopmental outcomes, remains to be defined. From a series of 164 survivors of neonatal cardiac surgery, 114 underwent developmental evaluation utilizing Bayley Scales of Infant Development II at 1 year of age [59]. Electrographic seizures occurred in 15 of 114 (13%) patients, but developmental outcomes were not different in patients with and without a history of seizures [59]. However, cEEG after cardiac surgery might help in delineating short-term outcomes. In a series of 723 adults who underwent cardiac surgery, neurological dysfunction within 24 h after surgery occurred in 12 patients: five did not regain consciousness after surgery, four had a clinical event suspicious for seizure, and three had neurological deficits [60]. Among the five patients who did not regain consciousness, two (40%) were in electrographic-only SE: one died during hospitalization, and the other received aggressive treatment for electrographic-only seizures and was discharged to an acute rehabilitation facility [60]. Among the 12 patients with neurological dysfunction, 5 (42%) patients died during the admission, 4 (33%) were discharged home, and 3 (25%) were discharged to an acute rehabilitation facility [60]. Numbers are small to evaluate whether cEEG results can reliably predict outcomes, but among the five patients with an EEG reactive to noxious stimuli, some were discharged home (three patients) or to an acute rehabilitation facility (two patients), while among the seven patients with a nonreactive EEG, five (71%) patients died [60]. It is likely that some of these poor outcomes can be attributed to relatively high frequency of stroke in children undergoing cardiac surgery [61, 62].

Outcome After Cardiac Arrest

Electrographic SE is common after cardiac arrest. A study of 101 adults on therapeutic hypothermia and cEEG following cardiac arrest found that electrographic SE occurred in 12 (12%) patients [63]. In this series, electrographic SE marked a poor prognosis with only 1 of 12 (8%) patients surviving—in a vegetative state [63]. In a study of children with therapeutic hypothermia after cardiac arrest, 9 of 19 (47.4%) children had electrographic seizures, of whom 6 had electrographic SE [64]. In this study five patients died: three with severely abnormal EEG backgrounds and electrographic seizures and two with mild/moderate EEG backgrounds and without seizures [64]. In a series of 106 adults on therapeutic hypothermia and cEEG after cardiac arrest, 33 (31%) patients had electrographic SE [65]. One year after cardiac arrest, 31 (29%) patients had favorable outcomes, and electrographic SE was the most relevant predictive factor of poor outcome [65]. cEEG helps to predict both good and poor outcome after cardiac arrest: in a series of 56 adults on therapeutic hypothermia and cEEG after cardiac arrest, 27 (48%) patients had a good neurological outcome, and 29 (52%) patients had a poor neurological outcome [66]. Low-voltage or isoelectric EEG patterns within 24 h of cardiac arrest predicted poor neurological outcome with a sensitivity of 40%, a specificity of 100%, a negative predictive value of 68%, and a positive predictive value of 100% [66]. Low-voltage or isoelectric EEG patterns predicted poor neurological outcome better than bilateral absent N20 responses with a sensitivity of 24%, a specificity of 100%, a negative predictive value of 55%, and a positive predictive value of 100% [66].

However, cEEG is resource-intensive. Therefore, reduced EEG montages and automated EEG analyses are being evaluated as a cheaper approach for outcome prediction after cardiac arrest [67]. Reduced versions of the EEG such as continuous amplitude-integrated EEG predict outcome as demonstrated by a series of 95 adults on therapeutic hypothermia, regular cEEG, and amplitude-integrated cEEG after cardiac arrest [68]. In this series, an initial flat amplitude-integrated EEG did not have prognostic value, but a continuous EEG pattern at the start of the recording was associated with recovery of consciousness in 87% of the patients, a continuous EEG pattern at normothermia was associated with recovery of consciousness in 90% of the patients, and suppression burst was always associated with eventual death [68]. Myoclonic SE after cardiac arrest has been classically considered incompatible with good outcome. However, in the era of therapeutic hypothermia, a growing body of evidence shows that some patients may recover after myoclonic SE following cardiac arrest [69–78].

Electrographic seizures, as well as abnormal EEG background patterns, may simply be a marker of severity for the underlying encephalopathy. However, some results suggest that electrographic seizures independently contribute to brain damage and worse outcomes. In an 85-year-old patient who underwent hypothermia and multimodality monitoring after cardiac arrest, 17 electrographic seizures were time-locked with reductions in brain tissue oxygen tension, increases in cerebral blood flow, and increases in brain temperature [79]. These metabolic derangements normalized during interictal periods and after AED treatment stopped the seizures [79]. Therefore, electrographic seizures may impose an increase metabolic demand which cannot be met in the already damaged brain leading to further tissue damage. More importantly, these findings suggest that timely treatment of seizures might halt additional damage.

Outcome in Tumors

Clinical seizures are one of the most common presenting symptoms of intracranial tumors. Seizures occur more frequently in slow-growing tumors than in aggressive tumors—hence the fact that seizures may sometimes be actually considered to be a marker of good prognosis in brain tumors [80]. Seizures are also a marker of tumor recurrence after surgical resection. In a series of 332 adults who underwent initial surgery for low-grade gliomas, 269 (81%) had at least one clinical seizure before surgery [81]. Seizure freedom after resective surgery occurred in 67% of patients and was more frequent among those with gross-total resection than after subtotal resection or biopsy [81]. Seizure recurrence after initial postoperative seizure control was a marker of tumor progression with a proportional hazard ratio of 3.8 (95% CI, 1.74–8.29) [81].

It is unclear how aggressive electrographic-only seizures should be treated. In a series of 947 EEGs in 658 patients with tumors, 26 episodes of electrographic SE were found in 25 patients [82]. Among these, 11 (44%) patients had a primary brain tumor, 12 (48%) patients had a systemic tumor, and 2 (8%) had both [82]. Fifteen of 25 (60%) patients with electrographic SE had a new intracranial lesion defined as progression of neoplastic disease or a new unrelated lesion [82]. In this series, 3 of 25 (12%) patients died during electrographic SE, but more aggressive AED treatment was not pursued as the patients received comfort care in a terminal disease [82]. Based on limited literature, electrographic seizures associated with tumors likely represent a marker of the underlying pathology and do not significantly alter outcome.

Pediatric Outcome

Electrographic seizures are frequent in critically ill children, occurring with a frequency of 7–46% depending on indications and clinical settings [8, 83–87]. However, it remains unclear whether electrographic seizures worsen outcome or they are mere biomarkers of a more severe underlying etiology. In a study of children in coma, 74 of 204 (36.3%) had electrographic seizures, and they independently predicted poor outcome with an OR of 15.4 (95% CI, 4.7–49.7) [88]. In a series of children who underwent cEEG, 84 of 200 (42%) had electrographic seizures, and 43 had electrographic SE [9]. In this study, electrographic seizures were not an independent predictor of mortality, but electrographic SE was with an OR of 5.1 (95% CI, 1.4–18) [9]. Therefore, the presence of SE may be independently associated with worse outcomes. In particular, in a series of 259 children with EEG monitoring, electrographic seizures occurred in 93 (35.9%) and electrographic SE in 23 patients [8]. Above a maximum seizure burden threshold of 20% — 12 min — per hour, both the probability and the magnitude of neurological decline rose sharply [8]. On multivariable analysis, the odds of neurological decline increased by 1.13 (95% CI, 1.05–1.21) for every 1% increase in maximum seizure burden per hour [8].

Seizure burden or severity is also associated with poor outcomes in newborns [5]. In a series of 77 term newborns at risk for hypoxic-ischemic brain injury, the presence and severity of clinical seizures was an independent predictor of motor and cognitive poor outcome [3]. In a series of 56 newborns treated with hypothermia, seizures occurred in 17 (32.7%) and electrographic SE in 5 [89]. Moderate to severe brain injury was more common in newborns with seizures with a relative risk of 2.9 (95% CI, 1.2–4.5), and electrographic-only seizures were associated with injury as electroclinical seizures [89]. In a series of 218 term infants with moderate to severe neonatal encephalopathy, children with no seizures on amplitude-integrated EEG had a higher incidence of death and severe neurodevelopmental disability at 18 months of age with an OR of 1.96 (95% CI, 1.02–3.74) [90].

Conclusions

Electrographic seizures are common (10–40%) in critically ill newborns, children, and adults, and most cannot be detected without an EEG. It remains unknown whether elec-trographic seizures worsen outcomes independently from the underlying cause, but available literature to date suggests an independent impact on outcome. Treatment may also have to be tailored taking underlying etiology into consideration.

References

1. Claassen J, Mayer SA, Kowalski RG, Emerson RG, Hirsch LJ. Detection of electrographic seizures with continuous EEG monitoring in critically ill patients. Neurology. 2004;62:1743–8.
2. Abend NS, Arndt DH, Carpenter JL, et al. Electrographic seizures in pediatric ICU patients: cohort study of risk factors and mortality. Neurology. 2013;81:383–91.
3. Glass HC, Glidden D, Jeremy RJ, Barkovich AJ, Ferriero DM, Miller SP. Clinical neonatal seizures are independently associated with outcome in infants at risk for hypoxic-ischemic brain injury. J Pediatr. 2009;155:318–23.
4. Lambrechtsen FA, Buchhalter JR. Aborted and refractory status epilepticus in children: a comparative analysis. Epilepsia. 2008;49:615–25.
5. McBride MC, Laroia N, Guillet R. Electrographic seizures in neonates correlate with poor neurodevelopmental outcome. Neurology. 2000;55:506–13.
6. Pisani F, Cerminara C, Fusco C, Sisti L. Neonatal status epilepticus vs recurrent neonatal seizures: clinical findings and outcome. Neurology. 2007;69:2177–85.
7. Gwer S, Idro R, Fegan G, et al. Continuous EEG monitoring in Kenyan children with non-traumatic coma. Arch Dis Child. 2012;97:343–9.
8. Payne ET, Zhao XY, Frndova H, et al. Seizure burden is independently associated with short term outcome in critically ill children. Brain. 2014;137:1429–38.
9. Topjian AA, Gutierrez-Colina AM, Sanchez SM, et al. Electrographic status epilepticus is associated with mortality and worse short-term outcome in critically ill children. Crit Care Med. 2013;41:215–23.
10. Claassen J, Albers D, Schmidt JM, et al. Nonconvulsive seizures in subarachnoid hemorrhage link inflammation and outcome. Ann Neurol. 2014;75:771–81.
11. Foreman B, Claassen J, Abou Khaled K, et al. Generalized periodic discharges in the critically ill: a case-control study of 200 patients. Neurology. 2012;79:1951–60.
12. Oddo M, Carrera E, Claassen J, Mayer SA, Hirsch LJ. Continuous electroencephalography in the medical intensive care unit. Crit Care Med. 2009;37:2051–6.
13. Ney JP, van der Goes DN, Nuwer MR, Nelson L, Eccher MA. Continuous and routine EEG in intensive care: utilization and outcomes, United States 2005–2009. Neurology. 2013;81:2002–8.
14. Sanchez SM, Carpenter J, Chapman KE, et al. Pediatric ICU EEG monitoring: current resources and practice in the United States and Canada. J Clin Neurophysiol. 2013;30:156–60.
15. Gavvala J, Abend N, LaRoche S, et al. Continuous EEG monitoring: a survey of neurophysiologists and neurointensivists. Epilepsia. 2014;55:1864–71.
16. Gutierrez-Colina AM, Topjian AA, Dlugos DJ, Abend NS. Electroencephalogram monitoring in critically ill children: indications and strategies. Pediatr Neurol. 2012;46:158–61.
17. Yang A, Arndt DH, Berg RA, et al. Development and validation of a seizure prediction model in critically ill children. Seizure. 2015;25:104–11.
18. Abend NS, Topjian AA, Williams S. How much does it cost to identify a critically ill child experiencing electrographic seizures? J Clin Neurophysiol. 2015;32:257–64.
19. Young GB, Jordan KG, Doig GS. An assessment of nonconvulsive seizures in the intensive care unit using continuous EEG

monitoring: an investigation of variables associated with mortality. Neurology. 1996;47:83–9.

20. Abend NS, Topjian AA, Williams S. Could EEG monitoring in critically ill children be a cost-effective neuroprotective strategy? J Clin Neurophysiol. 2015;32:486–94.

21. Abend NS, Wusthoff CJ, Goldberg EM, Dlugos DJ. Electrographic seizures and status epilepticus in critically ill children and neonates with encephalopathy. Lancet Neurol. 2013;12:1170–9.

22. Lynch NE, Stevenson NJ, Livingstone V, Murphy BP, Rennie JM, Boylan GB. The temporal evolution of electrographic seizure burden in neonatal hypoxic ischemic encephalopathy. Epilepsia. 2012;53:549–57.

23. Tsuchida TN, Wusthoff CJ, Shellhaas RA, et al. American clinical neurophysiology society standardized EEG terminology and categorization for the description of continuous EEG monitoring in neonates: report of the American Clinical Neurophysiology Society critical care monitoring committee. J Clin Neurophysiol. 2013;30:161–73.

24. Alldredge BK, Gelb AM, Isaacs SM, et al. A comparison of lorazepam, diazepam, and placebo for the treatment of out-of-hospital status epilepticus. N Engl J Med. 2001;345:631–7.

25. Tobochnik S, Gutierrez C, Jacobson MP. Characteristics and acute outcomes of ICU patients with initial presentation of seizure. Seizure. 2015;26:94–7.

26. Abend NS, Dlugos DJ, Hahn CD, Hirsch LJ, Herman ST. Use of EEG monitoring and management of non-convulsive seizures in critically ill patients: a survey of neurologists. Neurocrit Care. 2010;12:382–9.

27. O'Connor KL, Westover MB, Phillips MT, et al. High risk for seizures following subarachnoid hemorrhage regardless of referral bias. Neurocrit Care. 2014;21:476–82.

28. Hosokawa K, Gaspard N, Su F, Oddo M, Vincent JL, Taccone FS. Clinical neurophysiological assessment of sepsis-associated brain dysfunction: a systematic review. Crit Care. 2014;18:674.

29. Polito A, Eischwald F, Maho AL, et al. Pattern of brain injury in the acute setting of human septic shock. Crit Care. 2013;17:R204.

30. Kurtz P, Gaspard N, Wahl AS, et al. Continuous electroencephalography in a surgical intensive care unit. Intensive Care Med. 2014;40:228–34.

31. Vespa PM, Nuwer MR, Nenov V, et al. Increased incidence and impact of nonconvulsive and convulsive seizures after traumatic brain injury as detected by continuous electroencephalographic monitoring. J Neurosurg. 1999;91:750–60.

32. Arndt DH, Lerner JT, Matsumoto JH, et al. Subclinical early post-traumatic seizures detected by continuous EEG monitoring in a consecutive pediatric cohort. Epilepsia. 2013;54:1780–8.

33. O'Neill BR, Handler MH, Tong S, Chapman KE. Incidence of seizures on continuous EEG monitoring following traumatic brain injury in children. J Neurosurg Pediatr. 2015;16:167–76.

34. Vespa PM, McArthur DL, Xu Y, et al. Nonconvulsive seizures after traumatic brain injury are associated with hippocampal atrophy. Neurology. 2010;75:792–8.

35. Cantu D, Walker K, Andresen L, et al. Traumatic brain injury increases cortical glutamate network activity by compromising gabaergic control. Cereb Cortex. 2015;25:2306–20.

36. Vespa P, Prins M, Ronne-Engstrom E, et al. Increase in extracellular glutamate caused by reduced cerebral perfusion pressure and seizures after human traumatic brain injury: a microdialysis study. J Neurosurg. 1998;89:971–82.

37. Vespa PM, Miller C, McArthur D, et al. Nonconvulsive electrographic seizures after traumatic brain injury result in a delayed, prolonged increase in intracranial pressure and metabolic crisis. Crit Care Med. 2007;35:2830–6.

38. Vespa P, Tubi M, Claassen J, et al. Metabolic crisis occurs with seizures and periodic discharges after brain trauma. Ann Neurol. 2016;79:579–90.

39. Thompson K, Pohlmann-Eden B, Campbell LA, Abel H. Pharmacological treatments for preventing epilepsy following traumatic head injury. Cochrane Database Syst Rev. 2015;8:CD009900.

40. De Marchis GM, Pugin D, Meyers E, et al. Seizure burden in subarachnoid hemorrhage associated with functional and cognitive outcome. Neurology. 2016;86:253–60.

41. Riazi K, Galic MA, Kuzmiski JB, Ho W, Sharkey KA, Pittman QJ. Microglial activation and TNFalpha production mediate altered CNS excitability following peripheral inflammation. Proc Natl Acad Sci U S A. 2008;105:17151–6.

42. Greenhalgh AD, Brough D, Robinson EM, Girard S, Rothwell NJ, Allan SM. Interleukin-1 receptor antagonist is beneficial after subarachnoid haemorrhage in rat by blocking haem-driven inflammatory pathology. Dis Model Mech. 2012;5:823–33.

43. Claassen J, Hirsch LJ, Frontera JA, et al. Prognostic significance of continuous EEG monitoring in patients with poor-grade subarachnoid hemorrhage. Neurocrit Care. 2006;4:103–12.

44. Claassen J, Hirsch LJ, Kreiter KT, et al. Quantitative continuous EEG for detecting delayed cerebral ischemia in patients with poor-grade subarachnoid hemorrhage. Clin Neurophysiol. 2004;115:2699–710.

45. Szaflarski JP, Rackley AY, Kleindorfer DO, et al. Incidence of seizures in the acute phase of stroke: a population-based study. Epilepsia. 2008;49:974–81.

46. Vespa PM, O'Phelan K, Shah M, et al. Acute seizures after intracerebral hemorrhage: a factor in progressive midline shift and outcome. Neurology. 2003;60:1441–6.

47. Passero S, Rocchi R, Rossi S, Ulivelli M, Vatti G. Seizures after spontaneous supratentorial intracerebral hemorrhage. Epilepsia. 2002;43:1175–80.

48. Claassen J, Jette N, Chum F, et al. Electrographic seizures and periodic discharges after intracerebral hemorrhage. Neurology. 2007;69:1356–65.

49. Leira R, Davalos A, Silva Y, et al. Early neurologic deterioration in intracerebral hemorrhage: predictors and associated factors. Neurology. 2004;63:461–7.

50. Bladin CF, Alexandrov AV, Bellavance A, et al. Seizures after stroke: a prospective multicenter study. Arch Neurol. 2000;57:1617–22.

51. Camilo O, Goldstein LB. Seizures and epilepsy after ischemic stroke. Stroke. 2004;35:1769–75.

52. Garrett MC, Komotar RJ, Starke RM, Merkow MB, Otten ML, Connolly ES. Predictors of seizure onset after intracerebral hemorrhage and the role of long-term antiepileptic therapy. J Crit Care. 2009;24:335–9.

53. Messe SR, Sansing LH, Cucchiara BL, et al. Prophylactic antiepileptic drug use is associated with poor outcome following ICH. Neurocrit Care. 2009;11:38–44.

54. Waterhouse EJ, Vaughan JK, Barnes TY, et al. Synergistic effect of status epilepticus and ischemic brain injury on mortality. Epilepsy Res. 1998;29:175–83.

55. Goldstone AB, Bronster DJ, Anyanwu AC, et al. Predictors and outcomes of seizures after cardiac surgery: a multivariable analysis of 2,578 patients. Ann Thorac Surg. 2011;91:514–8.

56. Gofton TE, Chu MW, Norton L, et al. A prospective observational study of seizures after cardiac surgery using continuous EEG monitoring. Neurocrit Care. 2014;21:220–7.

57. Young GB, Sharpe MD, Savard M, Al Thenayan E, Norton L, Davies-Schinkel C. Seizure detection with a commercially available bedside EEG monitor and the subhairline montage. Neurocrit Care. 2009;11:411–6.

58. Naim MY, Gaynor JW, Chen J, et al. Subclinical seizures identified by postoperative electroencephalographic monitoring are common after neonatal cardiac surgery. J Thorac Cardiovasc Surg. 2015;150:169–78. discussion 178-180

59. Gaynor JW, Jarvik GP, Bernbaum J, et al. The relationship of post-operative electrographic seizures to neurodevelopmental outcome at 1 year of age after neonatal and infant cardiac surgery. J Thorac Cardiovasc Surg. 2006;131:181–9.

60. Marcuse LV, Bronster DJ, Fields M, Polanco A, Yu T, Chikwe J. Evaluating the obtunded patient after cardiac surgery: the role of continuous electroencephalography. J Crit Care. 2014;29:316.e1–5.

61. Chen J, Zimmerman RA, Jarvik GP, et al. Perioperative stroke in infants undergoing open heart operations for congenital heart disease. Ann Thorac Surg. 2009;88:823–9.

62. Domi T, Edgell DS, McCrindle BW, et al. Frequency, predictors, and neurologic outcomes of vaso-occlusive strokes associated with cardiac surgery in children. Pediatrics. 2008;122:1292–8.

63. Rittenberger JC, Popescu A, Brenner RP, Guyette FX, Callaway CW. Frequency and timing of nonconvulsive status epilepticus in comatose post-cardiac arrest subjects treated with hypothermia. Neurocrit Care. 2012;16:114–22.

64. Abend NS, Topjian A, Ichord R, et al. Electroencephalographic monitoring during hypothermia after pediatric cardiac arrest. Neurology. 2009;72:1931–40.

65. Legriel S, Hilly-Ginoux J, Resche-Rigon M, et al. Prognostic value of electrographic postanoxic status epilepticus in comatose cardiac-arrest survivors in the therapeutic hypothermia era. Resuscitation. 2013;84:343–50.

66. Cloostermans MC, van Meulen FB, Eertman CJ, Hom HW, van Putten MJ. Continuous electroencephalography monitoring for early prediction of neurological outcome in postanoxic patients after cardiac arrest: a prospective cohort study. Crit Care Med. 2012;40:2867–75.

67. Friberg H, Westhall E, Rosen I, Rundgren M, Nielsen N, Cronberg T. Clinical review: continuous and simplified electroencephalography to monitor brain recovery after cardiac arrest. Crit Care. 2013;17:233.

68. Rundgren M, Westhall E, Cronberg T, Rosen I, Friberg H. Continuous amplitude-integrated electroencephalogram predicts outcome in hypothermia-treated cardiac arrest patients. Crit Care Med. 2010;38:1838–44.

69. Accardo J, De Lisi D, Lazzerini P, Primavera A. Good functional outcome after prolonged postanoxic comatose myoclonic status epilepticus in a patient who had undergone bone marrow transplantation. Case Rep Neurol Med. 2013;2013:872127.

70. Hovland A, Nielsen EW, Kluver J, Salvesen R. EEG should be performed during induced hypothermia. Resuscitation. 2006;68:143–6.

71. Kaplan PW, Morales Y. Re: Status epilepticus: an independent outcome predictor after cerebral anoxia. Neurology. 2008;70:1295. author reply 1295–1296

72. Lucas JM, Cocchi MN, Salciccioli J, et al. Neurologic recovery after therapeutic hypothermia in patients with post-cardiac arrest myoclonus. Resuscitation. 2012;83:265–9.

73. Rossetti AO, Oddo M, Liaudet L, Kaplan PW. Predictors of awakening from postanoxic status epilepticus after therapeutic hypothermia. Neurology. 2009;72:744–9.

74. Rossetti AO, Oddo M, Logroscino G, Kaplan PW. Prognostication after cardiac arrest and hypothermia: a prospective study. Ann Neurol. 2010;67:301–7.

75. Ruijter BJ, van Putten MJ, Hofmeijer J. Generalized epileptiform discharges in postanoxic encephalopathy: quantitative characterization in relation to outcome. Epilepsia. 2015;56:1845–54.

76. Seder DB, Sunde K, Rubertsson S, et al. Neurologic outcomes and postresuscitation care of patients with myoclonus following cardiac arrest. Crit Care Med. 2015;43:965–72.

77. Sunde K, Dunlop O, Rostrup M, Sandberg M, Sjoholm H, Jacobsen D. Determination of prognosis after cardiac arrest may be more difficult after introduction of therapeutic hypothermia. Resuscitation. 2006;69:29–32.

78. Westhall E, Rundgren M, Lilja G, Friberg H, Cronberg T. Postanoxic status epilepticus can be identified and treatment guided successfully by continuous electroencephalography. Ther Hypothermia Temp Manag. 2013;3:84–7.

79. Ko SB, Ortega-Gutierrez S, Choi HA, et al. Status epilepticus-induced hyperemia and brain tissue hypoxia after cardiac arrest. Arch Neurol. 2011;68:1323–6.

80. Lote K, Stenwig AE, Skullerud K, Hirschberg H. Prevalence and prognostic significance of epilepsy in patients with gliomas. Eur J Cancer. 1998;34:98–102.

81. Chang EF, Potts MB, Keles GE, et al. Seizure characteristics and control following resection in 332 patients with low-grade gliomas. J Neurosurg. 2008;108:227–35.

82. Spindler M, Jacks LM, Chen X, Panageas K, DeAngelis LM, Avila EK. Spectrum of nonconvulsive status epilepticus in patients with cancer. J Clin Neurophysiol. 2013;30:339–43.

83. Abend NS, Gutierrez-Colina AM, Topjian AA, et al. Nonconvulsive seizures are common in critically ill children. Neurology. 2011; 76:1071–7.

84. Hosain SA, Solomon GE, Kobylarz EJ. Electroencephalographic patterns in unresponsive pediatric patients. Pediatr Neurol. 2005; 32:162–5.

85. Jette N, Claassen J, Emerson RG, Hirsch LJ. Frequency and predictors of nonconvulsive seizures during continuous electroencephalographic monitoring in critically ill children. Arch Neurol. 2006; 63:1750–5.

86. Saengpattrachai M, Sharma R, Hunjan A, et al. Nonconvulsive seizures in the pediatric intensive care unit: etiology, EEG, and brain imaging findings. Epilepsia. 2006;47:1510–8.

87. Shahwan A, Bailey C, Shekerdemian L, Harvey AS. The prevalence of seizures in comatose children in the pediatric intensive care unit: a prospective video-EEG study. Epilepsia. 2010;51:1198–204.

88. Kirkham FJ, Wade AM, McElduff F, et al. Seizures in 204 comatose children: incidence and outcome. Intensive Care Med. 2012;38: 853–62.

89. Glass HC, Nash KB, Bonifacio SL, et al. Seizures and magnetic resonance imaging-detected brain injury in newborns cooled for hypoxic-ischemic encephalopathy. J Pediatr. 2011;159:731–5. e731

90. Wyatt JS, Gluckman PD, Liu PY, et al. Determinants of outcomes after head cooling for neonatal encephalopathy. Pediatrics. 2007;119:912–21.

Diagnosing and Monitoring Seizures in the ICU: The Role of Continuous EEG for Detection and Management of Seizures in Critically Ill Patients, Including the Ictal-Interictal Continuum

Gamaleldin Osman, Daniel Friedman, and Lawrence J. Hirsch

Introduction

Nonconvulsive seizures (NCSzs) and nonconvulsive status epilepticus (NCSE) are increasingly recognized as a common occurrence in the ICU, where 6–59% of patients undergoing continuous EEG monitoring (cEEG) may have NCSz, depending on the study population [1–5] (Fig. 3.1). NCSz, as the term is used in this chapter, refers to electrographic seizures with little or no overt clinical manifestations. NCSE occurs when NCSzs are prolonged; a common definition is continuous or near-continuous electrographic seizures lasting at least 30 min [6–8]. Some experts included recurrent electrographic seizures occupying more than 30 min in any 1 h [9]. The Neurocritical Care Society guidelines on SE defined NCSE as any continuous electrographic seizure activity for ≥ 5 min [10]. More recently, ILAE taskforce defined SE as "a condition resulting from either the failure of mechanisms responsible for termination of seizures or from the initiation of mechanisms, which lead to abnormally prolonged seizures, after time point t_1. It is a condition, which can have long term consequences (after time point t_2) includ-

ing neuronal death, neuronal injury...." [11] For focal SE with impaired consciousness, the proposed t_1 (after which seizures need to be acutely treated) is estimated to be 10 min, while the proposed t_2 (after which more aggressive therapy may be justified) is >60 min [11]. Most patients with NCSz (about 75% averaging many studies) have purely electrographic seizures [1] (Fig. 3.2), but NCSz can be associated with other subtle signs such as face and limb twitching, nystagmus, eye deviation, pupillary abnormalities (including hippus), and autonomic instability [12–14]. None of these signs are highly specific for NCSz and are often seen under other circumstances in the critically ill patient; thus, cEEG is necessary to diagnose NCSz. In this chapter, we will discuss the implementation of cEEG in the critically ill and how to review the data, including available quantitative EEG (qEEG) tools that enable efficient review of the vast amount of raw EEG generated by prolonged monitoring. We will also review which patients are appropriate candidates for cEEG as well and the numerous EEG patterns that may be encountered. Finally, we will discuss future directions for cEEG and neurophysiological monitoring in the ICU.

How to Monitor

Obtaining high-quality cEEG recordings in the ICU is a challenge. Adequate technologist coverage is necessary to connect patients promptly, including off hours, and maintain those connections 24 h/day. Critically ill patients are frequently repositioned and transported to tests, which makes maintaining electrode integrity difficult. In both of our centers, we often employ collodion to secure disk electrodes and check the electrodes twice daily, usually supplemented by keeping the live recordings visible remotely to see which patients require electrode maintenance. Newer electrodes, such as subdermal wires, which may be more secure and lead to less skin breakdown, may be appropriate for comatose

G. Osman
Department of Neurology and Psychiatry, Ain Shams University, Cairo, Egypt

Comprehensive Epilepsy Center, Department of Neurology, Yale University, New Haven, CT, USA
e-mail: gamal-eldin.osman@yale.edu;
gamal_osman@med.asu.edu.eg

D. Friedman
Comprehensive Epilepsy Center, Department of Neurology, New York University, New York, NY, USA
e-mail: daniel.friedman@nyumc.org

L.J. Hirsch (✉)
Comprehensive Epilepsy Center, Department of Neurology, Yale University, New Haven, CT, USA
e-mail: lawrence.hirsch@yale.edu

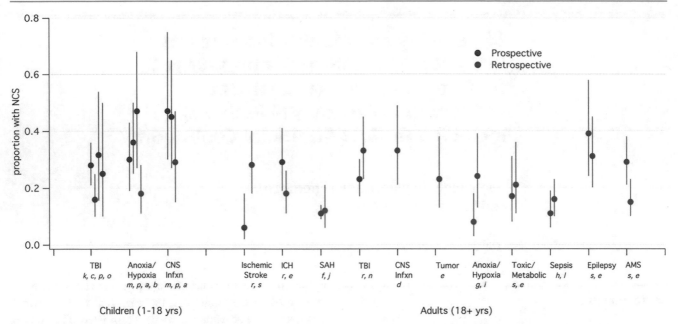

Fig. 3.1 Incidence of nonconvulsive seizures in different populations of critically ill children and adults. The confidence intervals were not reported by the studies, but were calculated based on the number of subjects in the study and the proportion of patients in whom nonconvulsive seizures were detected. Data is derived from (**a**) Abend NS, et al. Electrographic seizures in pediatric ICU patients: cohort study of risk factors and mortality. Neurology 2013; 81:383–391. (**b**) Abend NS, et al. Electroencephalographic monitoring during hypothermia after pediatric cardiac arrest. Neurology 2009; 72:1931–1940. (**c**) Arndt DH, et al. Subclinical early posttraumatic seizures detected by continuous EEG monitoring in a consecutive pediatric cohort. Epilepsia 2013; 54(10):1780–1788. (**d**) Carrera E, et al. Continuous electroencephalographic monitoring in critically ill patients with CNS infections. Arch Neurol 2008; 65 (12):1612–1618. (**e**) Claassen J, et al. Detection of electrographic seizures with continuous EEG monitoring in critically ill patients: Neurology 2004; 62:1743–1748. (**f**) Claassen J, et al. Electrographic seizures and periodic discharges after intracerebral hemorrhage. Neurology 2007; 69:1356–1365. (**g**) Crepeau AZ, et al. Value analysis of continuous EEG in patients during therapeutic hypothermia after cardiac arrest. Resuscitation 2014 (85):785–789. (**h**) Gilmore EJ, et al. Acute brain failure in severe sepsis: A prospective study in the medical intensive care unit utilizing continuous EEG monitoring. Intensive Care Med 2015; 41(4):686–694. (**i**) Mani R, et al. The frequency and timing of epileptiform activity on continuous electroencephalography in comatose post-cardiac- arrest syndrome patients

treated with therapeutic hypothermia. Resuscitation 2012 (83):840–847. (**j**) O'connor KL, et al. High risk for seizures following subarachnoid hemorrhage regardless of referral bias. Neurocrit Care 2014; 21:476–482. (**k**) O'neill BR, et al. Incidence of seizures on continuous EEG monitoring following traumatic brain injury in children. J Neurosurg Pediatr 2015; 16: 167–176. (**l**) Oddo M, et al. Continuous Electroencephalography in the medical intensive care unit. Crit Care Med 2009; 37 (6): 2051–2056. (**m**) Payne ET, et al. Seizure Burden is independently associated with short-term outcome in critically ill children. Brain 2014; 137: 1429–1438. (**n**) Ronne-Engstrom E , Winkler T. Continuous EEG monitoring in patients with traumatic brain injury reveals high incidence of epileptiform activity. Arch Neurol Scand 2006; 114: 47–53. (**o**) Schreiber JM, et al. Continuous video EEG monitoring for patients with acute encephalopathy in a pediatric intensive care unit. Neurocrit Care 2012; 17:31–38. (**p**) Topjian AA, et al. Electrographic status epilepticus is associated with mortality and worse short-term outcome in critically ill children. Crit Care Med 2013; 41 (1):210–213. (**q**) Vespa PM, et al. Nonconvulsive seizures after traumatic brain injury are associated with hippocampal atrophy. Neurology 2010; 75 (9):792–798. (**r**) Vespa PM, et al. Acute seizures after intracerebral hemorrhage: A factor in progressive midline shift and outcome. Neurology 2003; 60:1441–1446. (**s**) Westover B, et al. The probability of seizures during EEG monitoring in critically ill adults. Clinical Neurophysiology 2015; 126:463–471 (Published with kind permission from © Lawrence J. Hirsch, MD 2016. All Rights Reserved)

patients who are expected to undergo cEEG for many days to weeks [15]. While these electrodes may take more time to apply, they require less maintenance and are MRI and CT compatible (both safe and not affecting image interpretation), thereby saving substantial technologist time. Concerns for image artifacts and patient safety make it necessary to remove and then reapply standard disk electrodes when patients undergo brain MRIs, but there has been some progress in creating practical MRI- and CT-compatible electrodes [16], including conductive plastic electrodes. Figure 3.3 shows CT and MRI images taken with these electrodes in place displaying minimal image artifact and CT images in a

different patient with considerable image artifact caused by the electrodes. MRI-compatible disposable plastic cup electrodes are now commercially available and can be used in the ICU setting to minimize risk of transmitting infections [17].

There are numerous sources of artifact in the ICU environment that make cEEG challenging. Some are easily identified and filtered out such as 60 Hz (or 50 Hz in Europe) line noise from nearby electrical equipment. Others, however, such as pacemaker artifact, chest percussion, vibrating beds, ventilator activity, and intravenous drips, may be difficult to distinguish from seizures or other rhythmic or periodic cerebral activities [18–20] (Fig. 3.4). Simultaneous video

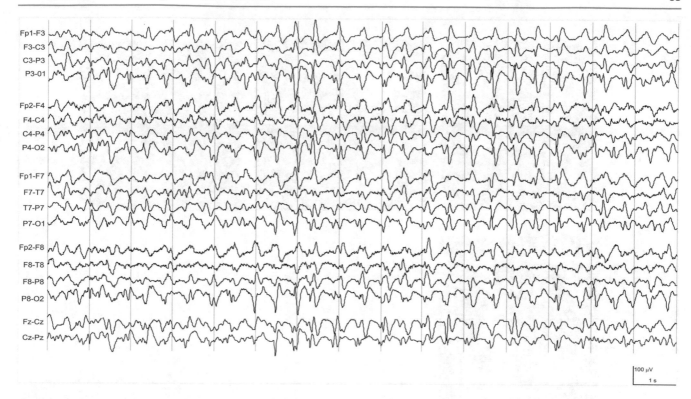

Fig. 3.2 Nonconvulsive status epilepticus. This is the EEG from a 29-year-old man with a history of liver transplantation and chronic immunosuppression who presented with convulsive status epilepticus due to encephalitis. He was treated with intravenous anticonvulsants and movements ceased, but he remained comatose. His EEG demonstrated electrographic seizure activity without clinical correlate. Low-frequency filter (LFF) = 1 Hz, high-frequency filter (HFF) = 70 Hz, notch off (Published with kind permission from © Lawrence J. Hirsch, MD 2013. All Rights Reserved)

recording is useful for distinguishing brain signals from artifact, especially rhythmic patterns such as those seen with chest percussion. In addition, video recording helps correlate EEG patterns with patient behaviors. In some cases, periodic EEG patterns can be determined to be ictal if they are time-locked to subtle patient movements [21]. In addition, some significant EEG patterns in the critically ill appear after the patient is stimulated, which is easily determined by reviewing the video [22, 23] (see below).

The number of electrodes used in cEEG studies varies considerably. In both our centers, we typically perform "full electrode" recordings using 16 or more active electrodes in addition to one or two reference electrodes and cardiac leads. Other authors have used reduced electrode configurations [24]. The advantage of a reduced electrode system is that it is faster to apply and easier to maintain. It is also easier to work around other neuro-monitoring devices, surgical wounds, or ventricular drains common in neuro-ICU patients. However, a full electrode configuration improves the ability to distinguish brain signals from artifact, aids in spatial localization of pathological activity, and provides a safety factor in case one or more leads fail, including allowing qEEG calculations and alarms to continue to function adequately [25]. In addition, reduced electrode methods,

especially when coupled to qEEG tools, may miss clinically significant events. For instance, Shellhaas et al. [26] found that neonatologists evaluating amplitude-integrated EEG (aEEG) using only two electrodes for seizure detection, a technique employed in purpose-built devices common in neonatal ICUs, detected only 12–38% of seizures identified using conventional electrode arrangements. Although emergent below-the-hairline EEG recordings have only moderate sensitivities and specificities [27], they are almost certainly better than no EEG at all; a full EEG should be done when possible to confirm or refute the results. Several disposable headpieces including pre-gelled electrodes are now available and can be utilized, allowing fast application by ICU nurses, house staff, and other staff not fully trained in EEG electrode application [28].

Data Analysis

Several days of cEEG generates gigabytes of data that, in its raw form, is time consuming for a neurophysiologist to review, especially if many patients are being monitored simultaneously. Furthermore, the raw EEG may be difficult for non-experts, such as ICU physicians and nurses, to inter-

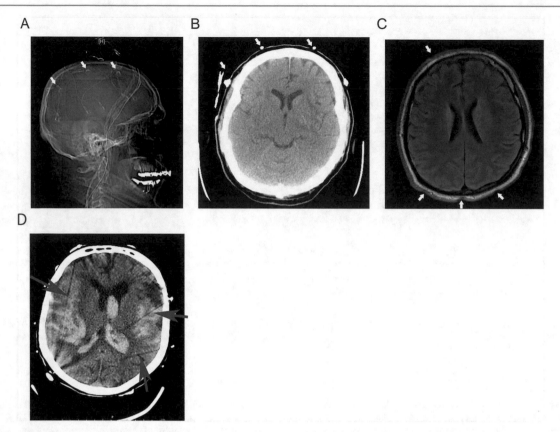

Fig. 3.3 CT- and MRI-compatible EEG electrodes. (**a**) A CT "scout" image demonstrating the placement of a full montage of conductive plastic electrodes (*white arrows*) on the scalp of a patient undergoing cEEG monitoring. (**b**) An axial image from the CT scan from the same patient demonstrates minimal artifact due to the electrodes (*white arrows*). Note there is no evidence of "streaking" common to head CT with conventional electrodes. (**c**) Axial FLAIR MRI performed 3 days later with electrodes in place. Note only minimal image artifact near the scalp (*white arrows*). (**d**) Axial CT in a different patient with multicompartmental intracranial hemorrhage showing beam hardening CT artifact caused by intact standard metal electrodes (*blue arrows*) (Modified with kind permission from © Lawrence J. Hirsch, MD 2013. All Rights Reserved)

pret at the bedside. Therefore, concerning electrographic events may not be noticed until several hours later, when the neurophysiologist reviews the file, unless real-time remote monitoring is performed continuously (currently available only in a minority of academic centers). Computing advances have enabled the use of qEEG algorithms to reduce the data and provide graphical representation of significant patterns and trends to speed review. Some of the commonly employed qEEG methods are discussed below (see [29] for a detailed review).

Many qEEG data reduction and trending tools are based on transforming the raw cEEG into a time-frequency series using algorithms such as short-time Fourier transform or continuous wavelet transform. Several hours of cEEG recordings can be reduced to a single screen of time-frequency values using a compressed spectral array or density spectral array. The time-frequency data can be averaged over scalp regions or hemispheres to further reduce the data. Using these techniques, the abrupt changes in cEEG spectral power in a relatively narrow frequency range during seizures are highlighted, allowing quick assessment of seizure frequency and duration (Fig. 3.5). Time-frequency transformation of the cEEG can be further manipulated to provide a single scalar value for each epoch of time. For instance, Claassen et al. [30] showed that the ratio of total hemispheric power in the alpha-frequency band (8–13 Hz) to the total power in the delta-frequency band (1–4 Hz) after maximal alerting, or poststimulation alpha-delta ratio (ADR), was the most useful qEEG parameter for detecting delayed cerebral ischemia in patients with high-grade subarachnoid hemorrhage (SAH) (see later). Hemispheric asymmetries in spectral power, computed as ratio of left and right total power for all EEG frequencies or as relative differences at each frequency, can be used to quickly identify focal seizures (e.g., Fig. 3.5). The greatest utility of reducing the cEEG to single scalar values is that these values can easily be displayed and interpreted on bedside monitors like heart rate and blood pressure. This could allow for early identification of neurophysiological events by the ICU staff and alarms to trigger patient examination and could lead to more responsive treatment. Another measure used as part of quantitative EEG trending analysis is the rhythmicity spectrogram. This

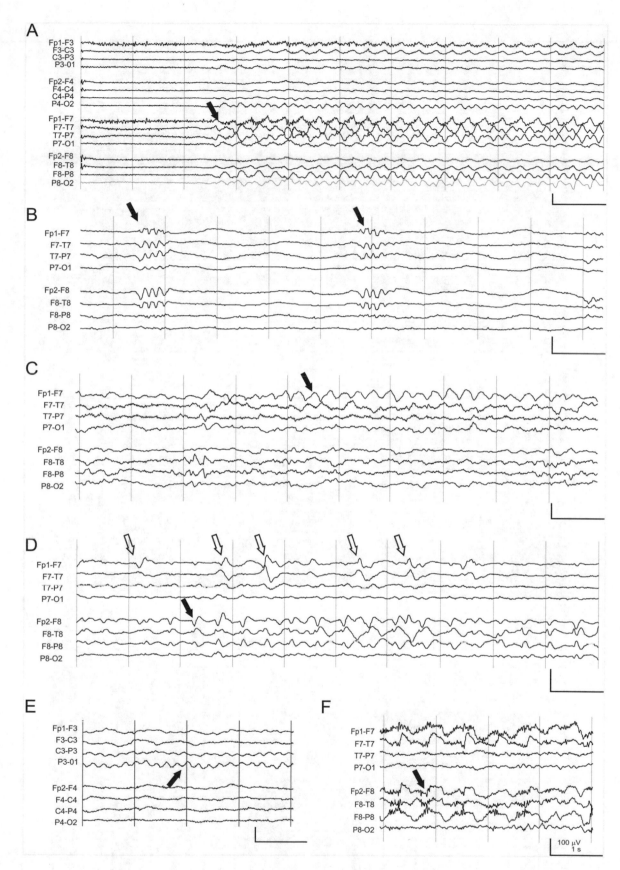

Fig. 3.4 Common ICU EEG artifacts. (**a**) Rhythmic bitemporal artifact due to chest compression in a medical ICU patient (*arrow*). (**b**) Respirator artifact due to fluid collecting in the tubing (*arrow*). These patterns are easily recognized on simultaneous video recording as they are synchronized with respirations. (**c**) *Left* temporal rhythmic waveforms (*arrow*) due to patting in an infant. This pattern is sometimes easy to confuse with seizures without video as it often shows a physiological field with evolution in frequency and amplitude. (**d**) Semirhythmic right temporal artifact (*black arrow*) due to chest percussion mimicking *right* LPDs or potentially ictal activity in a patient with true *left* hemisphere LPDs (*white arrows*). (**e**) Right occipital 6 Hz rhythmic artifact (*arrow*) due to automatic bed oscillation. (**f**) Rhythmic 1–1.5 Hz artifact (*arrow*) due to chewing in an edentulous patient. LFF = 1 Hz, HFF = 70 Hz, notch off (Published with kind permission from © Lawrence J. Hirsch, MD 2013. All Rights Reserved)

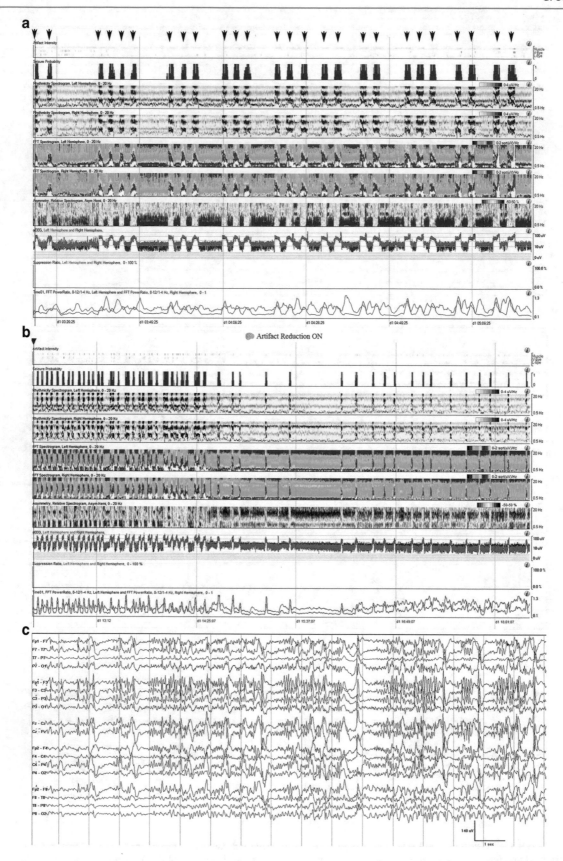

Fig. 3.5 qEEG trends (comprehensive panel view) from Persyst 12™ (Persyst. Inc.; San Diego, California) in a 24-year-old woman with SE. (**a**) 2 h qEEG page showing long-term trends: Artifact intensity (*first from top*) displays the amount of muscle artifact, vertical and lateral eye move-

ment present. The intensity of these artifacts may help determine the state of the patient. Seizure probability (*2nd from top*): Red bars display seizure probability on a scale from 0 to 1, as determined by Persyst seizure detection algorithm. Rhythmicity spectrogram for left and right measure highlights the rhythmic or periodic component of different frequencies, thus facilitating seizure identification. A diagonal pattern in particular is characteristic of seizures as it shows rhythmicity rapidly and consistently changing in frequency, a typical pattern of ictal evolution [29].

Other trending algorithms highlight amplitude measures, which can also be used to detect seizures. Amplitude-integrated EEG (aEEG) displays compressed, smoothed, and full-wave rectified EEG signal (Fig. 3.5). It is particularly useful for assessing background amplitude and burst suppression. aEEG is commonly used in commercial devices in neonatal ICUs [31] to assess the background EEG and occasionally as an initial screening tool for detecting seizures, although aEEG may be inadequately sensitive and is probably not specific enough for detecting seizures [26]. Envelope trend displays median amplitude of raw EEG background activity within a specified frequency range in a chosen time period, thus minimizing the effect of transient change in EEG signal created by artifacts, which are common in the ICU environment [32]. Multiple seizure detection algorithms are now available and can be utilized for automated seizure detection in the ICU setting [33]. Nonetheless, reliance on qEEG tools without the ability to review the raw EEG for non-cerebral signals can lead to false-positive seizure detections; thus, qEEG should only be interpreted in conjunction with the raw EEG wave forms and in conjunction with skilled electroencephalographers with special training in ICU EEG whenever possible [34].

Quantitative EEG tools can also calculate the degree of burst suppression of the EEG background to allow for easy titration of medications to induce coma, a common treatment of status epilepticus or refractory elevated intracranial pressure [35]. EEG-based monitors such as bispectral index [36], patient state index [37], Narcotrend [38] and entropy systems [38] have been in use in operating rooms and ICUs for nearly two decades to monitor depth of sedation. While these single-purpose devices use proprietary algorithms, evaluation of the raw cEEG or qEEG measures can also provide information about arousal in the paralyzed patient [39]. Data on the utility of these algorithms in those with underlying neurological issues is limited, as is the use of these devices to detect seizures; this should not be done without confirmation via review with expert review of raw EEG [40].

Several studies have evaluated the utility of qEEG trends analysis for seizure identification in critically ill individuals. Stewart et al. [41] investigated the sensitivity of qEEG for seizure identification in critically ill children by qEEG-naïve neurophysiologists and found that the median sensitivity of compressed spectral array (CSA) analysis was 83.3%, while that of aEEG was 81.5%. Missed seizures were more likely to be strictly focal, of low amplitude, or short duration [41]. In another larger study involving critically ill adults, 89% of seizures were identified utilizing CSA-guided review by qEEG-naïve neurology residents after receiving 2 h of qEEG training [42]. Another recent study evaluated the use of multiple qEEG panels for seizure identification and found that the overall sensitivity for seizure identification using these panels across all reviewer types was 84%, while the overall specificity was 69%. Interestingly, there was no statistically significant difference in sensitivities between the different reviewer groups (neurophysiologists, technologists, and neuroscience ICU nurses). Among four qEEG trends used in this study, rhythmicity spectrogram seemed to help the most in seizure identification [43]. These data further support the role for qEEG as a reliable tool for screening EEG and targeting raw EEG review by both experienced and non-experienced readers. qEEG-guided EEG review may save as much as 78% of EEG reading time without carrying a significant impact on sensitivity [44].

In our experience, no one qEEG tool is appropriate for all patients or even for the same patient at all times. Situations may occur where one tool is more susceptible to certain artifacts or is less sensitive to the seizures the individual patient may have. Instead, we employ multiple tools simultaneously to screen the initial cEEG record and focus particularly on reviewing the raw EEG data at times where there appear to be clear changes in the qEEG measures from baseline. Once the patient's seizure pattern is identified, the parameters of the qEEG tools can be further refined to highlight this pattern and improve the recognition of subsequent seizures.

Fig. 3.5 (continued) hemispheres (3rd and 4th from top, respectively) illustrates rhythmic components of different frequencies, darker colors being more rhythmic. FFT spectrogram for *left and right* hemispheres (*5th and 6th from top*, respectively) demonstrates power of different frequencies at different time periods. Time is displayed on *x*-axis, frequencies on *y*-axis, and amplitude of power of different frequencies as different colors on *z*-axis (see *color scale*). Relative asymmetry spectrogram (*7th from top*): illustrates comparison of power of different frequencies at homologous electrodes in each hemisphere (*blue* if higher power on *left*, *red* if on *right*). Suppression percentage (*8th from top*) displays the percent of the EEG record that is below a determined threshold amplitude (e.g., 10 μV). No EEG suppression is seen in this panel. aEEG (*9th from top*; combined *left* and *right* hemispheres; *left*, *blue*; *right*, *red*; *overlap*, *pink*): displays mean filtered and smoothed EEG amplitude (*y*-axis) across time (*x*-axis). FFT power ratio (*last from top*) illustrates alpha/delta ratio across time in both *left* (*blue*) and *right* (*red*) hemisphere. 26 seizures were detected in this 2 h page (*black arrow heads*), evidenced by surges in FFT power and aEEG, as well as evolving rhythmicity on rhythmicity spectral analysis. All of these seizures were also detected by seizure probability index (*red bars* on seizure probability index; *2nd panel from top*). (**b**) 6 h qEEG page for the same patient shows significant decline in the number of seizures in the second half of the page. Using longer time windows allows for greater appreciation of long-term trends and assists in monitoring response to therapy. (**c**) Raw EEG for one of the detected seizures. LFF = 1 Hz, HFF = 70 Hz, notch off (Published with kind permission from © Lawrence J. Hirsch, MD 2016. All Rights Reserved)

With Internet-based networking, it is now practical to monitor dozens of patients in multiple ICUs. If there is sufficient network capability in the hospital, cEEG can be streamed live over the network and can be interpreted in real-time if needed (and personnel are available). In addition, cEEG can be reviewed remotely from home or from a distant hospital site using virtual private networks and virtual network computing [25]. However, in current practice, cEEG is not yet truly real-time "monitoring" at most centers. In both our centers, records are routinely reviewed by neurophysiologists or technologists two-three times daily; ACNS guidelines suggest a minimum of twice daily [34]. All new records should be interpreted as soon as possible. Ongoing records should be reviewed more frequently than just a few times per day if there are suspicious clinical events or medications are being titrated. However, as most NCSzs have little or no detectable clinical correlate, they may go unrecognized for several hours with only intermittent review. It is clear that we need to move toward continuous real-time monitoring via use of quantitative EEG alarms and around-the-clock "neurotelemetrists" to respond to the alarms and review the long-term trends. Several academic centers are already doing this.

Who to Monitor

Recent studies using routine and continuous EEG monitoring have helped to identify which patients are at risk for NCSz and, therefore, may benefit from cEEG. The causes of NCSz and NCSE in ICU patients are similar to the causes of convulsive seizures in these patients. These include acute structural lesions, infections (including sepsis), metabolic derangements, toxins, withdrawal, and epilepsy, all common diagnoses in the critically ill patient [45]. It is important to stress that the majority of seizures in these critically ill patients are nonconvulsive and can only be diagnosed with EEG [1, 6, 46–48]. NCSzs are even more common in the pediatric population, especially in infants [1, 25, 49, 50]. There are many studies using cEEG that have identified the incidence of NCSz and NCSE in various patient populations. These studies are summarized in Fig. 3.1.

While it may not be surprising that patients with acute brain injuries [1, 51] and recent convulsive status epilepticus [52] have a high risk of NCSz, NCSzs are not uncommon in medical or surgical ICU patients, including in those without known structural brain injury. Critically ill medical and surgical patients are susceptible to many toxic, electrolyte, and metabolic abnormalities that may cause both mental status changes and seizures [7, 47]. 17–21% of patients with toxic-metabolic encephalopathy and impaired mental status had electrographic seizures on cEEG monitoring in two retrospective studies [1, 2]. Moreover, in one study of 201 medical ICU patients without known brain injury that

underwent cEEG monitoring, 22% of patients had periodic discharges (PDs) or seizures; sepsis and acute renal failure were significantly associated with both PDs and seizures [53]. A more recent prospective study found that among 100 episodes of sepsis in 98 patients without diagnosed acute primary neurological illness, periodic discharges were identified in 25 episodes; 11 of whom had nonconvulsive seizures [54]. Meanwhile, 16% of patients admitted to the surgical ICU undergoing cEEG monitoring had electrographic seizures in one recent study, while 29% had periodic discharges (PDs) [55].

The American Clinical Neurophysiology Society (ACNS) recently published an official guideline entitled "Consensus Statement on Continuous EEG in Critically Ill Adults and Children." The following are the proposed indications [56]:

1. Persistent alteration of mental state following generalized convulsive status epilepticus (GCSE)
2. Altered mental state in association with acute supratentorial brain injury
3. Unexplained alteration of mental status without evidence of acute brain injury
4. Periodic discharges on routine or emergent EEG
5. Pharmacological paralysis in patients at high risk for seizures
6. Paroxysmal events suspected to be seizures to determine ictal vs. non-ictal nature of these events

Other indications recommended by ACNS include monitoring response to treatment of seizures and SE. In addition, the ACNS taskforce suggested the use of continuous EEG monitoring for detection of cerebral ischemia in high risk individuals, as an adjunct to other methods [56]. Similar statements discussing indications of continuous EEG monitoring have been released by the European Society of Intensive Care Medicine (ESICM) [57], as well as the Neurocritical Care Society as part of recommendations on management of SE [10].

EEG Patterns Encountered During EEG Monitoring

The background, interictal, and ictal EEG patterns of the critically ill patient are significantly different from those encountered in ambulatory patients [58, 59]. Ictal patterns may include rhythmic epileptiform discharges or rhythmic waves at greater than 3 Hz (as with most seizures). However, in critically ill patients, rhythmic or periodic patterns occurring at a rate of less than three per second can be ictal as well. One set of criteria for defining NCSz are shown in Table 3.1. It should be noted that these criteria reflect expert consensus and there are periodic patterns common in critically ill

Table 3.1 Criteria for diagnosing nonconvulsive seizures

Patients without known epileptic encephalopathy:
• Epileptiform discharges (EDs) > 2.5 Hz
• EDs ≤ 2.5 Hz or rhythmic delta/theta activity >0.5 Hz and one of the following:
EEG and clinical improvement after IV AEDs
Subtle clinical ictal phenomena during the EEG pattern mentioned above
Typical spatiotemporal evolution
Patients with known epileptic encephalopathy:
• Increase in prominence or frequency of the features mentioned above when compared to baseline with observable change in clinical state
• Improvement of clinical and EEG features with IV AEDs

Adapted from Beniczky et al. [74], who modified the criteria of Kaplan [151]) (Published with kind permission from © Lawrence J. Hirsch, MD 2013. All Rights Reserved

Table 3.2 ACNS terminology for description of periodic and rhythmic patterns [63] (Published with kind permission from © Lawrence J. Hirsch, MD 2013. All Rights Reserved)

Main term A (for localization)	Main term B (pattern type)
Generalized (G)	Periodic discharge (PD)
Lateralized (L)	Rhythmic delta activity (RDA)
Bilateral independent (BI)	Spike-wave or sharp-wave complex (SW)
Multifocal (Mf)	

For L: Reporter has to specify whether the discharge is unilateral or bilateral asymmetric and lobe(s) or hemisphere most involved

For G: Reporter has to specify if the discharge is frontally predominant, occipitally predominant, midline predominant, or truly generalized (generalized NOS)

Modifiers are to be specified for each category. Modifiers specify prevalence, frequency, duration, number of phases, sharpness, amplitude, polarity, presence of stimulus-induced patterns, presence of evolving or fluctuating patterns, as well as presence of plus modifiers. Plus modifiers include +S (for sharply contoured waveforms or for rhythmic patterns superimposed by sharp waves), +F (for discharges superimposed by fast frequency activity), and +R (for superimposed rhythmic or quasi-rhythmic delta activity) or a combination of these plus modifiers (+FR or +FS). For more details, refer to [63]

patients where the relationship to seizures is unknown [60]. In practice, it is often difficult to determine whether periodic or rhythmic activity at 1–3 Hz in a comatose patient reflects seizure activity or a brain at risk for seizures or is merely a marker of severe brain injury. These patterns have been considered to lie along the ictal-interictal continuum [61]. Aiming to create common terminology for use by critical care electroencephalographers worldwide, the ACNS published standardized terminology for describing these patterns, initially proposed in 2005 and then revised and published as an official guideline in late 2012 [62, 63]. The current terminology is summarized in Table 3.2. In one recent study, the interrater reliability for ACNS terminology was near perfect for main terms (1) and (2), which describe

the location and the nature of the pattern, respectively. However, the interrater reliability for evolution and some of the other modifiers was not as good [64].

There is accumulating evidence that certain periodic discharges may reflect injured tissue at high risk for seizures such as lateralized periodic discharges (LPDs; previously called periodic lateralized epileptiform discharges (PLEDs)) and generalized periodic discharges (GPDs) (Fig. 3.6) [60]. There is convincing evidence to suggest that LPDs are sometimes ictal. For instance, LPDs can be time-locked to focal clonic movements in some patients with focal motor status epilepticus [21]. This seems to be more common in cases in which LPDs primarily involve Rolandic cortex (not surprisingly) [65]. Positron emission tomography in one patient with frequent LPDs demonstrated increased regional glucose metabolism similar to what is seen with focal seizures [66]. Single-photon emission CT (SPECT) imaging in patients with LPDs demonstrated increased regional cerebral perfusion in some patients that normalized when the LPDs resolved [67, 68]. In addition, frequent LPDs in elderly patients have been associated with a confusional state that resolves spontaneously or with diazepam treatment [69]. However, other studies have described cases where LPDs are clearly non-ictal such as in some epilepsy patients with chronic interictal LPDs [70]. In addition, when some patients with LPDs and acute brain injury demonstrate seizures, the EEG pattern is often faster and with different morphology [71]. Given the close association with seizures and the fact they are at times clearly associated with behavioral changes, some authors view LPDs as an unstable state in an "irritable" brain, lying along an ictal-interictal continuum [60, 72].

A common practice used to distinguish ictal from non-ictal periodic EEG patterns in the critically ill is to see if they are abolished by a trial of short-acting benzodiazepines (Table 3.3). However, almost all periodic discharges are attenuated by benzodiazepines [75]. Thus, unless there is clinical improvement accompanying the EEG change, the test is not helpful. Unfortunately, clinical improvement can take substantial time even if the activity represents NCSE and is aborted with benzodiazepines. However, a substantial portion of ICU patients with nonconvulsive seizures or NCSE will improve neurologically and usually within a day of treatment. For example, Hopp et al. [76] showed that 35% of patients with suspected NCSE receiving IV benzodiazepine (BZP) trial achieved positive clinical response. Moreover, positive clinical response correlated well with survival, recovery of consciousness, and achieving good functional outcome [76]. In order to avoid the confounding effect of sedation, we often use loading doses of nonsedating IV antiepileptic drugs (AEDs) such as valproate, lacosamide, levetiracetam, and phenytoin, for these diagnostic trials (see Table 3.3). One recent retrospective study evaluated clinical response to antiepileptic drug trial in patients with

Fig. 3.6 Periodic discharges in critically ill patients. (**a**) Right frontal LPDs occurring at 1 Hz (*arrow*) in an 82-year-old man after resection of a bifrontal meningioma. The patient subsequently developed *right frontal electrographic seizures*. (**b**) Generalized periodic discharges at 1–2 Hz in a 79-year-old patient with dementia, renal disease, and altered mental status. Although these waveforms have a triphasic morphology at times, the pattern subsequently evolved to 2.5–3 Hz GPDs consistent with NCSz and was associated with modest elevations in neuron-specific enolase to 14 (reference range 3.7–8.9). Low-frequency filter (LFF) = 1 Hz, HFF = 70 Hz, notch off (Published with kind permission from © Lawrence J. Hirsch, MD 2013. All Rights Reserved)

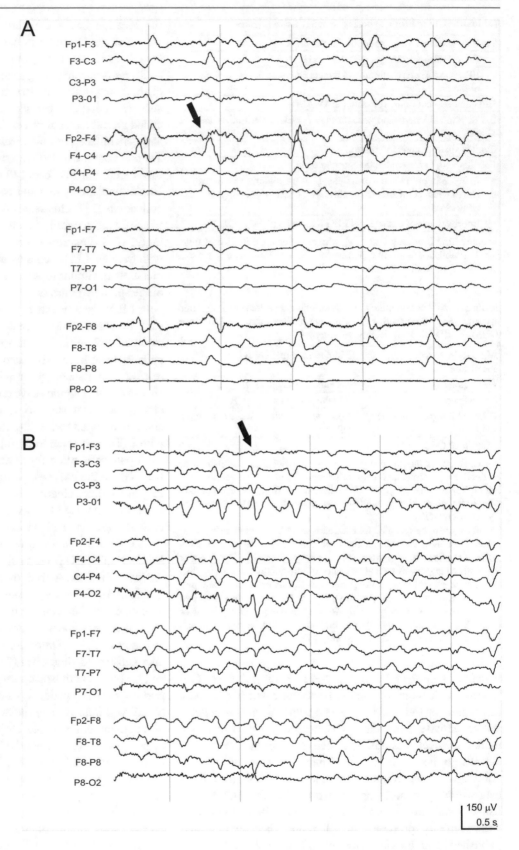

unexplained encephalopathy and triphasic wave pattern on EEG and found that 42.2% of patients receiving nonsedating IV AED trial achieved positive clinical response, whereas only 18.9% of patients receiving IV BZP trial did [77]. Our protocol for attempting to prove the presence of NCSE is shown in Table 3.3. It is important to recognize that lack of clinical improvement does not exclude NCSE—it simply does not help determine its presence or absence. This

Table 3.3 Antiepileptic drug trial for the diagnosis of nonconvulsive status epilepticus (adapted from Hirsch and Gaspard [73] with permission from Wolters Kluwer Health, Inc.)

Indication
Rhythmic or periodic focal or generalized epileptiform discharges on EEG with neurologic impairment

Contraindication
Patients who are heavily sedated or paralyzed

Monitoring
EEG, pulse oximetry, blood pressure, electrocardiography, respiratory rate with dedicated nurse

Antiepileptic drug trial
Sequential small doses of rapidly acting short-duration benzodiazepine such as midazolam at 1 mg/dose or nonsedating IV antiepileptic drug such as levetiracetam, valproate, fosphenytoin, or lacosamide
Between doses, repeated clinical and EEG assessment
Trial is stopped after any of the following:
1. Persistent resolution of the EEG pattern (and exam repeated)
2. Definite clinical improvement
3. Respiratory depression, hypotension, or other adverse effect
4. A maximum dose is reached (such as 0.2 mg/kg midazolam, though higher doses may be needed if the patient is on chronic benzodiazepines)

Interpretation
The test is considered positive ("definite NCSE") [74] if there is resolution of the potentially ictal EEG pattern *and* either an improvement in the clinical state or the appearance of previously absent normal EEG patterns (e.g., posterior-dominant "alpha" rhythm)
If EEG improves but patient does not, the result is equivocal ("possible NCSE") [74]
Nonictal patterns may disappear after administration of benzodiazepines (always without clinical improvement)
Administration of too high a dose of benzodiazepine might improve the EEG but also leads to sedation, preventing the ability to detect clinical improvement
Negative or equivocal response does not rule out nonconvulsive status epilepticus

situation (EEG improvement without clinical improvement) has been referred to as "possible NCSE" [74].

There is fairly consistent evidence that the presence of PDs and frequent nonconvulsive seizures are an independent risk factor for worse prognosis in ICH [78], SAH [79], and sepsis [53] and after GCSE [52, 80], even in patients without evidence of acute brain injury [81]. In addition, there is accumulating evidence that increased electrographic seizure burden is correlated with worse outcome in both pediatric and adult populations [9, 82, 83]. Both NCSzs and LPDs have been shown to be independently associated with later epilepsy as well [84]. Nonetheless, it is unclear whether these and other periodic discharges require treatment and how aggressive this treatment should be. Laboratory studies and computer modeling are beginning to probe the network mechanisms that mediate periodic discharges in the injured brain [85].

Another recently described pattern in critically ill patients is lateralized rhythmic delta activity (LRDA). This pattern was identified as an independent predictor of increased risk of acute seizures in critically ill individuals. It has been suggested that it carries similar implication as LPDs as regards risk of acute seizures [86]. One recent study suggested that LRDA is more likely to be associated with seizures if it occurs at a frequency of ≥ 1.5 Hz or is associated with a plus modifier [87]. On the other hand, the presence of generalized rhythmic delta activity (GRDA), even when sharply contoured or superimposed by sharp waves or fast frequency activity (GRDA + S or GRDA + F, respectively), doesn't seem to carry a significant increase in risk of electrographic seizures [87], at least based on the single retrospective study that has looked at this [87].

Epileptiform or rhythmic activity triggered by stimulation or arousal is also a common pattern in encephalopathic ICU patients. The evoked activity may be anywhere on the interictal-ictal spectrum and is collectively known as stimulus-induced rhythmic, periodic, or ictal discharges [22] (SIRPIDs). There is usually no clinical correlate, as with most ICU seizures, but a small portion of patients will have focal motor seizures consistently elicited by alerting stimuli [23]. On the other hand, there have been two case reports of SPECT-negative SIRPIDs, suggesting that some of these poststimulation discharges do not represent clear ictal phenomena or at least do not have the usual seizure-associated increased blood flow [88, 89]. SIRPIDs most likely occur as a result of hyperexcitable cortex that is activated by normal arousal pathways, which involve the upper brainstem, thalamus, and widespread thalamocortical projections. This epileptiform activity may become clinically apparent if it causes synchronous activation, propagates caudally in an organized fashion, and involves motor pathways. At both our centers, technologists stimulate patients twice daily to assess for state-dependent changes in the EEG including the appearance of SIRPIDs, but the relationship between ictal discharges and arousals raises the possibility that limiting unnecessary stimulation in patients with SIRPIDs may be beneficial. One recent study demonstrated that the presence of SIRPIDs was not independently associated with in-hospital mortality in critically ill patients [90]. Another study reported that the presence of SIRPIDs is a poor prognostic marker in postanoxic patients, particularly when recorded during therapeutic hypothermia [91]. The effect of SIRPIDs on long-term outcome in other settings as well as its therapeutic implication remains unclear. We treat stimulus-induced patterns the same as spontaneous patterns (other than potentially limiting stimulation) as there is no theoretical reason or evidence that they differ in their ability to cause neuronal injury.

Lastly, brief potentially ictal rhythmic discharges (B(I)RDs), a pattern previously described in neonates [92], has been recently reported in critically ill patients and shown to be associated with a high risk (75%) of acute seizures during continuous electroencephalography [93]. This pattern consists of focal rhythmic discharges that are 5 Hz or faster and last less than 10 s, whether evolving or not (often too short to determine); the most common form is sharply contoured rhythmic theta lasting a few seconds [93]. When seizures are successfully treated, B(I)RDs usually resolve. More research is needed to determine the exact prognostic implication and effect of treatment of these patterns [93].

Assessing response to treatment in status epilepticus is one of the indications for cEEG monitoring mentioned earlier in this chapter. Delorenzo et al. [52] found that 48% of patients with treated GCSE develop nonconvulsive seizures. Most authorities recommend monitoring for 24 h after the last electrographic seizure [10]. The optimum EEG end point of treatment of refractory status epilepticus (RSE) is not well established, but commonly used targets include seizure suppression, burst suppression, or in some cases complete EEG suppression to a nearly flat record. Two retrospective analyses demonstrated that achieving burst suppression is not correlated with outcome in patients with RSE [94, 95]. Another retrospective series [96] included 35 patients treated with pentobarbital infusion for RSE. Of the 35 assessed patients, 12 reached burst suppression pattern, 20 attained complete EEG suppression to a nearly flat record, and 3 became seizure free without needing to reach burst suppression or complete EEG suppression. 17/20 (85%) patients who had nearly flat records, 6/12 (50%) patients who reached burst suppression pattern, and 3/3 (100%) patients who became seizure free without attaining burst suppression or nearly flat EEG remained seizure free. All of the latter patients survived, while 12/20 (60%) patients reaching nearly flat EEG and 3/12 (25%) patients reaching burst suppression survived [96]. The key message from these limited data is that in some cases, good outcome may be achieved without reaching burst suppression, while in other cases, near-complete EEG suppression may be needed. The underlying etiology appears to be the most important prognostic determinant [94–96]. On the other hand, the duration of interburst suppression doesn't seem to correlate with outcome [97]. However, the presence of highly epileptiform bursts may indicate increased risk for seizure recurrence, suggesting the need for a more aggressive therapeutic end point [97, 98]. In general, we recommend treating to seizure suppression (not to a specific background pattern) as long as continuous EEG is being monitored. We often tolerate brief nonconvulsive seizures as well, especially in cases requiring prolonged iatrogenic coma.

Why Monitor

While NCSzs are common in the critically ill, the evidence that they worsen outcomes and require prompt identification and treatment is mixed [99, 100]. In several studies, the presence of NCSE and delay to diagnosis and treatment were each associated with significantly higher mortality [7, 101] though mortality in patients with NCSE may be most related to the underlying cause [102]. Recent evidence indicate that NCSE is more likely to be associated with worse outcome in critically ill children than NCSz [9] and that increased seizure burden is correlated with more significant degrees of neurological decline in that population [82]. One recent prospective study showed that increased seizure burden was associated with poor functional and cognitive outcome at 3 months following subarachnoid hemorrhage [83]. Nonetheless, while NCSE may be associated with poor prognosis in the critically ill elderly [103], one retrospective study from almost 20 years ago showed that aggressive treatment of NCSz and NCSE was associated with worse outcomes in this population [104]. In addition, three recent studies have shown that IV anesthetic use is correlated with poor outcome in status epilepticus [105–107]. This correlation was more significant in patients with complex partial status epilepticus in the latter study [107]. However, all of these studies failed to completely account for the severity and refractoriness of SE, and none of them included assessment of long-term cognitive or seizure outcomes [108]. Nevertheless, because of the conflicting outcome data, much of the justification for identifying and treating NCSz in the critically ill comes from human and animal data demonstrating that seizures can lead to neuronal injury. To date, there have been no prospective controlled trials to determine if treating NCSz or NCSE improves neurologic outcomes; this type of study may not be feasible as most neurologists and intensivists are not willing to leave seizures untreated based on the above evidence.

There is a large body of evidence that prolonged seizures in animals, even if nonconvulsive, can lead to neuronal damage. In a seminal study, Meldrum et al. [109] found that paralyzed and artificially ventilated baboons had hippocampal cell loss after treatment with a convulsant. Cell death occurred after 60 min of continuous electrographic seizures despite careful control of oxygenation, temperature, and metabolic status. In rodent models, electrical and chemoconvulsant-induced SE is associated with cell loss, free radical production, inflammation, gliosis, and synaptic reorganization [110]. Pathological changes can be seen in the absence of overt convulsions and can have profound long-term effects such as impaired performance on cognitive tasks after one episode of NCSE [111] and the development of epilepsy [112]. There is also some evidence from animal models that even single or multiple brief seizures may lead to cell death and cognitive impairment [113, 114]. Even in the absence of cell death, brief seizures in certain animal models can lead to alterations in gene expression [115]; impaired long-term potentiation, which is related to memory [116]; and reduced threshold for subsequent seizures [116]. SE in humans has also been associated with hippocampal cell loss in postmortem studies [117], and acute posttraumatic non-convulsive seizures have been shown to be associated with significant long-term hippocampal atrophy [3]. In hospitalized patients, SE is associated with neuronal injury as demonstrated by elevated levels of serum neuron-specific enolase (NSE), including in patients without detectable acute brain injury (e.g., from seizure activity alone) [118, 119]. While the sequelae of NCSz and NCSE are not as well understood, evidence suggests that they can lead to neuronal damage in humans. DeGiorgio et al. [120] showed that NSE levels, though elevated after all seizures, were especially high following NCSz and seizures of partial onset even in absence of acute brain injury. In addition to direct pathological effects of seizures themselves, seizures may also worsen the extent of injury from the inciting neurological injury. Seizures can place increased metabolic, excitotoxic, and oxidative stress on at-risk brain leading to irreversible injury. For instance, microdialysis studies in patients with TBI demonstrated increases of extracellular glutamate to excitotoxic levels following NCSz [121] as well as associated elevated lactate/pyruvate ratios and ICP [122]. Glycerol, a marker of cellular breakdown, has also been found to be elevated in the microdialysate after NCSz in TBI patients [123]. Compared to patients without NCSz that had similar injuries, impaired brain metabolism and increased intracranial pressure (ICP) could be seen up to 100 h after injury [122]. NCSzs in ICH were associated with increased mass effect on serial imaging, as well as worse NIHSS scores in one study [4] and expansion of hematoma size in another [78]; there was a trend toward worse outcomes in those with NCSzs in both studies. Seizures are also associated with increased metabolic demand that may worsen injury to ischemic brain, particularly the penumbra. NCSzs were associated with increased infarct volumes and higher mortality rates following middle cerebral artery occlusion in rats [124], and treatment resulted in reduced volumes [125]. In addition, even brief seizures can lead to hemodynamic changes, such as increased cerebral blood flow [126], which may lead to transient and potentially injurious elevations in ICP even in the absence of tonic-clonic activity [127, 128]. Finally, seizures are associated with peri-injury depolarizations, a process related to cortical spreading depression that seems to be very common and to contribute to secondary neuronal injury itself [129, 130].

How Long to Monitor

Several studies have addressed the duration of cEEG monitoring required to diagnose NCSz in critically ill patients. In their study of NICU patients, Pandian et al. [46] found that routine EEGs (30 min) detected seizures in only 11% of patients, while subsequent cEEG (mean duration of 2.9 days) detected seizures in 28%. In 110 critically ill patients with seizures detected by cEEG (92% of patients had purely nonconvulsive seizures), Claassen et al. [1] found that only half of patients had their first seizure within the first hour of monitoring. Although 95% of non-comatose patients had their first seizure within 24 h, only 80% of comatose patients had a seizure by this time. After 48 h of monitoring, the first seizure had occurred in 98% of non-comatose versus 87% of comatose patients. Coma and the presence of PDs predicted a delay in the time to first seizure (>24 h). Similarly, Jette et al. [50] found that 50% of 51 children with nonconvulsive seizures had their first seizure within 1 h and 80% within 24 h. Therefore, we feel monitoring for 24 h is probably sufficient to rule out NCSz in non-comatose patients without PDs, but longer periods may be required for comatose patients. However, recently it has been proposed that shorter monitoring may be sufficient in patients with no epileptiform abnormalities on EEG after 2 h of recording. One recent retrospective study evaluated time-dependent seizure probability in critically ill patients undergoing ≥18 h of recording and demonstrated that 72 h risk of seizures declined to less than 5% in patients with no epileptiform discharges in their initial 2 h of recording [2]. In addition, one study showed that the presence of generalized slowing as the sole finding on initial 30 min of EEG monitoring was predictive of low risk of electrographic seizures in patients undergoing at least 24 h of continuous EEG monitoring [5]. None of the 112 patients in this study with generalized slowing as the initial EEG finding developed electrographic seizures [43]. More studies are needed to confirm and refine these recommendations.

Cost-Effectiveness

Continuous EEG monitoring is labor intensive and requires substantial amount of resources. The main challenge is to prove that it actually leads to changes in management, that these changes in management improve outcome, and perhaps that the magnitude of these effects outweighs the cost of cEEG monitoring. One prospective study showed that continuous EEG monitoring led to significant changes in AED prescribing in 52% of critically ill adults [131]. A similar study in pediatric population showed that cEEG monitoring led to significant changes in management in 59% of critically ill children [132]. These changes include prescribing AEDs to patients not previously receiving them, as well as stopping unneeded medications for patients not having NCSz or rhythmic/periodic patterns on EEG monitoring, thus protecting them from side effects and toxicity of unnecessary medications. The question that remains elusive is: to what extent do these changes impact outcome? Observational data from

UCLA suggested that cEEG monitoring implementation led to significant decrease in hospital cost, via shortening of length of hospital stay, and improved recovery on discharge. In the meantime, cEEG monitoring contributed to only 1% of hospital cost [133]. However, these observations didn't control for other simultaneous changes in hospital protocols. More recently, Abend et al. [56] performed decision analysis to examine variables affecting the decision of whether or not to perform cEEG monitoring. They postulated that for 24 h cEEG monitoring to be considered a cost-effective measure, detection of NCSE/NCSz should lead to at least 3% improvement in outcome [56]. Nonetheless, data on the effect of cEEG monitoring on outcome remain scarce, and research in this field is of utmost importance to both practitioners in the field and healthcare administration.

Future Directions

In addition to detecting seizures, cEEG can be used to identify other changes in brain physiology. In recent years, there has been renewed interest in using cEEG for the detection of brain ischemia. It has been known for some time that EEG changes occur within seconds of reduction in cerebral blood flow (CBF) [134, 135], which is the basis for intraoperative EEG monitoring for ischemia during carotid endarterectomy [136–138]. In these patients, as CBF falls below 25–30 mL/100 g/min, there is a progressive loss of higher frequencies and prominent slowing of background EEG activity, yet cell death does not occur at this level. When CBF falls below 8–10 mL/100 g/min, low enough to cause irreversible cell death, all EEG frequencies are suppressed [139, 140]. Therefore, cEEG can detect a window where intervention can potentially prevent permanent brain injury.

Recent advances in computing have allowed for the real-time application of qEEG tools for extracting time-frequency data to measure changes in the background EEG rhythms. The ability to reduce EEG patterns usually identified by visual review to scalar values allows for prolonged use of cEEG monitoring in the ICU to detect cerebral hypoperfusion or other acute processes and is especially useful in comatose or sedated patients where clinical examination is limited. In a study of 32 primarily good-grade SAH patients, Vespa et al. [24] found that a reduction in the variability of relative alpha-frequency (a visual scoring of a tracing displaying 6–14 Hz expressed as a percentage of total power between 1 and 20 Hz) was 100% sensitive and 50% specific for vasospasm as detected by TCD or angiography. In the majority of patients, qEEG changes preceded the diagnosis of vasospasm by over 2 days. In a study of 34 poor-grade SAH patients (Hunt-Hess grades 4 and 5), Claassen et al. [141] found that the poststimulation alpha/delta ratio (ADR) was the most useful quantitative EEG parameter for detection of delayed cerebral ischemia (DCI): a reduction in the poststimulation ratio of alpha- to delta-frequency power of >10% relative to baseline in six consecutive epochs of cEEG was 100% sensitive and 76% specific for delayed cerebral ischemia. A reduction of >50% in a single epoch was 89% sensitive and 84% specific. Furthermore, in a recent prospective cohort study involving 20 patients with aneurysmal SAH, Rots et al. [142] found that ADR was the most reliable parameter in detecting DCI, showing the most significant change in patients with CT-detected DCI. Quantitative EEG changes preceded clinical diagnosis of DCI by a median of 7 h and preceded CT changes by a median of 44 h [142]. Further research is needed to determine the effect of early identification of DCI by qEEG on management and overall outcome.

Real-time application of cEEG monitoring—neurotelemetry—including using automated alarm systems at the bedside, as exists with cardiac telemetry in almost all hospitals today, is becoming an approachable goal. Reducing the raw cEEG to a few displayed variables using qEEG tools will make it a practical tool that can be interpreted by nurses and intensivists or by neurotelemetry technologists. In addition, trend and critical value alarms can be used to alert staff to potential changes in neurological status [143]. Computer algorithms have been successfully used to detect ongoing seizures in epilepsy monitoring unit patients [144]. Because seizure pattern in the critically ill are different from ambulatory patients, new algorithms must be designed to detect seizures in this patient population [143]. Refining techniques to help identify patterns of interest is an area of active research [145, 146]. Improvement is needed as many qEEG and data reduction tools are not sufficiently specific [147] and susceptible to contamination by artifact. While ICU staff can be trained to review raw cEEG traces for obvious artifacts and even pathological patterns [148], a neurophysiologist must still be available to verify the interpretation.

In parallel with these technical advancements, continued research is needed to confirm that real-time monitoring is a necessary goal. Further studies need to be performed in both laboratory models and in prospective clinical trials to examine if identifying and treating NCSz early improves outcomes. It is also necessary to determine the relationship of the different periodic and rhythmic EEG patterns in the critically ill to ongoing brain injury to identify targets for intervention [60]. Studies are also needed to determine whether using cEEG to detect ischemia improves patient outcomes and to identify the time window for intervention after a change is detected by cEEG.

Continuous EEG monitoring is just one of the modalities available to evaluate brain physiology in the ICU. Intracranial pressure monitoring using intraventricular catheters or intraparenchymal probes, brain tissue oxygenation monitors, CBF monitoring, and brain metabolism monitoring using

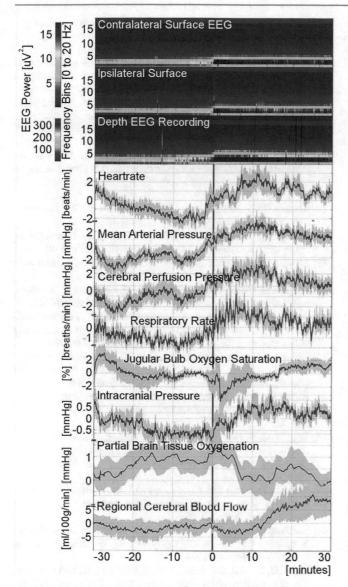

Fig. 3.7 Physiologic changes associated with intracortical seizures. Increase in HR, RR, MAP, and CPP is seen very early, correlating with increased spectral power on depth EEG recording. Rise in ICP is seen later. A transient decline in jugular bulb oxygen saturation is seen around 2 min after seizure onset, followed by a drop in partial brain tissue oxygenation. Regional cerebral blood flow increase is seen around 10 min after seizure onset (Reproduced from Claassen et al. [150] with permission from Wiley-Blackwell Publishing)

microdialysis probes [149] all provide critical data about brain physiology. The use of these methods in combination with cEEG may help further understand the complex relationships between cerebral blood flow, tissue oxygenation, cerebral metabolism, and neuronal activity in the injured brain. In addition, multimodal physiological monitoring (Fig. 3.7) offers critical information on physiological changes in response to seizures, e.g., changes in heart rate (HR), respiratory rate (RR), and mean arterial pressure (MAP) [150]. Recent evidence indicates that these physio-

logical changes may precede demonstrable EEG seizure onset on scalp EEG, often coinciding with intracortical seizure onset detected by mini-depth recording (Fig. 3.7) [150]. The combined use of these methods together may be able to compensate for some of the shortcomings of the individual methods. For instance, microdialysis and tissue oxygenation probes sample only the immediate area of the brain into which they are inserted and can miss new injury to a remote area of the brain that may be detected by cEEG because of the wide spatial coverage.

Finally, new research is examining the utility of electrophysiological monitoring beyond conventional scalp EEG. Recent studies in patients with severe TBI using subdural electrodes found episodes of cortical spreading depression, slow and prolonged peri-injury depolarizations lasting several minutes or longer, and near-injured brain [129]. In another recent study involving 48 patients with poor-grade aneurysmal SAH undergoing invasive EEG monitoring by mini-depth electrodes, 38% of patients had seizures on mini-depth recording. 43% of these seizures were only detected by mini-depth recording. Interestingly, 19% of intracortical seizures were associated with ictal-interictal continuum patterns on scalp EEG [150]. It is possible that many focal seizures occurring across the cerebral cortex, but not synchronized sufficiently to generate scalp EEG changes, may contribute to impaired consciousness in some comatose patients without evidence of seizures on cEEG. Whether targeting these events for therapy improves patient outcomes needs to be determined. When possible, physiology-driven data (such as the lactate/pyruvate ratio and glutamate on microdialysis) can be used to decide which EEG patterns require additional treatment and which do not.

Summary

Nonconvulsive seizures are common in brain-injured patients with altered mental status and even in critically ill patients without structural brain injury. Seizures can contribute to depressed level of consciousness and cause secondary neuronal injury. Therefore, in both of our centers, we recommend cEEG for all critically ill patients with acute brain injury and altered mental status and for patients with fluctuating or unexplained impaired mental status. Patients who are encephalopathic, but not comatose, are typically monitored for 24 h to exclude NCSz. However, patients who are comatose, who have PDs, or who are having sedation/AEDs withdrawn undergo at least 48 h of cEEG. Once NCSz or equivocal periodic patterns are identified, monitoring can continue for several days. If NCSzs are identified, cEEG is necessary to monitor the response to treatment and, more importantly, correlate improvement in the cEEG findings with improvement in the patient's clinical status. If the cEEG demonstrates periodic activity that is suspicious for, but not definitively, seizure activity, further monitoring can help the neurophysiologist gather additional evidence for or against the ictal nature of the pattern (e.g., to see if there are unequivocal seizures). This monitoring requires 24 h technologist coverage to connect patients and perform maintenance, appropriate information technology infrastructure, and available neurophysiologists to review the data and tools (quantitative EEG) to speed data review. While this requires a substantial amount of resources, it is feasible, and cEEG is routinely employed in many neuroscience ICUs around the world. In addition, cEEG has applications outside of NCSz detection that can expand the number of patients who may benefit from monitoring. Advances in the use of cEEG for ischemia detection and general brain function monitoring can make it a widely applicable tool for dynamic assessment of neurological function, in combination with other monitoring modalities, with the potential to detect brain injury moments after it occurs and even to prevent it.

References

1. Claassen J, Mayer SA, Kowalski RG, Emerson RG, Hirsch LJ. Detection of electrographic seizures with continuous EEG monitoring in critically ill patients. Neurology. 2004;62:1743–8.
2. Westover MB, Shafi MM, Bianchi MT, et al. The probability of seizures during EEG monitoring in critically ill adults. Clin Neurophysiol. 2015;126:463–71.
3. Vespa PM, McArthur DL, Xu Y, et al. Nonconvulsive seizures after traumatic brain injury are associated with hippocampal atrophy. Neurology. 2010;75:792–8.
4. Vespa PM, O'Phelan K, Shah M, et al. Acute seizures after intracerebral hdeemorrhage: a factor in progressive midline shift and outcome. Neurology. 2003;60:1441–6.
5. Swisher CB, Shah D, Sinha SR, Husain AM. Baseline EEG pattern on continuous ICU EEG monitoring and incidence of seizures. J Clin Neurophysiol. 2015;32:147–51.
6. Jordan K. Nonconvulsive status epilepticus in acute brain injury. J Clin Neurophysiol. 1999;16:332–40.
7. Young GB, Jordan KG, Doig GS. An assessment of nonconvulsive seizures in the intensive care unit using continuous EEG monitoring: an investigation of variables associated with mortality. Neurology. 1996;47:83–9.
8. Walker M, Cross H, Smith S, et al. Nonconvulsive status epilepticus: epilepsy research foundation workshop reports. Epileptic Dis. 2005;7:253–96.
9. Topjian AA, Gutierrez-Colina AM, Sanchez SM, et al. Electrographic status epilepticus is associated with mortality and worse short-term outcome in critically ill children*. Crit Care Med. 2013;41:215–23.
10. Brophy G, Bell R, Claassen J, et al. Guidelines for the evaluation and management of status epilepticus. Neurocrit Care. 2012;17:3–23.
11. Trinka E, Cock H, Hesdorffer D, et al. A definition and classification of status epilepticus—report of the ILAE task force on classification of status epilepticus. Epilepsia. 2015;56:1515–23.
12. Kaplan PW. Behavioral manifestations of nonconvulsive status epilepticus. Epilepsy Behav. 2002;3:122–39.
13. Husain AM, Horn GJ, Jacobson MP. Non-convulsive status epilepticus: usefulness of clinical features in selecting patients for urgent EEG. J Neurol Neurosurg Psychiatry. 2003;74:189–91.
14. Jirsch J, Hirsch LJ. Nonconvulsive seizures: developing a rational approach to the diagnosis and management in the critically ill population. Clin Neurophysiol. 2007;118:1660–70.
15. Young GB, Ives JR, Chapman MG, Mirsattari SM. A comparison of subdermal wire electrodes with collodion-applied disk electrodes in long-term EEG recordings in ICU. Clin Neurophysiol. 2006;117:1376–9.
16. Mirsattari SM, Lee DH, Jones D, Bihari F, Ives JR. MRI compatible EEG electrode system for routine use in the epilepsy monitoring unit and intensive care unit. Clin Neurophysiol. 2004;115:2175–80.
17. Alvarez V, Rossetti AO. Clinical use of EEG in the ICU: technical setting. J Clin Neurophysiol. 2015;32:481–5.
18. Young GB, Campbell VC. EEG monitoring in the intensive care unit: pitfalls and caveats. J Clin Neurophysiol. 1999;16:40.
19. Hirsch LJ. Continuous EEG monitoring in the intensive care unit: an overview. J Clin Neurophysiol. 2004;21:332–40.
20. Gaspard N, Hirsch LJ. Pitfalls in ictal EEG interpretation: critical care and intracranial recordings. Neurology. 2013;80:S26–42.
21. Snodgrass SM, Tsuburaya K, Ajmone-Marsan C. Clinical significance of periodic lateralized epileptiform discharges: relationship with status epilepticus. J Clin Neurophysiol. 1989;6:159–72.
22. Hirsch LJ, Claassen J, Mayer SA, Emerson RG. Stimulus-induced rhythmic, periodic, or ictal discharges (SIRPIDs): a common EEG phenomenon in the critically ill. Epilepsia. 2004;45:109–23.
23. Hirsch LJ, Pang T, Claassen J, et al. Focal motor seizures induced by alerting stimuli in critically ill patients. Epilepsia. 2008;49:968–73.
24. Vespa PM, Nuwer MR, Juhász C, et al. Early detection of vasospasm after acute subarachnoid hemorrhage using continuous EEG ICU monitoring. Electroencephalogr Clin Neurophysiol. 1997;103:607–15.
25. Kull LL, Emerson RG. Continuous EEG monitoring in the intensive care unit: technical and staffing considerations. J Clin Neurophysiol. 2005;22:107.
26. Shellhaas RA, Soaita AI, Clancy RR. Sensitivity of amplitude-integrated electroencephalography for neonatal seizure detection. Pediatrics. 2007;120:770–7.
27. Kolls BJ, Husain AM. Assessment of hairline EEG as a screening tool for nonconvulsive status epilepticus. Epilepsia. 2007;48:959–65.
28. StatNet™. (Accessed 17 Nov 2015, at http://www.hydrodot.net/Products/statnet.html.)
29. Hirsch LJ, Sinha SR. Continuous EEG monitoring in the intensive care unit. In: Ebersole JS, editor. Current practice of clinical electroencephalography. Philadelphia: LWW; 2014. p. 567.
30. Claassen J, Hirsch LJ, Kreiter KT, et al. Quantitative continuous EEG for detecting delayed cerebral ischemia in patients with poor-grade subarachnoid hemorrhage. Clin Neurophysiol. 2004;115:2699–710.
31. Toet MC, van der Meij W, de Vries LS, Uiterwaal CS, van Huffelen KC. Comparison between simultaneously recorded amplitude integrated electroencephalogram (cerebral function monitor) and standard electroencephalogram in neonates. Pediatrics. 2002;109:772–9.
32. Akman CI, Micic V, Thompson A, Riviello Jr JJ. Seizure detection using digital trend analysis: factors affecting utility. Epilepsy Res. 93:66–72.
33. Sackellares JC, Shiau DS, Halford JJ, LaRoche SM, Kelly KM. Quantitative EEG analysis for automated detection of nonconvulsive seizures in intensive care units. Epilepsy Behav. 2011;22(Suppl 1):S69–73.

34. Herman ST, Abend NS, Bleck TP, et al. Consensus statement on continuous EEG in critically ill adults and children, Part II: personnel, technical specifications, and clinical practice. J Clin Neurophysiol. 2015;32:96–108.

35. Eisenberg HM, Frankowski RF, Contant CF, Marshall LF, Walker MD. High-dose barbiturate control of elevated intracranial pressure in patients with severe head injury. J Neurosurg. 1988;69: 15–23.

36. Simmons LE, Riker RR, Prato BS, Fraser GL. Assessing sedation during intensive care unit mechanical ventilation with the bispectral index and the sedation-agitation scale. Crit Care Med. 1999;27:1499–504.

37. Prichep LS, Gugino LD, John ER, et al. The patient state index as an indicator of the level of hypnosis under general anaesthesia. Br J Anaesth. 2004;92:393–9.

38. Al-Kadi MI, Reaz MBI, Ali MAM. Evolution of electroencephalogram signal analysis techniques during anesthesia. Sensors (Basel, Switzerland). 2013;13:6605–35.

39. Roustan JP, Valette S, Aubas P, Rondouin G, Capdevila X. Can electroencephalographic analysis be used to determine sedation levels in critically ill patients? Anesth Analg. 2005;101:1141–51.

40. Bousselmi R, Lebbi A, Ferjani M. Bispectral index changes during generalised tonic-clonic seizures. Anaesthesia. 2013;68: 1084–5.

41. Stewart CP, Otsubo H, Ochi A, Sharma R, Hutchison JS, Hahn CD. Seizure identification in the ICU using quantitative EEG displays. Neurology. 2010;75:1501–8.

42. Williamson C, Wahlster S, Shafi M, Westover MB. Sensitivity of compressed spectral arrays for detecting seizures in acutely ill adults. Neurocrit Care. 2014;20:32–9.

43. Swisher CB, White CR, Mace BE, et al. Diagnostic accuracy of electrographic seizure detection by neurophysiologists and non-neurophysiologists in the adult ICU using a panel of quantitative EEG trends. J Clin Neurophysiol. 2015;32:324–30.

44. Moura LMVR, Shafi MM, Ng M, et al. Spectrogram screening of adult EEGs is sensitive and efficient. Neurology. 2014;83:56–64.

45. Abou Khaled KJ, Hirsch LJ. Advances in the management of seizures and status epilepticus in critically ill patients. Crit Care Clin. 2006;22:637–59. abstract viii

46. Pandian JD, Cascino GD, So EL, Manno E, Fulgham JR. Digital video-electroencephalographic monitoring in the neurological-neurosurgical intensive care unit: clinical features and outcome. Arch Neurol. 2004;61:1090–4.

47. Towne AR, Waterhouse EJ, Boggs JG, et al. Prevalence of nonconvulsive status epilepticus in comatose patients. Neurology. 2000;54:340–5.

48. Privitera M, Hoffman M, Moore JL, Jester D. EEG detection of nontonic-clonic status epilepticus in patients with altered consciousness. Epilepsy Res. 1994;18:155–66.

49. Clancy RR, Legido A, Lewis D. Occult neonatal seizures. Epilepsia. 1988;29:256–61.

50. Jette N, Claassen J, Emerson RG, Hirsch LJ. Frequency and predictors of nonconvulsive seizures during continuous electroencephalographic monitoring in critically ill children. Arch Neurol. 2006;63:1750–5.

51. Vespa P. Continuous EEG monitoring for the detection of seizures in traumatic brain injury, infarction, and intracerebral hemorrhage: "to detect and protect". J Clin Neurophysiol. 2005;22: 99–106.

52. DeLorenzo RJ, Waterhouse EJ, Towne AR, et al. Persistent nonconvulsive status epilepticus after the control of convulsive status epilepticus. Epilepsia. 1998;39:833–40.

53. Oddo M, Carrera E, Claassen J, Mayer SA, Hirsch LJ. Continuous electroencephalography in the medical intensive care unit. Crit Care Med. 2009;37:2051–6.

54. Gilmore EJ, Gaspard N, Choi HA, et al. Acute brain failure in severe sepsis: a prospective study in the medical intensive care unit utilizing continuous EEG monitoring. Intensive Care Med. 2015;41:686–94.

55. Kurtz P, Gaspard N, Wahl AS, et al. Continuous electroencephalography in a surgical intensive care unit. Intensive Care Med. 2014;40:228–34.

56. Herman ST, Abend NS, Bleck TP, et al. Consensus statement on continuous EEG in critically ill adults and children, part I: indications. J Clin Neurophysiol. 2015;32:87–95.

57. Claassen J, Taccone FS, Horn P, Holtkamp M, Stocchetti N, Oddo M. Recommendations on the use of EEG monitoring in critically ill patients: consensus statement from the neurointensive care section of the ESICM. Intensive Care Med. 2013;39:1337–51.

58. Young GB. The EEG in Coma. J Clin Neurophysiol. 2000;17:473.

59. Kaplan PW. The EEG in metabolic encephalopathy and coma. J Clin Neurophysiol. 2004;21:307–18.

60. Chong DJ, Hirsch LJ. Which EEG patterns warrant treatment in the critically ill? Reviewing the evidence for treatment of periodic epileptiform discharges and related patterns. J Clin Neurophysiol. 2005;22:79–91.

61. Claassen J, How I. Treat patients with EEG patterns on the ictal–interictal continuum in the neuro ICU. Neurocrit Care. 2009;11: 437–44.

62. Hirsch LJ, Brenner RP, Drislane FW, et al. The ACNS subcommittee on research terminology for continuous EEG monitoring: proposed standardized terminology for rhythmic and periodic EEG patterns encountered in critically ill patients. J Clin Neurophysiol. 2005;22:128–35.

63. Hirsch LJ, LaRoche SM, Gaspard N, et al. American clinical neurophysiology society's standardized critical care EEG terminology: 2012 version. J Clin Neurophysiol. 2013;30:1–27.

64. Gaspard N, Hirsch LJ, LaRoche SM, Hahn CD, Westover MB, the Critical Care EEGMRC. Interrater agreement for Critical Care EEG Terminology. Epilepsia. 2014;55:1366–73.

65. Sen-Gupta I, Schuele SU, Macken MP, Kwasny MJ, Gerard EE. "Ictal" lateralized periodic discharges. Epilepsy Behav. 2014;36: 165–70.

66. Handforth A, Cheng JT, Mandelkern MA, Treiman DM. Markedly increased mesiotemporal lobe metabolism in a case with PLEDs: further evidence that PLEDs are a manifestation of partial status epilepticus. Epilepsia. 1994;35:876–81.

67. Assal F, Papazyan JP, Slosman DO, Jallon P, Goerres GW. SPECT in periodic lateralized epileptiform discharges (PLEDs): a form of partial status epilepticus? Seizure. 2001;10:260–5.

68. Bozkurt MF, Saygi S, Erbas B. SPECT in a patient with postictal PLEDs: is hyperperfusion evidence of electrical seizure? Clin Electroencephalogr. 2002;33:171–3.

69. Terzano MG, Parrino L, Mazzucchi A, Moretti G. Confusional states with periodic lateralized epileptiform discharges (PLEDs): a peculiar epileptic syndrome in the elderly. Epilepsia. 1986;27:446–57.

70. Westmoreland BF, Klass DW, Sharbrough FW. Chronic periodic lateralized epileptiform discharges. Arch Neurol. 1986;43:494–6.

71. Brenner RP. Is it status? Epilepsia. 2002;43(Suppl 3):103–13.

72. Pohlmann-Eden B, Hoch DB, Cochius JI, Chiappa KH. Periodic lateralized epileptiform discharges—a critical review. J Clin Neurophysiol. 1996;13:519–30.

73. Hirsch LJ, Gaspard N. Status epilepticus. Continuum (Minneapolis, Minn). 2013;19:767–94.

74. Beniczky S, Hirsch LJ, Kaplan PW, et al. Unified EEG terminology and criteria for nonconvulsive status epilepticus. Epilepsia. 2013;54:28–9.

75. Fountain NB, Waldman WA. Effects of benzodiazepines on triphasic waves: implications for nonconvulsive status epilepticus. J Clin Neurophysiol. 2001;18:345–52.

76. Hopp JL, Sanchez A, Krumholz A, Hart G, Barry E. Nonconvulsive status epilepticus: value of a benzodiazepine trial for predicting outcomes. Neurologist. 2011;17:325–9.

77. O'Rourke D, Chen PM, Gaspard N, et al. Response rates to anticonvulsant trials in patients with triphasic-wave EEG patterns of uncertain significance. Neurocrit Care 2015.

78. Claassen J, Jette N, Chum F, et al. Electrographic seizures and periodic discharges after intracerebral hemorrhage. Neurology. 2007;69:1356–65.

79. Claassen J, Hirsch LJ, Frontera JA, et al. Prognostic significance of continuous EEG monitoring in patients with poor-grade subarachnoid hemorrhage. Neurocrit Care. 2006;4:103–12.

80. Jaitly R, Sgro JA, Towne AR, Ko D, DeLorenzo RJ. Prognostic value of EEG monitoring after status epilepticus: a prospective adult study. J Clin Neurophysiol. 1997;14:326–34.

81. Sainju RK, Manganas LN, Gilmore EJ, et al. Clinical correlates and prognostic significance of lateralized periodic discharges in patients without acute or progressive brain injury: a case–control study. J Clin Neurophysiol. 2015;32:495–500.

82. Payne ET, Zhao XY, Frndova H, et al. Seizure burden is independently associated with short term outcome in critically ill children. Brain. 2014;137:1429–38.

83. De Marchis GM, Pugin D, Meyers E, et al. Seizure burden in subarachnoid hemorrhage associated with functional and cognitive outcome. Neurology. 2015; Epub ahead of print23

84. Punia V, Garcia CG, Hantus S. Incidence of recurrent seizures following hospital discharge in patients with LPDs (PLEDs) and nonconvulsive seizures recorded on continuous EEG in the critical care setting. Epilepsy Behav. 2015;49:250–4.

85. Frohlich F, Bazhenov M, Sejnowski TJ. Pathological effect of homeostatic synaptic scaling on network dynamics in diseases of the cortex. J Neurosci. 2008;28:1709.

86. Gaspard N, Manganas L, Rampal N, Petroff OA, Hirsch LJ. Similarity of lateralized rhythmic delta activity to periodic lateralized epileptiform discharges in critically ill patients. JAMA Neurol. 2013;70:1288–95.

87. Rodriguez A, Vlachy J, Lee JW, et al. Periodic and rhythmic patterns in the critically ill: Characteristics associated with seizures. 69th Annual meeting of the American Epilepsy Society. Philadephia, PA, USA. 2015.

88. Zeiler SR, Turtzo LC, Kaplan PW. SPECT–negative SIRPIDs argues against treatment as seizures. J Clin Neurophysiol. 2011;28:493–6.

89. Smith CC, Tatum WO, Gupta V, Pooley RA, Freeman WD. SPECT-negative SIRPIDs: less aggressive neurointensive care? J Clin Neurophysiol. 2014;31:e6–e10.

90. Braksick A, Burkholder DB, Tsetsou S, et al. Stimulus-induced rhythmic, periodic or ictal discharges (SRIPIDs): associated factors and prognostic implications. 69th Annual meeting of the American Epilepsy Society. Philadelphia, PA, USA 2015.

91. Alvarez V, Oddo M, Rossetti AO. Stimulus-induced rhythmic, periodic or ictal discharges (SIRPIDs) in comatose survivors of cardiac arrest: characteristics and prognostic value. Clin Neurophysiol. 2013;124:204–8.

92. Tsuchida TN, Wusthoff CJ, Shellhaas RA, et al. American clinical neurophysiology society standardized EEG terminology and categorization for the description of continuous EEG monitoring in neonates: report of the American clinical neurophysiology society critical care monitoring committee. J Clin Neurophysiol. 2013;30:161–73.

93. Yoo J, Rampal N, Petroff OA, Hirsch LJ, Gaspard N. BRief potentially ictal rhythmic discharges in critically ill adults. JAMA Neurol. 2014;71:454–62.

94. Rossetti AO, Logroscino G, Bromfield EB. Refractory status epilepticus: effect of treatment aggressiveness on prognosis. Arch Neurol. 2005;62:1698–702.

95. Kang BS, Jung KH, Shin JW, et al. Induction of burst suppression or coma using intravenous anesthetics in refractory status epilepticus. J Clin Neurosci. 2015;22:854–8.

96. Krishnamurthy KB, Drislane FW. Depth of EEG suppression and outcome in barbiturate anesthetic treatment for refractory status epilepticus. Epilepsia. 1999;40:759–62.

97. Johnson E, Ritzl EK. EEG characteristics of successful burst suppression for status epilepticus. 69th Annual meeting of the American Epilepsy Society. Philadelphia, PA, USA. 2015.

98. Thompson SA, Hantus S. Highly epileptiform bursts are associated with seizure recurrence. J Clin Neurophysiol. 2015; Publish Ahead of Print

99. Aminoff MJ. Do nonconvulsive seizures damage the brain?–No. Arch Neurol. 1998;55:119–20.

100. Young GB, Jordan KG. Do nonconvulsive seizures damage the brain?–Yes. Arch Neurol. 1998;55:117–9.

101. Vespa PM, Nuwer MR, Nenov V, et al. Increased incidence and impact of nonconvulsive and convulsive seizures after traumatic brain injury as detected by continuous electroencephalographic monitoring. J Neurosurg. 1999;91:750–60.

102. Shneker BF, Fountain NB. Assessment of acute morbidity and mortality in nonconvulsive status epilepticus. Neurology. 2003;61:1066–73.

103. Bottaro FJ, Martinez OA, Pardal MM, Bruetman JE, Reisin RC. Nonconvulsive status epilepticus in the elderly: a case-control study. Epilepsia. 2007;48:966–72.

104. Litt B, Wityk RJ, Hertz SH, et al. Nonconvulsive status epilepticus in the critically ill elderly. Epilepsia. 1998;39:1194–202.

105. Kowalski RG, Ziai WC, Rees RN, et al. Third-line antiepileptic therapy and outcome in status epilepticus: The impact of vasopressor use and prolonged mechanical ventilation*. Crit Care Med. 2012;40:2677–84.

106. Sutter R, Marsch S, Fuhr P, Kaplan PW, Ruegg S. Anesthetic drugs in status epilepticus: risk or rescue? A 6-year cohort study. Neurology. 2014;82:656–64.

107. Marchi NA, Novy J, Faouzi M, Stahli C, Burnand B, Rossetti AO. Status epilepticus: impact of therapeutic coma on outcome. Crit Care Med. 2015;43:1003–9.

108. Hirsch LJ. Finding the lesser of two evils: treating refractory status epilepticus. Epilepsy Curr. 2015;15:313–6.

109. Meldrum BS, Vigouroux RA, Brierley JB. Systemic factors and epileptic brain damage. Prolonged seizures in paralyzed, artificially ventilated baboons. Arch Neurol. 1973;29:82–7.

110. Holmes GL. Seizure-induced neuronal injury: animal data. Neurology. 2002;59:S3–6.

111. Krsek P, Mikulecka A, Druga R, et al. Long-term behavioral and morphological consequences of nonconvulsive status epilepticus in rats. Epilepsy Behav. 2004;5:180–91.

112. Lothman EW, Bertram EH, Bekenstein JW, Perlin JB. Self-sustaining limbic status epilepticus induced by 'continuous' hippocampal stimulation: electrographic and behavioral characteristics. Epilepsy Res. 1989;3:107–19.

113. Cavazos JE, Das I, Sutula TP. Neuronal loss induced in limbic pathways by kindling: evidence for induction of hippocampal sclerosis by repeated brief seizures. J Neurosci. 1994;14:3106–21.

114. Kotloski R, Lynch M, Lauersdorf S, Sutula T. Repeated brief seizures induce progressive hippocampal neuron loss and memory deficits. Prog Brain Res. 2002;135:95–110.

115. Saffen DW, Cole AJ, Worley PF, Christy BA, Ryder K, Baraban JM. Convulsant-induced increase in transcription factor messenger RNAs in rat brain. Proc Natl Acad Sci U S A. 1988;85:7795–9.

116. Dube C, Chen K, Eghbal-Ahmadi M, Brunson K, Soltesz I, Baram TZ. Prolonged febrile seizures in the immature rat model enhance hippocampal excitability long term. Ann Neurol. 2000;47:336–44.

117. DeGiorgio CM, Tomiyasu U, Gott PS, Treiman DM. Hippocampal pyramidal cell loss in human status epilepticus. Epilepsia. 1992;33:23–7.

118. Rabinowicz AL, Correale J, Boutros RB, Couldwell WT, Henderson CW, DeGiorgio CM. Neuron-specific enolase is increased after single seizures during inpatient video/EEG monitoring. Epilepsia. 1996;37:122–5.

119. DeGiorgio CM, Gott PS, Rabinowicz AL, Heck CN, Smith TD, Correale JD. Neuron-specific enolase, a marker of acute neuronal injury, is increased in complex partial status epilepticus. Epilepsia. 1996;37:606–9.

120. DeGiorgio CM, Heck CN, Rabinowicz AL, Gott PS, Smith T, Correale J. Serum neuron-specific enolase in the major subtypes of status epilepticus. Neurology. 1999;52:746–9.

121. Vespa P, Prins M, Ronne-Engstrom E, et al. Increase in extracellular glutamate caused by reduced cerebral perfusion pressure and seizures after human traumatic brain injury: a microdialysis study. J Neurosurg. 1998;89:971–82.

122. Vespa PM, Miller C, McArthur D, et al. Nonconvulsive electrographic seizures after traumatic brain injury result in a delayed, prolonged increase in intracranial pressure and metabolic crisis. Crit Care Med. 2007;35(12):2830–6.

123. Vespa P, Martin NA, Nenov V, et al. Delayed increase in extracellular glycerol with post-traumatic electrographic epileptic activity: support for the theory that seizures induce secondary injury. Acta Neurochir Suppl. 2002;81:355–7.

124. Hartings JA, Williams AJ, Tortella FC. Occurrence of nonconvulsive seizures, periodic epileptiform discharges, and intermittent rhythmic delta activity in rat focal ischemia. Exp Neurol. 2003;179:139–49.

125. Williams AJ, Tortella FC, Lu XM, Moreton JE, Hartings JA. Antiepileptic drug treatment of nonconvulsive seizures induced by experimental focal brain ischemia. J Pharmacol Exp Ther. 2004;311:220–7.

126. Johnson DW, Hogg JP, Dasheiff R, Yonas H, Pentheny S, Jumao-as A. Xenon/CT cerebral blood flow studies during continuous depth electrode monitoring in epilepsy patients. AJNR Am J Neuroradiol. 1993;14:245–52.

127. Gabor AJ, Brooks AG, Scobey RP, Parsons GH. Intracranial pressure during epileptic seizures. Electroencephalogr Clin Neurophysiol. 1984;57:497–506.

128. Marienne JP, Robert G, Bagnat E. Post-traumatic acute rise of ICP related to subclinical epileptic seizures. Acta Neurochir Suppl (Wien). 1979;28:89–92.

129. Fabricius M, Fuhr S, Bhatia R, et al. Cortical spreading depression and peri-infarct depolarization in acutely injured human cerebral cortex. Brain. 2006;129:778–90.

130. Fabricius M, Fuhr S, Willumsen L, et al. Association of seizures with cortical spreading depression and peri-infarct depolarisations in the acutely injured human brain. Clin Neurophysiol. 2008;119:1973–84.

131. Kilbride RD, Costello DJ, Chiappa KH. How seizure detection by continuous electroencephalographic monitoring affects the prescribing of antiepileptic medications. Arch Neurol. 2009;66:723–8.

132. Abend N, Topjian A, Gutierrez-Colina A, Donnelly M, Clancy R, Dlugos D. Impact of continuous EEG monitoring on clinical management in critically ill children. Neurocrit Care. 2011;15:70–5.

133. Vespa PM, Nenov V, Nuwer MR. Continuous EEG Monitoring in the intensive care unit: early findings and clinical efficacy. J Clin Neurophysiol. 1999;16:1–13.

134. Sundt Jr TM, Sharbrough FW, Anderson RE, Michenfelder JD. Cerebral blood flow measurements and electroencephalograms during carotid endarterectomy. J Neurosurg. 1974;41:310–20.

135. Sundt Jr TM, Sharbrough FW, Piepgras DG, Kearns TP, Messick Jr JM, O'Fallon WM. Correlation of cerebral blood flow and electroencephalographic changes during carotid endarterectomy: with results of surgery and hemodynamics of cerebral ischemia. Mayo Clin Proc. 1981;56:533–43.

136. Sharbrough FW, Messick Jr JM, Sundt Jr TM. Correlation of continuous electroencephalograms with cerebral blood flow measurements during carotid endarterectomy. Stroke. 1973;4:674–83.

137. Zampella E, Morawetz RB, McDowell HA, et al. The importance of cerebral ischemia during carotid endarterectomy. Neurosurgery. 1991;29:727–30. discussion 30-1

138. Arnold M, Sturzenegger M, Schaffler L, Seiler RW. Continuous intraoperative monitoring of middle cerebral artery blood flow velocities and electroencephalography during carotid endarterectomy. A comparison of the two methods to detect cerebral ischemia. Stroke. 1997;28:1345–50.

139. Astrup J, Siesjo BK, Symon L. Thresholds in cerebral ischemia—the ischemic penumbra. Stroke. 1981;12:723–5.

140. Jordan KG. Emergency EEG and continuous EEG monitoring in acute ischemic stroke. J Clin Neurophysiol. 2004;21:341–52.

141. Claassen J, Hirsch LJ, Emerson RG, Mayer SA. Treatment of refractory status epilepticus with pentobarbital, propofol, or midazolam: a systematic review. Epilepsia. 2002;43:146–53.

142. Rots ML, van Putten MJAM, Hoedemaekers CWE, Horn J. Continuous EEG monitoring for early detection of delayed cerebral ischemia in subarachnoid hemorrhage: a pilot study. Neurocrit Care. 2015;24:207–16.

143. Scheuer ML, Wilson SB. Data analysis for continuous EEG monitoring in the ICU: seeing the forest and the trees. J Clin Neurophysiol. 2004;21:353–78.

144. Gotman J. Automatic detection of seizures and spikes. J Clin Neurophysiol. 1999;16:130.

145. Shah AK, Agarwal R, Carhuapoma JR, Loeb JA. Compressed EEG pattern analysis for critically Ill neurological-neurosurgical patients. Neurocrit Care. 2006;5:124–33.

146. Fürbass F, Hartmann MM, Halford JJ, et al. Automatic detection of rhythmic and periodic patterns in critical care EEG based on American Clinical Neurophysiology Society (ACNS) standardized terminology. Neurophysiol Clin. 2015;45:203–13.

147. Adams DC, Heyer EJ, Emerson RG, et al. The reliability of quantitative electroencephalography as an indicator of cerebral ischemia. Anesth Analg. 1995;81:80–3.

148. Jordan KG, Continuous EEG. Monitoring in the neuroscience intensive care unit and emergency department. J Clin Neurophysiol. 1999;16:14.

149. Wartenberg KE, Schmidt JM, Mayer SA. Multimodality monitoring in neurocritical care. Crit Care Clin. 2007;23:507–38.

150. Claassen J, Perotte A, Albers D, et al. Nonconvulsive seizures after subarachnoid hemorrhage: multimodal detection and outcomes. Ann Neurol. 2013;74:53–64.

151. Kaplan PW. EEG criteria for nonconvulsive status epilepticus. Epilepsia. 2007;48:39–41.

152. Bauerle K, Greim CA, Schroth M, Geisselbrecht M, Kobler A, Roewer N. Prediction of depth of sedation and anaesthesia by the NarcotrendTM EEG monitor. Br J Anaesth. 2004;92:841–5.

153. Zhou JL, Shatskikh TN, Liu X, Holmes GL. Impaired single cell firing and long-term potentiation parallels memory impairment following recurrent seizures. Eur J Neurosci. 2007;25:3667–77.

Seizures and Quantitative EEG

Jennifer A. Kim, Lidia M.V.R. Moura, Craig Williamson,
Edilberto Amorim, Sahar Zafar, Siddharth Biswal,
and M.M. Brandon Westover

Introduction

Continuous EEG (cEEG) monitoring has become increasingly utilized as high rates of nonconvulsive seizures (NCS) and nonconvulsive status epilepticus (NCSE) in ICU patients have become widely recognized. Diagnosis of NCS and NCSE requires continuous EEG monitoring [1–3]. Timely seizure recognition is important as it may lead to acute changes in therapy aimed at suppressing seizures and correcting potential precipitating factors [4, 5].

As continuous EEG monitoring has become more prevalent, the time-consuming review necessary by neurophysiology experts trained in evaluating these records has become taxing and in many cases difficult to maintain. Although demand for continuous EEG (cEEG) monitoring has increased dramatically, the number of EEG readers has remained stable [6]. Many facilities that could benefit from the availability of cEEG may not have skilled EEG interpreters to provide ongoing interpretation of cEEG in the ICU. Even when skilled EEG reviewers are available, if multiple patients simultaneously undergo prolonged cEEG monitoring, interpretation and communication of findings becomes fragmented, the problem of "continuous monitoring and intermittent care" and delayed intervention [7].

Routine evaluation of EEG consists of visual inspection of the data with an average review time of 20–30 min per 24-h study, with more detailed analysis taking more time [7]. Visual analysis of the raw EEG record may miss gradual trends in EEG that evolve over long periods of time [8]. To address these challenges, different quantitative methods to evaluate cEEG data have emerged. Advantages, hoped for, of quantitative EEG (qEEG) techniques include the ability to quantify information within the EEG signal, to compress the time scale and shorten the review time, to quickly identify events/periods of interest for closer analysis, and to make real-time monitoring more feasible. The main impetus for developing qEEG methods in ICU EEG has been to assist with rapidly identifying rare/occasional seizures in prolonged recordings without the need for exhaustive visual screening of each 10-s display window of raw EEG [9].

In summary, qEEG has the potential to improve efficiency of interpretation and communication in intensive medical care [10, 11]. However, qEEG remains a relatively new family of technologies, many of which are still in early stages of development, validation, and adoption. In this chapter we first provide a brief survey of qEEG methods that are in clinical use. We then provide a detailed treatment of one of the oldest and most clinically useful qEEG methods, "compressed spectral arrays" or spectrograms.

Overview of Quantitative EEG Methods

Amplitude-Based Methods

Amplitude-integrated EEG (aEEG) is a simplified bedside continuous EEG monitoring technology that has become widely used in the neonatal population over the past two decades to monitor for seizures and to assist with prognostication in neonates with hypoxic-ischemic encephalopathy [12]. aEEG is typically based on a limited number of

J.A. Kim (✉) • Lidia M.V.R. Moura • E. Amorim • S. Zafar
S. Biswal • M.M.B. Westover
Department of Neurology, Harvard Medical School,
Massachusetts General Hospital, Boston, MA 02114, USA
e-mail: jkim72@partners.org; lidia.moura@mgh.harvard.edu;
EAMORIM@mgh.harvard.edu; SFZAFAR@mgh.harvard.edu;
SBISWAL2@PARTNERS.ORG; MWESTOVER@mgh.harvard.edu

C. Williamson
Department of Neurology and Neurological Surgery, University of
Michigan, University Hospital, Ann Arbor, MI 48109, USA
e-mail: craigaw@umich.edu

© Springer International Publishing AG 2017
P.N. Varelas, J. Claassen (eds.), *Seizures in Critical Care*, Current Clinical Neurology, DOI 10.1007/978-3-319-49557-6_4

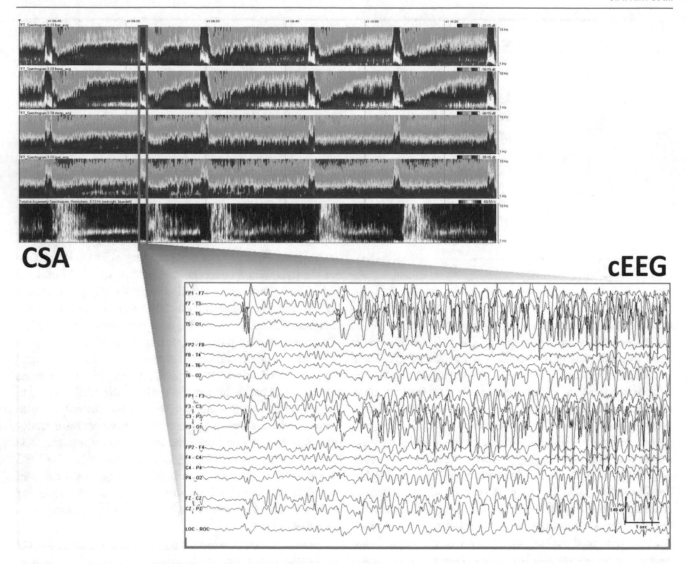

Fig. 4.1 An example compressed spectral array (CSA). Panels, *top to bottom*: left parietal average signal, left temporal average signal, right temporal average signal, right parietal average signal, relative asymmetry index. *Inset*: region CSA corresponding to the onset of a seizure as shown in the native EEG segment. This CSA is an example of *regular flame* pattern of seizures. Please see Sect. 5 and Table 4.1 for further details

recording channels, the data from which is filtered, rectified, and displayed on a semilogarithmic time- and amplitude-compressed scale [7]. Processed in this way, seizures are often evident as sudden increases and then decreases in EEG amplitude [13].

Envelope trend-based qEEG displays the median amplitude of all background activity over a specified time interval. Seizures can often be identified by an increase in median amplitude [9]. One study found that envelope trend analysis could accurately identify seizures lasting >1 min by experienced users with 88% sensitivity and few false positives [14].

Spectrograms

Various informative EEG displays may be created from the power spectrum as a function of time, also known as the compressed spectral array (CSA)) or spectrogram. By show-

ing relatively large stretches of data in a compressed format while making changes in background activity salient, spectrograms can be used to expedite EEG review (Fig. 4.1) [10]. The spectrogram is sometimes referred to as the "FFT of the EEG," though this is a misnomer, as explained in the section on the theory of spectrograms.

Displays Derived from Spectrograms

Asymmetry trends use comparisons in power between homologous electrodes in the right and left hemispheres to highlight power asymmetries between the hemispheres. The comparison can be made based on absolute or relative power. This may be helpful to identify lateralized or focal seizures.

Asymmetry spectrograms are shown in subsequent sections as the fifth panel in the case examples discussed in section "Case Vignettes with Example Spectrogram Patterns". In our case examples, red represents greater power in the right hemisphere and blue represents greater power in the left hemisphere (though in other systems, this color scheme may be reversed).

Methods for Monitoring Burst Suppression

Monitoring burst suppression in ICU patients is another area in which qEEG can be informative. Pharmacologically induced burst suppression is often used in the treatment of refractory status epilepticus. In these cases EEG monitoring is important to ensure that medications can be appropriately titrated in real time to ensure appropriate levels of burst suppression while avoiding over- and under-dosing. It is also helpful to have such monitoring capabilities in patients with pathologically generated burst suppression patterns, such as after severe hypoxic-ischemic injury, to assess for trends in this background pattern for prognostication.

Burst suppression can be quantified using the burst suppression ratio (BSR), defined as the percentage of time within an epoch spent in suppression [15], or as the burst suppression probability (BSP), defined as the instantaneous probability that the EEG is in the suppressed state [15, 16]. Under steady-state conditions, the BSR and BSP agree closely. However, the BSP algorithm is better suited for tracking the depth of burst suppression under dynamic conditions. An example of tracking the BSP in a patient with status epilepticus is shown in Fig. 4.2.

Automated Seizure Detection

One of the ultimate goals of qEEG is to offer the potential for automated detection of clinically significant events such as seizures and ischemia. Ictal patterns are highly variable and thus make the development of such detectors difficult. Features that have been used to develop seizure detectors include amplitude, frequency, rhythmicity, and degree of asymmetry [9]. Most of these algorithms have been designed for identification of classic seizure patterns in the setting of the epilepsy monitoring unit. However, seizures in ICU patients typically have different characteristics than those of the EMU population and thus are not as reliably detected with standard seizure detection algorithms [9]. Pitfalls in qEEG analysis include the high degree of false-positive detections due to common ICU artifacts in addition to false negatives from very brief, low amplitude of slowly evolving seizures. Because seizures occurring in critically ill patients frequently exhibit patterns of rhythmicity and evolution that are slower than those seen in epileptic patients, existing detection programs may be relatively insensitive to certain types of ICU ictal patterns [8]. Another challenge is that many ICU seizures tend to wax and wane with subtle onset and termination rather than the abrupt ictal onset and cessation patterns of seizures typically seen in the EMU.

Automated Detection of Other Epileptiform Patterns

Recently one group has developed software, called NeuroTrend, that attempts to detect patterns in the long-term scalp EEGs in the ICU using the standardized EEG

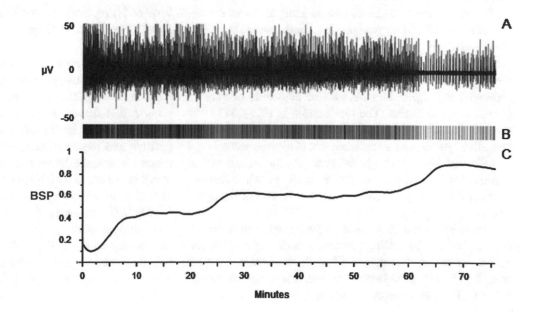

Fig. 4.2 Burst suppression probability (BSP)). (**a**) EEG signal compressed over 75 min. (**b**) Ticker plot representing each burst. (**c**) BSP increases over time as the periods of suppression become more frequent as the recording progresses

terminology [17]. Persyst Corp. has also recently developed an algorithm for identifying periodic discharges, available in version P13 of its software. Details from the algorithms from both NeuroTrend and Persyst Corp. are unpublished and proprietary. Rigorous external validation studies remain to be performed.

Fundamentals of Spectrograms

Motivation for Spectral Analysis

It is often natural to describe oscillatory signals like the EEG in the frequency domain. Indeed, this is reflected in the convention of describing clinical EEG recordings in terms of activity within frequency bands (e.g., delta, theta, alpha, and beta). In this section we briefly review key concepts from the mathematical analysis of frequency domain or spectral characteristics of signals. This overview will help the reader to better understand common features of spectrograms encountered in the ICU setting, reviewed in section "Interpretation of Spectrograms."

Spectral Decomposition: Fourier Transforms and the "FFT"

The basic problem of spectral estimation theory is: given a finite segment of a signal, *estimate* how the total power in the signal is distributed over a range of frequencies. The emphasis on estimation is because the EEG, like many other biological signals, is best regarded as composed of signal and noise. The noise must be suppressed in some way to obtain a clear view of the underlying spectral EEG characteristics that are of interest.

Before one can understand how to analyze stochastic signals like the EEG, one first needs to understand the principles underlying the more basic theory of spectral decomposition, which we will review now. Figure 4.3 shows the decomposition of a fairly complex 9-s long single-channel EEG signal into a series of sinusoids of varying phases and amplitudes. The black curve in Fig. 4.3a shows the original signal, consisting initially of a low-amplitude "baseline" period and an epileptiform discharge around $t = 4$ s, followed by a larger amplitude oscillating pattern at approximately 2 Hz that decays in amplitude while slowing in frequency to approximately 1 Hz by the end of the figure window.

The overlaid red curve is an approximation to the black curve, obtained by adding together a series of 50 sine and cosine waves or "components," with frequencies ranging from 0 to 35 Hz spaced evenly at intervals of approximately 0.7 Hz. The nine components which make the largest contribution to the approximation, i.e., the components with the largest amplitudes, sorted by frequency, are displayed in Fig. 4.3b.

For the most part, the sum of these sinusoidal components faithfully represents the original black signal. Careful scrutiny reveals that the approximation succeeds by a delicate series of constructive and destructive interferences of peaks and troughs. This remarkable balancing act is accomplished automatically by a mathematical formula known as the discrete Fourier series. In the examples shown in Figs. 4.3 and 4.4, the formula used is called the discrete Fourier transform, or DFT.

The amplitude spectrum for a signal is obtained by taking the geometric mean of the amplitudes of the sine-cosine pair for each frequency and plotting these amplitudes as a function of frequency, as shown in Fig. 4.3c.

For the most part, the red approximation or "reconstruction" is faithful to the original black signal. However, in places, the reconstruction is not accurate. These failures are instructive. Note particularly the epileptiform discharge or "spike" that occurs at approximately $t = 4$ s. Here, the reconstruction is smoother than the original signal. It fails to reproduce the abrupt rise in voltage and subsequent abrupt decrease that constitute the spike. This is because in this reconstruction we deliberately excluded sinusoids above 35 Hz from the reconstruction. The true bandwidth of the signal is evidently greater than 35 Hz. That is, higher frequency components are required in the Fourier sum to capture the more abrupt transitions or "sharper turns" that make up an epileptiform discharge. In this case, had we included components for all frequencies up to the Nyquist sampling rate (in this case, approximately 100 Hz), the reconstruction would have been essentially perfect.

Signal Sharpening Manifests as Amplitude Spectrum Broadening

We further illustrate the important relationship between "sharpness" and the presence of higher frequency components in the amplitude spectrum in Fig. 4.4. In Fig. 4.4a, we show a bell-shaped curve, reminiscent of an EEG "slow wave," together with the components in a frequency decomposition and the corresponding amplitude spectrum. As in the previous figure, there is an underlying black curve and an overlaid red curve which approximates the black curve as a sum of sinusoids with amplitudes calculated by the formula for the DFT. We see that, for a waveform with a blunted or non-sharp morphology, the amplitude spectrum is relatively narrow. By contrast, Fig. 4.4b shows a narrow, spikelike, bell-shaped curve, reminiscent of an epileptiform discharge. We see that a broader range of sinusoids extending to a much higher range of frequencies is required to faithfully represent

Fig. 4.3 Spectral decomposition. (**a**) Original signal (*black*) with superimposed approximation signal (*red*) composed of sine and cosine "components" making up the original signal. (**b**) Frequency decomposition—nine components which make up the largest contribution of the approximation. (**c**) Amplitude spectrum showing the distribution of frequencies contributing to the signal with higher amplitudes contributing more to the reconstructed signal

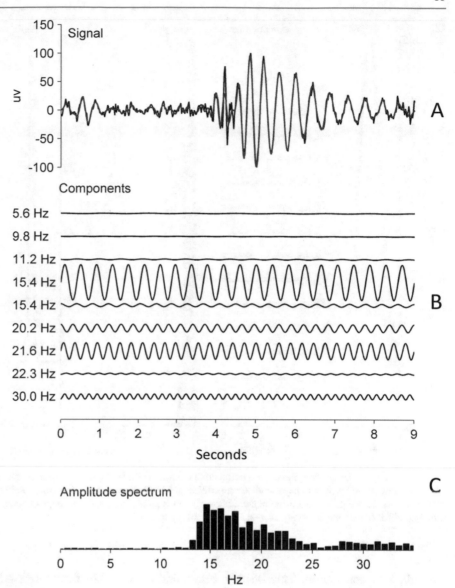

a spikelike transient. We will see that this observation, that signal "sharpness" manifests in the frequency domain as a broadening of the amplitude spectrum, is fundamental in interpreting spectrograms in ICU EEG monitoring.

From Spectra to Spectrograms

Though we have seen that it is possible to decompose complex signals into simple sinusoidal components, there is something unnatural about this decomposition for signals like the one shown in Fig. 4.3. In particular, the signal appears to change character over course of the 9 s shown. It would be more natural to break signals like this into smaller segments or windows, over which the signal characteristics are approximately constant. In statistical jargon, we desire to break the signal into segments that are statistically stationary.

Figure 4.5 shows an example of another signal that shows marked nonstationarity. This example shows a 3-min-long single-channel EEG signal. Figure 4.5b is the raw signal containing a seizure that begins around $t = 20$ s and ends around $t = 120$ s. The panels in Fig. 4.5a show the power spectrum (essentially, the amplitude spectrum squared, except for some smoothing—see next below) calculated from three different windows centered at $t = 20$, 60, and 130 s. The spectra within these three windows differ markedly, reflecting the evolution of signal characteristics that typify seizure activity.

Figure 4.5c shows the result of repeatedly calculating the spectrum of signals in 2-s windows, using a "sliding window" to obtain a new spectrum every 0.1 s. These spectra collectively form an image, or time-frequency spectrogram, formed by representing the power spectrum on a colormap. In this example, the power is shown in decibel (log) units,

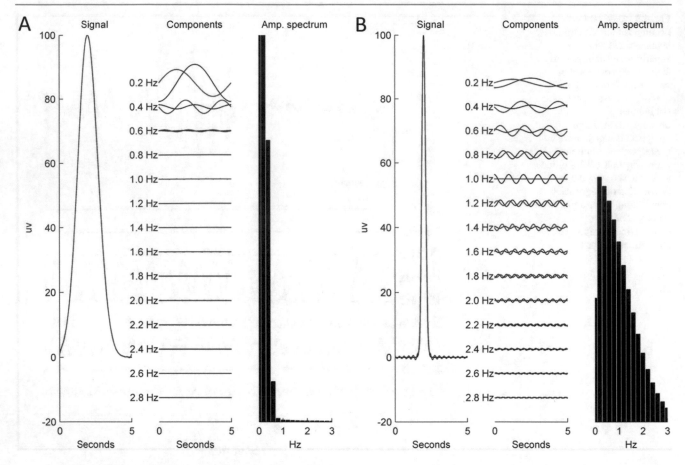

Fig. 4.4 Effect of signal "sharpness" on spectral components. (**a**) Bell-shaped "slow wave" with its frequency decomposition and amplitude spectrum. As with Fig. 4.3, the original signal (*black*) and approximation signal (*red*) are superimposed. Non-sharp morphology results in a narrow amplitude spectrum. (**b**) Narrow "spike-shaped" curve with the same functions plotted as in (**a**). This sharp morphology requires a broader range of sinusoids to approximate its signal

according to convention. This display convention allows simultaneous visualization of the signal power over a wide range of frequencies in one image, despite the fact that in human EEG the power at different physiologically relevant frequencies can vary by an order of magnitude or more. Representing this EEG signal as a spectrogram clearly brings out the salient dynamical features of the seizure, namely, an increase in the dominant frequency of oscillatory activity and a sharpening of the signal contour, followed by slowing down as the seizure ends. These features are not visible in the raw signal at this scale, though they are clearly evident when examining the signal within a more conventional 10-s window used for clinical review of EEG data. By contrast, these dynamics are clearly evident in the spectrogram despite the "large" 3-min window. The ability of spectrograms to display salient features of the EEG at a zoomed out or "compressed" scale is a major reason that spectrograms are useful in ICU EEG. Further examples at more compressed scales (2 h) will be discussed in subsequent sections.

Understanding Spectrograms: Cardinal Patterns from Synthetic Signals

The principles of spectral analysis described above are exploited to interpret patterns that occur commonly in spectrograms from cEEG recordings in the ICU setting. We illustrate these patterns using synthetic data in Fig. 4.5, before turning to real examples. Figure 4.6a shows a simple signal, a "monotonous" or unchanging low-amplitude sinusoid of 2 Hz. The corresponding spectrogram has a single peak at 2 Hz within every time window that manifests in the spectrogram as a red line at 2 Hz. This signal is reminiscent of the common ICU EEG pattern of "delta slowing" seen in patients with encephalopathy. Figure 4.6b shows a sinusoidal signal with a frequency that begins at 2 Hz, then increases following a linear ramp to 5 Hz while increasing also in amplitude, and then drops abruptly back to 2 Hz. The evolving portion of this pattern is manifest in the spectrogram as an upsloping line. This example is reminiscent of the classic pattern of

Fig. 4.5 Nonstationarity of a
3-min EEG signal containing
a seizure. (**a**) Power spectra
calculated at three different
time windows of the
recording (*t* = 20, 60, 130 s).
(**b**) Raw EEG signal
compressed over a 3-min
interval, with *box insets*
corresponding to the time
windows plotted in (**a**). (**c**)
Spectrogram of EEG signal
from (**b**) using two sliding
windows, box insets
correspond to the time
windows plotted in (**a**)

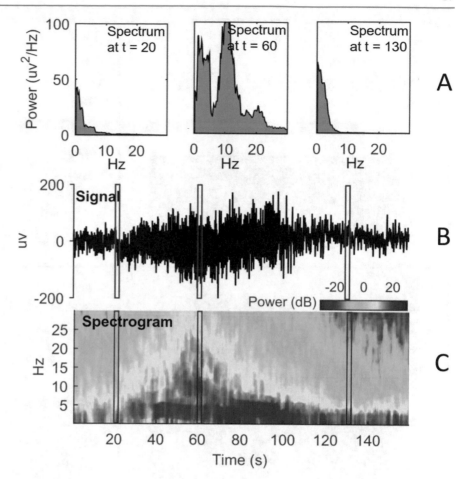

evolution characteristic of many epileptic seizures and typifies what we will refer to in a subsequent section as a "flame"-type seizure.

Figure 4.6c shows a more complex synthetic signal, consisting of a series of sharp discharges of randomly varying amplitudes, occurring in a regular or periodic fashion at 1 Hz. The spectrogram in this case shows high power not only at 1 Hz, reflecting the periodicity of the repeating pattern, but also a broadening of the spectrum up to approximately 5 Hz and beyond. This broadband character of the spectrogram reflects the fact that the morphology of the discharges is sharp and thus has a broad amplitude or power spectrum, as discussed previously in connection with Fig. 4.4b. Figure 4.6d shows another more extreme example, a sawtooth wave.

In both Fig. 4.6c, d, the pattern can be characterized as *broadband monotonous*, referring to the repetitive periodic nature combined with the relatively broadband of high power due to the sharpness of the underlying discharges. As will be seen in the real examples below, the *broadband-monotonous* pattern typifies the spectrogram when the underlying EEG is in a state of either periodic epileptiform discharges or certain closely related states of status epilepticus.

Technical Considerations: Trade-Offs in Spectral Estimation

Our discussion regarding spectral estimation has glossed over many important technical details that are critical in certain applications of spectral estimation. We touch briefly on two important fundamental issues that affect the quality of spectrograms.

Trade-Off Between Temporal and Spectral Resolution

Consider again the example of a seizure and its spectrogram shown in Fig. 4.5. In that example we chose to make the window size 2 s. This choice in turn dictated a limit to the level of detail with which we were able to resolve temporal features in the EEG, so that the spectrogram has a certain degree of blurring or smoothness across time. If we attempt to obtain higher temporal resolution by making the analysis windows progressively smaller, we would at the same time see that we progressively lose the ability to distinguish detail in the frequency domain. This is because decreasing the signal

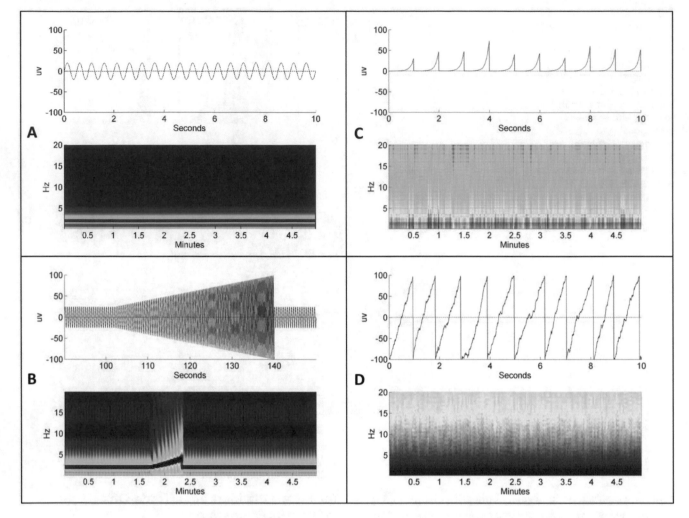

Fig. 4.6 Four simulated EEG patterns converted to CSAs. (**a**) Sinusoidal signal at 2 Hz without variation, reminiscent of "delta slowing." CSA shows a *red line*, representing a consistent peak at 2 Hz. (**b**) Sinusoidal signal with linear ramp from 2 to 5 Hz followed by an abrupt termination, modeling an evolving seizure. CSA shows a rise in the power of frequencies up to 5 Hz corresponding to the linear ramp seen in the sinusoidal signal and a return back to 2 Hz. (**c**) Synthetic model of periodic sharp discharges at 1 Hz. CSA shows a high-power band at 1 Hz with a broadening of the spectrogram reflecting the sharpness of the discharges as described in Fig. 4.4. (**d**) Synthetic model of extreme sawtooth pattern, which best exemplifies the *broadband-monotonous* pattern described in Table 4.1

segment length (keeping the sampling rate constant) reduces the number of frequency components and increases the spacing between components in the DFT. In effect, nearby peaks in the spectrum become single peaks, in the same way that creating a histogram using wide bins can smooth together and obscure peaks in a distribution that has multiple modes.

This consideration highlights a fundamental trade-off that exists between the maximal spectral resolution (the level of detail with which we can calculate the spectrum, i.e., the spacing between frequency components) and the maximal temporal resolution (the smallest window over which we can perform spectral analysis on a signal). The mathematical reasons behind the trade-off between temporal and spectral resolution are in fact identical to those that describe the well-known "Heisenberg uncertainty principle," which describes the inverse relationship between the precision with which one can simultaneously measure the position and velocity of a particle.

Trade-Off Between Bias and Variance

A second fundamental trade-off arises from the fact that the EEG, like many other naturally occurring signals, is best regarded as stochastic, containing an underlying signal of interest that is corrupted by noise. Consequently, the spectrum and hence the spectrogram need to be estimated. This fact gives rise to a trade-off between bias and variance.

The bias-variance trade-off in spectral estimation is illustrated in Fig. 4.7. In Fig. 4.7a, we show a sample of a stochastic signal generated by a model with a known power spectrum, shown as a red curve in Fig. 4.7b–e. This spectrum has two peaks, at approximately 11 and 14 Hz. Let us assume that we have already chosen a window size for our spectral estimates, based on either the maximum window length over which the signal can be considered to be statistically station-

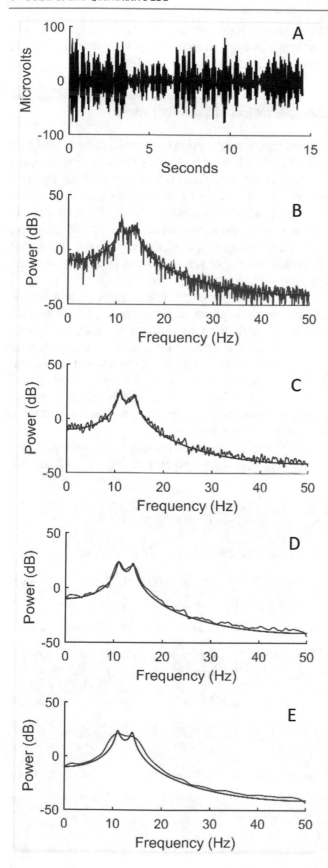

Fig. 4.7 The bias-variance trade-off. (**a**) A stochastic signal generated by a model with a known power spectrum (*red curves*, **b–e**). (**b–e**) Test of varying time windows used for estimating the discrete Fourier transform. Short time windows (**b**) result in noisy estimations, while broad windows (**e**) smooth the data so much as to make peaks indistinguishable

ary or the desired level of temporal resolution. In this case we have chosen a window size of 15 s.

Given the chosen window length, a common but suboptimal way to obtain a spectral "estimate" from this finite-length signal is simply to calculate the discrete Fourier transform, usually using a fast algorithm known as the "fast Fourier transform" (FFT), and to then take the squared amplitude of the result as an estimate of the power spectrum. The result is shown as the blue line in Fig. 4.7b. The spectrum appears very noisy. This is not surprising when one considers that what we have done amounts to "estimating" a quantity using only a single sample. Estimates obtained in this way are sometimes called "periodograms." (We have passed over the fact that, technically, to calculate the periodogram, one usually multiplies the signal by a windowing function or "data taper" before computing the FFT to reduce an effect known as spectral leakage. All spectral estimates shown in this chapter have been computed with appropriate data tapers.)

Under the right conditions in a laboratory, it might be possible to obtain numerous repeated sample segments of the same signal. Given enough repeated samples, we could obtain an accurate estimate of the underlying true spectrum by averaging periodograms. However, in ICU EEG monitoring, we of course do not have the luxury of holding the patient's state constant to obtain repeated samples. We are thus forced to resort to methods of reducing the variance of the spectral estimates, i.e., of making the spectrogram smoother. Figure 4.7c–e show progressively more aggressive smoothing of the original signal. Smoothing necessarily blurs together fine spectral details, as evidenced by the fact that beyond a certain point the spectral peaks in this example become indistinguishable (Fig. 4.7e).

We operationally define the spectral resolution of the estimated power spectrum as the minimum distinguishable difference between two narrow peaks that can be distinguished in the estimated spectrum. Judging by eye, the approximate spectral resolution in Fig. 4.7c–e is <1 Hz, 2 Hz, and 5 Hz, respectively. The optimal trade-off between variance reduction (smoothness) and spectral resolution in this example appears to be most closely achieved in Fig. 4.6d. Note that the spectral resolution is thus usually lower than the maximal spectral resolution discussed in the preceding subjection. The maximal spectral resolution depended on the window width rather than on statistical considerations.

The most appropriate degree of spectral smoothing clearly depends on the spectral characteristics and intrinsic smoothness of the underlying processes which generate the signal and thus varies depending on the application. In clinical ICU EEG monitoring, a spectral resolution of approximately 0.75 Hz is usually adequate and allows for sufficient spectral smoothing to obtain high-quality spectral estimates. This is the resolution used for the spectrogram in Fig. 4.5 and in the examples shown later.

Numerous approaches to spectral smoothing have been proposed. Common methods include averaging spectra from consecutive neighboring windows ("weighted overlapping segment averaging," WOSA) or replacing the amplitudes in a "noisy" spectrum obtained from an appropriately computed discrete Fourier transform by locally weighted averages of neighboring values. Various window functions or "kernels" can be used for this "kernel smoothing" method. The current state of the art, however, is the method called multitaper spectral estimation algorithm (MTSA), which involves averaging together the amplitude spectra of multiple discrete Fourier-transformed segments that have been pre-multiplied by a specific series of windowing functions or "tapers," known as the discrete prolate spheroidal sequences (DPSS). While the technical details of MTSA are beyond the score of this chapter, it suffices for our purposes to know that MTSA is the solution to a mathematically well-defined optimization problem, designed to achieve a balance between spectral resolution (bias) and the variance of spectral estimates. Surprisingly, though it was invented in the early 1980s, MTSA is not yet in wide use. In fact spectral estimation routines implemented in many commercial products produce relatively poor-quality spectrograms, very often simply "computing the FFT" [18–20].

As with all smoothing methods, MTSA has adjustable parameters that allow one to decide precisely how to balance the bias against variance. In the remaining figures shown in this chapter, spectrograms are computed with a moving window length of 4 s, with overlapping windows shifting by 0.1 s, and a spectral resolution of 0.75 Hz.

Interpretation of Spectrograms

We now turn from theory to the interpretation of ICU EEG recordings. While there is no single pattern on a spectrogram that is invariably associated with seizures or other abnormal periodic patterns, many events of interest fall into a small number of recognizable patterns. In this section we briefly review some of the most common spectral patterns associated with pathological ICU EEG events. In the next section, we review a series of actual cases to gain experience with spectrogram interpretation.

The most easily recognizable seizures present with an abrupt increase in power across a range of frequencies that stands out clearly from the surrounding background. Given the red and white color typically used to indicate high power on a color density spectrogram and the shape of these events in the spectrogram, these abrupt changes resemble small flames (e.g., Fig. 4.1). We refer to this pattern as *regular flame*, to distinguish it from the less clear-cut pattern of *choppy flame* (see below).

Cyclic seizures are also often easy to recognize as a series of repeating *regular flame* events (e.g., Figs. 4.1, 4.8, and 4.9).

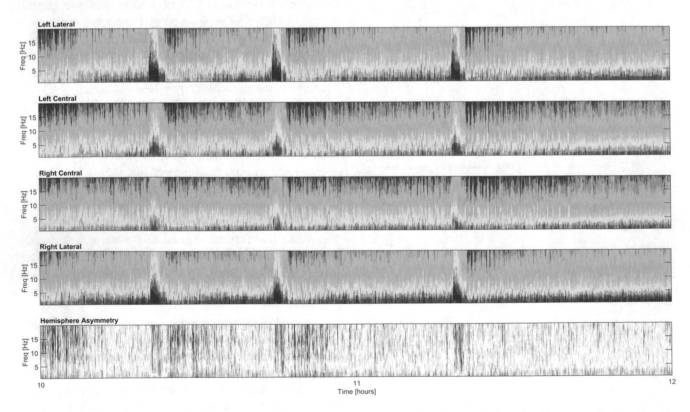

Fig. 4.8 Cyclic seizures (Case 1). This example is typical of the *regular flame* morphology. For Figs. 4.8–4.23, the 2-h CSA panels are displayed as follows (from top): left lateral, left central, right central, right lateral, and hemisphere asymmetry (a.k.a. relative asymmetry). For the top four panels, high power is in *red* and low power in deep *blue*. The hemisphere asymmetry panel assesses where spectral power of the right > left hemisphere (*red*), left > right hemisphere (*blue*), or both are equal (*white*)

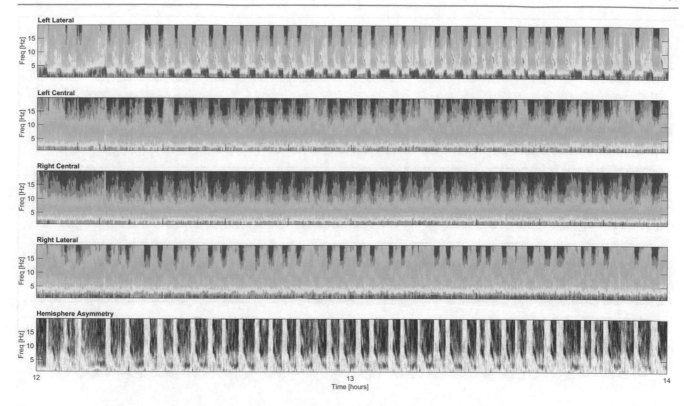

Fig. 4.9 Frequent cyclic seizures (Case 2). Again, this shows the *regular flame* morphology

Once a cyclic seizure has been verified by review of the raw EEG, further seizures can often easily be identified by review of the spectrogram alone. It may even be possible for inexperienced users at the bedside, such as nurses or residents, to detect recurrent seizures in these cases.

State changes and decreased sedation may also cause relatively abrupt increases in power that may mimic flame-type seizure patterns. However, these changes will often have a choppier or more irregular appearance than when an actual seizure is present; hence we refer to these as *choppy flames* (e.g., Fig. 4.10). However, in practice, differentiating seizures from other changes without review of the raw EEG can be challenging.

Similarly, longer-lasting nonconvulsive seizures or periodic discharges often manifest with a spectral signature that is high power across a broadband of frequencies, extending from delta up to theta or higher. These patterns are often unchanging or "monotonous" over long periods or exhibit only changes in their spectral signatures, without a clear beginning or end. We refer to these patterns as "broadband monotonous." The broadband-monotonous patterns are high power because of their typically high amplitude. They are broadband because of the regularity and sharpness of the underlying waveforms, as was explained in the synthetic examples shown in Fig. 4.6c, d. Other examples are shown in the cases that follow (e.g., Figs. 4.11 and 4.12).

As opposed to the broadband-monotonous pattern, diffuse nonrhythmic slowing as is commonly seen in patients with encephalopathy who are not having seizures typically produces a spectral pattern that is monotonous and relatively restricted to the low-frequency part of the power spectrum. We refer to this pattern as "narrowband monotonous" (e.g., Fig. 4.18).

A final easily recognizable common spectral pattern in ICU EEG is that of burst suppression. Burst suppression typically appears as a series of colored "stripes," representing the bursts, alternating with a blue (low-power) background, corresponding to the suppression periods (e.g., Fig. 4.14).

Very brief or very focal seizures may be missed by spectrogram review alone [10, 11]. Because spectrograms compress EEG data and display long periods of time on a single screen, very brief seizures may not result in an identifiable change. Similarly, as spectrograms typically average across a number of leads, very focal seizures may also be impossible to visualize.

Case Vignettes with Example Spectrogram Patterns

In this section, we show several examples of common patterns encountered in EEG spectrograms of ICU patients, including seizures, periodic discharges, and artifact. Where possible, we will describe these patterns using the categories introduced above: *regular flame, choppy flame, broadband*

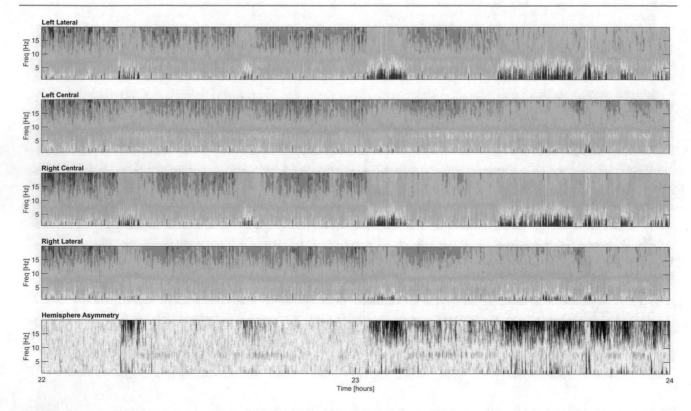

Fig. 4.10 *Irregular flame* morphology (Case 3). This pattern often represents seizures, but can correspond to waxing and waning periodic discharges or artifacts

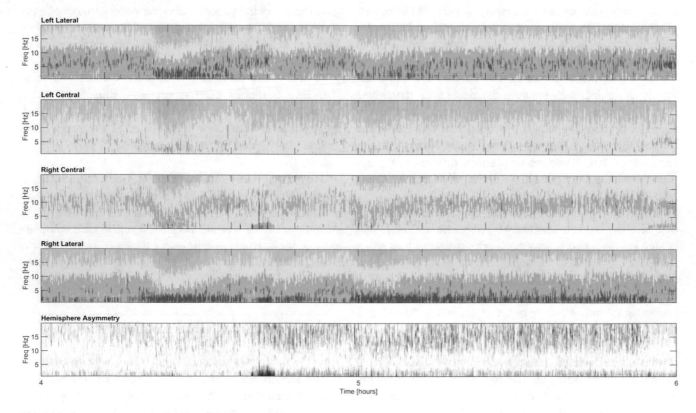

Fig. 4.11 Postanoxic status epilepticus (Case 4). A striking example of the *broadband-monotonous* pattern, often seen with status epilepticus or with periodic discharges

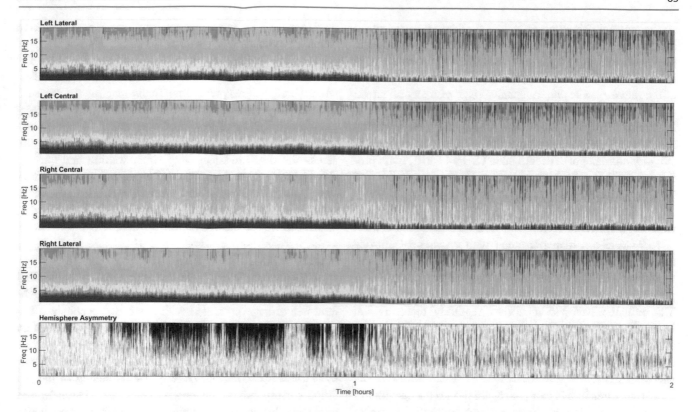

Fig. 4.12 Nonconvulsive status epilepticus (Case 5). A more typical example of the *broadband-monotonous* pattern

Table 4.1 Proposed nomenclature for common spectrographic patterns

Spectrogram pattern	Description	Example(s)
Regular flame	Sudden rise and subsequent fall in power across a broad range of frequencies in a brief period reminiscent of a candle flame This is the most common seizure pattern observed	Fig. 4.8 Fig. 4.9
Choppy flame	Discrete events that stand out against the background, but each event is not as well formed and solid as in the *regular flame* pattern. The flames are more "wispy" This most often reflects seizures, but can correspond to periodic discharges or artifacts	Fig. 4.10
Broadband monotonous	High-power band over a broad range of frequencies across time. Appears as a thick band across the spectrogram This is seen either in status epilepticus or with periodic discharges or less often in high-amplitude rhythmic delta activity	Fig. 4.11 Fig. 4.12
Narrowband monotonous	High-power band over a narrow range of frequencies across time. Appears as a thin band across the spectrogram This is most commonly seen in focal or generalized slowing	Fig. 4.13
Burst suppression	Repetitive dark blue vertical stripes, corresponding to "suppression segments," alternating with brighter (higher power) stripes representing high-power "bursts"	Fig. 4.14

monotonous, *narrowband monotonous*, and *burst suppression* (Table 4.1). We note that while the authors have found these terms helpful, they are not presently part of any officially recognized or validated nomenclature.

Basic Patterns

Case 1: (Fig. 4.8)

A 75-year-old woman with a history of dementia and anticoagulation for deep venous thrombosis presented with seizures in the setting of a left frontoparietal hemorrhage secondary to cerebral amyloid angiopathy. Her cEEG showed 3–5 electrographic nonconvulsive seizures per hour and left centrotemporal and posterior lateralized periodic discharges (LPDs).

In this spectrogram one sees three generalized electrographic seizures with clearly defined discrete starting and ending points. This example is very similar to the example in Figs. 4.1 and 4.5. The sudden rise and subsequent fall in power across a broad range of frequencies in these discrete intervals is reminiscent of a candle flame. This is an example of the *regular flame* pattern characteristic of many seizures.

The background EEG between seizures showed generalized periodic epileptiform discharges. The corresponding spectrogram, not surprisingly, falls into the *broadband-monotonous* category (described in Cases 4 and 5), with prolonged periods lasting more than 10 min at a time of high-power activity extending above 5 Hz.

Case 2: (Fig. 4.9)

A 75-year-old man presented with a syncopal episode resulting in a left frontoparietal skull fracture and an underlying parenchymal contusion. His hospital course was complicated by intracranial hypertension and status epilepticus. The patient developed repetitive, regularly recurring left hemisphere seizures. Seizures started abruptly with 10–12-Hz low-amplitude (<20-mV) discharges and had no clinical correlate. A diagnosis of nonconvulsive status epilepticus was made.

The seizures in this example again fit into the category of *regular flame* seizures. The repetitive, periodic nature of these events demonstrates a spectrographic pattern of left hemisphere cyclic seizures.

The background in the right lateral, left central, and right central regions had a *narrowband-monotonous pattern* (described in Case 6), corresponding to diffuse slowing in these regions on the raw EEG.

Case 3: (Fig. 4.10)

A 70-year-old woman with a history of stroke, subarachnoid hemorrhage, and seizures presented with status epilepticus in the setting of bilateral subdural hematomas. After treatment with anticonvulsants, her cEEG revealed bilateral independent multifocal sharp waves and recurrent discrete nonconvulsive left centrotemporal seizures.

The seizures in this case have a different spectrographic thumbprint from the preceding cases. There are still discrete events that stand out against the background, but each event is not as well formed and solid as in the prior two cases. These "flames" are more "wispy," perhaps reminiscent of flames generated by an electric fireplace. We have termed this the *choppy flame* spectrographic pattern. While this pattern often reflects seizures as in this case, it can also correspond to waxing and waning periodic discharges or artifacts more often than the *regular flame* pattern.

Case 4: (Fig. 4.11)

A 36-year-old woman with a history of alcohol abuse presents with coma after cardiac arrest. Despite undergoing therapeutic hypothermia, she developed generalized periodic discharges at 5 Hz consistent with postanoxic nonconvulsive status epilepticus.

This is a striking example of a spectrogram where the power is relatively high over a broad range of frequencies, which changes slowly with time. In the spectrogram one sees a thick orange band going across the left hemisphere spectrogram and a lighter yellow band over the right hemisphere regions. The thickness of this band remains relatively stable across the displayed recording time, waxing and waning slowly. Given these features, this pattern can be described as *broadband monotonous*. This pattern can be seen with either status epilepticus (as in this case) or with periodic discharges, as discussed in connection with Fig. 4.6c, d.

Case 5: (Fig. 4.12)

A 50-year-old female with developmental delay, familial transthyretin amyloidosis, and non-aneurysmal subarachnoid hemorrhage presented with acute hydrocephalus. The patient had near continuous seizures that persisted until an intravenous propofol infusion was initiated.

This is a more typical example of the *broadband-monotonous* spectrogram pattern. The widening of the red stripe corresponds to increased power and sharpness and reflects in this case continuous nonconvulsive seizure activity. The power then shifts back to the lower frequencies as propofol is uptitrated. Near the end of the 2-h epoch, the EEG has entered a state of *burst suppression*, as reflected by the appearance of a striped pattern in the spectrogram (compare with Case 7, Fig. 4.14).

Case 6: (Fig. 4.13)

An 83-year-old man with a history of end-stage renal disease, coronary artery bypass grafts, hypertension, and hyperlipidemia presented with aphasia and poor mental status. He was found to have a left middle cerebral artery stroke. He had some intermittent staring spells, which were concerning for seizures, so cEEG monitoring was performed. His EEG showed diffuse slowing without any epileptiform abnormalities.

Here, one can appreciate a thin yellow-orange band that continues through the displayed record in the low (<3-Hz)-frequency range. Unlike the broadband-monotonous pattern, this *narrowband-monotonous pattern* is most commonly associated with focal or generalized slowing observed on cEEG, rather than periodic discharges or seizures.

Case 7: (Fig. 4.14)

A 33-year-old man with history of severe traumatic brain injury and meningitis status-post ventriculoperitoneal shunting presented with status epilepticus due to shunt malfunction. His EEG showed evidence of recurrent right frontotemporal 2–3-Hz sharp waves evolving to 3–4-Hz lateralized periodic discharges, unresponsive to second-line

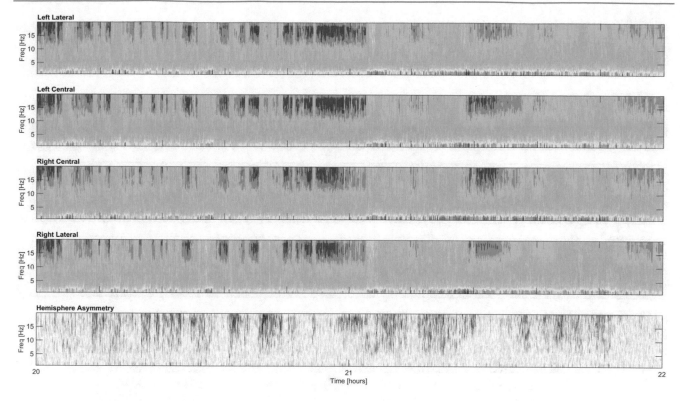

Fig. 4.13 Diffuse slowing (Case 6). This is an example of the *narrowband-monotonous* pattern, often seen in focal or diffuse slowing

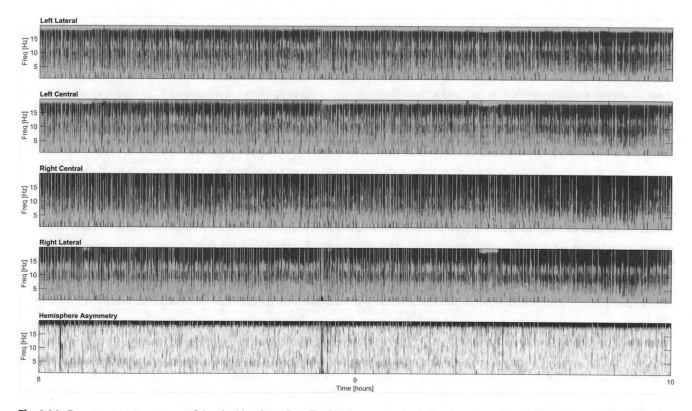

Fig. 4.14 Burst suppression on propofol and midazolam (Case 7). Here is an example of what *burst suppression* patterns look like on CSA

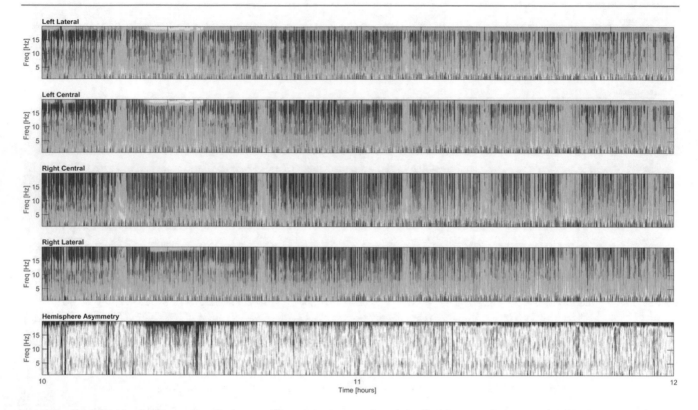

Fig. 4.15 Lifting sedation after burst suppression (Case 7, continued). Here is a continuation of the CSA in Fig. 4.14, showing the *burst suppression* pattern lightening and the emergence of *regular flame*-shaped seizures

intravenous anticonvulsants. He was diagnosed with refractory status epilepticus and treated with intravenous propofol and midazolam.

This is an example of a *burst suppression* on a spectrogram. There are repetitive dark blue vertical stripes throughout the record. The dark blue stripes correspond to the "suppression" segments and the light blue stripes with associated small red-orange bases represent the higher power "bursts."

Case 7, continued: (Fig. 4.15)

This is the succeeding epoch of the same case vignette above. Here, one can again appreciate dark and light blue stripes representing the signature pattern for *burst suppression*. However, during this displayed epoch, sedation was lightened. As *burst suppression* lightens, one can appreciate that the density of the dark blue stripes lessens. One can also appreciate the emergence of at least four *regular flame*-shaped seizures "breaking through" as sedation lightens.

Combination Patterns

Case 8: (Figs. 4.16–4.18)

An 83-year-old man with a medical history significant for chronic kidney disease and atrial fibrillation developed status

epilepticus after cardiac arrest. The cEEG showed diffuse background attenuation associated with generalized periodic discharges and myoclonic movements. Sedation was increased and the seizures resolved, albeit gradually.

This case example illustrates three different patterns. The first (Fig. 4.16) shows very frequent cyclic seizures of the *regular flame* pattern, which become less frequent toward the end of the first 2-h window, with further reduction in seizure frequency in Fig. 4.17. The seizures stop approximately 24 min into Fig. 4.17. The spectrogram pattern then changes to a *broadband-monotonous* pattern and then finally *narrowband monotonous* by the third 2-h epoch (Fig. 4.18).

Case 9: (Figs. 4.19–4.20)

A 38-year-old man with alcoholic cirrhosis presented with variceal hemorrhage complicated by sepsis and renal failure, managed with ciprofloxacin and meropenem. He developed NCSE during his hospitalization. The cEEG showed seizures consisting of abrupt onset of beta activity every 2–5 min without clinical correlate.

This case example is illustrated across two consecutive 2-h epochs. In the first epoch (Fig. 4.19), there are *regular flame* seizures in a cyclic pattern that increase in frequency and ultimately fuse into a *broadband-monotonous* pattern, consistent with status epilepticus. The patient receives antiseizure medication, and the status epilepticus converts into a

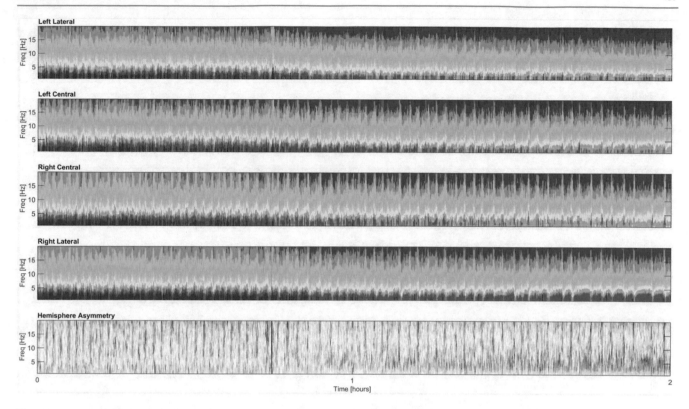

Fig. 4.16 Frequent *regular flame*-shaped seizures consistent with status epilepticus (Case 8)

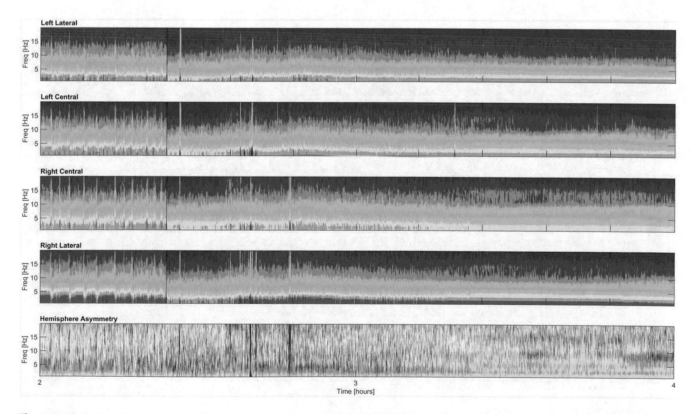

Fig. 4.17 Evolution of seizures as sedation increased (Case 8, continued). The CSA begins with *regular flame* seizures continued from Fig. 4.16, with a reduction in frequency followed by a transition to a *broadband-monotonous* pattern

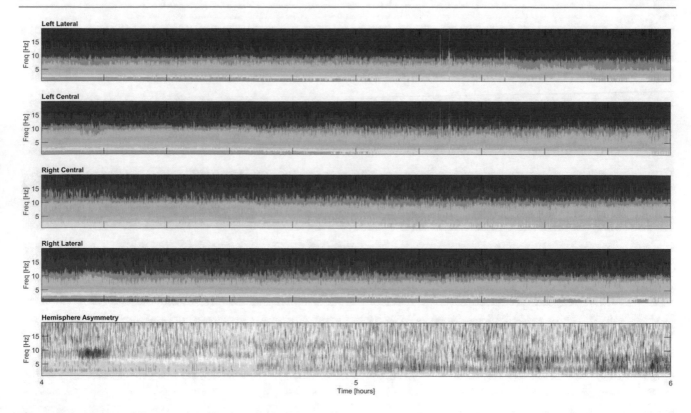

Fig. 4.18 Evolution to diffuse slowing (Case 8, continued). A continuation of Fig. 4.17, the CSA now shows a *narrowband-monotonous* pattern suggestive of diffuse slowing

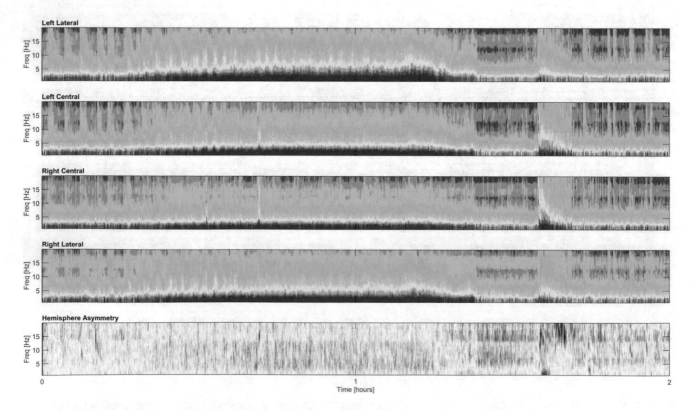

Fig. 4.19 *Regular flame* seizures evolving into *broadband-monotonous* status epilepticus (Case 9)

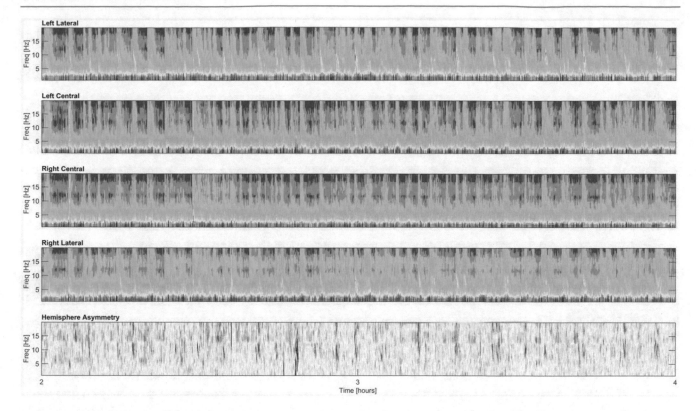

Fig. 4.20 Antiepileptic drug administration prompting the transition from status epilepticus back to *regular flame* seizures with a *narrowband-monotonous*, diffuse slowing background (Case 9, continued)

cyclic seizure pattern with less frequent *regular flame* seizures, on a *narrowband-monotonous* background pattern, corresponding to generalized slowing on the underlying EEG (Fig. 4.20).

Artifacts:

No qEEG method can escape the inherent limitations of scalp EEG and this is particularly true in the ICU environment. Frequent interventions and the use of multiple technologies make differentiating seizures and other patterns of interest from artifact sometimes challenging. We present a few examples to illustrate common artifacts seen on spectrograms in ICU patients.

Case 7, continued: (Fig. 4.21)

This spectrogram is from a later 2-h epoch of Case 7 (Figs. 4.14–4.15). Please refer back to Case 7 for the clinical vignette.

At the beginning of the epoch, the spectrogram shows a uniform deep blue, reflecting near-complete suppression of the EEG background. In this case the suppression is not due to pharmacological intervention, but rather reflects the end stage of severe diffuse anoxic brain injury. Near the end of the 2-h epoch, we see an abrupt change from very low to very high, full-bandwidth power, which manifests as a red color across the entire bandwidth of the spectrogram. This is a typical pattern for disconnection artifact. This pattern

occurs when the EEG shows high-amplitude voltages due to amplifier saturation, due to either disconnection of the electrodes from the scalp or disconnection of all the electrodes from the headbox, as in this example.

Case 10: (Fig. 4.22)

A 51-year-old man presented with subarachnoid hemorrhage secondary to aneurysm rupture. An EEG was performed for vasospasm monitoring.

The background spectrographic pattern is intermediate between *narrowband* and *broadband monotonous*, raising the possibility of periodic discharges, although in this case in fact the background showed generalized high amplitude slowing. Interrupting this background pattern intermittently, one can see high-power red stripes that span the entire frequency range. Unlike the above example of disconnection artifact, these stripes are of much shorter duration suggesting very brief high-amplitude, high-frequency artifact such as is generated by movements leading to amplifier saturation or temporary EEG disconnection.

Case 11: (Fig. 4.23)

A 70-year-old man with a history of laryngeal cancer treated with radiation developed a delayed right common carotid artery rupture requiring carotid artery ligation. A cEEG was performed for cerebral perfusion monitoring in

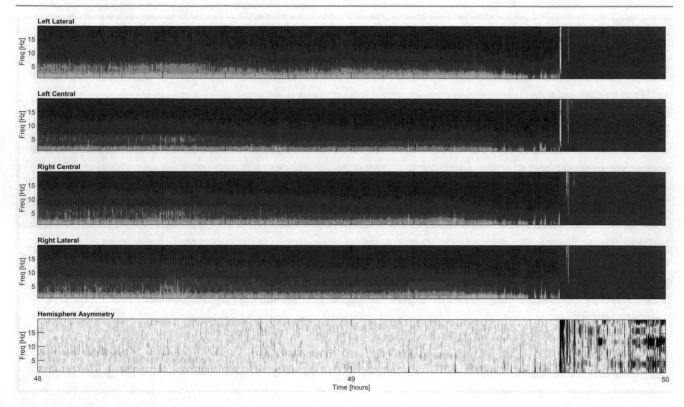

Fig. 4.21 Disconnection artifact (Case 7, continued). Seen as abrupt change in CSA from low power to sudden high-amplitude voltages due to amplifier saturation

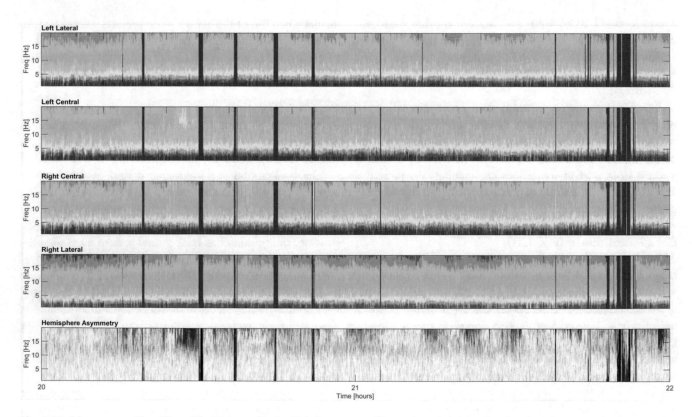

Fig. 4.22 Movement artifact (Case 10). High-amplitude, high-frequency artifacts of much briefer duration than those seen in disconnection artifact

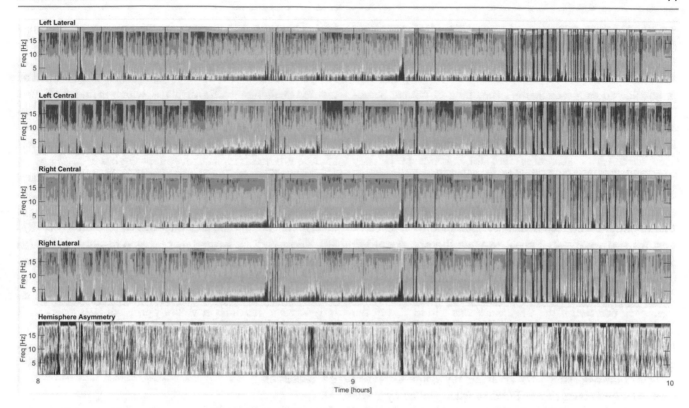

Fig. 4.23 Movement artifact (Case 11). Such artifacts can sometimes be mistaken for *regular flame* seizures

the setting of a drug-induced hypertension trial. There was no deterioration of neurological exam despite carotid ligation and withdrawal of hypertension-inducing medications. His EEG showed right frontotemporal slowing but no epileptiform discharges.

This spectrogram represents another typical example of frequent movement artifacts. One can imagine how the artifacts in the middle of the 2-h epoch might be mistaken for a *regular flame* pattern.

Case 6, continued: (Fig. 4.13)

On reexamination of the spectrogram in Fig. 4.13 from Case 6, in addition to the *narrowband-monotonous* pattern that constitutes the background, we note that there are transient bursts of yellow at higher frequencies. These events are sometimes described as looking like falling rain, rays of sunshine, or stalactites hanging from a cave ceiling. This pattern is typical of myogenic artifact. A similar myogenic artifact event is evident near the beginning of the epoch in Fig. 4.12, in the left lateral, right central, and right lateral regions.

There are many other types of artifacts that can give rise to unusual spectrogram patterns. For example, oscillating beds are characterized by the well-demarcated appearance of a high-power band that corresponds to the frequency at which the bed is oscillating. Electrical artifact at 55 Hz or 60 Hz caused by the numerous devices present in an ICU

occurs at higher frequencies than are routinely displayed on spectrograms. Patient cleaning and repositioning may result in artifact that appears similar to the movement artifacts illustrated above. For patients undergoing active cooling following cardiac arrest, shivering – even minute shivering that is not clearly visible – can result in high-frequency movement and myogenic artifact. Some commercially available quantitative EEG software includes algorithms to identify and reduce artifact or to exclude leads with significant artifact from quantitative analysis and display.

Clinical Utility Of Quantitative EEG and Spectrograms

Determining the validity and utility of qEEG for clinical use is important to the continued use and optimization of these tools for patient care. Multiple studies have evaluated the sensitivity and specificity of various qEEG methods, though the most commonly evaluated has been spectrograms, usually by the terms CSA or DSA in the existing literature.

In a study of qEEG for pediatric ICU EEG data, one group compared the diagnostic accuracy of CSA and amplitude-integrated EEG for seizure identification [21]. For pediatric data, they found that sensitivity was relatively similar for CSA vs. aEEG (83 vs. 81%). However, overall, more seizures were completely missed when using CSA (21%) vs. aEEG (14%). The most commonly missed seizures were those with low-amplitude, short and focal seizures. Other authors have also confirmed that CSA-guided review in many different protocols can support sensitive screening of critical pathological information in cEEG recordings [10, 12, 14, 21–25].

One study focusing on qEEG for interpretation of adult ICU EEG recordings concluded that spectrograms could be used as sensitive screening tool for seizures [11]. They trained two *non*-expert electrophysiology reviewers (neurology residents) to assess CSA signals for the presence or absence of seizures or other clinically important patterns. The reviewers were blinded to the presence or absence of seizures and were not allowed to view the primary cEEG data. An independent experienced electroencephalographer reviewed the raw EEG within 60 s on either side of each mark and recorded any seizures. Seizures were considered to have been detected if the CSA mark was within 60 s of the seizure. The CSA reviewers in this study achieved high seizure detection rates, but the study design deliberately allowed high false-positive rates to do so.

In a follow-up study, by allowing reviewers to review selected segments of raw cEEG data when guided by CSA-based screening (see Fig. 4.1), the authors hypothesized that the time required for review would be significantly less than required for conventional review of the entire raw cEEG without compromising the sensitivity for seizures or other critical pathologies [10]. This method also mirrors the way spectrograms are typically used in actual clinical practice by EEG experts, i.e., as an addition and aid for reviewing the raw EEG. In this study CSA-guided cEEG review identified all patients with seizures and detected 87% of all individual seizures among the cohort. Using this method, they were also able to detect period epileptiform discharges, rhythmic delta activity, focal slowing, and generalized slowing in >95% of patients. Using this method, they found CSA-guided screening identified the vast majority of seizures and other abnormal patterns while cutting review times by nearly 75% and missing only rare, brief, highly localized, nonconvulsive seizures. The authors concluded that the correlation of CSA patterns with the underlying EEG was critical in achieving high sensitivity and efficiency.

Given that one of the major limitations of cEEG is the limited availability of expert neurophysiologists, it would be optimal if qEEG methods could be interpreted by a broader audience. Several groups have explored the possibility of training non-neurophysiologists to utilize qEEG trends for seizure detection. One group evaluated the diagnostic accuracy of electrographic seizure detection by neurophysiologists and non-neurophysiologists using qEEG trend panels. They found that in isolated review of a qEEG panel, there was an overall sensitivity of 84% and specificity of 69% for all reviewer types for the detection of the presence of seizures

[26]. These results were corroborated by other groups that evaluated critical care nurses, residents, and fellows [27]. They found that accuracy was not different between nurses and physicians after a short training program. Amorim et al. favored challenging CSA displays, which included seizures (50%) and periodic discharges (35%), a much higher frequency than commonly seen in patients monitored in a neurological ICU [28]. The false-alarm rate for nurses in this study was twice as high as for epileptologists in cases involving periodic discharges without seizures. The false-alarm rate in CSA displays with periodic discharges was not systematically reported in other studies; however, the number of displays containing seizures was comparable (30–66%) [27–30]. These findings suggest that in cases in which separation of seizures from periodic discharges is challenging, non-expert review of CSA would likely benefit from combined CSA and raw EEG correlation by neurophysiologists, similarly to what was done in Moura's protocol [10].

Quantitative EEG Outside the Realm of Seizures

Quantitative ICU EEG also has clinical applications outside the realm of seizures and status epilepticus, particularly for ischemia detection. Delayed cerebral ischemia (DCI), a major complication that occurs after aneurysmal SAH, can be seen in up to 50% of patients [31, 32]. Currently, transcranial Doppler ultrasonography (TCD) to assess blood flow velocity in the major cerebral arteries is most commonly used, but is operator dependent and done at most once per day. cEEG can potentially provide continuous real-time data for DCI monitoring.

The two features of qEEG that are commonly used to detect ischemia are the alpha-delta ratio and the relative alpha variability [33]. As cerebral blood flow decreases, predominantly slower oscillations are seen in the EEG, and there is a sequential loss of alpha followed by delta frequencies and subsequent suppression [33]. The alpha-delta ratio (ADR) is the ratio of the sum of the power within the alpha band (8–13 Hz) and delta band (1–4 Hz). The ADR is typically displayed as a moving average or histogram. Figure 4.24 shows an example of how a relative drop in alpha frequency power compared to delta frequency power results in a decrease in the ADR. Foreman and Claassen showed changes in the ADR with changes in GCS, neurological exam, and treatment [33]. ADR was found to have a strong association with DCI in a retrospective study that looked at qEEG in 34 high-grade (Hunt and Hess IV and V) SAH patients with high sensitivity (100%) and relatively good specificity (76%) [34]. Relative alpha variability (RAV) is the other commonly used qEEG parameter to detect early ischemia. This method uses the alpha-to-total power ratio (8–12 vs. 1–20 Hz). One

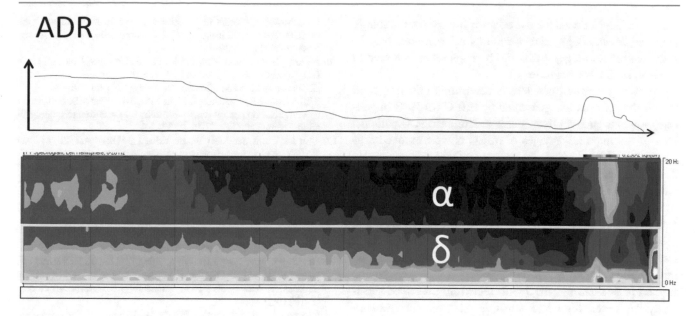

Fig. 4.24 Alpha-delta ratio (ADR). As the alpha power in a spectrogram decreases relative to delta frequency power, there is a decrease in the alpha-delta ratio

study evaluated RAV on a poor to excellent scale of 1–4, respectively [35]. A decrease in RAV by 1 in at least one channel was correlated risk of impending DCI.

Quantitative EEG is also increasingly used to help determine prognosis in post-cardiac arrest patients with anoxic brain injury. The burst suppression ratio, response entropy, state entropy, and wavelet sub-band entropy are some of the qEEG features that have been investigated in patients with anoxic brain injury [36]. The Cerebral Recovery Index (CRI) is a recently introduced prognostic index that combines power, Shannon entropy, alpha-to-delta ratio, "regularity," and coherence in the delta band. An initial pilot study found that higher CRI correlates with better outcomes [37].

Summary

qEEG can be a useful tool to augment evaluation of raw cEEG data in the ICU setting. Properly used, qEEG methods can reduce review time while maintaining adequate sensitivity. qEEG may reduce the burden of raw EEG review by expert encephalographers as well, since studies have shown that at least some qEEG trends can be evaluated by novices with minimal training to identify seizures and other patterns of interest. The increased employment of qEEG could potentially make tele-EEG review more feasible, thereby increasing the availability of EEG data at institutions which would not otherwise have these resources. Most importantly, the use of existing qEEG tools can facilitate real-time monitoring, which is vital to optimizing care of patients in the ICU setting.

There are still limitations with using existing qEEG technology that have proven challenging to overcome thus far. One of the most prominent limitations is that unlike EMU populations, seizures in critically ill patients frequently exhibit patterns of rhythmicity and evolution that are slower and may be harder to identify based on current algorithms [8]. Additionally, because of the variation in patterns seen in ICU patients, it is often difficult to have high expert interrater reliability in review of the raw EEG [38]. Thus, some of the limitations in sensitivities of qEEG methods may be related to this inherent inconsistency. There is also some concern that the false-positive rates for seizure identification are of concern as patients may be exposed to anticonvulsive therapy or anesthetics unnecessarily. Furthermore, some argue that these false-positive identifications may increase the burden of electroencephalographers to review the raw data and communicate misidentified events to the clinical providers. At present, it is still important to avoid using qEEG in isolation. Instead, it is best used as an adjunct to review of the raw EEG.

There are many directions in which qEEG can advance in the near future. A useful first step would be to develop standardized terminology with which to describe the most common physiologic and artifactual spectrogram patterns observed. By cataloging the common patterns and standardizing terminology, studies can better develop and cross-validate the sensitivity and specificity of these qEEG patterns to the raw EEG patterns. It may also help in the development of more uniform training modules for non-electrophysiology expert staff members who become involved in monitoring qEEG data at the bedside. In this chapter, we introduced the use of some informal terminology (*regular flame, choppy flame, broadband monotonous, narrowband monotonous*) that could perhaps serve as a seed to develop such nomenclature.

Another important problem is determining the degree to which the information generated by qEEG (or EEG in general) impacts intervention and/or outcome in ICU patients. One of the main advantages of qEEG is the improved efficiency by which data can be reviewed. Does this or can this faster evaluation impact real-time clinical decision making? Are patients being clinically reexamined or scanned or receiving increased interventions based upon the information conveyed, and if so, does this lead to net benefit? A related topic is whether such efficiency can be improved by training a wider variety of staff members. The studies discussed above have shown that non-expert reviewers can be trained in evaluating qEEG with relatively preserved sensitivity. However, high false-positive rates remain problematic. Would this lead to overtreatment in certain cases? Alternatively, would the burden of cross-checking by neurophysiologists outweigh any benefit of training non-expert readers? Improved training programs for using qEEG technology will likely improve the clinical utility of qEEG, as will the development of a well-calibrated standardized terminology.

These issues are vital to the future of qEEG since these methods are meant to improve the delivery of care and hopefully patient outcomes. There has already been an exponential growth of interest in qEEG. This will likely continue as the field strives to improve qEEG algorithms and increase its integration into the real-time assessment of ICU patients.

References

1. Claassen J, Mayer SA, Kowalski RG, Emerson RG, Hirsch LJ. Detection of electrographic seizures with continuous EEG monitoring in critically ill patients. Neurology. 2004;62:1743–8.
2. Towne AR, Waterhouse EJ, Boggs JG, Garnett LK, Brown AJ, Smith JR, RJ DL. Prevalence of nonconvulsive status epilepticus in comatose patients. Neurology. 2000;54:340.
3. Claassen J, Vespa P. Electrophysiologic monitoring in acute brain injury. Neurocrit Care. 2014;21(Suppl. 2):S129–47.
4. Bassin S, Smith TL, Bleck TP. Clinical review: status epilepticus. Crit Care. 2002;6:137–42.
5. Niligan A, Shorvon S. Frequency and prognosis of convulsive status epilepticus of different causes: a systematic review. Arch Neurol. 2010;67:931–40.
6. Powers L, Shepard KM, Craft K. Payment reform and the changing landscape in medical practice: implications for neurologists. Neurol Clin Pract. 2012;2:224–30.
7. Sinha SR. Quantitative EEG basic principles. In: Handbook of ICU EEG monitoring; 2013. Demos Medical Publishing. New York, NY. p. 221–8.
8. Scheuer ML, Wilson SB. Data analysis for continuous eeg monitoring in the ICU: seeing the forest and the trees. J Clin Neurophysiol. 2004;21:353–78.
9. Laroche SM. Quantitative EEG for seizure detection. In:Handbook of ICU EEG monitoring. In; 2013. Demos Medical Publishing. New York, NY. p. 229–38.
10. Moura LMVR, Shafi MM, Ng M, Pati S, Cash SS, Cole AJ, Hoch DB, Rosenthal ES, Westover MB. Spectrogram screening of adult EEGs is sensitive and efficient. Neurology. 2014;83:56–64.
11. Williamson CA, Wahlster S, Shafi MM, Westover MB. Sensitivity of compressed spectral arrays for detecting seizures in acutely ill adults. Neurocrit Care. 2014;20:32–9.
12. Toet MC, van der Meij W, de Vries LS, Uiterwaal CSPM, van Huffelen KC. Comparison between simultaneously recorded amplitude integrated electroencephalogram (cerebral function monitor) and standard electroencephalogram in neonates. Pediatrics. 2002;109:772–9.
13. Prior PF, Virden RS, Maynard DE. An EEG device for monitoring seizure discharges. Epilepsia. 1973;14:367–72.
14. Abend NS, Dlugos D, Herman S. Neonatal seizure detection using multichannel display of envelope trend. Epilepsia. 2008;49:349–52.
15. Brandon Westover M, Shafi MM, Ching S, Chemali JJ, Purdon PL, Cash SS, Brown EN. Real-time segmentation of burst suppression patterns in critical care EEG monitoring. J Neurosci Methods. 2013;219:131–41.
16. Chemali J, Ching S, Purdon PL, Solt K, Brown EN. Burst suppression probability algorithms: state-space methods for tracking EEG burst suppression. J Neural Eng. 2013;10:056017.
17. Herta J, Koren J, Fürbass F, Hartmann M, Kluge T, Baumgartner C, Gruber A. Prospective assessment and validation of rhythmic and periodic pattern detection in NeuroTrend: a new approach for screening continuous EEG in the intensive care unit. Epilepsy Behav. 2015;49:273–9.
18. Thomson DJ. Spectrum estimation and harmonic analysis. Proc IEEE. 1982;70:1055–96.
19. Bokil H, Purpura K, Schoffelen JM, Thomson D, Mitra P. Comparing spectra and coherences for groups of unequal size. J Neurosci Methods. 2007;159:337–45.
20. Bokil H, Andrews P, Kulkarni JE, Mehta S, Mitra PP. Chronux: a platform for analyzing neural signals. J Neurosci Methods. 2010;192:146–51.
21. Stewart CP, Otsubo H, Ochi A, Sharma R, Hutchison JS, Hahn CD. Seizure identification in the ICU using quantitative EEG displays. Neurology. 2010;75:1501–8.
22. Shah DK, Mackay MT, Lavery S, Watson S, Harvey AS, Zempel J, Mathur A, Inder TE. Accuracy of bedside electroencephalographic monitoring in comparison with simultaneous continuous conventional electroencephalography for seizure detection in term infants. Pediatrics. 2008;121:1146–54.
23. Shellhaas RA, Soaita AI, Clancy RR. Sensitivity of amplitude-integrated electroencephalography for neonatal seizure detection. Pediatrics. 2007;120:770–7.
24. Rennie JM, Chorley G, Boylan GB, Presslet P, Nguyen Y, Hooper R. Non-expert use of the cerebral function motinor for neonatal seizure detection. Arch Dis Child Fetal Neonatal. 2004;89:37–41.
25. Bourez-Swart MD, van Rooij L, Rizzo C, de Vries LS, Toet MC, Gebbink TA, AGJ E, van Huffelen AC. Detection of subclinical electroencephalographic seizure patterns with multichannel amplitude-integrated EEG in full-term neonates. Clin Neurophysiol. 2009;120:1916–22.
26. Swisher CB, Shah D, Sinha SR, Husain AM. Baseline EEG Pattern on continuous ICU EEG monitoring and incidence of seizures. J Clin Neurophysiol. 2015;32:147–51.
27. Dericioglu N, Yetim E, Bas DF, Bilgen N, Caglar G, Arsava EM, Topcuoglu MA. Non-expert use of quantitative EEG displays for seizure identification in the adult neuro-intensive care unit. Epilepsy Res. 2015;109:48–56.
28. Amorim E, Williamson CA, Moura LMVR, Shafi MM, Gaspard N, Rosenthal ES, Guanci MM, Rajajee V, Westover MB. Performance

of spectrogram-based seizure identification of adult EEGs by critical care nurses and neurophysiologists. J Clin Neurophysiol. 2016:1. doi:10.1097/wnp.0000000000000368.

29. Topjian AA, Fry M, Jawad AF, Herman ST, Nadkarni VM, Ichord R, Berg RA, Dlugos DJ, Abend NS. Detection of electrographic seizures by critical care providers using color density spectral array after cardiac arrest is feasible. Pediatr Crit Care Med. 2015;16: 461–7.

30. Swisher CB, White CR, Mace BE, Dombrowski KE, Husain AM, Kolls BJ, Radtke RR, Tran TT, Sinha SR. Diagnostic accuracy of electrographic seizure detection by neurophysiologists and non-neurophysiologists in the adult ICU using a panel of quantitative EEG trends. J Clin Neurophysiol. 2015;32:324–30.

31. Claassen J, Bernardini GL, Kreiter K, Bates J, Du YE, Copeland D, Connolly ES, Mayer SA. Effect of cisternal and ventricular blood on risk of delayed cerebral ischemia after subarachnoid hemorrhage: the Fisher scale revisited. Stroke. 2001;32: 2012–20.

32. Roos YB, de Haan RJ, Beenen LF, Groen RJ, Albrecht KW, Vermeulen M. Complications and outcome in patients with aneurysmal subarachnoid haemorrhage: a prospective hospital based cohort study in The Netherlands. J Neurol Neurosurg Psychiatry. 2000;68:337–41.

33. Foreman B, Claassen J. Quantitative EEG for the detection of brain ischemia. Crit Care. 2012;16:216.

34. Claassen J, Hirsch LJ, Kreiter KT, Du EY, Connolly ES, Emerson RG, Mayer SA. Quantitative continuous EEG for detecting delayed cerebral ischemia in patients with poor-grade subarachnoid hemorrhage. Clin Neurophysiol. 2004;115:2699–710.

35. Vespa PM, Nuwer MR, Juhász C, Alexander M, Nenov V, Martin N, Becker DP. Early detection of vasospasm after acute subarachnoid hemorrhage using continuous EEG ICU monitoring. Electroencephalogr Clin Neurophysiol. 1997;103:607–15.

36. Wennervirta JE, Ermes MJ, Tiainen SM, et al. Hypothermia-treated cardiac arrest patients with good neurological outcome differ early in quantitative variables of EEG suppression and epileptiform activity. Crit Care Med. 2009;37:2427–35.

37. Tjepkema-Cloostermans MC, van Meulen FB, Meinsma G, van Putten MJAM. A Cerebral Recovery Index (CRI) for early prognosis in patients after cardiac arrest. Crit Care. 2013;17:R252.

38. Jirsch J. Computer-assisted interpretation of EEG for the ICU: monitoring made palatable. Clin Neurophysiol. 2011;122:1901–3.

Spreading Depolarizations and Seizures in Clinical Subdural Electrocorticographic Recordings

Gajanan S. Revankar, Maren K.L. Winkler, Sebastian Major, Karl Schoknecht, Uwe Heinemann, Johannes Woitzik, Jan Claassen, Jed A. Hartings, and Jens P. Dreier

Introduction

Spreading depolarization (SD) is the generic term for pathologic events of abrupt, near-complete breakdown of the neuronal intra-/extracellular ion gradients associated with sustained near-complete depolarization [1, 2]. It is observed as a large negative direct current (DC) shift in subdural and intracortical electrocorticographic (ECoG) recordings (DC frequency range, <0.05 Hz) (Fig. 5.1a) [3]. SD typically propagates as a wave in the brain's gray matter with a velocity of 2–9 mm/min [4] and induces spreading depression of spontaneous activity [5]. SD originates in neurons [6, 7], while astrocytes support the recovery of the neuronal ion gradients and protect from SD [8, 9]. Also astrocytes show marked depolarization during SD [10]. The astrocytic depolarization is presumably produced passively by the decline in the potassium transmembrane gradient following the rise in extracellular potassium concentration. The depolarization implicates a flux of negatively charged chloride ions into the astrocyte. Because of the chloride influx, the membrane potential remains more negative than the new potassium equilibrium potential, and this attracts potassium to follow chloride into the astrocyte.

The other important pathological network event in the brain is epileptiform activity (Fig. 5.1b). The so-called paroxysmal depolarization shift (PDS) characterizes interictal or preictal epileptiform activity on the cellular level. This is a synchronous event resulting from a giant excitatory postsynaptic potential that usually lasts for 80–200 ms [11]. The giant excitatory postsynaptic potential seems to be the consequence of a synchronous activation of recurrent excitatory paths. In ECoG and scalp electroencephalography (EEG)

G.S. Revankar • M.K.L. Winkler
Center for Stroke Research Berlin, Charité University Medicine Berlin, Berlin 10117, Germany
e-mail: gajanan.revankar@charite.de; maren.winkler@charite.de

S. Major • J.P. Dreier (✉)
Center for Stroke Research Berlin, Charité University Medicine Berlin, Charitéplatz 1, Berlin 10117, Germany

Department of Neurology, Charité University Medicine Berlin, Charitéplatz 1, Berlin 10117, Germany

Department of Experimental Neurology, Charité University Medicine Berlin, Charitéplatz 1, Berlin 10117, Germany
e-mail: sebastian.major@charite.de; jens.dreier@charite.de

K. Schoknecht
Center for Stroke Research Berlin, Charité University Medicine Berlin, Berlin 10117, Germany

Department of Neurology, Charité University Medicine Berlin, Charitéplatz 1, Berlin 10117, Germany

Department of Neurology, Charité University Medicine Berlin, Berlin 10117, Germany

Neuroscience Research Center, Charité University Medicine Berlin, Charitéplatz 1, Berlin 10117, Germany
e-mail: karl.schoknecht@charite.de

U. Heinemann
Neuroscience Research Center, Charité University Medicine Berlin, Charitéplatz 1, Berlin 10117, Germany
e-mail: uwe.heinemann@charite.de

J. Woitzik
Department of Neurosurgery, Charité University Medicine Berlin, Berlin 12200, Germany
e-mail: johannes.woitzik@charite.de

J. Claassen
Neurocritical Care, Columbia University College of Physicians and Surgeons, New York, NY 10032, USA

Division of Critical Care and Hospitalists Neurology, Department of Neurology, Columbia

University Medical center, New York Presbyterian Hospital, New York, NY, USA
e-mail: jc1439@columbia.edu

J.A. Hartings
Department of Neurosurgery, University of Cincinnati College of Medicine, Cincinnati, OH 45267, USA

Mayfield Clinic, Cincinnati, OH 45209, USA
e-mail: jed.hartings@uc.edu

© Springer International Publishing AG 2017
P.N. Varelas, J. Claassen (eds.), *Seizures in Critical Care*, Current Clinical Neurology, DOI 10.1007/978-3-319-49557-6_5

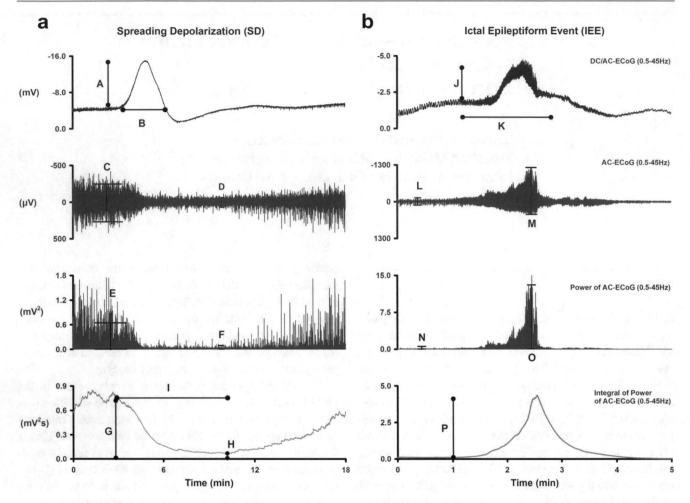

Fig. 5.1 SD and IEE. (**a**) SD is observed as a large negative DC shift (first trace, full-band recording between 0 and 45 Hz). (*A*) shows the amplitude and (*B*) the duration of the negative DC shift. SD is associated with spreading depression of spontaneous activity (second trace, frequency range from 0.5 to 45 Hz; third trace, power of the spontaneous activity; fourth trace, integral of the power of the spontaneous activity). (*C*) gives the mean amplitude of the spontaneous activity before and (*D*) during SD. Note the amplitude reduction (= silencing = depres-

sion) during SD. Analogously, (*E*)–(*H*) display the amplitudes of the power and integral of the power of spontaneous activity before and during SD. Note the decreases. Depression durations of SD were scored beginning at the initial decrease in the integral of the power of the AC-ECoG and ending at the start of the recovery phase (*I*). (**b**) The IEE is analyzed accordingly (*J*–*P*). Note that the IEE shows a smaller DC shift than the SD, and the amplitudes of spontaneous activity, power, and integral of the power increase during IEE in contrast to SD

traces, its extracellular correlate is the interictal or preictal spike [12]. Ictal epileptiform events (IEEs) result from longer cellular depolarizations, which seem to be the consequence of melting PDS [13]. Clinical correlates of IEE are convulsive and nonconvulsive epileptic seizures.

From a thermodynamic perspective, IEE and SD represent two different levels of free energy between the physiological state of neurons and dead tissue. This concept has been based on the free energy contained in the electrochemical gradients across the neuronal membranes [10]. These gradients reach robust, characteristic ceiling levels during IEE and SD [14–18]. Table 5.1 shows the typical stepwise changes of electrical, sodium, calcium, and potassium transmembrane gradients in animals from the physiological state to IEE to SD. According to these changes, IEE is closer to the physiological state, while SD is closer to dead tissue. In fact, SD is the largest known disruption of viable cerebral gray matter. Nonetheless, cortical tissue spontaneously recovers from SD except under condi-

tions of severe pathology or energy deprivation when long-lasting depolarization can lead to cell death or infarction.

Among the many variables reflecting this thermodynamic hierarchy, the negative DC shift is the one most readily measurable in humans. Here, we performed a direct comparison between DC amplitudes of IEE and SD in the human brain for the first time. The changes were similar to those previously observed in other mammals.

Methods

General

We describe four consecutive patients with aneurysmal subarachnoid hemorrhage (aSAH) who showed both IEE and SD on subdural ECoG monitoring during intensive care. The patients were prospectively enrolled at two participating

Table 5.1 Comparison between physiological state, IEE, and SD based on animal experiments [75]

Variable	Physiology	IEE	SD
Sustained negative neuronal membrane potential (mV)	60–70	40–45	1–17
Negative intracortical extracellular DC shift (mV)	–	1–4	5–30
Size of extracellular space (%)	18–22	14	5–9
Intra-/extracellular sodium concentration (mM)	10/146–154	16/135–143	35/57–59
Intra-/extracellular calcium concentration (μM)	0.06/1200–1300	0.13/800–1000	25/80
Intra-/extracellular potassium concentration (mM)	134/2.3–3.1	126/10–12	106/35–60
Free energy content in the electrochemical gradients across the cellular membranes of neurons (J/l) (10)	21.9–24.4	19.1–21.6	2.4–2.5

centers of the Co-Operative Study on Brain Injury Depolarizations (COSBID), Campus Benjamin Franklin, and Campus Virchow-Klinikum (Charité University Medicine Berlin, Berlin, Germany). Inclusion criteria were (1) age ≥ 18 years, (2) World Federation of Neurosurgical Societies (WFNS) grades I–V, (3) ruptured saccular aneurysm proven by computed tomography (CT) angiography (CTA) or digital subtraction angiography, and (4) either surgical treatment of the aneurysm via craniotomy or, in coiled patients, burr hole trepanation for placement of a ventricular drain or oxygen sensor, which allows the simultaneous placement of a subdural electrode strip [19–21]. Exclusion criteria were subarachnoid hemorrhage due to other causes (e.g., trauma, fusiform, or mycotic aneurysm), admission in a clinical state with unfavorable prognosis (e.g., wide, nonreactive pupils for more than 1 h), bleeding diathesis or pregnancy, unavailability of the monitoring equipment, and refusal of the patient or legal representative to participate in the study. The research protocol was approved by the local ethics committee of the Charité University Medicine Berlin. Either informed consent or surrogate informed consent was obtained for all patients. Research was conducted in accordance with the Declaration of Helsinki.

Aneurysmal SAH was diagnosed by assessment of CT scans. Hemorrhage was graded according to the original Fisher scale [22, 23], and clinical presentation on admission according to the WFNS scale. A study neurologist or neurosurgeon performed a neurological and general medical evaluation on admission. Baseline demographic data and clinical signs and symptoms of the initial hemorrhage were recorded. The aneurysm was assessed using four-vessel digital subtraction angiography or a more restricted study when indicated.

After treatment of the aneurysm, all patients were transferred to the neurocritical care unit where the continuous neuromonitoring data were acquired for up to 15 days. Glasgow Coma Score, blood gases, glucose, and electrolytes were documented at least every 6 h. A thorough neurological examination was performed at least daily. Oral nimodipine was given prophylactically. Transcranial Doppler sonography was performed daily as described previously [24]. Delayed ischemic neurological deficit (DIND) was defined as the occurrence of focal neurological impairment (such as hemiparesis, aphasia, apraxia, hemianopia, or neglect) or a decrease of at least two points on the Glasgow Coma Scale (either on the total score or on one of its individual components (eyes, motor on either side, verbal) >72 h after aSAH onset). Moreover, the diagnosis of a DIND required that the neurological deficit not to have been present immediately after aneurysm occlusion lasted for at least 1 h and could not have been attributed to other causes such as hydrocephalus or rebleeding by means of clinical assessment or imaging studies of the brain and appropriate laboratory investigations [24–26]. Whenever necessary, serial CT scans were performed at times of clinical deterioration. Patients were diagnosed to have delayed cerebral ischemia (DCI) when they showed a DIND and/or a neuroimaging-proven delayed ischemic stroke [26]. Patients with DCI were treated with hyperdynamic therapy (hypertension, hypervolemia) [27]. Angioplasty or intra-arterial therapy was not performed. At the conclusion of the monitoring period, the electrode strip was removed at the bedside by gentle traction.

Recording of the Neuromonitoring Data

For the continuous ECoG recordings, a linear, six-contact platinum electrode strip (Wyler, 5 mm diameter; Ad-Tech Medical, Racine, Wisconsin, USA) was placed on cerebral cortex accessible through craniotomy during aneurysm surgery as described previously [20]. Ground was provided by a subdermal platinum needle ipsilateral to the recording strip (Technomed Europe, Maastricht, Netherlands). Full-band ECoG, including both DC and alternating current (AC) components, was recorded in six active channels from the six-contact linear electrode array (interelectrode distance 1 cm) with a subdermal platinum needle serving as reference. Monopolar recordings were acquired with a BrainAmp amplifier (Brain Products GmbH, Munich, Germany) as reported previously [20, 28]. Data were sampled at 200 Hz and recorded, filtered (0–45 Hz), and analyzed with a PowerLab 16/SP analog/digital converter and Chart-7 software (ADInstruments, New South Wales, Australia). Intracranial pressure (ICP) was monitored via ventricular drainage catheter or ICP transducer (Codman or Camino systems). The systemic arterial pressure was continuously recorded via a catheter in the radial artery. Mean arterial pressure (MAP) and cerebral perfusion pressure (CPP) were calculated according to standard practice.

Analysis of Neuromonitoring Data

In accordance with the analytical framework and characteristics described previously [24, 29, 30], SD was observed in the DC-ECoG (bandpass, 0–0.05 Hz) as the consecutive onset of a large negative DC shift in neighboring ECoG channels.

In contrast to DC changes that define the phenomenon of SD, spontaneous and evoked electrical activity of the brain is observed in the AC range of the ECoG above ~0.5 Hz. In electrically active tissue, SD typically causes spreading depression of spontaneous activity. This is observed in neighboring ECoG channels as a rapidly developing reduction in amplitude, power, and integral of the power of the AC-ECoG activity (bandpass, 0.5–45 Hz) as shown in Fig. 5.1a [31].

Depression durations of SD were scored beginning at the initial decrease in the integral (60 s decay time constant) of the power of the AC-ECoG and ending at the start of the recovery phase as described previously and shown in Fig. 5.1a [31].

IEEs were defined as any spikes, sharp waves, or sharp-and-slow-wave complexes lasting for 10 s or more at either a frequency of at least 3/s or a frequency of at least 1/s with clear evolution in frequency, morphology, or recording sites of the electrode strip. IEE are typically associated with an increase in the AC-ECoG power and integral of the power [24, 32, 33] and were analyzed as shown in Fig. 5.1b.

Statistics

First, the median of each variable was calculated within a given patient. Based on this, median, first, and third quartile of each variable was then calculated for the four patients. All SDs or, respectively, all IEEs within one patient were in other words treated as dependent. $P \le 0.05$ was accepted as statistically significant. Further details of the statistical analysis are given in the "Results" section.

Results

Case Reports

All patients had both aSAH and a large intracerebral hematoma. The clinical variables are summarized in Table 5.2.

Patient 1 showed a DIND characterized by altered consciousness, diplopia, left facial palsy, and left arm paresis. She was treated with hyperdynamic therapy. In addition, lorazepam was given during this time period because she reported anxiety and agitation. No clinical seizures were observed. She slowly improved after day 10 without evidence of a delayed infarct on follow-up neuroimaging.

Patient 2 showed neither DIND nor delayed infarct. However, early in the course, he developed hydrocephalus, which was initially treated with extraventricular drainage. Later on, a ventriculoperitoneal shunt was established. Chest x-ray was significant for pneumonia on day 4. Pneumonia and a urinary tract infection were treated with antibiotics. On day 12, the nurses noted spells associated with breath-holding that were interpreted as epileptic seizures, since the ECoG showed IEE. The patient was treated with levetiracetam. After discharge, he developed posthemorrhagic epilepsy.

Patient 3 had a history of migraine with olfactory auras for over 20 years. During the monitoring phase, she had two typical migraine attacks, but developed neither DIND nor delayed infarct. There was no clinical evidence of epileptic seizures. She did not receive any anticonvulsant medication.

Patient 4 had neither DIND nor delayed infarct nor clinical seizures. Pulmonary function was severely compromised, and the patient progressively developed a severe hepatorenal syndrome. She died on day 12.

Comparison Between SD and IEE

A total of 215 SDs and 371 IEEs were observed and analyzed during a total ECoG recording time of 771.8 h in these four patients. Figures 5.2–5.5 display the typical electrophysiological signatures and Fig. 5.6 the time courses of SD and IEE for each patient including the time points of treatment with anticonvulsant drugs. The electrophysiological variables are summarized in Table 5.2.

The median amplitude of the negative DC shift of SD was 14 times larger than that of IEE (8.4 (6.2, 10.9) mV (first quartile, third quartile) versus 0.6 (0.2, 0.9) mV, $P = 0.029$, $n = 4$ patients, Mann-Whitney Rank Sum Test). The median duration of the negative DC shift of SD was 153 (136, 169) s ($n = 4$ patients), and the median monopolar depression duration of SD was 503 (475, 505) s ($n = 4$ patients). The depression duration always exceeded the duration of the negative DC shift. During spreading depressions, the power fell from 100 to 35 (16, 57) % and the integral of power from 100 to 26 (16, 39) % ($n = 4$ patients). The median duration of IEE was 158 (99, 243) s ($n = 4$ patients). During IEE, the power increased from 100 to 395 (242, 817) % and the integral of power from 100 to 318 (194, 679) % ($n = 4$ patients). Overall,

Table 5.2 Cases and electrophysiological variables

	Patient 1	Patient 2	Patient 3	Patient 4
Age	48	71	42	78
Sex	F	M	F	F
History of epilepsy	No	No	No	No
Location of aneurysm	MCA	ACoA	MCA	ACoA
WFNS grade	1	5	4	4
Fisher grade	3	4	3	3
ICH (largest $\emptyset$, cm)	5	6	3.5	5
Surgical intervention	Clip ligation	Clip ligation	Clip ligation	Clip ligation
Total recording time of monopolar DC/AC recordings (h)	138.6	226.8	195.6	210.8
Number of SDs in the monopolar DC/AC recordings	58	114	28	15
Median amplitude of the negative DC shift of SD (mV) (n = local measurements)	6.3 (4.8, 7.6) (n = 158)	5.7 (3.9, 8.0) (n = 261)	11.9 (8.2, 3.5) (n = 90)	10.5 (7.6, 12.7) (n = 30)
Median duration of the negative DC shift of SD, minimum and maximum duration (s)	146 (116, 179) 52–418	159 (129, 111) 59–359	198 (157, 215) 108–361	104 (93, 123) 67–154
Median monopolar depression duration in the integral of power (s)	505 (345, 675)	501 (251, 909)	505 (332, 720)	397 (321, 611)
Depression of AC-ECoG power during SD in percent of baseline (=100%)	11 (6, 22)	70 (35, 87)	18 (10, 29)	52 (31, 81)
Depression of the AC-ECoG integral of power during SD in percent of baseline (=100%)	11 (4, 20)	58 (37, 75)	18 (9, 31)	33 (24, 37)
Recording sites involved in SD	Up to 4	Up to 3	Up to 4	Up to 3
Median of mean MAP during SD (mmHg)	98 (93, 105)	97 (92, 101)	95 (88, 104)	81 (78, 86)
Median of mean ICP during SD (mmHg)	1 (1, 1)	15 (11, 18)	12 (8, 16)	11 (8, 15)
Median of mean CPP during SD (mmHg)	98 (92, 104)	82 (76, 87)	80 (75, 93)	71 (65, 74)
Number of IEEs in the monopolar DC/AC recordings	15	34	127	195
Median amplitude of the negative DC shift of IEE (mV) (n = local measurements)	0.2 (0.0, 1.0) (n = 30)	1.0 (0.5, 1.6) (n = 71)	0.9 (0.6, 1.2) (n = 219)	0.0 (0.0, 0.3) (n = 319)
Median duration of IEE (s)	201 (94, 278)	367 (241, 434)	55 (34, 82)	114 (77, 153)
Increase of AC-ECoG power during IEE in percent of baseline (=100%)	204 (166, 272)	1659 (727, 2865)	254 (169, 359)	536 (377, 834)
Increase of the AC-ECoG integral of power during IEE in percent of baseline (=100%)	203 (169, 231)	1418 (627, 2197)	165 (140, 223)	433 (292, 688)
Recording sites involved in IEE	Up to 2	Up to 4	Up to 3	Up to 2
Median of mean MAP during SD (mmHg)	100 (98, 104)	99 (94, 104)	92 (89, 96)	80 (78, 86)
Median of mean ICP during SD (mmHg)	1 (0, 1)	15 (12, 19)	17 (14, 19)	13 (9, 15)
Median of mean CPP during SD (mmHg)	100 (97, 103)	84 (76, 88)	75 (72, 79)	68 (64, 74)

ACoA anterior communicating artery, *MCA* middle cerebral artery
The numbers in parentheses represent the first and third quartiles

the analysis of percent changes in the integral of power was less robust (more artifact laden) than the analysis of percent changes in the power (SD, 370 versus 494 successful measurements at different electrodes; IEE, 624 versus 634). In the pooled analysis of all SD and IEE, linear regression found that the changes in power and integral of power significantly correlated with each other during both SD and IEE (SD, adjusted R^2 = 0.613, P < 0.001, n = 349 local measurements; IEE, adjusted R^2 = 0.470, P < 0.001, n = 622 local measurements). No significant differences in mean MAP, mean ICP, or mean CPP were found between SD and IEE (n = 4 patients) (Table 5.2).

Discussion

Comparison of IEE and SD

On the surface of the human brain, we observed that the median amplitude of the negative DC shift was 14 times larger during SD than during IEE. This corresponds well to recordings in animals in vivo and in brain slices [2, 34–36]. Full-band recordings using platinum electrodes were already performed previously to measure the large DC shift of SD on the surface of the human brain [20, 28–30, 37], and the

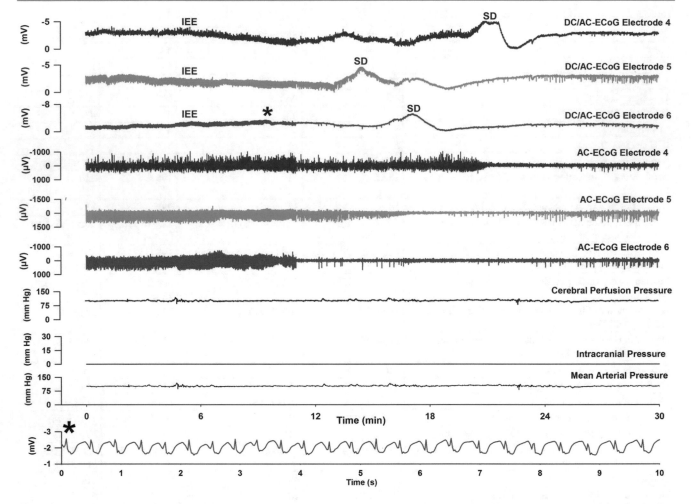

Fig. 5.2 Example traces of SD and IEE in patient 1. IEE with 3/s spike-wave activity followed by SD. The star in the third trace marks the time period which is shown in the lowest trace at higher temporal resolution

results presented here were similar. However, such recordings have not yet been performed in patients during IEE to our knowledge. Gross and colleagues used an amplifier with a high-pass filter of 0.01 Hz and stainless steel subdural electrodes [38], which are characterized by worse low-frequency recording properties than platinum electrodes [39]. These authors did not observe low-frequency shifts with most IEEs. Ikeda and colleagues used platinum electrodes similar to us and found low-frequency shifts with most IEEs, but the amplifier was yet equipped with a high-pass filter in contrast to the present study [40]. Such a filter distorts the DC signal and causes an artificial reduction in amplitude [41].

In general, noise and movement artifacts limited the interpretation of SD and IEE in a similar fashion in the present study. However, our results suggest that it should be easier for neurophysiologists and neurointensivists to learn the assessment of SD than the assessment of IEE, given the size and the duration of the events and the more restricted number of SD versus IEE variants. Admittedly, this may sound

paradoxical in view of the previous difficulties to record SD and the resulting debates of the past whether or not SD occurs in the human brain at all [42].

The difference in DC shift amplitudes between SD and IEE reported here roughly reflects the differences in ionic concentration changes and free energy between these two types of pathological network events (Table 5.1). However, there are not only quantitative but also qualitative differences in the generation of DC shifts between IEE and SD. Accordingly, SD was associated in hippocampal slices with a very large current sink located in the layer of apical dendrites, maximal among the proximal segment of dendrites, to which the cell body layer served as a source [43]. By contrast, a sink limited to the cell body layer was observed throughout the duration of IEE. It is assumed that the DC shift of IEE reflects, in particular, longitudinal and transmembrane current loops between the glial syncytium and the extracellular space, which are largely driven by the inhomogeneous distribution of the extracellular potassium concentration [44]. Further, somatodendritic neuronal dipoles are

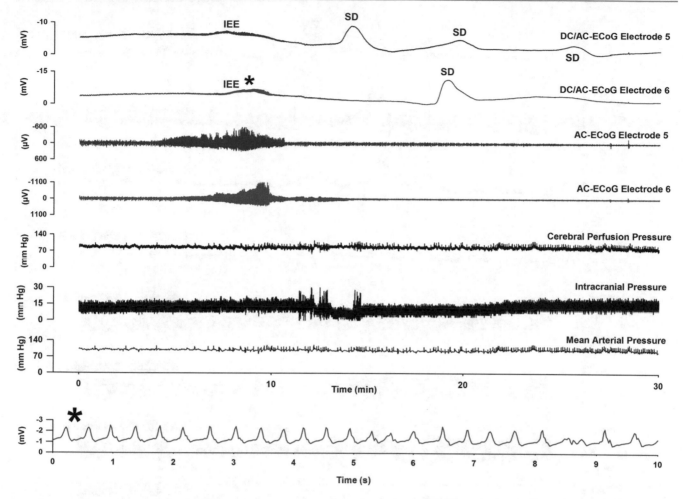

Fig. 5.3 Example traces of SD and IEE in patient 2. IEE with rhythmic 2.5/s delta activity followed by SD. The star in the second trace marks the time period which is shown in the lowest trace at higher temporal resolution

involved due to transmitter-dependent and excitation-dependent depolarization [45]. During SD, regional depolarization in single neurons seems to be the predominant factor. Following the core conductor theory, the regional depolarization establishes longitudinal gradients of neuronal depolarization and transmembrane current loops that sum up in the extracellular space to build the negative DC shift of SD [46]. This is possible because pyramidal cells are tightly arranged in parallel, thus optimizing the extracellular addition of currents and the spatial matching of single cell to population events with subcellular accuracy.

In addition to neurons and glial cells, the blood-brain barrier (BBB) is another source of DC potentials in the brain. For example, CO_2-dependent DC deflections are generated across the BBB [47, 48]. However, BBB-generated DC deflections show a homogeneous laminar profile throughout cortex and white matter unlike the steep zonal gradients observed in the cortex during IEE or SD [49–51]. Another argument for either no or only a small contribution of the BBB to intracortical DC shifts of IEE or, respectively, SD is

that they are remarkably similar between brain slices, which lack an intact BBB, and the brain in vivo [34, 35, 52].

SD also differs in its binary, all-or-nothing nature from IEE. Thus, SD is always observed as a large negative DC shift; both depolarization and breakdown of ion homeostasis are always near complete; and the depolarization always lasts for at least ~30 s. Depending on the local tissue energy status, the polarization state and ion homeostasis then either recover or not. By contrast, epileptiform activity shows an interictal-ictal continuum between physiology and full-blown IEE. This interictal-ictal continuum has been clinically defined as repetitive generalized or focal spikes, sharp waves, spike-and-wave or sharp-and-slow-wave complexes lasting for 10 s or more with a frequency between 1/s and 3/s without clear evolution in frequency, morphology, or location [32, 33].

The most conspicuous point of contrast between IEE and SD is the opposite nature of the associated changes in spontaneous activity. Spontaneous activity is produced by rapid extracellular field potential changes associated with

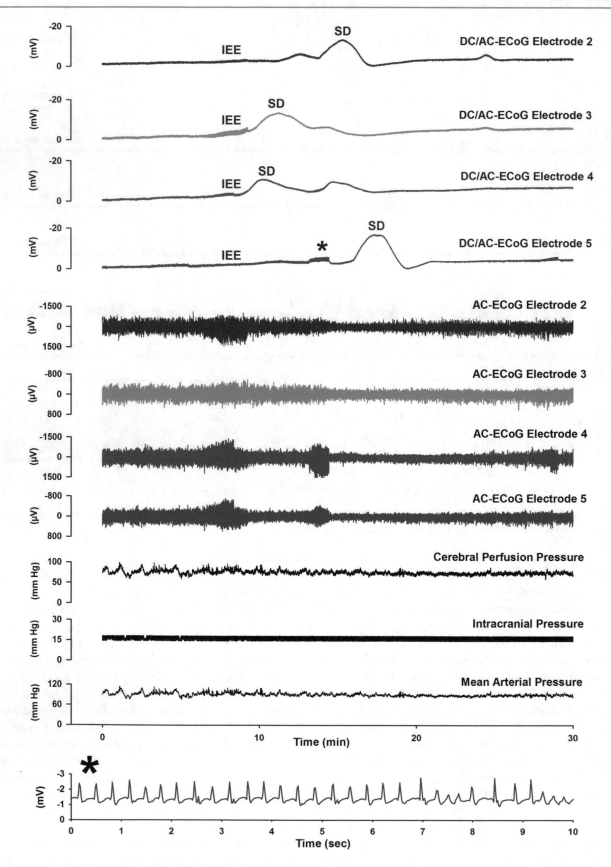

Fig. 5.4 Example traces of SD and IEE in patient 3. IEE with rhythmic 3/s spikes followed by SD. The star in the fourth trace marks the time period which is shown in the lowest trace at higher temporal resolution

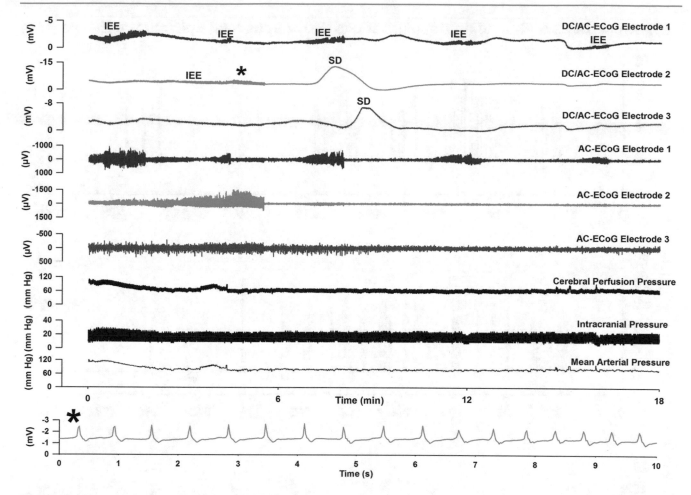

Fig. 5.5 Example traces of SD and IEE in patient 4. IEE with rhythmic 1.7/s spikes followed by SD. The star in the second trace marks the time period which is shown in the lowest trace at higher temporal resolution

postsynaptic potentials in cortical neurons. The summation of these potentials causes measurable changes in the ECoG frequency range above ~0.5 Hz. Notably, the sustained depolarization underlying IEE remains below the inactivation threshold for the action potential-generating channels in distal axons. This allows for continuous, synchronous, highly frequent firing of neurons, superimposed on the moderate sustained depolarization. In contrast to IEE, SD causes depression of spontaneous activity [5]. This is because the sustained depolarization exceeds the inactivation threshold for the action potential-generating channels [53]. However, the depression of activity is longer-lasting than the actual SD process, suggesting that it is maintained by other mechanisms that affect synaptic function such as intracellular zinc, calcium and/or adenosine accumulation, and activation of the electrogenic sodium pump [54–57]. In the AC-ECoG power and integral of the power, these changes of IEE and SD are reflected by large increases and decreases, respectively, in amplitude [24]. The present study demonstrated that for both IEE and SD, the AC-ECoG power and integral of the power are more or less inter-

changeable, but the integral of power was slightly more artifact laden. Nonetheless, visual assessment of the duration of the SD-induced depression period has been more robust using the integral of power [31].

Synergism of IEE and SD

Both IEE and SD co-occur spontaneously in experimental models of acute hyperexcitability such as the low-magnesium [56, 58] or high-potassium models [52, 59] in rodent and human brain slices, models of electrical stimulation in juvenile hippocampal slice cultures [57], or models of GABA$_A$ receptor [60, 61] or sodium pump inhibition [52, 62]. Moreover, SD can be initiated in a susceptible area by a single discharge of an epileptic focus termed spike-triggered SD [63]. Repeated SD may enhance epileptiform activities [64] by selective suppression of GABAergic function [65]. Therefore, it is not surprising that IEE and SD also co-occur in patients with acute cerebral injuries, although SD is more predominant. The estimated incidence of IEE in continuous

DC-Amplitudes of Spreading Depolarizations (SD) versus Ictal Epileptiform Events (IEE)

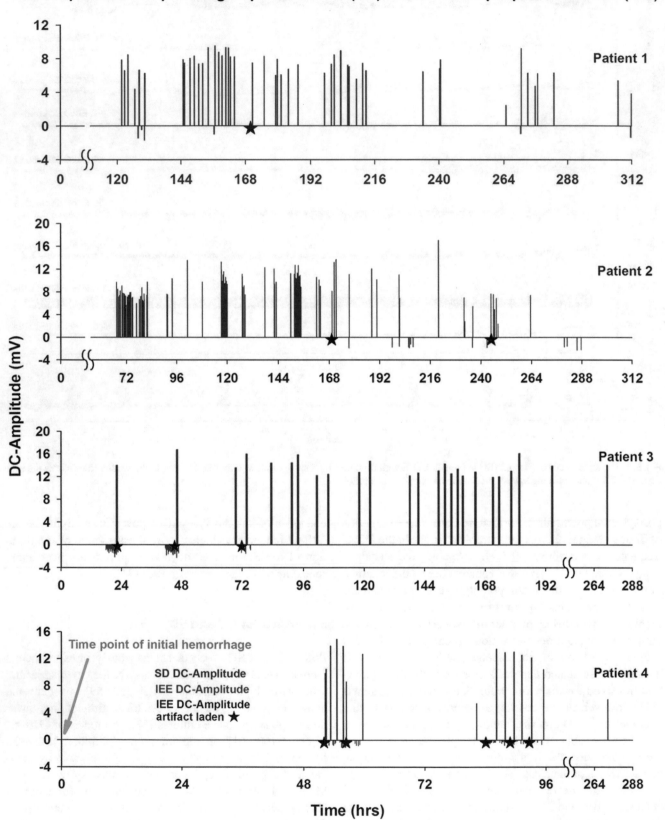

Fig. 5.6 Occurrences of SD and IEE over time in patients 1–4. Note the predominance of SD over IEE in all patients

EEG or ECoG recordings during the first week after the initial insult can be as high as 23% in traumatic brain injury (TBI) [66], 38% in aSAH [24, 33, 67], 31% in intracerebral hemorrhage (ICH) [68], and 27% in ischemic stroke [69]. SD in the acute and subacute period was recorded in about 56% of patients with TBI [70, 71], 60–70% of patients with ICH [72, 73], 70–80% of patients with aSAH [24, 31], and practically 100% of patients with malignant hemispheric stroke (MHS) [4, 74].

Further, there seems to be a clinical overlap between syndromes of epilepsy and migraine aura, one of the clinical manifestations of SD [75]. For all three genes associated with familial hemiplegic migraine, there are carriers of the mutations who also had epilepsy [76–78]. In a large cohort of participants with non-acquired generalized and focal epilepsy, a shared genetic susceptibility to migraine with aura and epilepsy was demonstrated [79]. Moreover, after acute cerebral injury, early SD may be a risk factor for the development of late epilepsy. In a pilot study, the peak SD number early after aSAH was significantly higher in patients who later developed posthemorrhagic epileptic seizures [24]. In the course of epileptogenesis, the propensity to SD may, however, decline, while the propensity to spontaneous IEE increases. The potassium threshold for SD was increased in neocortical slices both from patients who had undergone surgery for intractable epilepsy and from rats that had chronic epilepsy following pilocarpine-induced status epilepticus [35]. By contrast, brain slices from age-matched healthy control rats showed a significantly lower threshold. In a similar fashion, the propensity to SD was reduced following epileptogenesis in the course of BBB disruption and pentylenetetrazol kindling in rats [80, 81]. Speculatively, the decreased propensity to SD in chronically epileptic tissue could result from the decline in neuron density [82] or from upregulation of yet unknown defense mechanisms.

Perspective on Injury and Plasticity

Our findings add another argument that the signal characteristics and fundamental processes of IEE and SD have been highly conserved in the phylogenesis of the central nervous system across lissencephalic and gyrencephalic species, including humans. This conservation could be interpreted in two radically different ways: (1) features pushing the brain toward cutting-edge neural processing, such as denser packaging of neurons and speeding of synaptic transmission, could represent phylogenetic advantages for the healthy individual but may carry the risk of greater network instability that permits IEE and SD under pathological conditions or (2) IEE and SD could have long-term advantages after cerebral injury that outweigh their adverse effects in the short term.

Ample evidence from experimental studies demonstrates, in particular, that SD mediates infarct development in metabolically compromised tissue in the short term through prolonged ionic breakdown and spreading ischemia [75]. Although less well established, IEE might be unfavorable as well [33]. Nonetheless, mid- and long-term effects of IEE and SD could, potentially, be beneficial. Objects of debate include such effects as preconditioning [83–85], immunological modifications [86–88], and promotion of plasticity [89] or regeneration [90, 91]. However, the lack of susceptibility to SD of the neonatal brain may be mentioned as a developmental argument against the notion that SD shows an overall benefit for the injured brain [92]. Indeed, if SD evolved as a process protecting neurons from injury, the brain should be very prone to generate SD during birth since birth is the point in life cycle at which the statistical risk for hypoxia is maximal. By contrast, maximal susceptibility to both IEE and SD is found in childhood when the learning capacity is maximal and the risk of cerebral injury is low [35, 61, 93, 94]. A link between learning, kindling, seizures, and SD was already suggested previously in relationship with N-methyl-D-aspartate (NMDA) receptors because they are crucially involved in all of these phenomena [95, 96] and show characteristic modifications in subunit composition during postnatal development [97, 98]. These opposing hypotheses deserve further study in the context of acute cerebral injury, treatments that target SD and IEE, and adaptive (rehabilitation) and maladaptive (epileptogenesis) long-term plasticity.

Disclosure/Conflict of Interest The authors state that they have no relevant financial or nonfinancial relationships to disclose.

Acknowledgments This is supported by the Bundesministerium für Bildung und Forschung (Center for Stroke Research Berlin, 01 EO 0801; BCCN 01GQ1001C B2) and Era-Net Neuron 01EW1212 to Dr. Dreier, Deutsche Forschungsgemeinschaft (DFG DR 323/5-1) to Dr. Dreier and Dr. Woitzik, NeuroCure SESAH (EXC 257/2) to Dr. Dreier and Dr. Heinemann, and Mayfield Education and Research Foundation to Dr. Hartings.

References

1. Dreier JP. The role of spreading depression, spreading depolarization and spreading ischemia in neurological disease. Nat Med. 2011;17:439–47.
2. Somjen GG. Mechanisms of spreading depression and hypoxic spreading depression-like depolarization. Physiol Rev. 2001;81(3):1065–96.
3. Canals S, Makarova I, Lopez-Aguado L, Largo C, Ibarz JM, Herreras O. Longitudinal depolarization gradients along the somatodendritic axis of CA1 pyramidal cells: a novel feature of spreading depression. J Neurophysiol. 2005;94(2):943–51.

4. Woitzik J, Hecht N, Pinczolits A, Sandow N, Major S, Winkler MK, et al. Propagation of cortical spreading depolarization in the human cortex after malignant stroke. Neurology. 2013;80(12):1095–102.

5. Leão AAP. Spreading depression of activity in the cerebral cortex. J Neurophysiol. 1944;7:359–90.

6. Peters O, Schipke CG, Hashimoto Y, Kettenmann H. Different mechanisms promote astrocyte Ca^{2+} waves and spreading depression in the mouse neocortex. J Neurosci. 2003;23(30):9888–96.

7. Chuquet J, Hollender L, Nimchinsky EA. High-resolution in vivo imaging of the neurovascular unit during spreading depression. J Neurosci. 2007;27(15):4036–44.

8. Largo C, Cuevas P, Somjen GG, Martin del Rio R, Herreras O. The effect of depressing glial function in rat brain in situ on ion homeostasis, synaptic transmission, and neuron survival. J Neurosci. 1996;16(3):1219–29.

9. Largo C, Cuevas P, Herreras O. Is glia disfunction the initial cause of neuronal death in ischemic penumbra? Neurol Res. 1996;18(5):445–8.

10. Dreier JP, Isele T, Reiffurth C, Offenhauser N, Kirov SA, Dahlem MA, et al. Is spreading depolarization characterized by an abrupt, massive release of Gibbs free energy from the human brain cortex? Neuroscientist. 2013;19(1):25–42.

11. Ayala GF, Dichter M, Gumnit RJ, Matsumoto H, Spencer WA. Genesis of epileptic interictal spikes. New knowledge of cortical feedback systems suggests a neurophysiological explanation of brief paroxysms. Brain Res. 1973;52:1–17.

12. Matsumoto H, Marsan CA. Cortical cellular phenomena in experimental epilepsy: interictal manifestations. Exp Neurol. 1964;9:286–304.

13. Matsumoto H, Marsan CA. Cortical cellular phenomena in experimental epilepsy: ictal manifestations. Exp Neurol. 1964;9:305–26.

14. Heinemann U, Lux HD. Ceiling of stimulus induced rises in extracellular potassium concentration in the cerebral cortex of cat. Brain Res. 1977;120(2):231–49.

15. Kraig RP, Nicholson C. Extracellular ionic variations during spreading depression. Neuroscience. 1978;3(11):1045–59.

16. Vyskocil F, Kritz N, Bures J. Potassium-selective microelectrodes used for measuring the extracellular brain potassium during spreading depression and anoxic depolarization in rats. Brain Res. 1972;39(1):255–9.

17. Hansen AJ, Zeuthen T. Extracellular ion concentrations during spreading depression and ischemia in the rat brain cortex. Acta Physiol Scand. 1981;113(4):437–45.

18. Windmuller O, Lindauer U, Foddis M, Einhaupl KM, Dirnagl U, Heinemann U, et al. Ion changes in spreading ischaemia induce rat middle cerebral artery constriction in the absence of NO. Brain. 2005;128(Pt. 9):2042–51.

19. Eross L, Bago AG, Entz L, Fabo D, Halasz P, Balogh A, et al. Neuronavigation and fluoroscopy-assisted subdural strip electrode positioning: a simple method to increase intraoperative accuracy of strip localization in epilepsy surgery. J Neurosurg. 2009;110(2):327–31.

20. Dreier JP, Major S, Manning A, Woitzik J, Drenckhahn C, Steinbrink J, et al. Cortical spreading ischaemia is a novel process involved in ischaemic damage in patients with aneurysmal subarachnoid haemorrhage. Brain. 2009;132(Pt. 7):1866–81.

21. Bruce DA, Bizzi JW. Surgical technique for the insertion of grids and strips for invasive monitoring in children with intractable epilepsy. Childs Nerv Syst. 2000;16(10–11):724–30.

22. Fisher CM, Kistler JP, Davis JM. Relation of cerebral vasospasm to subarachnoid hemorrhage visualized by computerized tomographic scanning. Neurosurgery. 1980;6(1):1–9.

23. Bretz JS, von Dincklage F, Woitzik J, Winkler MKL, Major S, Dreier JP, et al. The Hijdra scale has a significant prognostic value for the functional outcome of Fisher grade 3 patients with subarachnoid hemorrhage. Clin Neuroradiol. 2016. doi:10.1007/s00062-016-0509-0.

24. Dreier JP, Major S, Pannek HW, Woitzik J, Scheel M, Wiesenthal D, et al. Spreading convulsions, spreading depolarization and epileptogenesis in human cerebral cortex. Brain. 2012;135(Pt. 1):259–75.

25. Drenckhahn C, Brabetz C, Major S, Wiesenthal D, Woitzik J, Dreier JP. Criteria for the diagnosis of noninfectious and infectious complications after aneurysmal subarachnoid hemorrhage in DISCHARGE-1. Acta Neurochir Suppl. 2013;115:153–9.

26. Vergouwen MD, Vermeulen M, van Gijn J, Rinkel GJ, Wijdicks EF, Muizelaar JP, et al. Definition of delayed cerebral ischemia after aneurysmal subarachnoid hemorrhage as an outcome event in clinical trials and observational studies: proposal of a multidisciplinary research group. Stroke. 2010;41(10):2391–5.

27. van Gijn J, Rinkel GJ. Subarachnoid haemorrhage: diagnosis, causes and management. Brain. 2001;124(Pt. 2):249–78.

28. Oliveira-Ferreira AI, Milakara D, Alam M, Jorks D, Major S, Hartings JA, et al. Experimental and preliminary clinical evidence of an ischemic zone with prolonged negative DC shifts surrounded by a normally perfused tissue belt with persistent electrocorticographic depression. J Cereb Blood Flow Metab. 2010;30:1504–19.

29. Hartings JA, Watanabe T, Bullock MR, Okonkwo DO, Fabricius M, Woitzik J, et al. Spreading depolarizations have prolonged direct current shifts and are associated with poor outcome in brain trauma. Brain. 2011;134:1529–40.

30. Drenckhahn C, Winkler MKL, Major S, Scheel M, Kang EJ, Pinczolits A, et al. Correlates of spreading depolarizations in human scalp electroencephalography. Brain. 2012;135:853–68.

31. Dreier JP, Woitzik J, Fabricius M, Bhatia R, Major S, Drenckhahn C, et al. Delayed ischaemic neurological deficits after subarachnoid haemorrhage are associated with clusters of spreading depolarizations. Brain. 2006;129(Pt. 12):3224–37.

32. Chong DJ, Hirsch LJ. Which EEG patterns warrant treatment in the critically ill? Reviewing the evidence for treatment of periodic epileptiform discharges and related patterns. J Clin Neurophysiol. 2005;22(2):79–91.

33. Claassen J, Perotte A, Albers D, Kleinberg S, Schmidt JM, Tu B, et al. Nonconvulsive seizures after subarachnoid hemorrhage: multimodal detection and outcomes. Ann Neurol. 2013;74(1):53–64.

34. Dreier JP, Heinemann U. Regional and time dependent variations of low Mg^{2+} induced epileptiform activity in rat temporal cortex slices. Exp Brain Res. 1991;87(3):581–96.

35. Maslarova A, Alam M, Reiffurth C, Lapilover E, Gorji A, Dreier JP. Chronically epileptic human and rat neocortex display a similar resistance against spreading depolarization in vitro. Stroke. 2011;42(10):2917–22.

36. Lapilover EG, Lippmann K, Seda S, Maslarova A, Dreier JP, Heinemann U, et al. Peri-infarct blood-brain barrier dysfunction facilitates induction of spreading depolarization associated with epileptiform discharges. Neurobiol Dis. 2012;48:495–506.

37. Hartings JA, Wilson JA, Look AC, Vagal A, Shutter LA, Dreier JP, et al. Full-band electrocorticography of spreading depolarizations in patients with aneurysmal subarachnoid hemorrhage. Acta Neurochir Suppl. 2013;115:131–41.

38. Gross DW, Gotman J, Quesney LF, Dubeau F, Olivier A. Intracranial EEG with very low frequency activity fails to demonstrate an advantage over conventional recordings. Epilepsia. 1999;40(7):891–8.

39. Tallgren P, Vanhatalo S, Kaila K, Voipio J. Evaluation of commercially available electrodes and gels for recording of slow EEG potentials. Clin Neurophysiol. 2005;116(4):799–806.

40. Ikeda A, Taki W, Kunieda T, Terada K, Mikuni N, Nagamine T, et al. Focal ictal direct current shifts in human epilepsy as studied by subdural and scalp recording. Brain. 1999;122(Pt. 5):827–38.

41. Hartings JA, Watanabe T, Dreier JP, Major S, Vendelbo L, Fabricius M. Recovery of slow potentials in AC-coupled electrocorticography: application to spreading depolarizations in rat and human cerebral cortex. J Neurophysiol. 2009;102(4):2563–75.

42. Oliveira-Ferreira AI, Winkler MKL, Reiffurth C, Milakara D, Woitzik J, Dreier JP. Spreading depolarization, a pathophysiological mechanism of stroke and migraine aura. Future Neurol. 2012;7: 45–64.

43. Wadman WJ, Juta AJ, Kamphuis W, Somjen GG. Current source density of sustained potential shifts associated with electrographic seizures and with spreading depression in rat hippocampus. Brain Res. 1992;570(1–2):85–91.

44. Dietzel I, Heinemann U, Lux HD. Relations between slow extracellular potential changes, glial potassium buffering, and electrolyte and cellular volume changes during neuronal hyperactivity in cat brain. Glia. 1989;2(1):25–44.

45. Speckmann EJ, Elger C. Introduction to the neurophysiological basis of the EEG and DC potentials. In: Niedermeyer E, Lopes da Silva F, editors. Electroencephalography: basic principles, clinical applications and related fields. Baltimore, MD: Williams and Wilkins; 1999. p. 15–27.

46. Makarova J, Makarov VA, Herreras O. Generation of sustained field potentials by gradients of polarization within single neurons: a macroscopic model of spreading depression. J Neurophysiol. 2010;103(5):2446–57.

47. Voipio J, Tallgren P, Heinonen E, Vanhatalo S, Kaila K. Millivolt-scale DC shifts in the human scalp EEG: evidence for a nonneuronal generator. J Neurophysiol. 2003;89(4):2208–14.

48. Kang EJ, Major S, Jorks D, Reiffurth C, Offenhauser N, Friedman A, et al. Blood-brain barrier opening to large molecules does not imply blood-brain barrier opening to small ions. Neurobiol Dis. 2013;52:204–18.

49. Caspers H, Speckmann EJ, Lehmenkuhler A. DC potentials of the cerebral cortex. Seizure activity and changes in gas pressures. Rev. Physiol., Biochem. Pharmacol. 1987;106:127–178.

50. O'Leary JL, Goldring S. D–C potentials of the brain. Physiol Rev 1964;44:91–125.

51. Wurtz RH. Physiological correlates of steady potential shifts during sleep and wakefulness. II. Brain temperature, blood pressure, and potential changes across the ependyma. Electroencephalogr Clin Neurophysiol. 1967;22(1):43–53.

52. Major S, Petzold GC, Reiffurth C, Windmüller O, Foddis M, Lindauer U, et al. A role of the sodium pump in spreading ischemia in rats. J Cereb Blood Flow Metab. 2016; doi:10.1177/0271678x16639059.

53. Kager H, Wadman WJ, Somjen GG. Conditions for the triggering of spreading depression studied with computer simulations. J Neurophysiol. 2002;88(5):2700–12.

54. Carter RE, Seidel JL, Lindquist BE, Sheline CT, Shuttleworth CW. Intracellular Zn^{2+} accumulation enhances suppression of synaptic activity following spreading depolarization. J Neurochem. 2013;125(5):673–84.

55. Lindquist BE, Shuttleworth CW. Adenosine receptor activation is responsible for prolonged depression of synaptic transmission after spreading depolarization in brain slices. Neuroscience. 2012;223: 365–76.

56. Mody I, Lambert JD, Heinemann U. Low extracellular magnesium induces epileptiform activity and spreading depression in rat hippocampal slices. J Neurophysiol. 1987;57(3):869–88.

57. Pomper JK, Haack S, Petzold GC, Buchheim K, Gabriel S, Hoffmann U, et al. Repetitive spreading depression-like events result in cell damage in juvenile hippocampal slice cultures maintained in normoxia. J Neurophysiol. 2006;95(1):355–68.

58. Avoli M, Drapeau C, Louvel J, Pumain R, Olivier A, Villemure JG. Epileptiform activity induced by low extracellular magnesium in the human cortex maintained in vitro. Ann Neurol. 1991;30(4): 589–96.

59. Gabriel S, Njunting M, Pomper JK, Merschhemke M, Sanabria ER, Eilers A, et al. Stimulus and potassium-induced epileptiform activity in the human dentate gyrus from patients with and without hippocampal sclerosis. J Neurosci. 2004;24(46): 10416–30.

60. Köhling R, Koch UR, Hagemann G, Redecker C, Straub H, Speckmann EJ. Differential sensitivity to induction of spreading depression by partial disinhibition in chronically epileptic human and rat as compared to native rat neocortical tissue. Brain Res. 2003;975(1–2):129–34.

61. Hablitz JJ, Heinemann U. Alterations in the microenvironment during spreading depression associated with epileptiform activity in the immature neocortex. Brain Res Dev Brain Res. 1989;46(2): 243–52.

62. Vaillend C, Mason SE, Cuttle MF, Alger BE. Mechanisms of neuronal hyperexcitability caused by partial inhibition of Na^+-K^+-ATPases in the rat CA1 hippocampal region. J Neurophysiol. 2002;88(6):2963–78.

63. Koroleva VI, Bures J. Cortical penicillin focus as a generator of repetitive spike-triggered waves of spreading depression in rats. Exp Brain Res. 1983;51(2):291–7.

64. Gorji A, Speckmann EJ. Spreading depression enhances the spontaneous epileptiform activity in human neocortical tissues. Eur J Neurosci. 2004;19(12):3371–4.

65. Kruger H, Luhmann HJ, Heinemann U. Repetitive spreading depression causes selective suppression of GABAergic function. Neuroreport. 1996;7(15–17):2733–6.

66. Vespa PM, McArthur DL, Xu Y, Eliseo M, Etchepare M, Dinov I, et al. Nonconvulsive seizures after traumatic brain injury are associated with hippocampal atrophy. Neurology. 2010;75(9):792–8.

67. Claassen J, Hirsch LJ, Frontera JA, Fernandez A, Schmidt M, Kapinos G, et al. Prognostic significance of continuous EEG monitoring in patients with poor-grade subarachnoid hemorrhage. Neurocrit Care. 2006;4(2):103–12.

68. Vespa PM, O'Phelan K, Shah M, Mirabelli J, Starkman S, Kidwell C, et al. Acute seizures after intracerebral hemorrhage: a factor in progressive midline shift and outcome. Neurology. 2003;60(9): 1441–6.

69. Jordan KG. Emergency EEG and continuous EEG monitoring in acute ischemic stroke. J Clin Neurophysiol. 2004;21(5):341–52.

70. Fabricius M, Fuhr S, Bhatia R, Boutelle M, Hashemi P, Strong AJ, et al. Cortical spreading depression and peri-infarct depolarization in acutely injured human cerebral cortex. Brain. 2006;129(Pt. 3):778–90.

71. Hartings JA, Bullock MR, Okonkwo DO, Murray LS, Murray GD, Fabricius M, et al. Spreading depolarisations and outcome after traumatic brain injury: a prospective observational study. Lancet Neurol. 2011;10(12):1058–64.

72. Lauritzen M, Dreier JP, Fabricius M, Hartings JA, Graf R, Strong AJ. Clinical relevance of cortical spreading depression in neurological disorders: migraine, malignant stroke, subarachnoid and intracranial hemorrhage, and traumatic brain injury. J Cereb Blood Flow Metab. 2011;31(1):17–35.

73. Helbok R, Schiefecker AJ, Friberg C, Beer R, Kofler M, Rhomberg P, et al. Spreading depolarizations in patients with spontaneous intracerebral hemorrhage: association with perihematomal edema progression. J Cereb Blood Flow Metab. 2016. doi:10.1177/0271678x16651269

74. Dohmen C, Sakowitz OW, Fabricius M, Bosche B, Reithmeier T, Ernestus RI, et al. Spreading depolarizations occur in human ischemic stroke with high incidence. Ann Neurol. 2008;63(6):720–8.

75. Dreier JP, Reiffurth C. The stroke-migraine depolarization continuum. Neuron. 2015;86(4):902–22.

76. Haan J, Terwindt GM, van den Maagdenberg AM, Stam AH, Ferrari MD. A review of the genetic relation between migraine and epilepsy. Cephalalgia. 2008;28(2):105–13.

77. Castro MJ, Stam AH, Lemos C, de Vries B, Vanmolkot KR, Barros J, et al. First mutation in the voltage-gated Nav1.1 subunit gene SCN1A with co-occurring familial hemiplegic migraine and epilepsy. Cephalalgia. 2009;29(3):308–13.

78. Costa C, Prontera P, Sarchielli P, Tonelli A, Bassi MT, Cupini LM, et al. A novel ATP1A2 gene mutation in familial hemiplegic migraine and epilepsy. Cephalalgia. 2013;34:68–72.

79. Winawer MR, Connors R. Evidence for a shared genetic susceptibility to migraine and epilepsy. Epilepsia. 2013;54(2):288–95.

80. Tomkins O, Friedman O, Ivens S, Reiffurth C, Major S, Dreier JP, et al. Blood-brain barrier disruption results in delayed functional and structural alterations in the rat neocortex. Neurobiol Dis. 2007;25(2):367–77.

81. Koroleva VI, Vinogradova LV, Bures J. Reduced incidence of cortical spreading depression in the course of pentylenetetrazol kindling in rats. Brain Res. 1993;608(1):107–14.

82. Lehmenkuhler A, Sykova E, Svoboda J, Zilles K, Nicholson C. Extracellular space parameters in the rat neocortex and subcortical white matter during postnatal development determined by diffusion analysis. Neuroscience. 1993;55(2):339–51.

83. Matsushima K, Hogan MJ, Hakim AM. Cortical spreading depression protects against subsequent focal cerebral ischemia in rats. J Cereb Blood Flow Metab. 1996;16(2):221–6.

84. Kobayashi S, Harris VA, Welsh FA. Spreading depression induces tolerance of cortical neurons to ischemia in rat brain. J Cereb Blood Flow Metab. 1995;15(5):721–7.

85. Muramatsu H, Kariko K, Welsh FA. Induction of tolerance to focal ischemia in rat brain: dissociation between cortical lesioning and spreading depression. J Cereb Blood Flow Metab. 2004;24(10):1167–71.

86. Kunkler PE, Hulse RE, Kraig RP. Multiplexed cytokine protein expression profiles from spreading depression in hippocampal organotypic cultures. J Cereb Blood Flow Metab. 2004;24(8): 829–39.

87. Jander S, Schroeter M, Peters O, Witte OW, Stoll G. Cortical spreading depression induces proinflammatory cytokine gene expression in the rat brain. J Cereb Blood Flow Metab. 2001;21(3):218–25.

88. Gehrmann J, Mies G, Bonnekoh P, Banati R, Iijima T, Kreutzberg GW, et al. Microglial reaction in the rat cerebral cortex induced by cortical spreading depression. Brain Pathol. 1993;3(1):11–7.

89. Berger M, Speckmann EJ, Pape HC, Gorji A. Spreading depression enhances human neocortical excitability in vitro. Cephalalgia. 2008;28(5):558–62.

90. Yanamoto H, Miyamoto S, Tohnai N, Nagata I, Xue JH, Nakano Y, et al. Induced spreading depression activates persistent neurogenesis in the subventricular zone, generating cells with markers for divided and early committed neurons in the caudate putamen and cortex. Stroke. 2005;36(7):1544–50.

91. Urbach A, Brueckner J, Witte OW. Cortical spreading depolarization stimulates gliogenesis in the rat entorhinal cortex. J Cereb Blood Flow Metab. 2015;35(4):576–82.

92. Somjen GG. Irreversible hypoxic (ischemic) neuron injury. In: Somjen GG, editor. Ions in the brain. New York, NY: Oxford University Press; 2004. p. 338–72.

93. Kotsopoulos IA, van Merode T, Kessels FG, de Krom MC, Knottnerus JA. Systematic review and meta-analysis of incidence studies of epilepsy and unprovoked seizures. Epilepsia. 2002;43(11):1402–9.

94. Menyhart A, Makra P, Szepes BE, Toth OM, Hertelendy P, Bari F, et al. High incidence of adverse cerebral blood flow responses to spreading depolarization in the aged ischemic rat brain. Neurobiol Aging. 2015;36(12):3269–77.

95. Morris RG, Anderson E, Lynch GS, Baudry M. Selective impairment of learning and blockade of long-term potentiation by an N-methyl-D-aspartate receptor antagonist, AP5. Nature. 1986;319(6056):774–6.

96. Baudry M. Long-term potentiation and kindling: similar biochemical mechanisms? Adv Neurol. 1986;44:401–10.

97. Bar-Shira O, Maor R, Chechik G. Gene expression switching of receptor subunits in human brain development. PLoS Comput Biol. 2015;11(12):e1004559.

98. Liu XB, Murray KD, Jones EG. Switching of NMDA receptor 2A and 2B subunits at thalamic and cortical synapses during early postnatal development. J Neurosci. 2004;24(40):8885–8895.

Multimodality Monitoring Correlates of Seizures

Jens Witsch, Nicholas A. Morris, David Roh, Hans-Peter Frey, and Jan Claassen

Abbreviations

cEEG   Continuous EEG
dEEG   Depth/intracortical EEG
EEG   Electroencephalography
MMM   Multimodality monitoring
sEEG   Surface EEG

Neuro ICU Monitoring Modalities

In the context of the neurological intensive care unit and as discussed below the term multimodality monitoring (MMM) usually implies both non-invasive and invasive diagnostic tools. Non-invasive ones include neuroimaging, continuous scalp EEG, extra- and transcranial duplex and Doppler exams, evoked potentials, and near infrared spectroscopy (NIRS). Commonly used invasive monitors measure and record intracranial pressure (ICP), cerebral oxygenation (partial brain tissue oxygenation, PbtO2), regional cerebral blood flow (rCBF), intracranial EEG, cortical spreading depressions, and cerebral chemistry via microdialysis (MD). By subtracting the ICP from the mean arterial pressure (MAP), the cerebral perfusion pressure (CPP) can be approximated. It is important to be aware of strengths and limitations of each monitoring modality in order to optimize their utility, especially in the context of seizures. In the following chapter we will first briefly introduce the main intracranial monitoring techniques (for an in-depth discussion of cortical spreading depression please refer to Chap. 20), followed by an overview of the physiologic signal detected from invasive monitoring devices during seizures.

Intracranial Pressure

ICP measurements may be achieved via pressure sensors located within the ventricle (external ventricular drain, EVD), with the advantage that CSF can also be drained from the ventricle in order to lower the pressure [1, 2]. The disadvantage is that most commercially available EVDs either drain CSF or measure ICP at a given time but are unable to perform both functions simultaneously. In contrast, intraparenchymal ICP monitors provide a constant account of the ICP with similar reliability and accuracy [3].

ICP values higher than 20–25 mmHg are usually a trigger for treatment interventions in clinical practice [4]. At the same time, there is broad consensus that this cutoff is somewhat arbitrary and that the interpretation of ICP depends on the clinical context and duration of ICP elevation [5, 6]. Although an association between response to ICP-lowering treatment and outcome has been shown [7–9], there is a paucity of high quality data showing that the current practice of ICP management improves outcomes in patients with acute brain injury [10, 11]. In defense of ICP monitoring it may be argued that, rather than absolute ICP values, ICP changes over time and cumulative ICP burden may contain valuable diagnostic information [10, 12–17]. In addition, the ICP waveform contains information on intracranial compliance and autoregulation and may influence blood pressure management [18, 19]. In the context of MMM, ICP monitoring is indispensable as it may herald newly developing intracerebral masses or impending herniation, and is necessary to calculate cerebral perfusion pressure (CPP) [20–22].

J. Witsch • N.A. Morris • D. Roh • H.-P. Frey
Division of Critical Care and Hospitalist Neurology, Department of Neurology, Columbia University Medical Center, New York Presbyterian Hospital, New York, NY 10032, USA
e-mail: jensjulianwitsch@gmail.com; Nicholas.Morris@umm.edu; dr2753@cumc.columbia.edu; hf2289@cumc.columbia.edu

J. Claassen (✉)
Neurocritical Care, Columbia University College of Physicians and Surgeons, New York, NY, USA

Division of Critical Care and Hospitalist Neurology, Department of Neurology, Columbia

University Medical Center, New York Presbyterian Hospital, New York, NY, USA
e-mail: jc1439@cumc.columbia.edu

P.N. Varelas, J. Claassen (eds.), *Seizures in Critical Care*, Current Clinical Neurology, DOI 10.1007/978-3-319-49557-6_6

Cerebral Perfusion Pressure and Regional Cerebral Blood Flow

Brain perfusion can be estimated globally through CPP calculation (MAP-ICP) or locally. Local measurements are possible via laser Doppler flowmetry [23], or via insertion of a thermal dilution probe into the brain parenchyma, which then measures regional cerebral blood flow (rCBF) in an area of approximately 3 cm^2 surrounding the probe [24]. Furthermore Xenon CT and Perfusion CT provide snapshot measures of brain perfusion, but these techniques will not be reviewed here.

CPP is considered normal at values between 55 and 70 mmHg [25], but as with MAP and ICP, the clinical interpretation of CPP is very much context-dependent and absolute values are limited as targets of therapeutic interventions [22, 26, 27].

A given CPP value's validity as therapeutic target is dependent on intact cerebrovascular autoregulation. Autoregulation refers to the ability of arterioles in the brain to adjust diameter over a range of CPP in order to maintain constant end-organ blood flow. Thus, with intact autoregulation, the measure of CPP is independent of the rCBF [28]. However, patients with acute brain injury often have impaired autoregulation, which is why in these patients' MAP increases may cause ICP increases, and CPP and rCBF may be linearly correlated [21].

The pressure reactivity index (PRx) is a reflection of autoregulation that takes into account both individual variability among patients and temporal perfusion dynamics within individuals [29, 30]. PRx measures the degree of correlation between MAP and ICP and is calculated over a sliding time window of several minutes. Poor correlation corresponds to intact and strong correlation to absent autoregulation. Absent autoregulation also implies that the therapeutic regulation of CPP is paramount since in this situation CPP directly determines rCBF in the brain [31]. For most patients, plotting the CPP against the PRx yields an optimal CPP or CPPopt, where the brain is best protected from hypo- and hyperperfusion. While in TBI patients with impaired autoregulation both low CPP and high CPP have been associated with poor outcomes [13, 22, 28], the more individualized approach of CPPopt-driven blood pressure regulation has not been established as clearly beneficial so far. Feasibility studies have shown improved outcomes in patients who remain at their individual CPPopt during the first 48 h [26, 32], but prospective phase III intervention studies reproducing these results are not available so far [33].

The most commonly used intraparenchymal probe to estimate brain perfusion uses thermal dilution principles measuring the convection and heat conduction properties of the surrounding brain tissue. These rCBF values are comparable to those obtained by Xenon-CT [24]. Widely accepted ranges defining normal and abnormal rCBF remain to be established [4]. An averaged approximation to a normal value is 50 ml/100 mg/min, with white matter being less perfused on average (20 ml/100 mg/min) than grey matter (80 ml/100 mg/min). Major measurement artifacts are introduced through periodic recalibration of the temperature sensor. Moreover, the technique is considered less reliable in patients with elevated body temperature. However, despite methodological limitations, relative changes in conjunction with other monitoring modalities—especially quantification of metabolic demand through MD—may aid the detection of impending tissue ischemia or seizure activity [34]. Currently there is no evidence that rCBF-targeted treatment of patients with acute brain injury leads to better outcomes [4].

Brain Tissue Oxygenation

There are two invasive methods to measure brain parenchyma oxygenation locally, the Licox system (Integra Neurosciences) and the Neurovent-PTO System (Raumedic), which yield comparable results [35]. The Neurovent-PTO system measures oxygen tension by means of a fluorescence sensor. The Licox system consists of a Clark-type polarographic probe coated by a semi permeable membrane [36, 37]. Oxygen probes are commonly coupled with a temperature probe (in the Licox system temperature is measured by the same probe) or with temperature and ICP probes (Raumedic) [38, 39] (Fig. 6.1). Similar to rCBF partial brain tissue oxygen pressure (PbtO2) should be interpreted in synthesis with other parameters, such as CPPopt [40, 41]. Moreover low PbtO2 values can easily be "improved" by increasing the fraction of inspiratory oxygen, which, however, does not necessarily improve brain metabolism.

The physiologic PbtO2 range is still a matter of debate. Based on data obtained in patients undergoing elective neurosurgical procedures and in patients with acute brain injuries, 20–35 mmHg can be considered normal, <20 mmHg moderate hypoxia, and <10 mmHg severe hypoxia [42–44]. There is an abundance of data showing that very low PbtO2 values correlate with poor outcome, in both TBI and SAH patients [45–48]. Further evidence for the physiologic plausibility of PbtO2 measurement was provided by a study correlating PbtO2 and regional cerebral blood flow [49] and by a study showing that PbtO2 in brain dead patients is zero mmHg [50]. So far, PbtO2-targeted therapy and its impact on outcome have only been studied in small patient cohorts but with some promising results [51].

Cerebral Microdialysis

MD allows the determination of interstitial molecule concentrations in the brain, by insertion of a catheter–with attached tubing system for filtering and passage of the dialysate–into the white matter [52, 53]. The dialysate is then

Fig. 6.1 Invasive multimodality monitoring "bundle" in a patient in the neurointensive care unit. (**a**) External view of the patient's head with microdialysis and rCBF probes in the foreground and the Licox probe (PbtO2, Temperature, ICP) in the background. (**b**) X-ray skull survey with right frontal insertion of probes shown in (**a**). (**c**) CT head without contrast showing the tips of the probes (*red arrow*) immediately next to each other. (**d**) Conventional Angiography showing MMM probes in relation to the cerebral vasculature in the right frontal ACA/MCA territory. *rCBF* regional cerebral blood flow, *PbtO2* partial brain oxygen pressure, *ICP* intracranial pressure, *MMM* multimodality monitoring, *ACA* anterior cerebral artery, *MCA* middle cerebral artery

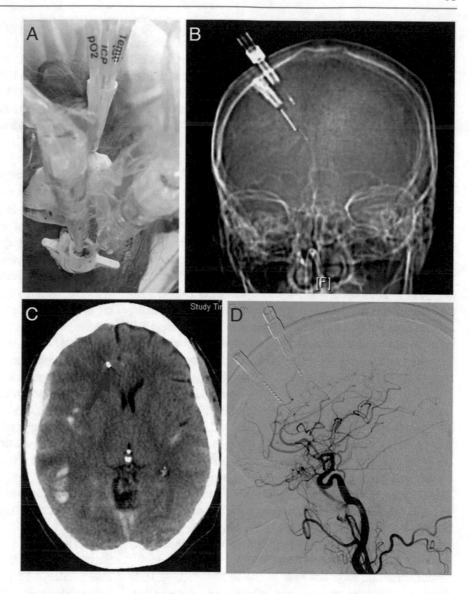

typically analyzed at the bedside [54]. The maximal sampling frequency is limited to approximately 6 times per hour due to the time needed for equilibration of the chemical molecule gradient across the microdialysis membrane. Most institutions that use MD on a routine basis sample the catheter fluid once per hour, which may be a limitation when MD parameters are to be compared to other monitoring modalities with higher time resolution.

Molecules of interest include brain glucose, the glycolysis products lactate and pyruvate, as well as markers of excitotoxicity or cell damage, such as glutamate and glycerol [55]. The lactate-pyruvate ratio (LPR) rather than the two parameters in isolation is believed to be associated with tissue energy failure. A low interstitial brain glucose concentration in combination with a high LPR can be indicative of hypoxia/ischemia. However, elevation of the LPR alone may indicate an accelerated brain metabolism and is not necessarily associated with brain damage. MD-values need to be

interpreted in context; the comparison with PbtO2 and rCBF has been shown to provide a meaningful first approach to evaluate the metabolic state of the brain tissue [56, 57].

Normal glucose values range between 1.5 and 2 mM. LPR values of greater than 25 and 40, respectively, have been described as a marker of injury [58–60]. Normal ranges of glycerol and glutamate—markers of brain cell membrane break down and excitotoxicity—are less well established. Generally glutamate concentrations <10 mM and glycerol concentrations <50 mM are considered normal [54, 61–63].

Both low glucose and high LPR are associated with poor outcome [17, 56, 57]. Moreover high interstitial glutamate in SAH patients has been shown to indicate delayed cerebral ischemia [64]. In a large observational study including 223 patients with TBI, glucose and LPR contralateral to traumatic injury were each independently associated with 6-month mortality [59].

Although brain glucose metabolism can be altered by systemic interventions [65], to date, no interventional studies using MD-values as treatment targets to improve clinical outcome have been conducted. However, MD with PbtO2 measurements have been used to identify optimal MAP/ICP and hemoglobin values, which may indirectly impact clinical outcome [26, 66, 67].

EEG as a Component of Multimodality Monitoring

Surface EEG

In the neuro ICU several methods of EEG recording can be applied to obtain EEG data from patients with acute brain injury, among them spot EEG, repeated short EEG recordings, continuous surface EEG, and depth EEG (dEEG). All of these modes of EEG recording can be enhanced by using quantitative EEG (see Chap. 20 for details). Surface EEG (sEEG), as one of the oldest and most intensely studied techniques of monitoring the brain, has its unquestioned diagnostic value in seizure detection, monitoring the depth of sedation, and in prognostication [68]. Open questions in the neuro ICU context include the choice of EEG technique (or combination of techniques) and duration of EEG recording that produces the highest diagnostic yield in a given disease entity and patient [69]. In recent years, technical advancements have made digital transformation of the analog EEG signal, storage, and—at least partly—the automated analysis of large amounts of EEG data possible. Nevertheless, continuous EEG (cEEG) recordings still require a substantial amount of manpower at significant cost, which is why research on effective use is warranted.

Both through modifications of the EEG recording technique and through development of data analysis methods researchers have tried to improve the applicability of sEEG in the neuro ICU [70].

Quantitative EEG (for an Extensive Discussion on qEEG Please Refer to Another Chapter of the Book)

A relatively new development in the neuro ICU is the use of quantitative EEG (qEEG) to aid in the timely extraction of diagnostic information from the large amounts of cEEG data. Various algorithms are available to analyze and visualize qEEG data. After undergoing Fast Fourier Transformation the raw EEG data can either be represented as total power, ratios of power (e.g., alpha delta ratio), or spectrograms. Spectrograms in turn can be graphed as numbers, compressed spectral arrays (CSA), staggered arrays, or histograms [71, 72]. The analogous interpretation of raw EEG data is too time consuming to be feasible by a neurointensive care physician alone whose responsibilities will only grow

with the technical progress in the field of neurocritical care, leaving less time for EEG review. The alternative, employment of full time electrophysiologists, is a financial and logistic challenge that most hospitals are not able to afford. In the future, qEEG will hopefully offer efficient screening and alarm mechanisms indicating clinically concerning EEG trends, in order to make big EEG data accessible and useful at the bedside [73].

Automated Seizure Detection Algorithms

Another approach to master the task of extracting relevant information from large amounts of raw EEG recordings is the development of seizure detection software. For such software to detect seizures with reasonable sensitivity and specificity, seizures should ideally have a clear on- and offset and should be clearly distinguishable from the EEG background. While this is often the case in a relatively noise-free environment, such as epilepsy monitoring units, it is rarely the case in neurointensive care units that have many ambient sources of noise [74, 75]. Moreover, muscle artifacts and periodic discharges are more common in the NICU. The latter share many electrographic features with seizures and are therefore difficult to distinguish by automated seizure detection software [76, 77]. Indeed there is ongoing debate regarding the clinical relevance of periodic discharges that fall along the ictal-interictal spectrum lacking the discrete on–offset of events that are universally recognized as ictal. Seizure detection algorithms using intracortical EEG data have not been tested so far, but are promising given the overall high signal to noise ratio of dEEG.

Depth EEG

Surface EEG has the advantage of providing a global electrophysiological signal covering most parts of the cerebral cortex. However, sEEG electrodes are separated from the source of the EEG signal originating from the brain tissue by several structures: skin, hair, the skull, as well as the meninges and any pathologic material (blood, pus, etc.) that may lie within. Distant from the source of the signal, sEEG is also close to sources of noise. Sources of noise include poor electrode contact and—particularly in the neuro ICU–surrounding electronic devices, which may cause artifacts distorting the EEG signal. Another major source of artifact is the electrical signal generated by muscle and movement. These disadvantages may be overcome by the local insertion of intracortical electrodes, which allows at least local—not global—EEG recordings with minimal artifact and a high signal to noise ratio.

Invasive EEG monitoring as a diagnostic modality arose in the context of seizure focus localization in patients with treatment-refractory focal epilepsy. It is typically achieved either by subdural/epidural grid placement or by implantation of intracortical strip or depth electrodes [78], which share a similar risk profile with other invasive monitoring techniques [79]. Despite comparatively poor spatial resolution, intracortical electrodes may prove to be a valuable diagnostic addition to sEEG monitoring in neurointensive care units that routinely use depth electrodes [79, 80].

EEG and Multimodality Monitoring

The concurrent use of EEG with other MMM techniques provides the opportunity to get a more complete picture of ongoing brain physiology, during major pathologic events like seizures, delayed cerebral ischemic events after SAH, or during waves of cortical spreading depression [81–83].

Apart from a few recent studies data are lacking using a combined EEG/MMM methodology [80, 84–86]. One of the most promising areas of research is the characterization of ongoing physiology during seizures, which may potentially help find treatment targets beyond administration of anticonvulsant drugs, with the goal to improve physiology. Seizures in ICU populations are both very common and associated with worse outcomes [85, 87], which is why the characterization of the physiologic signature of seizures through the use of MMM is very promising. With the use of cEEG electrographic seizures have been detected in up to 15% of patients with spontaneous SAH [87, 88], in 15% of patients with post-cardiac arrest syndrome [89], in around one quarter of patients with intracerebral hemorrhage [90, 91], in up to one third of patients with TBI [92, 93] and in one third of patients with CNS infections [94]. By the same token, 16 and 10% of patients in surgical and medical ICU populations are found to have electrographic only seizures [95, 96]. Better understanding of the underlying pathophysiological processes occurring during acute brain injury seizures may allow identification of seizures that deserve more or less aggressive treatment. Lastly, through the combined use of EEG and MMM the so-called ictal-interictal continuum might be characterized further, distinguishing EEG patterns that warrant treatment from those that do not [97].

Multimodality Monitoring Signature of Seizures

The detection of electrographic seizures is important because studies suggest a negative influence of seizures on clinical outcome [85, 87, 98]. A study in 479 SAH patients, undergoing cEEG monitoring using sEEG electrodes in the vast majority of cases, suggested a vicious cycle between seizures, inflammation, and poor outcome following acute brain injury [98]. However, the changes of physiology and metabolism of brain tissue during seizures remain poorly characterized, which is why treatment of seizures is restricted to administration of anticonvulsant drugs. MMM during seizures has the potential to generate a more complete picture of brain tissue changes and eventually open up new therapeutic options that target restoring physiology rather than seizure cessation.

Animal Studies

In animal models researchers have investigated the MMM signature of seizures for decades using varying techniques to measure ICP, CPP, cerebral blood flow, brain oxygen, and cerebral metabolites before, during, and after seizures [99]. Animal models have the advantage of being "clean" models of seizure physiology in contrast to human patients in the neurointensive care unit who tend to have a severe underlying brain pathology and systemic effects such as pneumonia or sepsis to account for [100]. Despite variability among studies regarding the type of animal model, the mode of seizure induction, and the methods employed (including variable sites of MD catheter placement) some comparable results can be extracted, indicating a potential common MMM signature of seizures.

As early as 1939, Penfield and co-workers described an increase of cerebral blood flow during seizures [101] and this finding has been reproduced quite consistently across animal species and seizure models using different types of intraparenchymal probes to measure rCBF [102–105].

Conversely brain tissue oxygen tension eventually decreases with ongoing seizure activity, sometimes following an initial increase of local oxygen tension, indicating a possible initial compensatory effort which eventually ends with decompensation of oxygen delivery [106–109].

Although not consistently reproduced across different disease processes, there are some animal studies showing that prolonged seizures may cause ICP elevations [110, 111]. Consequently CPP may be reduced during seizure activity, unless increased blood pressure during the event compensates the ICP elevation. However CPP is also influenced by various other factors such as presence or absence of functioning autoregulation; therefore, CPP changes during seizures are difficult to investigate and have not been systematically studied in animal models [84].

During experimentally induced status epilepticus initially marked increases in extracellular glucose and lactate levels have been observed, indicating increased energy demand and turnover [112]. This hypermetabolic situation may eventually lead to energy failure as indicated by decreases of extracellular glucose and increases in the LPR after 20–40 minutes of ongoing status epilepticus, as observed in the L-homocysteine induced seizure model in rats [113]. Marked increases of extracellular glutamate and glycerol after prolonged seizure activity have been interpreted as indicative of cell death as a consequence of prolonged status epilepticus [112, 114–118].

Studies in Humans

MMM studies in humans often face criticism because data is heterogeneous and not always conclusive, perhaps not surprising as most studies include heterogeneous disease processes and disease severities. In clinical practice all efforts are being made to terminate seizures as early as possible. However, a clear picture of MMM changes during seizure activity can often only be seen after prolonged status epilepticus, as evident from the animal studies described above. Figure 6.2 illustrates typical changes of brain oxygen and perfusion preceding, during, and after a prolonged electrographic seizure in a patient with a high-grade spontaneous subarachnoid hemorrhage (Fig. 6.2).

Apart from the dynamics of MMM parameters, secondarily developing lesions are often encountered following acute brain injury such as ischemic and hemorrhagic lesions and will affect the recorded brain physiology. Pathophysiologic changes of primary injury may at times be difficult to differentiate from secondary events. Moreover, variable disease severity at baseline is likely reflected in different baseline MMM values which is hypothetically the reason why pooled data is less likely to produce statistically significant results than comparison of within-subject changes [81, 85]. Despite these "real life" limitations a decent body of scientific evidence has been generated describing MMM changes during seizure activity in human patients.

Ictal hyperperfusion is a well-studied phenomenon, and has been seen in numerous studies using positron emission tomography, CT perfusion, MR perfusion, and Xenon CT in patients with and without acute brain injury, but studies using invasive rCBF measurement are sparse [119, 120]. In line with animal data, one study found that rCBF during seizures increases with continuous seizure activity, after approximately 10 minutes [85]. Also consistent with the animal data, PbtO2 has been found to decrease during seizures prior to the increase of rCBF, suggesting that perfusion may increase as a compensatory reaction to hypoxia [85]. In a group of 10 TBI patients with seizures compared to a matched control group of TBI patients without seizures, the occurrence of seizures correlated with a prolonged sustained increase of ICP [121]. In the study by Claassen et al. electrographic seizures were accompanied by an immediate increase of ICP, CPP, heart rate, MAP, respiratory rate, and minute ventilation [85]. These changes in cardiovascular parameters are common in partial and generalized epilepsies and are consistent with previous studies [122, 123].

Few studies are available evaluating brain MD changes during seizure activity in humans. In 30 subjects with TBI the occurrence of electrographic seizures coincided with a decrease of extracellular glucose concentrations [124] and this finding was reproduced in a recent study in 29 TBI patients in whom extracellular glucose concentrations during seizures were significantly lower than at baseline (mean 0.8 vs. 1.7 mmol/l) [81]. Administration of systemic insulin lowers both systemic and brain extracellular glucose concentrations and correlates with markers of metabolic stress in the brain, namely increased LPR and increased glutamate concentrations [65, 125]. The few available studies investigating lactate and LPR during seizures are in line with these findings. A study by During and colleagues investigated the effect of spontaneously occurring seizures in (otherwise healthy) patients with treatment-refractory complex partial seizures, after bilateral implantation of MD catheters in both hippocampi. Partial seizures with secondary generalization were accompanied by a mean 90% lactate increase in the first 60–90 minutes after seizure onset. This increase was restricted to the side of seizure initiation [126]. Pyruvate concentrations were not determined in this study.

MD changes may last beyond seizure cessation. In a study of non-convulsive seizures in TBI, Vespa et al. found prolonged and significantly higher LPR values in the seizure group compared to the group without seizures. This effect lasted beyond 100 hours after admission [121]. However, this finding was not reproduced in the study by Claassen et al., who did not find significant changes of MD parameters related to the occurrence of electrographic seizures. The discrepancy between both papers is possibly due to the statistical methods employed or due to the different entities studied (TBI versus SAH) [127]. In a recent study in patients with severe TBI undergoing MMM including MD, the comparison of 12 patients with seizures and 8 patients without seizures showed a numerically higher hourly LPR burden in the seizure group (as quantified using the area under the curve). This finding was not statistically significant in a pooled analysis but reached significance using a within-subject-design analyzing LPR changes of single patients on an hour by hour basis [81].

Extracellular glutamate is a key factor in abnormal neuronal discharges and has been implicated in triggering and maintaining seizures, and in kindling epilepsy [128]. MD studies in patients with temporal lobe epilepsy have shown chronically increased extracellular glutamate concentrations on the side of the epileptic focus leading to excitotoxicity, which hypothetically entertains the increased likelihood of further seizures [129]. Ronne-Engström and colleagues investigated extracellular amino acid levels during seizures and during the period immediately following the seizures in seven patients with epilepsy of focal origin by implanting a MD device into the epileptic focus. Extracellular glutamate concentrations rose approximately sevenfold during spontaneously occurring seizures, but normalized immediately after [130]. In patients with TBI, seizures were associated with the occurrence of transient extracellular glutamate increases [84].

Glycerol is an essential ingredient of cell membranes and serves—even more so than the LPR—as a direct marker of

Fig. 6.2 Multimodality monitoring signature of an electrographic seizure. (**a**) rCBF, PbtO2, CPP, and HR relative to the onset of a seizure, detected on both surface and depth EEG. The background colors in (**a**) indicate (1) *white* = no seizure activity, (2) *lgiht grey* = ictal-interictal continuum, (3) *dark grey* = seizure. B1–B3, Raw EEG clips (16 s each) corresponding to the phases shown in (**a**). Panel B1 shows no seizure activity, B2 ictal-interictal continuum, B3 seizure. *rCBF* regional cerebral blood flow, *PbtO2* partial brain oxygen tension, *CPP* cerebral perfusion pressure, *HR* heart rate

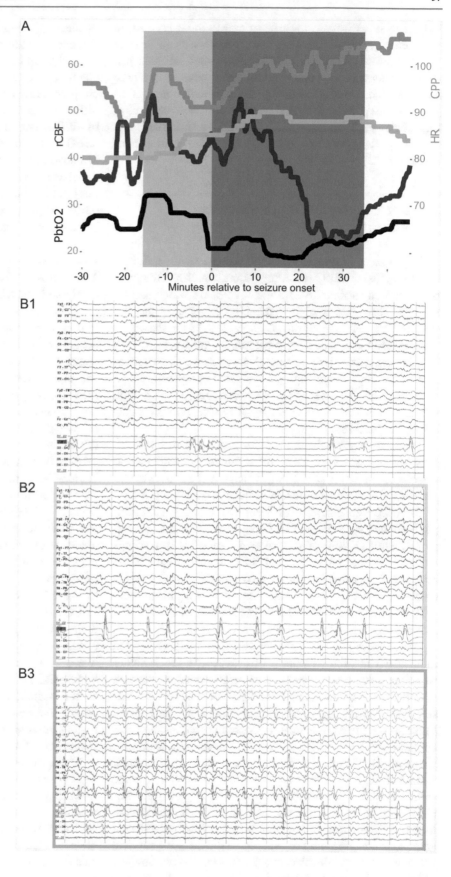

cell damage. However, the role of extracellular glycerol in the context of neurointensive care patients with seizures is poorly studied [131]. One of the few studies included just two patients with TBI and electrographic seizures in whom MD detected a higher mean glycerol concentration in comparison with patients who had no seizures. These concentrations, however, were average concentrations during days 1–3 and 7–9 post-injury and not time-locked to the occurrence of seizures [132].

Seizure Activity on Depth Electrode Recordings

Ideally seizure detection would be achieved with sufficient sensitivity using sEEG recordings alone, which as a diagnostic technique carries the advantages of being widely implemented. However, a high percentage of seizures are not detected by sEEG recordings, as suggested by studies in which dEEG and sEEG were recorded simultaneously [80, 85]. In fact, particularly recent advances in the characterization of the physiologic signature of seizures were only possible through the use of dEEG recordings, since a high percentage of seizures detected by dEEG had no visible correlate on sEEG [80, 81, 85, 98].

In a study by Waziri et al. in 14 patients with subarachnoid hemorrhage, 6 patients with seizures on dEEG had no seizure correlate on sEEG [80]. Claassen et al. included 48 patients with subarachnoid hemorrhage in their study. A total of 77 new onset seizures were identified. In this patient sample 38% had seizures on dEEG, whereas only 8% had seizures on sEEG. 43% of seizure events on dEEG recordings had no correlate on sEEG [85]. In their recent publication Vespa et al. reported the combined detection rate for periodic discharges and electrographic seizures in 34 patients with TBI, and found that 43% of seizures and PDs were only visible on dEEG, not on sEEG [81].

Apart from the much higher seizure and PD detection rate, dEEG has the advantage of providing a much higher signal to noise ratio, which opens up a myriad of research options, such as more detailed analyses of seizure onset/offset, spike morphology, and seizure evolution. The greatest limitation of dEEG, however, is its poor spatial resolution in comparison with sEEG. Moreover, despite a justifiable safety profile [79], it is an invasive technique, and insertion, maintenance, and safety control require specifically trained staff. sEEG, on the other hand, provides a global electrophysiological signature of the brain with higher spatial resolution, is non-invasive, can be removed before and replaced after neuroimaging studies, and demands no prior surgical training for electrode placement. To date, despite obvious additional diagnostic information, the use of dEEG is confined to few large academic centers, and continuous sEEG

monitoring remains the diagnostic mainstay of seizure detection and monitoring in patients with acute brain injury [68].

Design and reporting of studies on dEEG so far have emphasized advantages of dEEG over sEEG, not focusing on information contained in sEEG which is not reflected in dEEG. The goal of future studies cannot be to replace sEEG by dEEG, but to help define clinical scenarios, in which dEEG constitutes a reasonable diagnostic addition. Moreover, it may be worthwhile exploring sEEG correlates of seizures, primarily detected only on dEEG. Advances in this direction might have a more immediate and direct impact on clinical practice, since continuous sEEG—unlike dEEG— is increasingly available at many centers around the world.

The Clinical Significance of Depth and Surface EEG Seizures

In patients with spontaneous SAH it has been shown that the occurrence of seizures is associated with worse clinical outcome. This holds true in studies in which seizure detection was undertaken using sEEG, and in those studies that used predominantly dEEG. De Marchis et al. studied 402 patients with spontaneous SAH, almost exclusively undergoing sEEG monitoring. 50 (12%) had electrographic seizures on cEEG. Seizures were both qualitatively (presence/absence of seizures) and quantitatively (sum of seizure duration, seizure "burden") independently associated with worse outcome at 3 months follow up. No significant differences were found between seizure and non-seizure patient groups regarding overall disease severity and other established outcome predictors (Hunt and Hess grade on admission, modified Fisher grade on admission, etc.). Moreover, seizure burden, but not presence of seizures per se, correlated with cognitive performance at 3 months follow up [87].

Claassen et al. included 48 high-grade SAH patients in their study, who were undergoing both sEEG and dEEG. Surprisingly, patients with dEEG-only seizures had worse functional outcome at 3 months than patients with both sEEG and dEEG seizures (50% versus 25% death or severe disability, respectively) [85]. The authors speculate that the failure of seizures to propagate to sufficiently large regions of cortex so as to be seen on sEEG may reflect more severe cortical or subcortical injury.

The question whether seizures on dEEG carry clinical significance and demand treatment is unanswered at this point. It is unclear whether dEEG seizures are an epiphenomenon indicative of severe brain damage (and thus associated with worse outcomes), or if they are causing further brain injury. However, the available evidence on physiologic changes during dEEG seizures with the eventual depletion of energy substrates and brain tissue oxygen, and with the increase of metabolic stress markers, provides good arguments that dEEG seizures are not essentially different from sEEG seizures and therefore should probably be treated [81, 85]. Another study in 479 patients with spontaneous SAH tested the hypothesis of a causal link between post-SAH inflammation and seizures. Patients with seizures compared to patients without seizures on cEEG had higher Systemic Inflammatory Response Syndrome (SIRS) scores. It was furthermore shown that the concentrations of several serum biomarkers of inflammation were higher in patients with seizures. The authors also conducted a mediation analysis showing a potentially causal link between inflammatory response post-SAH and poor long-term outcome mediated by seizures [98].

Future research should establish frequency and significance of dEEG seizures in forms of brain injury. To avoid oversimplifications by assuming causal relationships between coincidental or associated observations, mediation analysis might be a useful tool to approach the difficult problem of causality [133]. Ultimately such efforts serve the purpose of defining the most promising treatment target to improve clinical outcomes after acute brain injury.

Acknowledgements J.W.'s work was supported by Deutsche Forschungsgemeinschaft (Research Fellowship Wi 4300/1-1).

References

1. Rajshekhar V, Harbaugh RE. Results of routine ventriculostomy with external ventricular drainage for acute hydrocephalus following subarachnoid haemorrhage. Acta Neurochir. 1992;115: 8–14.
2. Hasan D, Vermeulen M, Wijdicks EF, Hijdra A, van Gijn J. Management problems in acute hydrocephalus after subarachnoid hemorrhage. Stroke. 1989;20:747–53.
3. Lescot T, Reina V, Le Manach Y, Boroli F, Chauvet D, Boch A-L, et al. In vivo accuracy of two intraparenchymal intracranial pressure monitors. Intensive Care Med. 2011;37:875–9.
4. Le Roux P, Menon DK, Citerio G, Vespa P, Bader MK, Brophy G, et al. The International Multidisciplinary Consensus Conference on Multimodality Monitoring in Neurocritical Care: a list of recommendations and additional conclusions: a statement for healthcare professionals from the Neurocritical Care Society and the European. Neurocrit Care. 2014;21(Suppl. 2):S282–96.
5. Sahjpaul R, Girotti M. Intracranial pressure monitoring in severe traumatic brain injury–results of a Canadian survey. Can J Neurol Sci. 2000;27:143–7.
6. Stocchetti N, Penny KI, Dearden M, Braakman R, Cohadon F, Iannotti F, et al. Intensive care management of head-injured patients in Europe: a survey from the European brain injury consortium. Intensive Care Med. 2001;27:400–6.
7. Le Roux PD, Elliott JP, Newell DW, Grady MS, Winn HR. Predicting outcome in poor-grade patients with subarachnoid hemorrhage: a retrospective review of 159 aggressively managed cases. J Neurosurg. 1996;85:39–49.
8. Ransom ER, Mocco J, Komotar RJ, Sahni D, Chang J, Hahn DK, et al. External ventricular drainage response in poor grade aneurysmal subarachnoid hemorrhage: effect on preoperative grading and prognosis. Neurocrit Care. 2007;6:174–80.
9. Badri S, Chen J, Barber J, Temkin NR, Dikmen SS, Chesnut RM, et al. Mortality and long-term functional outcome associated with intracranial pressure after traumatic brain injury. Intensive Care Med. 2012;38:1800–9.
10. Chesnut RM, Temkin N, Carney N, Dikmen S, Rondina C, Videtta W, et al. A trial of intracranial-pressure monitoring in traumatic brain injury. N Engl J Med. 2012;367:2471–81.
11. Sykora M, Czosnyka M, Liu X, Donnelly J, Nasr N, Diedler J, et al. Autonomic impairment in severe traumatic brain injury: a multimodal neuromonitoring study. Crit Care Med. 2016;44:1173.
12. Forsyth RJ, Raper J, Todhunter E. Routine intracranial pressure monitoring in acute coma. Cochrane Database Syst Rev. 2015;11:CD002043.
13. Helbok R, Olson DM, Le Roux PD, Vespa P. Intracranial pressure and cerebral perfusion pressure monitoring in non-TBI patients: special considerations. Neurocrit Care. 2014;21(Suppl. 2): S85–94.
14. Heuer GG, Smith MJ, Elliott JP, Winn HR, LeRoux PD. Relationship between intracranial pressure and other clinical variables in patients with aneurysmal subarachnoid hemorrhage. J Neurosurg. 2004;101:408–16.
15. Lv Y, Wang D, Lei J, Tan G. Clinical observation of the time course of raised intracranial pressure after subarachnoid hemorrhage. Neurol Sci. 2015;36:1203–10.
16. Magni F, Pozzi M, Rota M, Vargiolu A, Citerio G. High-resolution intracranial pressure burden and outcome in subarachnoid hemorrhage. Stroke. 2015;46:2464–9.
17. Nagel A, Graetz D, Schink T, Frieler K, Sakowitz O, Vajkoczy P, et al. Relevance of intracranial hypertension for cerebral metabolism in aneurysmal subarachnoid hemorrhage. J Neurosurg. 2009;111:94–101.
18. Hickey JV, Olson DM, Turner DA. Intracranial pressure waveform analysis during rest and suctioning. Biol Res Nurs. 2009;11: 174–86.
19. Olson DM, Andrew Kofke W, O'Phelan K, Gupta PK, Figueroa SA, Smirnakis SM, et al. Global monitoring in the neurocritical care unit. Neurocrit Care. 2015;22:337–47.
20. Kolias AG, Kirkpatrick PJ, Hutchinson PJ. Decompressive craniectomy: past, present and future. Nat Rev Neurosci. 2013;9: 405–15.
21. Zweifel C, Lavinio A, Steiner LA, Radolovich D, Smielewski P, Timofeev I, et al. Continuous monitoring of cerebrovascular pressure reactivity in patients with head injury. Neurosurg Focus. 2008;25:E2.
22. Steiner LA, Czosnyka M, Piechnik SK, Smielewski P, Chatfield D, Menon DK, et al. Continuous monitoring of cerebrovascular pressure reactivity allows determination of optimal cerebral perfusion pressure in patients with traumatic brain injury. Crit Care Med. 2002;30:733–8.
23. Gesang D, Zhang D, Zhao J, Wang S, Zhao Y, Wang R, et al. Laser Doppler flowmeter study on regional cerebral blood flow in early stage after standard superficial temporal artery-middle cerebral artery bypass surgery for moyamoya disease. Chin Med J. 2009; 122:2412–8.
24. Vajkoczy P, Roth H, Horn P, Lucke T, Thomé C, Hubner U, et al. Continuous monitoring of regional cerebral blood flow: experimental and clinical validation of a novel thermal diffusion microprobe. J Neurosurg. 2000;93:265–74.
25. Bratton SL, Chestnut RM, Ghajar J, McConnell Hammond FF, Harris OA, Hartl R, et al. Guidelines for the management of severe traumatic brain injury. IX. Cerebral perfusion thresholds. J Neurotrauma. 2007;24(Suppl. 1):S59–64.
26. Schmidt JM, Ko S-B, Helbok R, Kurtz P, Stuart RM, Presciutti M, et al. Cerebral perfusion pressure thresholds for brain tissue hypoxia and metabolic crisis after poor-grade subarachnoid hemorrhage. Stroke. 2011;42:1351–6.

27. Diedler J, Santos E, Poli S, Sykora M. Optimal cerebral perfusion pressure in patients with intracerebral hemorrhage: an observational case series. Crit Care. 2014;18:R51.
28. Czosnyka M, Miller C. Monitoring of cerebral autoregulation. Neurocrit Care. 2014;21(Suppl. 2):S95–102.
29. Barth M, Woitzik J, Weiss C, Muench E, Diepers M, Schmiedek P, et al. Correlation of clinical outcome with pressure-, oxygen-, and flow-related indices of cerebrovascular reactivity in patients following aneurysmal SAH. Neurocrit Care. 2010;12:234–43.
30. Bijlenga P, Czosnyka M, Budohoski KP, Soehle M, Pickard JD, Kirkpatrick PJ, et al. "Optimal cerebral perfusion pressure" in poor grade patients after subarachnoid hemorrhage. Neurocrit Care. 2010;13:17–23.
31. Howells T, Elf K, Jones PA, Ronne-Engström E, Piper I, Nilsson P, et al. Pressure reactivity as a guide in the treatment of cerebral perfusion pressure in patients with brain trauma. J Neurosurg. 2005;102:311–7.
32. Rasulo FA, Girardini A, Lavinio A, De Peri E, Stefini R, Cenzato M, et al. Are optimal cerebral perfusion pressure and cerebrovascular autoregulation related to long-term outcome in patients with aneurysmal subarachnoid hemorrhage? J Neurosurg Anesthesiol. 2012;24:3–8.
33. Depreitere B, Güiza F, Van den Berghe G, Schuhmann MU, Maier G, Piper I, et al. Pressure autoregulation monitoring and cerebral perfusion pressure target recommendation in patients with severe traumatic brain injury based on minute-by-minute monitoring data. J Neurosurg. 2014;120:1451–7.
34. Frontera J, Ziai W, O'Phelan K, Leroux PD, Kirkpatrick PJ, Diringer MN, et al. Regional brain monitoring in the neurocritical care unit. Neurocrit Care. 2015;22:348–59.
35. Dengl M, Jaeger M, Renner C, Meixensberger J. Comparing brain tissue oxygen measurements and derived autoregulation parameters from different probes (Licox vs. Raumedic). Acta Neurochir Suppl. 2012;114:165–8.
36. Maas AI, Fleckenstein W, de Jong DA, van Santbrink H. Monitoring cerebral oxygenation: experimental studies and preliminary clinical results of continuous monitoring of cerebrospinal fluid and brain tissue oxygen tension. Acta Neurochir Suppl (Wien). 1993;59:50–7.
37. Purins K, Enblad P, Sandhagen B, Lewén A. Brain tissue oxygen monitoring: a study of in vitro accuracy and stability of Neurovent-PTO and Licox sensors. Acta Neurochir. 2010;152:681–8.
38. Stewart C, Haitsma I, Zador Z, Hemphill JC, Morabito D, Manley G, et al. The new Licox combined brain tissue oxygen and brain temperature monitor: assessment of in vitro accuracy and clinical experience in severe traumatic brain injury. Neurosurgery. 2008;63:1159–64. discussion 1164–5
39. Orakcioglu B, Sakowitz OW, Neumann J-O, Kentar MM, Unterberg A, Kiening KL. Evaluation of a novel brain tissue oxygenation probe in an experimental swine model. Neurosurgery. 2010;67:1716–22. discussion 1722–3
40. Dengler J, Frenzel C, Vajkoczy P, Wolf S, Horn P. Cerebral tissue oxygenation measured by two different probes: challenges and interpretation. Intensive Care Med. 2011;37:1809–15.
41. Dengler J, Frenzel C, Vajkoczy P, Horn P, Wolf S. The oxygen reactivity index and its relation to sensor technology in patients with severe brain lesions. Neurocrit Care. 2013;19:74–8.
42. Pennings FA, Schuurman PR, van den Munckhof P, Bouma GJ. Brain tissue oxygen pressure monitoring in awake patients during functional neurosurgery: the assessment of normal values. J Neurotrauma. 2008;25:1173–7.
43. Chen HI, Stiefel MF, Oddo M, Milby AH, Maloney-Wilensky E, Frangos S, et al. Detection of cerebral compromise with multimodality monitoring in patients with subarachnoid hemorrhage. Neurosurgery. 2011;69:53–63. discussion 63

44. Väth A, Kunze E, Roosen K, Meixensberger J. Therapeutic aspects of brain tissue pO_2 monitoring after subarachnoid hemorrhage. Acta Neurochir Suppl. 2002;81:307–9.
45. Ang BT, Wong J, Lee KK, Wang E, Ng I. Temporal changes in cerebral tissue oxygenation with cerebrovascular pressure reactivity in severe traumatic brain injury. J Neurol Neurosurg Psychiatry. 2007;78:298–302.
46. Stiefel MF, Udoetuk JD, Spiotta AM, Gracias VH, Goldberg A, Maloney-Wilensky E, et al. Conventional neurocritical care and cerebral oxygenation after traumatic brain injury. J Neurosurg. 2006;105:568–75.
47. Kett-White R, Hutchinson PJ, Al-Rawi PG, Gupta AK, Pickard JD, Kirkpatrick PJ. Adverse cerebral events detected after subarachnoid hemorrhage using brain oxygen and microdialysis probes. Neurosurgery. 2002;50:1213–21. discussion 1221–2
48. Oddo M, Bösel J. Monitoring of brain and systemic oxygenation in neurocritical care patients. Neurocrit Care. 2014;21(Suppl. 2):S103–20.
49. Bouzat P, Marques-Vidal P, Zerlauth J-B, Sala N, Suys T, Schoettker P, et al. Accuracy of brain multimodal monitoring to detect cerebral hypoperfusion after traumatic brain injury. Crit Care Med. 2015;43:445–52.
50. Palmer S, Bader MK. Brain tissue oxygenation in brain death. Neurocrit Care. 2005;2:17–22.
51. Bohman L-E, Pisapia JM, Sanborn MR, Frangos S, Lin E, Kumar M, et al. Response of brain oxygen to therapy correlates with long-term outcome after subarachnoid hemorrhage. Neurocrit Care. 2013;19:320–8.
52. Ungerstedt U. Microdialysis–principles and applications for studies in animals and man. J Intern Med. 1991;230:365–73.
53. Hillered L, Vespa PM, Hovda DA. Translational neurochemical research in acute human brain injury: the current status and potential future for cerebral microdialysis. J Neurotrauma. 2005;22:3–41.
54. Unterberg AW, Sakowitz OW, Sarrafzadeh AS, Benndorf G, Lanksch WR. Role of bedside microdialysis in the diagnosis of cerebral vasospasm following aneurysmal subarachnoid hemorrhage. J Neurosurg. 2001;94:740–9.
55. Hutchinson PJ. Microdialysis in traumatic brain injury–methodology and pathophysiology. Acta Neurochir Suppl. 2005;95:441–5.
56. Andrews PJD, Citerio G, Longhi L, Polderman K, Sahuquillo J, Vajkoczy P. NICEM consensus on neurological monitoring in acute neurological disease. Intensive Care Med. 2008;34:1362–70.
57. Bellander B-M, Cantais E, Enblad P, Hutchinson P, Nordström C-H, Robertson C, et al. Consensus meeting on microdialysis in neurointensive care. Intensive Care Med. 2004;30:2166–9.
58. Persson L, Valtysson J, Enblad P, Warme PE, Cesarini K, Lewen A, et al. Neurochemical monitoring using intracerebral microdialysis in patients with subarachnoid hemorrhage. J Neurosurg. 1996;84:606–16.
59. Timofeev I, Carpenter KLH, Nortje J, Al-Rawi PG, O'Connell MT, Czosnyka M, et al. Cerebral extracellular chemistry and outcome following traumatic brain injury: a microdialysis study of 223 patients. Brain. 2011;134:484–94.
60. Hutchinson PJ, Jalloh I, Helmy A, Carpenter KLH, Rostami E, Bellander B-M, et al. Consensus statement from the 2014 International Microdialysis Forum. Intensive Care Med. 2015;41:1517–28.
61. Nilsson OG, Brandt L, Ungerstedt U, Säveland H. Bedside detection of brain ischemia using intracerebral microdialysis: subarachnoid hemorrhage and delayed ischemic deterioration. Neurosurgery. 1999;45:1176–84. discussion 1184–5
62. Reinstrup P, Ståhl N, Mellergård P, Uski T, Ungerstedt U, Nordström CH. Intracerebral microdialysis in clinical practice: baseline values for chemical markers during wakefulness,

anesthesia, and neurosurgery. Neurosurgery. 2000;47:701–9. discussion 709–10

63. Hlatky R, Valadka AB, Goodman JC, Contant CF, Robertson CS. Patterns of energy substrates during ischemia measured in the brain by microdialysis. J Neurotrauma. 2004;21:894–906.

64. Sarrafzadeh A, Haux D, Sakowitz O, Benndorf G, Herzog H, Kuechler I, et al. Acute focal neurological deficits in aneurysmal subarachnoid hemorrhage: relation of clinical course, CT findings, and metabolite abnormalities monitored with bedside microdialysis. Stroke. 2003;34:1382–8.

65. Helbok R, Schmidt JM, Kurtz P, Hanafy KA, Fernandez L, Stuart RM, et al. Systemic glucose and brain energy metabolism after subarachnoid hemorrhage. Neurocrit Care. 2010;12:317–23.

66. Ko S-B, Choi HA, Parikh G, Helbok R, Schmidt JM, Lee K, et al. Multimodality monitoring for cerebral perfusion pressure optimization in comatose patients with intracerebral hemorrhage. Stroke. 2011;42:3087–92.

67. Oddo M, Milby A, Chen I, Frangos S, MacMurtrie E, Maloney-Wilensky E, et al. Hemoglobin concentration and cerebral metabolism in patients with aneurysmal subarachnoid hemorrhage. Stroke. 2009;40:1275–81.

68. Claassen J, Vespa P. Electrophysiologic monitoring in acute brain injury. Neurocrit Care. 2014;21:129.

69. Moura LMVR, Shafi MM, Ng M, Pati S, Cash SS, Cole AJ, et al. Spectrogram screening of adult EEGs is sensitive and efficient. Neurology. 2014;83:56–64.

70. Tanner AEJ, Särkelä MOK, Virtanen J, Viertiö-Oja HE, Sharpe MD, Norton L, et al. Application of subhairline EEG montage in intensive care unit: comparison with full montage. J Clin Neurophysiol. 2014;31:181–6.

71. Suzuki A, Mori N, Hadeishi H, Yoshioka K, Yasui N. Computerized monitoring system in neurosurgical intensive care. J Neurosci Methods. 1988;26:133–9.

72. Agarwal R, Gotman J, Flanagan D, Rosenblatt B. Automatic EEG analysis during long-term monitoring in the ICU. Electroencephalogr Clin Neurophysiol. 1998;107:44–58.

73. Claassen J, Hirsch LJ, Kreiter KT, Du EY, Connolly ES, Emerson RG, et al. Quantitative continuous EEG for detecting delayed cerebral ischemia in patients with poor-grade subarachnoid hemorrhage. Clin Neurophysiol. 2004;115:2699–710.

74. Murray DM, Boylan GB, Ali I, Ryan CA, Murphy BP, Connolly S. Defining the gap between electrographic seizure burden, clinical expression and staff recognition of neonatal seizures. Arch Dis Child Fetal Neonatal Ed. 2008;93:F187–91.

75. Sackellares JC, Shiau D-S, Halford JJ, LaRoche SM, Kelly KM. Quantitative EEG analysis for automated detection of nonconvulsive seizures in intensive care units. Epilepsy Behav. 2011;22(Suppl. 1):S69–73.

76. Stewart CP, Otsubo H, Ochi A, Sharma R, Hutchison JS, Hahn CD. Seizure identification in the ICU using quantitative EEG displays. Neurology. 2010;75:1501–8.

77. Akman CI, Micic V, Thompson A, Riviello JJ. Seizure detection using digital trend analysis: factors affecting utility. Epilepsy Res. 2011;93:66–72.

78. Behrens E, Zentner J, van Roost D, Hufnagel A, Elger CE, Schramm J. Subdural and depth electrodes in the presurgical evaluation of epilepsy. Acta Neurochir. 1994;128:84–7.

79. Stuart RM, Schmidt M, Kurtz P, Waziri A, Helbok R, Mayer SA, et al. Intracranial multimodal monitoring for acute brain injury: a single institution review of current practices. Neurocrit Care. 2010;12:188–98.

80. Waziri A, Claassen J, Stuart RM, Arif H, Schmidt JM, Mayer SA, et al. Intracortical electroencephalography in acute brain injury. Ann Neurol. 2009;66:366–77.

81. Vespa P, Tubi M, Claassen J, Blanco M, McArthur D, Velazquez AG, et al. Metabolic crisis occurs with seizures and periodic discharges after brain trauma. Ann Neurol. 2016;79:579.

82. Sandsmark DK, Kumar MA, Park S, Levine JM. Multimodal monitoring in subarachnoid hemorrhage. Stroke. 2012;43:1440–5.

83. Sakowitz OW, Santos E, Nagel A, Krajewski KL, Hertle DN, Vajkoczy P, et al. Clusters of spreading depolarizations are associated with disturbed cerebral metabolism in patients with aneurysmal subarachnoid hemorrhage. Stroke. 2013;44:220–3.

84. Vespa P, Prins M, Ronne-Engstrom E, Caron M, Shalmon E, Hovda DA, et al. Increase in extracellular glutamate caused by reduced cerebral perfusion pressure and seizures after human traumatic brain injury: a microdialysis study. J Neurosurg. 1998;89:971–82.

85. Claassen J, Perotte A, Albers D, Kleinberg S, Schmidt JM, Tu B, et al. Nonconvulsive seizures after subarachnoid hemorrhage: multimodal detection and outcomes. Ann Neurol. 2013;74:53–64.

86. Nangunoori R, Maloney-Wilensky E, Stiefel M, Park S, Andrew Kofke W, Levine JM, et al. Brain tissue oxygen-based therapy and outcome after severe traumatic brain injury: a systematic literature review. Neurocrit Care. 2012;17:131–8.

87. De Marchis GM, Pugin D, Meyers E, Velasquez A, Suwatcharangkoon S, Park S, et al. Seizure burden in subarachnoid hemorrhage associated with functional and cognitive outcome. Neurology. 2016;86:253 60.

88. Claassen J, Hirsch LJ, Frontera JA, Fernandez A, Schmidt M, Wittman J, et al. Prognostic significance of continuous eeg monitoring in patients with poor-grade subarachnoid hemorrhage. Neurocrit Care. 2006;4:103–12.

89. Rossetti AO, Urbano LA, Delodder F, Kaplan PW, Oddo M. Prognostic value of continuous EEG monitoring during therapeutic hypothermia after cardiac arrest. Crit Care. 2010;14:R173.

90. Claassen J, Jetté N, Chum F, Green R, Schmidt M, Choi H, et al. Electrographic seizures and periodic discharges after intracerebral hemorrhage. Neurology. 2007;69:1356–65.

91. Vespa PM, O'Phelan K, Shah M, Mirabelli J, Starkman S, Kidwell C, et al. Acute seizures after intracerebral hemorrhage: a factor in progressive midline shift and outcome. Neurology. 2003;60:1441–6.

92. Vespa PM, Nuwer MR, Nenov V, Ronne-Engstrom E, Hovda DA, Bergsneider M, et al. Increased incidence and impact of nonconvulsive and convulsive seizures after traumatic brain injury as detected by continuous electroencephalographic monitoring. J Neurosurg. 1999;91:750–60.

93. Ronne-Engstrom E, Winkler T. Continuous EEG monitoring in patients with traumatic brain injury reveals a high incidence of epileptiform activity. Acta Neurol Scand. 2006;114:47–53.

94. Carrera E, Claassen J, Oddo M, Emerson RG, Mayer SA, Hirsch LJ. Continuous electroencephalographic monitoring in critically ill patients with central nervous system infections. Arch Neurol. 2008;65:1612–8.

95. Kurtz P, Gaspard N, Wahl AS, Bauer RM, Hirsch LJ, Wunsch H, et al. Continuous electroencephalography in a surgical intensive care unit. Intensive Care Med. 2014;40:228–34.

96. Oddo M, Carrera E, Claassen J, Mayer SA, Hirsch LJ. Continuous electroencephalography in the medical intensive care unit. Crit Care Med. 2009;37:2051.

97. Chong DJ, Hirsch LJ. Which EEG patterns warrant treatment in the critically ill? Reviewing the evidence for treatment of periodic epileptiform discharges and related patterns. J Clin Neurophysiol. 2005;22:79–91.

98. Claassen J, Albers D, Schmidt JM, De Marchis GM, Pugin D, Falo CM, et al. Nonconvulsive seizures in subarachnoid hemorrhage link inflammation and outcome. Ann Neurol. 2014;75:771–81.

99. Snyder JV, Nemoto EM, Carroll RG, Safar P. Global ischemia in dogs: intracranial pressures, brain blood flow and metabolism. Stroke. 6:21–7.

100. Oddo M, Villa F, Citerio G. Brain multimodality monitoring: an update. Curr Opin Crit Care. 2012;18:111–8.

101. Penfield W, von Sántha K, Cipriani A. Cerebral blood flow during induced epileptiform seizures in animals and man. J Neurophysiol. 1939;2:257–67.

102. Meldrum BS, Nilsson B. Cerebral blood flow and metabolic rate early and late in prolonged epileptic seizures induced in rats by bicuculline. Brain. 1976;99:523–42.

103. Suzuki R, Nitsch C, Fujiwara K, Klatzo I. Regional changes in cerebral blood flow and blood-brain barrier permeability during epileptiform seizures and in acute hypertension in rabbits. J Cereb Blood Flow Metab. 1984;4:96–102.

104. Choy M, Wells JA, Thomas DL, Gadian DG, Scott RC, Lythgoe MF. Cerebral blood flow changes during pilocarpine-induced status epilepticus activity in the rat hippocampus. Exp Neurol. 2010;225:196–201.

105. Meldrum BS, Vigouroux RA, Brierley JB. Systemic factors and epileptic brain damage. Prolonged seizures in paralyzed, artificially ventilated baboons. Arch Neurol. 1973;29:82–7.

106. Freund TF, Buzsáki G, Prohaska OJ, Leon A, Somogyi P. Simultaneous recording of local electrical activity, partial oxygen tension and temperature in the rat hippocampus with a chamber-type microelectrode. Effects of anaesthesia, ischemia and epilepsy. Neuroscience. 1989;28:539–49.

107. Kreisman NR, Sick TJ, Rosenthal M. Concepts of brain oxygen sufficiency during seizures. Adv Exp Med Biol. 1984;180: 381–92.

108. Kreisman NR, Sick TJ, LaManna JC, Rosenthal M. Local tissue oxygen tension-cytochrome a,a3 redox relationships in rat cerebral cortex in vivo. Brain Res. 1981;218:161–74.

109. Gonzalez H, Hunter CJ, Bennet L, Power GG, Gunn AJ. Cerebral oxygenation during postasphyxial seizures in near-term fetal sheep. J Cereb Blood Flow Metab. 2005;25:911–8.

110. Goitein KJ, Shohami E. Intracranial pressure during prolonged experimental convulsions in cats. J Neurol. 1983;230:259–66.

111. Zweckberger K, Simunovic F, Kiening KL, Unterberg AW, Sakowitz OW. Anticonvulsive effects of the dopamine agonist lisuride maleate after experimental traumatic brain injury. Neurosci Lett. 2010;470:150–4.

112. Imran I, Hillert MH, Klein J. Early metabolic responses to lithium/pilocarpine-induced status epilepticus in rat brain. J Neurochem. 2015;135:1007–18.

113. Blennow G, Folbergrova J, Nilsson B, Siesjö BK. Cerebral metabolic and circulatory changes in the rat during sustained seizures induced by DL-homocysteine. Brain Res. 1979;179:129–46.

114. Millan MH, Obrenovitch TP, Sarna GS, Lok SY, Symon L, Meldrum BS. Changes in rat brain extracellular glutamate concentration during seizures induced by systemic picrotoxin or focal bicuculline injection: an in vivo dialysis study with on-line enzymatic detection. Epilepsy Res. 1991;9:86–91.

115. Nahorski SR, Roberts DJ, Stewart GG. Some neurochemical aspects of pentamethylenetetrazole convulsive activity in rat brain. J Neurochem. 1970;17:621–31.

116. Nilsson P, Ronne-Engström E, Flink R, Ungerstedt U, Carlson H, Hillered L. Epileptic seizure activity in the acute phase following cortical impact trauma in rat. Brain Res. 1994;637:227–32.

117. Liu Z, Stafstrom CE, Sarkisian MR, Yang Y, Hori A, Tandon P, et al. Seizure-induced glutamate release in mature and immature animals: an in vivo microdialysis study. Neuroreport. 1997;8:2019–23.

118. Stephens ML, Pomerleau F, Huettl P, Gerhardt GA, Zhang Z. Real-time glutamate measurements in the putamen of awake rhesus monkeys using an enzyme-based human microelectrode array prototype. J Neurosci Methods. 2010;185:264–72.

119. Kuhl DE, Engel J, Phelps ME, Selin C. Epileptic patterns of local cerebral metabolism and perfusion in humans determined by emission computed tomography of ^{18}FDG and ^{13}NH$_3$. Ann Neurol. 1980;8:348–60.

120. Rostami E, Engquist H, Enblad P. Imaging of cerebral blood flow in patients with severe traumatic brain injury in the neurointensive care. Front Neurol. 2014;5:114.

121. Vespa PM, Miller C, McArthur D, Eliseo M, Etchepare M, Hirt D, et al. Nonconvulsive electrographic seizures after traumatic brain injury result in a delayed, prolonged increase in intracranial pressure and metabolic crisis. Crit Care Med. 2007;35:2830–6.

122. Devinsky O. Effects of seizures on autonomic and cardiovascular function. Epilepsy Curr. 2004;4:43–6.

123. Sutherland GR, Ross BD, Lesiuk H, Peeling J, Pillay N, Pinsky C. Phosphate energy metabolism during domoic acid-induced seizures. Epilepsia. 34:996–1002.

124. Vespa PM, McArthur D, O'Phelan K, Glenn T, Etchepare M, Kelly D, et al. Persistently low extracellular glucose correlates with poor outcome 6 months after human traumatic brain injury despite a lack of increased lactate: a microdialysis study. J Cereb Blood Flow Metab. 2003;23:865–77.

125. Vespa P, Boonyaputthikul R, McArthur DL, Miller C, Etchepare M, Bergsneider M, et al. Intensive insulin therapy reduces microdialysis glucose values without altering glucose utilization or improving the lactate/pyruvate ratio after traumatic brain injury. Crit Care Med. 2006;34:850–6.

126. During MJ, Fried I, Leone P, Katz A, Spencer DD. Direct measurement of extracellular lactate in the human hippocampus during spontaneous seizures. J Neurochem. 1994;62:2356–61.

127. Dienel GA. Lactate shuttling and lactate use as fuel after traumatic brain injury: metabolic considerations. J Cereb Blood Flow Metab. 2014;34:1736–48.

128. Meldrum BS. The role of glutamate in epilepsy and other CNS disorders. Neurology. 1994;44:S14–23.

129. Cavus I, Kasoff WS, Cassaday MP, Jacob R, Gueorguieva R, Sherwin RS, et al. Extracellular metabolites in the cortex and hippocampus of epileptic patients. Ann Neurol. 2005;57:226–35.

130. Ronne-Engström E, Hillered L, Flink R, Spännare B, Ungerstedt U, Carlson H. Intracerebral microdialysis of extracellular amino acids in the human epileptic focus. J Cereb Blood Flow Metab. 1992;12:873–6.

131. Ungerstedt U, Rostami E. Microdialysis in neurointensive care. Curr Pharm Des. 2004;10:2145–52.

132. Vespa P, Martin NA, Nenov V, Glenn T, Bergsneider M, Kelly D, et al. Delayed increase in extracellular glycerol with post-traumatic electrographic epileptic activity: support for the theory that seizures induce secondary injury. Acta Neurochir Suppl. 2002;81:355–7.

133. Pearl J. Interpretation and identification of causal mediation. Psychol Methods. 2014;19:459–81.

Christa B. Swisher and Aatif M. Husain

Introduction

Seizures are a common occurrence in critically ill patients, especially those with acute neurologic injury. The vast majority of seizures in critically ill patients are nonconvulsive, therefore continuous electroencephalography (cEEG) monitoring is required for the diagnosis and to guide medication management. The emergent treatment of seizures with benzodiazepines and subsequent treatment with non-sedating antiepileptic drugs (AEDs) will be discussed in this chapter. The use of intravenous sedating AEDs for seizure management will be discussed in another chapter.

It has been well established that generalized convulsive status epilepticus (GCSE) is a medical emergency that requires immediate and aggressive treatment due to its high morbidity and mortality. However, the urgency of treatment for nonconvulsive seizures (NCS) and nonconvulsive status epilepticus (NCSE) is less certain. Since there is a relative paucity of data for the treatment of NCS and NCSE, the treatment of NCS and NCSE has reflected that of GCSE. This practice may be leading to over-treatment with intravenous sedating medications and potentially adverse outcomes. The concept of "appropriately aggressive treatment" has arisen from the notion that seizure types such as NCS and NCSE are less damaging to the brain than GCSE, and therefore may not need to be as aggressively. A clinical trial has recently been completed that provides a comparison between two

treatments for NCS. Ongoing advances in the field of seizure management in critically ill patients will hopefully lead to improved treatment paradigms for NCS and NCSE.

Definitions

Convulsive Seizures

Convulsive seizures include any seizure type that presents with an obvious clinical manifestation. These are the easiest type of seizures to recognize, however, these represent only a minority of seizures in patients with acute neurologic illness. In a study by Claassen et al., only 8% of seizures seen in critically ill patients were classified as convulsive [1]. The clinical manifestations of convulsive seizures in critically ill patients can be similar to those seen in patients with epilepsy (generalized tonic-clonic seizures, clonic seizures, tonic seizures, complex partial seizures, myoclonic seizures, partial-onset seizures evolving to secondarily generalized seizures, and simple partial seizures).

Generalized Convulsive Status Epilepticus

Status epilepticus (SE) is classified by the type of onset (partial or generalized) and primary motor function (tonic, clonic, atonic, etc.) [2]. A common type of convulsive status epilepticus (CSE) is GCSE. The definition of GCSE has evolved since it was first defined in the 1960s by the International League Against Epilepsy (ILAE) as a "seizure [that] persists for a sufficient length of time or is repeated enough to produce a fixed and enduring epileptic condition" [3]. Since this definition did not include guidelines of the time limitation to differentiate GCSE, the Working Group on Status Epilepticus modified the definition of GCSE as follows: continuous, generalized seizure activity lasting longer than 30 min or ≥2 generalized seizures within a 30-min period without full recovery of consciousness between

C.B. Swisher
Department of Neurology, Duke University Medical Center, Durham, NC 27710, USA
e-mail: christa.swisher@duke.edu

A.M. Husain (✉)
Department of Neurology, Duke University Medical Center, Durham, NC 27710, USA

Neurodiagnostic Center, Department of Veterans Affairs Medical Center, Durham, NC 27705, USA
e-mail: aatif.husain@duke.edu

© Springer International Publishing AG 2017
P.N. Varelas, J. Claassen (eds.), *Seizures in Critical Care*, Current Clinical Neurology, DOI 10.1007/978-3-319-49557-6_7

seizures [4]. Because most seizures have spontaneous cessation within 5 min [5, 6] and since animal data shows permanent neuronal injury before 30 min of continuous seizure activity has occurred [7], the revised definition of GCSE proposed by the Neurocritical Care Society is as follows: a single seizure lasting longer than 5 min or recurrent, discrete seizures without clinical recovery in between [8]. GCSE is a neurological emergency because it is associated with significant morbidity and mortality. The goal of the revised definition is to encourage more aggressive initial therapy for GCSE, reduce the number of refractory GCSE cases, and reduce the number of patients with recurrent GCSE.

Nonconvulsive Seizures

Up to 92% of seizures in patients with acute brain injury are nonconvulsive [1]. Nonconvulsive seizures (NCS) are diagnosed only with electroencephalography (EEG) and are defined as seizures lasting at least 10 s that have either no clinical manifestations or subtle clinical manifestations (such as facial or limb twitching, nystagmus, sustained gaze deviation, catatonia and psychosis) [9]. The EEG criteria for the diagnosis of NCS is made by the presence of one of the following: (1) repetitive generalized or focal epileptiform discharges at a rate of ≥ 3 Hz or (2) repetitive generalized or focal epileptiform discharges at a rate of < 3 Hz and the presence of the secondary criterion (significant improvement in the clinical state or appearance of the previously absent normal EEG patterns in response to acute administration of a rapid-acting AED, such as a benzodiazepine) or (3) sequential rhythmic, periodic, or quasiperiodic waves at >1 Hz and unequivocal evolution in frequency, morphology, or spatial extent [10]. NCS that continue despite adequate first- and second-line therapy (but do not meet the definition for NCSE) are considered refractory NCS. In the literature, the term electrographic seizure (ESz) is used interchangeably with NCS.

Nonconvulsive Status Epilepticus

The two phenotypes of nonconvulsive status epilepticus (NCSE) include (1) patients with new-onset epileptic phenomenon or patients with chronic epileptic syndromes that present to the emergency department as "wandering confused" patients or (2) patients that have an acute critical illness and have clinical manifestations of impairment in mental status with or without subtle motor movements [8] (described in NCS section above). Patients with NCSE may have subtle motor manifestations and this clinical condition is sometimes referred to as "subtle status epilepticus."

There have been several proposals to define NCSE among various organizations. The definition of SE as proposed by the Neurocritical Care Society includes 5 or more minutes of continuous electrographic seizure activity and/or recurrent electrographic seizure activity without recovery between seizures [8]. However, it is very difficult to assess clinical recovery between seizures in critically ill patients with acute neurologic injury.

A unified definition of NCSE was proposed in 2013 at the 4th London-Innsbruck Status Epilepticus Colloquium and has been widely adopted. For patients without known epileptic encephalopathy, NCSE is defined as (1) epileptiform discharges >2.5 Hz, OR (2) epileptiform discharges ≤ 2.5 Hz OR rhythmic delta/theta activity (>0.5 Hz) AND one of the following: (a) EEG and clinical improvement after IV AED, OR (b) subtle clinical ictal phenomena during the EEG patterns mentioned above, OR (c) typical spatiotemporal evolution. For patients with known epileptic encephalopathy, NCSE is defined as: (1) an increase in prominence or frequency of the features mentioned above, when compared to baseline with observable change in clinical state, OR (2) improvement of clinical and EEG features with IV AEDs. It is noted in the definition that "if EEG improvement occurs without clinical improvement, or if fluctuation without definite evolution, this should be considered possible NCSE." The definition of typical spatiotemporal evolution is defined as "incrementing onset (increase in voltage and change in frequency), or evolution in pattern (change in frequency >1 Hz or change in location), or decrementing termination (voltage or frequency)" [11].

It should be noted that another commonly used clinical and research definition for the diagnosis of NCSE is electrographic seizure activity lasting >30 min per hour of continuous electroencephalography (cEEG) recording [12]. This definition is criticized by experts because it introduces bias against NCSE morbidity, by suggesting that NCSE requires less urgent treatment than CSE, which is defined by seizure activity >5 min. This issue is discussed in more detail in the "Concept of appropriately aggressive treatment" section of this chapter.

Established Status Epilepticus

For patients presenting in SE, the standard, first-line treatment is administration of a benzodiazepine. However, in approximately 30% of patients with CSE, seizures will persist despite adequate doses of benzodiazepines, and these patients are therefore labeled as having established status epilepticus (ESE). ESE is also known as benzodiazepine-resistant SE.

Refractory Convulsive and Nonconvulsive Status Epilepticus

The definition of refractory status epilepticus (RSE) as proposed by the Neurocritical Care Society is defined as "SE that does not respond to the standard treatment regimens, such as an initial benzodiazepine followed by another AED" [8]. This definition is the same for refractory CSE and NCSE.

Super refractory Status Epilepticus

Super refractory status epilepticus (SRSE) is typically treated with intravenous anesthetic medications, although this practice has recently been questioned. SRSE is defined as "status epilepticus that continues 24 h or more after the onset of anesthesia, including those cases in which the status epilepticus recurs on the reduction or withdrawal of anesthesia" [13, 14]. This definition was created for patients that initially presented with convulsive SE. However, the same definition is widely accepted for patients that initially present with NCSE while admitted to the intensive care unit (ICU) that go on to develop SRSE after IV anesthetic AEDs fail.

Incidence of Critical Care Seizures

Based on several retrospective and prospective studies, it has been well established that approximately 20% of critically ill patients undergoing cEEG monitoring have NCS or NCSE [1, 15]. Of patients that are found to have nonconvulsive seizure activity on cEEG monitoring, one study found that approximately 75% will have NCS and 25% will have NCSE [15]. Seizures in the critically ill patient population tend to be nonconvulsive (92%) rather than convulsive (8%) [1]. The rate of NCS for critically ill patients undergoing cEEG monitoring depends on the underlying etiology: subdural hematoma approximately 43%, central nervous system infection 25–33%, postoperative from a neurosurgical procedure 18–29%, hypoxic-ischemic encephalopathy 20–54%, brain tumor 17–54%, epilepsy-related 24–56%, ischemic stroke 6–25%, traumatic brain injury (TBI) 8–28%, subarachnoid hemorrhage (SAH) 13–19%, and intracerebral hemorrhage (ICH) 13–28% [15]. Nonconvulsive seizures are often encountered in critically ill patients without known neurologic injury. A 2009 study of patients in the medical ICU without known neurologic injury undergoing cEEG monitoring found that 10% of patients have NCS [16].

Principles of Seizure Management in Critically Ill Patients

Concept of Appropriately Aggressive Treatment

NCS, refractory NCS, and NCSE are often discussed together in treatment paradigms with little differentiation between the different entities. This is further complicated by the fact that there is debate regarding specific definitions and criteria for these classifications. Assimilation of data from previous studies is difficult because outcomes of patients with SE are reported without differentiating between GCSE, NCSE, SRSE (either nonconvulsive or convulsive), and refractory NCS. Despite this, neurointensivists and neurophysiologists widely accept that there is a spectrum of severity starting with NCS at the lowest end of the spectrum and with convulsive SRSE at the highest end of the morbidity spectrum. The concept of "appropriately aggressive treatment" has arisen from the notion that the aggressiveness of therapy should depend on the degree of neuronal injury that is ongoing [12, 17, 18].

Intravenous anesthetic drugs (IVADs) are often used in patients with SE after initial benzodiazepine and a first-line AED therapy have failed. The use of IVADs necessitates intubation and mechanical ventilation due to respiratory depression. A 2009 survey of 273 neurologists, neurophysiologists, and neurointensivists revealed that more respondents were likely to suggest intubation for patients that had NCSE as opposed to NCS [19]. Additionally, respondents favored the use of non-sedating AEDs over IVADs for the treatment of NCS [19]. A retrospective analysis of 126 patients with mostly CSE found that the administration of IVADs was associated with poorer outcomes [20]. In a study of 171 patients with SE, patients treated with IVADs had more infections during SE and had a 2.9-fold relative risk of death [21]. This higher risk of death with IVAD use was independent of other clinical confounders, including different grades of SE severity and etiology. These findings have led to a heightened awareness of the adverse risks of aggressive therapy with IVADs.

The goal of AED treatment in patients with seizures is seizure cessation and prevention of neuronal injury. It is widely accepted that after 30 minutes of GCSE, there is reduction in cerebral oxygenation, cerebral glucose levels, and cerebral blood flow culminating in cerebral injury [2, 5, 22]. Due to the relatively sparse amount of data for NCSE as opposed to GCSE, it is unclear if the degree of neuronal injury in NCSE is comparable to the degree of neuronal injury in GCSE. Although initially challenged, there is accumulating evidence that NCSE leads to brain injury. Patients with NCSE (without other neurologic injury) have been found to have elevated serum neuron-specific enolase [23], a marker of neuronal injury. Additionally, NCS in patients with TBI were found to be associated with markers of metabolic distress [24]. Furthermore, the impact of NCS on clinical outcomes and mortality for adults is unknown since ethical concerns prevent placebo-controlled trials evaluating the treatment (or lack thereof) of NCS. Without knowing the degree of ongoing neuronal injury for patients with varying degrees of NCS and NCSE, it is likely that a "one-size-fits-all" treatment paradigm for patient with NCS and NCSE is not justifiable. With increasing evidence that IVADs may be detrimental for patients with NCS/NCSE, it is imperative that providers consider the concept of "appropriately aggressive therapy" by weighing the risks and benefits for individualized patients.

Stages of Treatment

Historically, guidelines for the acute treatment of seizures termed 1st, 2nd, 3rd, and 4th line therapy as the phases of management. Because this did not reflect the emergent need for SE control, the Neurocritical Care Society revised the traditional SE treatment paradigm to include the stages of SE treatment as follows: emergent initial therapy, urgent control therapy, and refractory therapy [8]. There have been no published guidelines regarding recommendations for the treatment of NCS. Although the incidence of NCS in critically ill patients has been established, there is limited data regarding recommendations for NCS management. Since there is a paucity of data for the treatment of NCS, the treatment of NCS largely reflects that of GCSE and NCSE. However, as mentioned previously, recent studies showing poorer outcomes with the use of sedating IVADs have raised the concern that aggressive treatment paradigms for NCS reflecting the treatment of GCSE may be harmful.

Emergent Initial Therapy

Per the recommendations by the Neurocritical Care Society, benzodiazepines (BDZs) (lorazepam, midazolam, or diazepam) should be the agent of choice for emergent initial treatment of SE (CSE, GCSE, or NCSE) [8]. These BDZs are discussed in more detail below. For IV administration, lorazepam is the preferred BDZ. There are no controlled trials that have allowed the determination of the optimal BDZ dosing for SE, therefore dosing guidelines discussed below are based on observational data and expert opinion. Emergent initial AED therapy should be administered within 0–5 min of seizure onset. First-line anticonvulsants fail to terminate GCSE in 31–50% of cases [25–27].

Urgent Control Therapy

The Neurocritical Care Society recommends that all patients presenting with SE receive additional AEDs for urgent control therapy after the administration of short acting BDZs. The goal of urgent control therapy for patients that have seizure cessation after emergent initial therapy with BDZs is rapid achievement of serum AED levels and continued AED therapy to maintain seizure cessation.

Patients in SE that have continued seizures despite acceptable doses of BZDs (approximately one third of patients) are considered to have ESE. The goal of urgent control therapy for patients with ESE is seizure cessation. Currently, there are no class I trials comparing the efficacy of various AEDs for the treatment of ESE. The Established Status Epilepticus Treatment Trial (ESETT) is a multi-center, randomized, double-blind study comparing the effectiveness of fosphenytoin, levetiracetam, and valproic acid for the treatment of ESE in adults and pediatric patients >2 years old [28, 29]. This study is currently underway. The following IV AEDs are recommended by the Neurocritical Care Society for urgent control therapy: valproic acid and phenytoin/fosphenytoin have Class IIa recommendations and midazolam infusion, phenobarbital and levetiracetam have Class IIB recommendations [8]. Urgent control AED therapy should be administered within 5–10 min of seizure onset.

Refractory Status Epilepticus Therapy

If seizures persist despite emergent initial therapy and urgent control therapy, the diagnosis of RSE is made (either CSE based on clinical exam or NCSE based on cEEG monitoring). After the diagnosis of RSE is made, clinicians can re-bolus the AED used for urgent control therapy (if dosing has not been maximized) or additional AEDs can be administered. The following AEDs are recommended by the Neurocritical Care Society for treatment of refractory SE: midazolam infusion, propofol infusion, pentobarbital/thiopental, valproic acid, levetiracetam, phenytoin/fosphenytoin, lacosamide, topiramate, and phenobarbital [8]. If seizures persist beyond this time-point, the diagnosis of SRSE is made.

IVADs are often used for the treatment of SRSE, whether convulsive or nonconvulsive. Due to the known complications of IVADs [30], ongoing studies are being performed that are evaluating various new treatments for SRSE. Treatment of RSE and SRSE will be discussed in further detail in another chapter.

General Medical Care

General medical care should be continuously provided to patients with any type of seizure or SE. Management and assessment of the patient's airway is extremely important.

For both convulsive seizures and NCS, the initial treatment protocol should consist of attention to the ABCs (airway, breathing, and circulation) while ensuring adequate IV access. Obtaining IV access in a patient with convulsive seizures may not be possible. In this circumstance, other methods of medication administration should be considered, such as intraosseous, buccal, intranasal, rectal, and intramuscular. After convulsive seizure activity cessation, peripheral, or central IV access should be obtained as clinically indicated.

If seizures are accompanied by respiratory failure, the patient should be intubated for airway protection. If neuromuscular blockade is necessary for intubation, the use of a short acting paralytic such as cisatricurium (0.2 mg/kg IV) or rocuronium (0.6 mg/kg IV) is preferable so that ongoing clinical seizure activity will not be masked. Vecuronium is not recommended since the active metabolite may accumulate in renal insufficiency. Cisatricurium and rocuronium do not have active metabolites. Succinylcholine is not recommended due to side effect of hyperkalemia (especially in the setting of convulsive seizures with acidosis) and risk of causing elevated intracranial pressure.

Close hemodynamic monitoring of oxygenation, blood pressure, and heart rate should be performed. Oxygen should be administered via nasal cannula or high-oxygen flow mask and oxygen saturation should be continuously monitored in the ICU. Hypotension (SBP<90 or MAP<65) may occur due to the seizures themselves, the treatment with benzodiazepines, or other AEDs or due to the underlying cause of the seizures (such as infection or sepsis). Clinicians should initiate vasopressor support if hypotension is observed despite adequate fluid resuscitation. Conversely, hypertension may be observed in conjunction with seizures (for example, in the setting of posterior reversible encephalopathy syndrome) and require treatment with IV antihypertensives. Nicardipine, clevidipine, or labetalol infusions are preferable due to attractive side effect profiles. Clevidipine is an ultra-short acting calcium channel blocker that can be rapidly titrated. Since patients with SE can have severe hemodynamic instability, medications that can be rapidly titrated are preferable. Nitroprusside should be avoided due to the risk of cyanide toxicity that may be seen as early as 4 h. Additionally, nitroprusside can result in a reduction in cerebral perfusion due to vasodilation. Esmolol and nitroglycerin infusions should be used with caution due to the potential risk of propylene glycol toxicity, which may accentuate the hyperlactatemia induced by seizures.

A thorough diagnostic assessment should be performed; however, this should not result in delay of seizure treatment. There are numerous causes of seizures, especially in critically ill patients (Table 7.1). A thorough history, physical, laboratory evaluation, and imaging will often yield an explanation for the acute presentation of seizures. The vast majority of seizures encountered in critically ill patients will be

Table 7.1 Etiologies of seizures in critically ill patients

History of epilepsy	Medication-related
Breakthrough seizures	Antibiotics (penicillins,
Low AED level	fluoroquinolones, imipenem)
Acute or chronic	Analgesics
cerebrovascular disease	Antidepressants (buproprion
Ischemic stroke	and TCAs)
ICH, SAH, SDH, EDH	Antineoplastic agents
Venous sinus thrombosis	Antipsychotics (lower
Malignancy	incidence with atypical
Solid neoplasm (primary or	antipsychotics)
metastatic)	Bronchial agents
Leptomeningeal	(theophylline)
carcinomatosis	General and local anesthetics
Paraneoplastic disease	Sympathomimetics
Traumatic brain injury	Other (amphetamines,
Hypoxic-ischemic	anticholinergics,
encephalopathy	antihistamines, iodinated
CNS infection	contrast, baclofen)
Meningitis or encephalitis	Substance-related
Cerebral abscess	Cocaine, heroin, PCP, ecstasy
Prion disease	Withdrawal (alcohol, BZD,
Autoimmune/inflammatory	opioid, barbiturates)
Autoimmune encephalitis	Sepsis
(i.e. anti-NMDA receptor	Metabolic
encephalitis)	Hypomagnesemia
Neurosarcoidosis	Hypoglycemia
Primary CNS vasculitis	Hypocalcemia
Systemic lupus erythematosus	Hyper- and hyponatremia
Hashimoto's encephalopathy	Uremia
	Eclampsia or hypertensive
	encephalopathy
	Posterior reversible
	encephalopathy syndrome

AED antiepileptic drug, *ICH* intracerebral hemorrhage, *SAH* subarachnoid hemorrhage, *SDH* subdural hematoma, *EDH* epidural hematoma, *CNS* central nervous system, *NMDA* N-methyl-D-aspartic acid, *TCA* tricyclic antidepressant, *PCP* phencyclidine; BZD: benzodiazepine

related to their initial presentation (i.e., TBI, SDH, SAH, ICH, etc.). Laboratory evaluation of patients with seizures should include AED levels if the patient is known to take AEDs and tests for etiology of seizures if underlying diagnosis is unknown.

Additional diagnostic testing (Table 7.2) should be performed to assess for the systemic complications of seizures, especially seen in GCSE. Arterial blood gas (ABG) is important to assess for the presence of acidosis, hypoxia, and hypercarbia. Patients will need to be intubated if ABG testing reveals hypoxia, hypercarbia, and/or respiratory acidosis. Bicarbonate may be indicated to treat acidosis, particularly if the patient's pH is <7.0. If the patient is found to have hypoglycemia, initiation of IV thiamine prior to glucose administration should be ensured to avoid precipitation of Wernicke's encephalopathy. Hyperglycemia should be avoided as it can worsen neurologic injury in GCSE. Hyperthermia is seen in up to 79% of patients with GCSE and can also worsen neurologic injury with GCSE. Intravascular or surface cooling may be indicated. Judicious use of IV fluids should be used

Table 7.2 Laboratory evaluation to assess secondary complications of seizures

Test	Complication of seizures
Telemetry	Tachycardia, arrhythmias
Blood pressure	Hypotension or hypertension
Pulse oximetry	Hypoxia
Temperature	Hyperthermia
Arterial blood gas	Acidosis, hypoxia, hypercarbia
Serum creatine kinase	Rhabdomyolysis
Serum troponin	Cardiac ischemia
Electrocardiogram	Cardiac ischemia
Lactate level	Lactic acidosis
Basic metabolic panel	Acute renal failure, hyperkalemia
Intracranial pressure	Intracranial hypertension
Echocardiogram	Heart failure
Fingerstick glucose	Hypoglycemia

in GCSE, if rhabdomyolysis is detected, while taking cardiac function into consideration [31].

After the patient has reached hemodynamic stability and seizures or SE are under control, brain imaging should be performed by computerized tomography (CT) and/or magnetic resonance imaging (MRI) to evaluate for acute intracranial processes, such as ICH, mass lesions, and infection. Brain CT or MRI may reveal a chronic lesion (such as a prior ischemic stroke) that could be a possible cause of seizures. Depending on the clinical presentation, sampling of the cerebrospinal fluid with a lumbar puncture may be indicated to evaluate for conditions such as SAH, meningitis, encephalitis, or carcinomatous meningitis. However, a lumbar puncture may be contraindicated if brain CT or MRI reveals a mass lesion that may be susceptible to herniation in the presence of a pressure gradient caused by a lumbar puncture (for example, when non-communicating hydrocephalus is present).

CEEG monitoring is an extremely important component of the diagnostic evaluation of critically ill patients with seizures since 92% of seizures in the critically ill patient population are nonconvulsive [1]. As recommended by the Neurocritical Care Society, the following are indications for cEEG monitoring: (1) recent clinical seizure or SE without return to baseline >10 min, (2) coma, including post-cardiac arrest, (3) epileptiform activity or periodic discharges on initial 30-min EEG, (4) intracranial hemorrhage including TBI, SAH, ICH, and (5) suspected NCS in patients with altered mental status [8]. The intensivist and ICU nursing staff should remember that the EEG leads may need to be removed before neuroimaging due to artifacts (CT) or non-compatibility (MRI) and, depending on the status of the patient, replaced after the test. Newer MRI compatible leads are not widely available.

Medications Used to Control ICU Seizures

The initial benzodiazepine treatment of seizures and SE (convulsive or nonconvulsive) in critically ill patients will be discussed in this chapter. Additionally, this chapter will discuss the use of non-sedating AEDs commonly used in the ICU. The use of sedating AEDs and less common treatment options for refractory seizures will be discussed in another chapter. A typical SE treatment algorithm is shown in the (Fig 7.1). An overview of the AEDs used to treat seizures in critically ill patients is outlined in Table 7.3. It should be noted that in the ICU setting, IV formulations of AEDs, if available, are preferable.

Benzodiazepines

It is widely accepted that BDZs are first-line therapy for the treatment of GCSE, although other AEDs have been studied as first-line therapy [8]. The mechanism of action of BDZs is enhancement of GABA-ergic neurotransmission at $GABA_A$ receptors. This results in more frequent opening of the chloride ion channel, thus hyperpolarizing the neuron. Due to the internalization of GABA receptors with ongoing seizure activity, BDZs are most effective when given very early during SE. They have broad-spectrum and potent anticonvulsant effects.

Bolus dosing of BDZs can result in hypotension and respiratory depression, therefore clinicians must be prepared with vasopressors, fluid boluses, and the tools needed for intubation and mechanical ventilation. Respiratory depression may also be caused by GCSE itself. One study showed that the risk of respiratory depression is highest in patients with GCSE that receives placebo as compared with patients that received BDZs [32].

The VA Cooperative Study, published in 1998, attempted to identify optimal GCSE treatment. The four treatment arms were (1) IV diazepam followed by phenytoin, (2) IV lorazepam, (3) IV phenobarbital, and (4) IV phenytoin. It showed that lorazepam was more effective than phenytoin (65% vs 44%), but not more effective than phenobarbital (58%) or the combination of diazepam and phenytoin (56%) for seizure cessation [25]. Based on the results of this study and the longer half-life, lorazepam is the preferred BDZ for the treatment of SE. However, if IV access is not available, midazolam is the BDZ of choice when the BDZ must be administered via the IM route. IM absorption is most reliable with midazolam as compared with the other BDZs. If IV access is absent and if IM midazolam is contraindicated, diazepam is the BDZ of choice for rectal administration [8]. Clonazepam is not used

Table 7.3 Medications used to treat critical care seizures

AED	Dosing	NCS treatment	Mechanism of action	Adverse reactions
Diazepam	0.15 mg/kg IV with rate not to exceed 5 mg/min	Emergent treatment	GABA agonist	Respiratory depression, hypotension, and sedation
Lorazepam	0.1 mg/kg IV with rate not to exceed 2 mg/min	Emergent treatment	GABA agonist	Respiratory depression, hypotension, and sedation
Midazolam[a]	0.2 mg/kg IM (maximum 10 mg in adults)	Emergent, urgent, or refractory treatment	GABA agonist	Respiratory depression, hypotension, and sedation
Phenytoin	Load 20 mg/kg IV then 5–8 mg/kg/day divided TID	Emergent, urgent, or refractory treatment	Sodium channel modulator	Drug rash, eosinophilia, purple-glove syndrome, irritative thrombophlebitis, and arrhythmias
Fosphenytoin	20 PE/kg then 5–8 PE/kg/day divided TID (PE = phenytoin equivalent)	Emergent or urgent treatment	Sodium channel modulator	Hypotension. Lower risk of infusion reaction than with phenytoin
Valproic acid	Load 20–40 mg/kg IV (max rate 6 mg/kg/min) then 10–15 mg/kg/day divided BID or TID	Emergent, urgent, or refractory treatment	Sodium channel inhibition, GABA potentiation, NMDA inhibition	Pancreatitis, hyperammonemia, thrombocytopenia, and encephalopathy
Levetiracetam	1000–3000 mg IV then daily dosing up to 4 gm/day divided BID	Emergent, urgent, or refractory treatment	Binds to synaptic vesicle-binding protein SV2A	Typically none but drowsiness and irritability can occur
Lacosamide	400 mg IV then daily dosing of 200 mg IV BID	Refractory treatment	Enhances slow inactivation of voltage-gated sodium channels	Drowsiness, PR prolongation, hypotension
Phenobarbital	Load 20 mg/kg IV then 1–4 mg/kg/day divided BID-TID	Emergent, urgent, or refractory treatment	Enhances GABA inhibition by modulating chloride currents	Long half-life (4 days), hypotension, respiratory depression, and sedation
Pregabalin	150–400 mg/day NG/PO	N/A	Binds to voltage-gated calcium channels	Dizziness, drowsiness
Gabapentin	Too limited data to suggest dosing for critically ill patients with seizures	N/A	Binds to voltage-gated calcium channels	Dizziness, drowsiness, ataxia, fatigue
Topiramate	200–400 mg/day NG/PO	Refractory treatment	Acts on sodium, GABA, and AMPA/kainate receptors	Non-anion gap metabolic acidosis, hyperammonemia, nephrolithiasis, and lethargy
Clobazam	Too limited data to suggest dosing for critically ill patients with seizures	N/A	GABA agonist	Drowsiness

Abbreviations: *AED* antiepileptic drug, *GABA*: gamma-Aminobutyric acid, *NMDA* N-methyl-D-aspartic acid, *AMPA* α-amino-3-hydroxy-5-methyl-4-isoxazolepropionic acid, *IV* intravenous, *PE* phenytoin equivalents
aMidazolam dosing for continuous infusion is discussed in another chapter. This table also does not include sedating anesthetic medications and other treatment options for RSE and SRSE

for the acute management of seizures in the USA due to the lack of an available IV formulation.

Diazepam

Diazepam is a long acting, highly lipid-soluble BDZ with a half-life of 20–100 h. It is available in PO, IV, IM, and PR formulations. The onset of action is 1–5 min after IV administration. It is rapidly absorbed and then rapidly enters the brain. The duration of peak effect is 15–60 min. Although its half-life is long, the duration of antiepileptic effect is relatively short due to its rapid redistribution to other body tissues (adipose tissue and muscle). Therefore, even after the fall of diazepam levels in the brain, the sedative effects persist. With repeated administration of diazepam, there is accumulation

within adipose tissue, thereby prolonging the systemic side effects of the medication. Diazepam has an active metabolite. The recommended IV dose is 0.15 mg/kg (up to 10 mg) at a rate of ≤5 mg/min [8]. This dose can be repeated in 5 min if seizures persist. IV administration of diazepam can result in local tissue irritation, venous phlebitis or thrombosis, and injection site pain. The use of diazepam for prolonged IV administration is covered in another chapter.

Rectal diazepam can be considered for ICU patients if IV access has been lost. The recommended PR dose for adults is 0.2 mg/kg, for children 6–11 years is 0.3 mg/kg, and for children 2–5 years is 0.5 mg/kg. Diazepam has a Class IIa, level A recommendation from the Neurocritical Care Society for emergent management of SE.

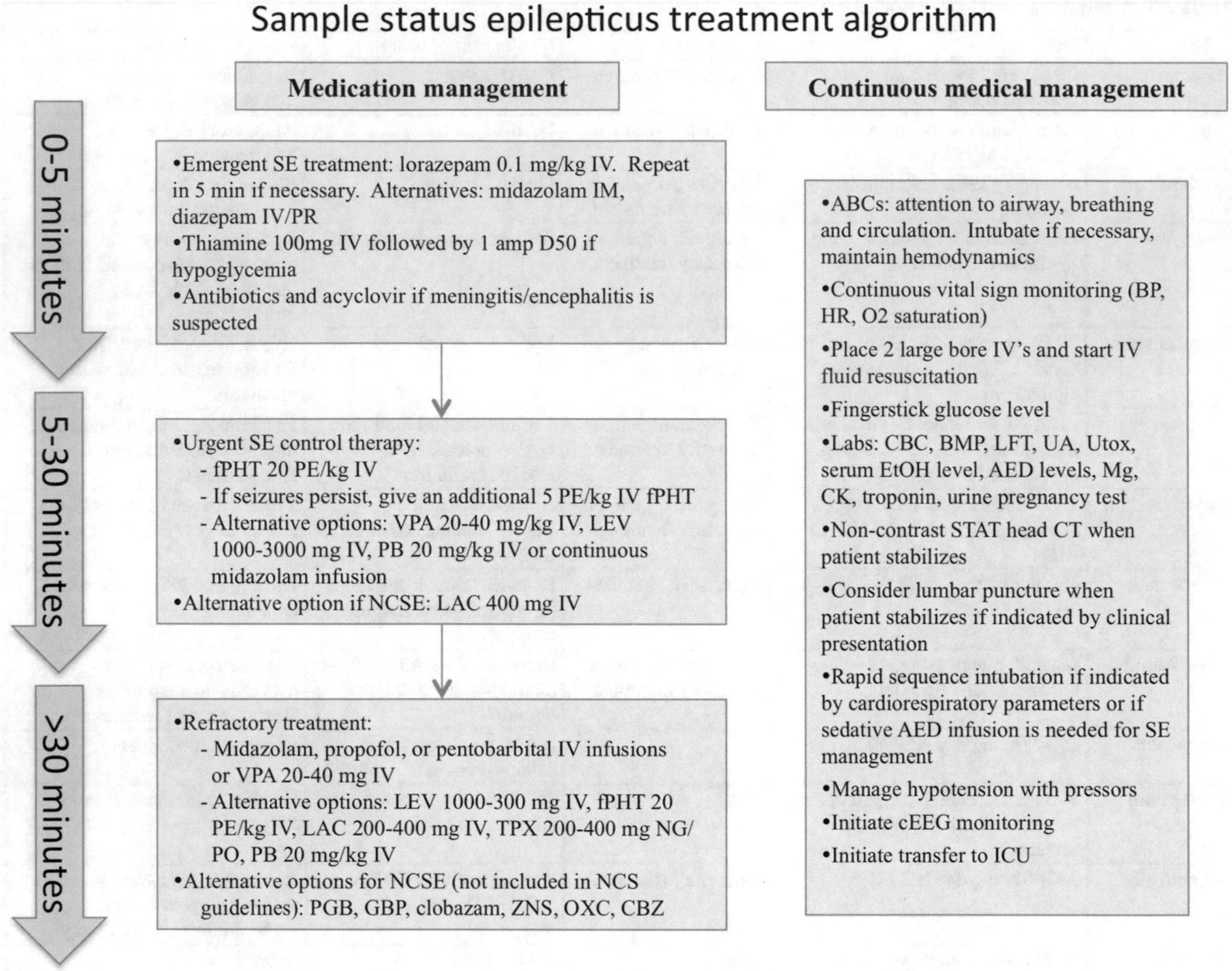

Sample status epilepticus treatment algorithm

| **Medication management** | **Continuous medical management** |

0–5 minutes

•Emergent SE treatment: lorazepam 0.1 mg/kg IV. Repeat in 5 min if necessary. Alternatives: midazolam IM, diazepam IV/PR
•Thiamine 100mg IV followed by 1 amp D50 if hypoglycemia
•Antibiotics and acyclovir if meningitis/encephalitis is suspected

•ABCs: attention to airway, breathing and circulation. Intubate if necessary, maintain hemodynamics
•Continuous vital sign monitoring (BP, HR, O2 saturation)
•Place 2 large bore IV's and start IV fluid resuscitation
•Fingerstick glucose level
•Labs: CBC, BMP, LFT, UA, Utox, serum EtOH level, AED levels, Mg, CK, troponin, urine pregnancy test
•Non-contrast STAT head CT when patient stabilizes
•Consider lumbar puncture when patient stabilizes if indicated by clinical presentation
•Rapid sequence intubation if indicated by cardiorespiratory parameters or if sedative AED infusion is needed for SE management
•Manage hypotension with pressors
•Initiate cEEG monitoring
•Initiate transfer to ICU

5–30 minutes

•Urgent SE control therapy:
  - fPHT 20 PE/kg IV
  - If seizures persist, give an additional 5 PE/kg IV fPHT
  - Alternative options: VPA 20–40 mg/kg IV, LEV 1000–3000 mg IV, PB 20 mg/kg IV or continuous midazolam infusion
•Alternative option if NCSE: LAC 400 mg IV

>30 minutes

•Refractory treatment:
  - Midazolam, propofol, or pentobarbital IV infusions or VPA 20–40 mg IV
  - Alternative options: LEV 1000–300 mg IV, fPHT 20 PE/kg IV, LAC 200–400 mg IV, TPX 200–400 mg NG/PO, PB 20 mg/kg IV
•Alternative options for NCSE (not included in NCS guidelines): PGB, GBP, clobazam, ZNS, OXC, CBZ

Fig. 7.1 Sample status epilepticus treatment algorithm. Abbreviations: *SE* status epilepticus, *fPHT* fosphenytoin, *VPA* valproic acid, *LEV* levetiracetam, *PB* phenobarbital, *LAC* lacosamide, *TPX* topiramate, *NCSE* non-convulsive status epilepticus, *PBG* pregabalin, *GBP* gabapentin, *ZNS* zonisamide, *OXC* oxcarbazepine, *CBZ* carbamazepine

Lorazepam

Lorazepam is a high-potency BDZ and is the drug of choice for the emergent management of seizures. Because it is less lipid-soluble than diazepam (and thus subject to less redistribution to body tissues) and has a high degree of protein binding, there is a longer duration of peak effect than diazepam. It is available in PO, IM, and IV formulations. The half-life is 10–20 h, with an anticonvulsant effect of 6–12 h. Due to its longer anticonvulsant effect, lorazepam is the drug of choice for alcohol withdrawal seizures.

Lorazepam is recommended as a Class I, level A medication for the initial management of SE by the Neurocritical Care Society [8]. The recommended dose is 0.1 mg/kg (rate of 2 mg/min IV push) with a maximum dose of 4 mg per dose. A second dose can be repeated in 5–10 min if seizures persist [8]. The use of lorazepam for prolonged IV administration is covered in another chapter. As with any BDZ, serious adverse effects can include respiratory depression and hypotension. The IV formulation of lorazepam contains the solvent, propylene glycol, which is known to cause hypotension and arrhythmias. Propylene glycol toxicity (arrhythmias, hypotension, and a clinical picture similar to sepsis) is a concern with prolonged high-dose administration of lorazepam. Lorazepam has an active metabolite. With mild-to-moderate renal or hepatic impairment, lorazepam should be used with caution. There is a tendency for tolerance to develop with BDZ treatment, therefore it is recommended that long term maintenance AEDs be administered in addition to BDZs.

In the VA Cooperative Study, the success rate for IV lorazepam was 65% for the control of overt GCSE [25]. In a randomized, double-blinded, placebo-controlled trial, IV lorazepam resulted in seizure control in 89% vs. 76% with IV diazepam for patients presenting with "convulsive, absence, partial elementary or partial complex status epilepticus" [33]. Although lorazepam has been associated with a lower risk of cardiac and respiratory depression than diazepam, this study showed similar rates of adverse cardiopulmonary complications (lorazepam 10.6% vs. diazepam 10.1%). In a study of treatment for out-of-hospital SE, lorazepam was more effective than diazepam or placebo for termination of SE (59% vs. 43% and 21%, respectively) [32]. Lorazepam has also been shown to be effective in pediatric SE. In 2008, a Cochrane Review of drug management of GTC seizures, including GCSE, in the pediatric population found that IV lorazepam is as effective as IV diazepam (70% vs. 65%, respectively), but has fewer side effects [34].

The body of literature for the treatment of NCS and NCSE with lorazepam is limited. A 2011 survey of neurologists found that lorazepam is used as first-line treatment of NCSE by 44% of respondents and by 28% of respondents for NCS [35], highlighting the observation that NCSE is typically treated more aggressively than NCS.

Midazolam

Midazolam is a short acting BDZ (half-life of 1–4 h) that is available in IV, IM, and transmucosal (nasal, buccal, and rectal) formulations. Midazolam is highly water soluble, leading to rapid absorption when administered by the IV and IM routes. Due to its water-solubility, it is unlikely to cause thrombophlebitis with IV administration and makes midazolam the most attractive BDZ for IM administration. Unlike lorazepam, propylene glycol is not a component for midazolam formulations; therefore, arrhythmias are not encountered with midazolam administration. Midazolam is metabolized in the liver by the cytochrome P450 (CYP450) system [36]. Other medications used in ICU patients that are also metabolized by the CYP450 system can affect the metabolism of midazolam. Midazolam is 96% protein-bound and undergoes renal excretion. Due to rapid redistribution after absorption, IV midazolam has a very short anticonvulsant effect of <5 min, leading to a high probability of seizure recurrence with bolus dosing. However, patients in the ICU may have an expanded volume of distribution, resulting in a longer half-life of midazolam, especially in liver dysfunction [37]. IM midazolam has a longer anticonvulsant effect (2 h). Due to the short anticonvulsant effect of midazolam, other BDZs (lorazepam and diazepam) are more often used for the emergent treatment of seizures in the ICU.

A double blind, randomized controlled trial of IM midazolam versus IV lorazepam in prehospital treatment of adult and pediatric SE by paramedics found that IM midazolam was statistically superior to IV lorazepam (73% vs. 63% seizure cessation, respectively) [38]. The rate of respiratory depression requiring intubation was similar between groups. Although there is a faster onset of action with lorazepam, the requirement for IV placement by paramedics offset the delayed onset of action of IM midazolam.

There is little data supporting the use of bolus dosing of midazolam in NCS and NCSE in critically ill patients. A 2010 survey of neurologists found that only 3% of respondents use midazolam for first-line treatment of NCS and 7% for first-line treatment of NCSE. In the ICU, midazolam is used more commonly as an infusion for coma induction for the treatment of refractory NCS and NCSE [35].

The Neurocritical Care Society has given IM midazolam a Class I, level A recommendation for the emergent treatment of SE [39]. The recommended dosing is 0.2 mg/kg IM (maximum 10 mg IM) in adults. For pediatrics, the recommended dosing as follows: 10 mg IM for >40 kg and 5 mg IM for 13–40 kg. Intranasal and buccal administration of midazolam is not encountered in the ICU. The dosing of midazolam for prolonged IV administration and the advantages of midazolam over other BDZs for prolonged infusions is covered in another chapter. Patients should be monitored closely for respiratory depression and hypotension after administration of IM midazolam. For patients in the ICU without IV access, IM midazolam can be considered for first-line therapy for convulsive or nonconvulsive seizures or SE.

Clonazepam

Although clonazepam is a potent BDZ with a high affinity for the $GABA_A$ receptor, it is rarely used in the ICU for seizure management due to the lack of an available IV formulation in the USA. It is highly lipid-soluble, therefore resulting in rapid anticonvulsant effects and has a longer half-life (10–20 h) than all other BDZs previously discussed. Clonazepam does not have a recommendation by the Neurocritical Care Society for the treatment of SE.

Phenytoin and Fosphenytoin

Phenytoin (PHT) has been used for the treatment of seizures for decades. It is FDA approved for the treatment of generalized tonic-clonic SE. The mechanism of action of PHT is stabilization of neuronal membranes and dose-dependent inhibition of sodium channels. It is available in IV and PO formulations. Phenytoin is insoluble in water and therefore, the parenteral formulation contains 40% propylene glycol to maintain solubility. PHT is highly caustic to veins, and a serious adverse effect of IV PHT is phlebitis due to extravasation of the medication. Due to this complication, it is recommended that IV PHT be administered via a central line if possible. Purple glove syndrome (PGS) (incidence of 6%) is characterized by limb discoloration associated with pain and edema distal to the peripheral infusion site. The pathophysiology of PGS is poorly understood and likely involves various mechanisms. It should be noted that PHT extravasation is not uniformly present in PGS, and extravasation of PHT may or may not result in PGS. Cardiovascular complications are attributable to both propylene glycol and PHT itself. There is a risk of hypotension (28–50%) and arrhythmias (2%) with the administration of parenteral PHT, with more side effects seen in patients older than 50 and patients with cardiac disease [5].

The recommended dose of PHT is 20 mg/kg ideal body weight (IBW) with a maximum rate of administration of 50 mg/min. Obese patients have prolonged PHT elimination half-life, greater total metabolic clearance of PHT, and prolonged PHT half-life. A recommended formula for PHT dosing in obese patients is 20 mg/kg IBW + (1.33 x excess weight over IBW) [40]. Of note, a common practice has been the administration of 1000 mg IV PHT to all patients regardless of weight; however, this "one-size-fits-all" dosing will result in insufficient dosing in many adults. There is a fast onset of action as brain concentrations of PHT are close to maximal when the loading dose of PHT is finished (typically 20–25 min) [5]. PHT is highly protein-bound (90–95%) and competes with other medications that are also highly protein-bound. For patients with low albumin levels (as is frequently encountered in critically ill patients) free PHT levels should be checked in addition to total PHT levels. The following formula can be used to calculate the approximate total PHT level in patients with hypoalbuminemia: corrected PHT = measured total PHT / [(0.2 × albumin) + 0.1]. The half-life of PHT is 6–24 h. PHT is metabolized in the liver and excreted in the urine.

Fosphenytoin is a water-soluble disodium phosphate ester of PHT and is often used preferentially over PHT for the acute treatment of seizures because propylene glycol is not needed as a vehicle. The dosing of fPHT is expressed as the amount of PHT delivered (PE, phenytoin equivalents). The recommended loading dose of fPHT is 20 mgPE/kg IBW. For obese patients, the loading dose can be calculated as 20 mgPE/kg IBW + (1.33 × the excess weight over IBW) [40]. This can be followed by an additional 5 mgPE/kg IV 10 min after the initial loading is finished if seizures persist [8]. The maintenance dose of fPHT/PHT is 5 mg/kg/day divided three times a day. The risk of local irritation at the site of injection is less with fPHT than PHT and therefore can be infused more rapidly (up to 150 mgPE/min IV). Slower infusion rates can be used in less urgent situations to minimize adverse reactions. The absence of propylene glycol makes fPHT compatible with common IV solutions and is safer to administer than PHT. Since fPHT is water-soluble, it can be given IM if IV access is unavailable. IM dosing of fPHT is the same as IV dosing. The risk of hypotension and arrhythmia is similar between PHT and fPHT [5].

fPHT is rapidly converted to PHT by hydrolysis by serum phosphatases. Therapeutic serum concentrations of PHT are achieved within 10–15 min of IV fPHT administration at the maximum rate. Total and free PHT serum concentrations should be measured after full conversion of fPHT to PHT is complete (approximately 1–1.5 h). The reference range of therapeutic total PHT level is 10–20 µg/mL and free PHT of 1–2.5 µg/mL. However, the term "therapeutic level" is misleading since a patient may be seizure free with a level of <10 µg/mL or a patient may require levels >20 µg/mL to obtain seizure control. The measure of clinical efficacy should be seizure cessation and prevention of seizure recurrence while minimizing side effects. Adverse side effects can be seen at all serum concentrations, but are more common with total PHT levels >20 µg/mL. Serum total PHT levels >30 µg/mL are considered toxic and may be epileptogenic. Patients with levels >40 µg/mL are likely to be lethargic or stuporous and may need aggressive supportive measures.

The most common CNS side effects seen with fPHT/PHT are nystagmus, somnolence, ataxia, and headache. Additional adverse effects of PHT/fPHT include hepatotoxicity, leukopenia, thrombocytopenia, pancytopenia, and hepatic enzyme induction. Contraindications to use of PHT/fPHT include hypersensitivity to class, sinus bradycardia, sinoatrial block, 2nd or 3rd degree atrioventricular block, and Adam–Stokes syndrome. The main drug interactions occur with CYP450 inducers.

The Neurocritical Care Society has given PHT/fPHT a Class IIa, level B evidence recommendation for the emergent and urgent management of SE [8]. Although PHT/fPHT has been studied as first-line therapy for the treatment of SE in the VA Cooperative Study showing an efficacy of 44%, the combination of diazepam and PHT was superior with an efficacy rate of 56% [25]. fPHT/PHT is typically used to maintain seizure cessation after seizures have stopped with typical first-line therapy of BDZs or to gain seizure cessation when first-line AEDs have failed. There have been numerous trials evaluating the efficacy of PHT/fPHT for the treatment of convulsive seizures and GCSE with variable results. A meta-analysis found that the overall efficacy of PHT for the treatment of CSE after BDZ failure was 50% (95% CI: 34–66%), compared with higher efficacy rates for valproic acid, phenobarbital, and levetiracetam. Despite the common practice of using fPHT/PHT as first-line therapy for SE after BDZ failure, the authors of this meta-analysis suggested that the evidence does not support the first-line use of fPHT/PHT [41]. However, the results should be interpreted with caution since most studies are observational and retrospective and complicated by bias and heterogeneity.

The efficacy and use of PHT/fPHT for NCS and NCSE are less studied as compared with convulsive seizures and SE. Based on the results of a survey of neurologists, PHT/fPHT is the most common first-line treatment of NCS (40% of respondents). For NCSE, survey respondents were also most likely to use PHT/fPHT as second-line therapy (43% of respondents). Only 32% of respondents reported they recommend PHT/fPHT for first-line therapy of NCSE (as compared with 44% that would recommend lorazepam as first-line therapy) [8].

Valproic Acid

Valproic acid (VPA) is a branched, short-chain fatty acid AED with broad-spectrum antiepileptic activity. It is FDA approved for the treatment of complex partial seizures and absence seizures, but is often used off-label to treat SE. Because VPA is available in an IV formulation in addition to PO formulations, it is commonly used in the ICU. It is thought that the antiepileptic effect of VPA is mediated through GABA-related actions, NMDA receptor antagonism, and histone-deacetylase inhibition. VPA has a half-life of 10–16 h and is extensively protein-bound. Protein binding is reduced in patients with renal insufficiency, chronic liver disease, or receiving other medications that are highly protein-bound, which are all common scenarios in the ICU. Because VPA is highly protein-bound, numerous drug–drug interactions have been reported with VPA. There are multiple routes of VPA metabolism with hepatic glucuronidation and beta oxidation in the mitochondria accounting for the majority of VPA metabolism. VPA is an inhibitor of the CYP450 system. Patients already receiving enzyme-inducing AEDs will require higher doses of VPA to achieve therapeutic levels. Additionally, VPA co-administration with PHT/fPHT will result in higher free PHT levels. Therefore close serum monitoring and dose adjustments are needed when VPA is co-administered with PHT/fPHT. It is important to note that the relationship between the administration dose of VPA and serum concentration is not linear.

Although VPA is generally safe and well tolerated there is black box warning by the FDA for life-threatening adverse drug reactions including hepatotoxocity, pancreatitis, and teratogenicity. The patient population that is particularly at risk for fatal VPA-induced hepatotoxicity are children <2 years old treated with multiple AEDs who have other medical or neurological conditions [42]. Therefore, careful monitoring of hepatic function is recommended. It is relatively contraindicated in patients with cirrhosis and hepatic failure due to the concern of accumulation and additional hepatic injury. It is also contraindicated in patients with hypersensitivity to drug class, urea cycle disorders, mitochondrial disorders, and pregnancy.

Common side effects that may be seen after initiation include tremor, nausea, and vomiting. VPA is typically less favorable than fPHT/PHT in patients in the Neuroscience ICU for two reasons. VPA can cause adverse hematologic side effects (thrombocytopenia, platelet dysfunction, and coagulopathy). The other main concern of VPA use in the ICU is the side effect of elevated ammonia resulting in altered mental status, further complicating the clinical picture of patients with acute neurologic injury. However, these theoretical side effects of VPA have not been reported in patients with SE [41]. Unlike lorazepam, diazepam, midazolam, phenobarbital, and PHT/fPHT, cardiopulmonary depression is not seen with VPA [43].

A meta-analysis reported the efficacy of VPA for the treatment of BDZ-resistant SE was 76% (95% CI: 64–85%) which was superior to the efficacy of PHT (50%) [41]. Since VPA is a broad-spectrum AED, it has been shown to have efficacy for various types of SE. It is preferred over fPHT/PHT for the treatment of SE due to generalized epilepsy disorders. VPA has a Class IIa, level A recommendation from the Neurocritical Care Society for the emergent and urgent treatment of SE [8].

Although commonly used, VPA has not been FDA approved for the treatment of SE. The recommended loading dose of VPA is 20–40 mg/kg IV at a rate of 6 mg/kg/min [8]. It is well-tolerated in the setting of high dosage (100 mg/kg) [41]. If seizures persist beyond 10 minutes after the loading dose, an additional re-bolus dose of 20 mg/kg can be considered. The standard maintenance dose is 10–15 mg/kg/day divided 2–3 times a day. Serum VPA levels can be obtained immediately after the loading dose [44].

Levetiracetam

Levetiracetam (LEV) is an AED that is FDA approved for the treatment of myoclonic seizures, partial-onset seizures, and primary generalized tonic-clonic seizures. LEV is commonly used off-label in the ICU due to availability of an IV formulation, minimal side effects, and drug to drug interactions. Although the exact mechanism of the antiepileptic action is unknown, LEV has been shown to inhibit N-type calcium channels, facilitate GABA-ergic inhibitory transmission, reduce delayed rectifier potassium current, bind to synaptic vesicle glycoprotein 2A (SV2A) and, thus, modulate neurotransmitter release. LEV is available in IV and PO formulations. It is rapidly absorbed, which is a desirable quality for medications used in the emergent management of seizures. LEV is only partially protein-bound (<10%). It is partially metabolized by enzymatic hydrolysis resulting in metabolites that are inactive. The elimination half-life is 6–8 h. Levetiracetam undergoes renal excretion with the majority excreted unchanged in the urine. Renal elimination of levetiracetam is affected by renal clearance, and therefore dose adjustments are needed in renal insufficiency and renal failure.

LEV is commonly used off-label for the treatment of SE and NCS/NCSE. There are no known interactions with other medications, including other AEDs, and no cardiovascular side effects [45], which have resulted in widespread use of LEV in critically ill patients. Common side effects include nausea, somnolence, dizziness, headache, irritability, depression, and psychosis. Blood levels of LEV can be obtained but are typically not helpful in the management of seizures in critically ill patients.

LEV has a Class IIb, level C recommendation from the Neurocritical Care Society for the treatment of SE [8]. The recommended initial dosing of LEV in SE is 1000–3000 mg IV [8]. Daily dosing is typically no more than 3000 mg/day since it has been shown that dosing > 3000 mg/day did not provide any additional benefit for patients with SE [46]. A meta-analysis of the efficacy of AEDs in BDZ-resistant convulsive SE found that LEV has an overall efficacy of 69% (95% CI: 56–79%) with individual doses of 1000–3000 mg iv or 20 mg/kg [41]. In this meta-analysis, LEV was less effective than phenobarbital and VPA but more effective than PHT. The efficacy of LEV for the treatment of NCS and refractory NCS is unknown since the majority of published data is for CSE and NCSE. In the author's experience, 16.1% of patients with NCS and refractory NCS will respond to LEV (unpublished data). There have been no randomized, controlled trials evaluating the efficacy of LEV for NCS or NCSE.

Lacosamide

Lacosamide (LCM) is a newer AED that is gaining popularity in the ICU, since an IV formulation is available in addition to a PO formulation. The exact antiepileptic mechanism of action is unknown, however, it is thought that LCM inhibits repetitive neuronal firing by enhancing the slow inactivation of voltage-gated sodium channels. LCM is FDA approved for use in partial-onset seizures and is gaining popularity for the off-label treatment of NCS, NCSE, and CSE. The half-life of LCM is 13 h, the time to peak effect is 1–4 h. LCM undergoes hepatic metabolism via the CYP3A4, CYP2C9, CYP2C19 pathways (with inactive metabolite formed) and is excreted in the urine. Dose adjustments are recommended in patients with renal or hepatic insufficiency and LCM is not recommended for use in patients with severe hepatic impairment.

Although the rate of adverse events with LCM is low, the most common adverse event reported with the use of LCM in critically ill patients is mild sedation. Additional adverse events that have been reported in the ICU patient population

are angioedema, allergic skin reaction, hypotension, and pruritus. There has been one patient reported to develop third-degree atrioventricular block and paroxysmal asystole [47]. LCM has been reported to have cardiovascular side effects with PR interval prolongation in addition to second- and third-degree heart blocks. Therefore, LCM should be used with caution in patients with conduction abnormalities, myocardial infarction, heart failure, and structural heart disease. In addition, LCM should be used with caution when given in conjunction with other medications that prolong the PR interval.

LCM has a Class IIb, level C recommendation for the treatment of refractory CSE or NCSE by the Neurocritical Care Society [8]. In a prospective, observational study of patients with CSE or NCSE, LCM was effective in 57% of patients with SE (70% of patients with CSE and 47% of patients with NCSE), when used as first-, second-, third-, or fourth-line therapy [48]. In a recent review, LCM was found to have an overall success rate of 56% for CSE or NCSE [47]. The first trial to compare AEDs for the treatment of NCS in critically ill patients was the Treatment of Recurrent Electrographic Nonconvulsive Seizures (TRENdS) trial. This was a randomized, controlled trial comparing the efficacy of fPHT vs. LCM for the treatment of NCS [12, 17]. Final results of this study are pending.

The loading dose of LCM in the TRENdS trial was 400 mg IV and maintenance dosing was 200 mg IV twice a day [12, 17]. The IV formulation has the same bioavailability as the PO formulation, therefore dose adjustments are not needed when switching between IV or PO formulations.

Phenobarbital

Phenobarbital (PHB) is a potent antiepileptic agent that also has sedative and hypnotic properties. PHB exerts its antiepileptic effect on $GABA_A$ receptors by prolonging the duration of GABA-mediated opening of chloride ion channels. This results in neuronal hyperpolarization. PO and IV formulations are available. However, the IV formulation is highly alkaline and may cause local irritation. After IV administration of PHB, onset of action is seen within 5 min and the peak effect is seen in about 30 min. The duration of action of IV PHB is 4–10 h. PHB is not extensively protein-bound (20–45%) and is 70–90% absorbed. Metabolism is primarily performed by liver CYP system and 25% is excreted unchanged in the urine. It is important to note that PHB is a potent inducer of the CYP system, which has numerous implications for drug–drug interactions. Concurrent medications that are metabolized by the CYP450 system will have decreased effectiveness due to their faster clearance. PHB may worsen VPA-induced hyperammonemia. It has a very long half-life of 2–7 days [36].

The side effects of PHB are numerous. Common side effects of acute administration of PHB include confusion, irritability, sedation, coma, respiratory depression, and hypotension. Respiratory depression and hypotension will be augmented if PHB is administered to patients that have already received BDZs. In children, paroxysmal hyperkinetic reactions can occur. The recommended loading dose is 20 mg/kg at a rate of 50–100 mg/min [8] followed by a maintenance dose of 1–4 mg/kg/day typically divided 2–3 times a day. Maintenance dosing adjustments can be made based on serum PHB levels. In adults, the typical therapeutic range of PHB is 20–40 mcg/mL. Symptoms seen with mild PHB toxicity (>40 mcg/mL) include slowness, ataxia, and nystagmus. Serum PHB concentration >65 mcg/mL can result in coma with brainstem reflexes and >100 mcg/mL will result in coma without brainstem reflexes. Some dosage forms may contain propylene glycol. Large amounts of PHB can lead to propylene glycol toxicity (hyperosmolality, lactic acidosis, seizures, and respiratory depression).

The Neurocritical Care Society has given PHB a Class IIb, level A recommendation for the emergent treatment of CSE and NCSE. In addition, there is a Class IIb, level C recommendation for both urgent treatment and refractory treatment of CSE and NCSE [8]. PHB does have FDA approval for the treatment of SE. In the VA Cooperative Study, the efficacy of phenobarbital was 58% for cessation of GCSE [25]. A meta-analysis reported the efficacy of PHB for the treatment of BDZ-resistant SE was 74% (95% CI: 58–85%) [41]. Although this study found that the efficacy of PHB was similar to that of LEV and VPA and superior to PHT, in practice PHB is rarely used as first-line therapy for the treatment of BDZ-resistant CSE or NCSE given its adverse side effect profile and potential for drug–drug interactions. For the management of NCS in critically ill patients, other non-sedating AEDs are preferable over PHB. A 2010 survey of neurologists reported only 2% of respondents used PHB as the first-line AED for NCS. Additionally, only 2% of respondents utilized PHB for the first-line therapy for NCSE. Neurologists were more likely to use PHB as third-line therapy for NCS or NCSE, rather than first or second-line therapy [19].

Options for Add-on Therapy

Pregabalin

Pregabalin (PGB) is an AED that is used to treat seizures, neuropathic pain, postherpetic neuralgia, and generalized anxiety disorder. It is FDA approved for the adjunctive treatment of partial-onset seizures. PGB is not FDA approved for the treatment of NCS and NCSE, but is sometimes used as add-on therapy for refractory NCS and NCSE.

PGB binds to the alpha$_2$-delta subunit of voltage-gated calcium channels and inhibits excitatory neurotransmitter release (glutamate, norepinephrine, serotonin, dopamine, substance P, and calcitonin gene-related peptide) [49]. Although PGB is only available in PO formulation, it can be administered via a nasogastric tube. It has almost complete gastrointestinal absorption and reaches peak levels within 1 h. Steady state is achieved within 24–48 h. The mean elimination half-life of PGB is 6 h. PGB is not protein-bound and is excreted unchanged in the urine. PGB does not undergo hepatic metabolism and has no effect on the CYP450 system, resulting in an absence of drug–drug interactions. PGB lacks idiosyncratic side effects and does not require titration [50].

Because of its predictable pharmacokinetics, lack of drug–drug interactions, and unique mechanism of action, PGB is an attractive option for add-on therapy for refractory NCS and NCSE. In a retrospective study, PGB was found to be efficacious in stopping NCS and NCSE is 52% of patients within 24 h of initiation [51]. In this study, PGB was mostly used as third or fourth-line therapy when other AEDs failed. PGB was more effective in stopping NCS than NCSE. Patients with brain tumors may respond better to PGB than patients with NCS or NCSE from other etiologies [51, 52]. Another retrospective study found the efficacy of PGB to be 45% for definite seizure cessation within 24 h of initiation for patients with various types of CSE [53]. The Neurocritical Care Society does not include PGB in their recommendations for the treatment of CSE and NCSE. When used to treat NCS and NCSE in critically ill patients, standard dosage is 150–400 mg/day divided 2–3 times a day. The median daily dose was 375 mg/day in one study [52]. Dizziness and drowsiness are the most common side effects seen in critically ill patients receiving PGB [51]. Dose adjustments are necessary in patients with renal insufficiency.

Gabapentin

Gabapentin (GBP) is an AED, but is more often used to treat pain syndromes (postherpetic neuralgia, neuropathic pain, fibromyalgia) and restless leg syndrome. GBP has a structural relationship to GABA, but has little to no action on the GABA receptor. Its exact mechanism of action is unknown, but it appears likely that GBP binds to voltage-gated calcium channels that possess the alpha-2-delta-1 subunit (a presynaptic channel). GBP may modulate the release of excitatory neurotransmitters. Like PGB, GBP is FDA approved for the treatment of partial-onset seizures, but is sometimes used off-label for add-on therapy for the treatment of refractory NCS and NCSE.

GBP is only available in a PO formulation and has variable absorption. The time to peak effect is 2–4 h. It is not protein-bound and does not undergo any metabolism. It is excreted in the urine as unchanged drug. GBP does not undergo hepatic metabolism and has no effect on the CYP450 system, resulting in an absence of drug–drug interactions. The half-life of GBP in adults is 5–7 h, with prolongation in renal insufficiency. Conversely, the half-life is reduced (4 h) in patients receiving hemodialysis. The most common side effects are dizziness, drowsiness, ataxia, and fatigue.

There have been two case reports for the successful treatment of SE with adjunctive GBP in patients with porphyria [54, 55]. Therefore, GBP can be considered for add-on therapy for patients with refractory SE who are presenting with an acute porphyria exacerbation. There have been no published studies reporting the efficacy of GBP for the treatment of NCS and NCSE. The Neurocritical Care Society does not include GBP in their recommendations for the treatment of CSE and NCSE.

Topiramate

Topiramate (TPM) is FDA approved for the treatment of epilepsy (monotherapy or adjunctive therapy) and migraine. Although it is only available in PO formulation, it has been used off-label for the treatment of RSE in adults. TPM is thought to exert its antiepileptic effect by blocking voltage-gated sodium channels, enhancing $GABA_A$ activity, antagonizing AMPA/kainate glutamate receptors, and inhibiting carbonic anhydrase. TPM undergoes rapid absorption, reaches a peak effect in 1–4 h, and has an elimination half-life of 21 h. TPM is partially protein-bound (15–41%). Small amounts of TPM are metabolized in the liver, but the majority (70%) is excreted as unchanged drug in the urine.

Because TPM can be administered via a nasogastric tube and can be rapidly titrated, there have been several case reports, case series, and retrospective reports for its use in RSE. The efficacy of TPM appears to be between 18 and 71% in the largest retrospective studies [56–58]. For the treatment of refractory CSE and refractory NCSE, TPM appears to be well-tolerated [56–59]. Reported adverse effects in this patient population are slight non-anion gap metabolic acidosis, hyperammonemia, nephrolithiasis, and lethargy. One concern about the use of high doses of TPM in critically ill patients is the development of hyperchloremic, non-anion gap, metabolic acidosis [60]. This is due to inhibition of carbonic anhydrase enzymes. Patients who had seizure cessation with TPM typically received doses of <800 mg/day, but doses as high as 1600 mg/day were reported. In one study, the most common dosing was 100 mg every 4–6 h [58]. The Neurocritical Care Society recommends initial dosing of 200–400 mg/day [8]. TPM has also been reported to be safe and effective for the treatment of pediatric RSE. The Neurocritical Care Society has given TPM a Class IIb, level C recommendation for the treatment of refractory CSE and NCSE [8].

Clobazam

Clobazam is a 1,5 BDZ that is FDA approved for the adjunctive treatment of seizures in Lennox–Gastaut syndrome, but is often used off-label to treat other types of seizure disorders, including NCS and refractory CSE and NCSE. The binding of clobazam to the ω_2 site on the postsynaptic $GABA_A$ receptor is thought to result in an antiepileptic effect by increasing neuronal permeability to chloride ions. Because clobazam has a lower affinity for allosteric ω_1 site on GABA receptors, clobazam has an improved safety and tolerability profile compared with other 1,4 BDZs [61]. Since it is insoluble in water, clobazam is only available in PO formulation. It is rapidly and extensively absorbed with a peak time of 0.5–4 h. The elimination half-life is 36–42 h. There is significant protein binding (80–90%). Clobazam is metabolized via the hepatic CYP3A4 (and to a lesser extent, the CYP2C19 and 2B6 system) with active metabolites. The active metabolite, N-desmethylclobazam has a half-life of 71–82 h. Despite the fact that clobazam is metabolized in the liver, there are no meaningful interactions with other AEDs metabolized in the liver [64].

In a case series of 17 patients with RSE (11 with prior history of epilepsy and most with focal SE), 13 patients (76%) had a successful response to clobazam after a median of 3 failed AEDs. The authors stated that clobazam averted the need for anesthetic infusions in 5 patients. Sedation was the only side effect seen (38% of patients), however, the authors noted that since the patients were receiving other AEDs, it is not clear if sedation could be attributed solely to clobazam [63]. The mean initial dosage was 15.8 mg/day and the mean maintenance dosage used in this study was 22.4 mg/day. Other case reports and case series have shown clobazam to be safe and well tolerated for the treatment as add-on therapy for RSE [64, 65]. There is no data regarding the efficacy of clobazam for the treatment of NCS. Additional prospective studies are needed to establish the efficacy of clobazam for the treatment of NCS and refractory CSE or NCSE. The Neurocritical Care Society does not include clobazam in their recommendations for the treatment SE. However, given the favorable pharmacokinetic profile, clobazam warrants further investigation as a treatment of refractory NCS and NCSE since traditional therapy with IVADs has been associated with poorer outcomes [20, 21].

Other Medications

Zonisamide (ZNS), carbamazepine (CBZ), and oxcarbazepine (OXC) are other AEDs that are often used in the outpatient management of epilepsy. ZNS blocks sodium and calcium channels. CBZ and OXC block voltage-sensitive sodium channels, NMDA receptor-activated sodium, and calcium influx and cause stabilization of the cell membrane. OXC has fewer side effects than CBZ by using non-oxidative metabolization pathway, as opposed to the CYP450-mediated metabolism of CBZ. One case series found an efficacy rate of 61% for OXC for the treatment of RSE (mostly remote symptomatic and mostly nonconvulsive). Hyponatremia was seen in 23% of patients with OXC [66]. Since ZNS, CBZ, and OXC lack the fast onset of action needed in the ICU for the acute treatment of NCS, CSE, and NCSE, and the side effect profile may be worse than with other AEDs, these medications are not typically used for the treatment of seizures in critically ill patients.

Antiepileptic Medication Discontinuation

All AEDs should not be discontinued abruptly due to the risk of worsening seizures. If AED withdrawal is indicated, ideally, all AEDs should be gradually tapered to curtail the risk of withdrawal seizures. However, in some circumstances, such as severe or life-threatening adverse reactions, AEDs must be stopped abruptly due to safety concerns.

AED tapering (early or late) has not been studied for patients with seizures secondary to acute brain injury. There is lack of data regarding optimal management of AEDs after seizure cessation is obtained. Patients with refractory NCS or NCSE are often treated with numerous antiepileptic medications. During the course of their hospitalization, patients receiving multiple AEDs may experience adverse side effects such as dizziness, fatigue, sedation, and cognitive dysfunction in addition to the potential of drug–drug interactions with other medications that are administered. At our institution, it is not uncommon to begin AED tapering in the days/weeks after we ensure seizure cessation in attempt to minimize adverse side effects of AED polytherapy. However, there is a risk of recurrent seizures with AED tapering, thus the risks and benefits of an AED taper must be weighed. It is likely that the number of AEDs, EEG findings, clinical exam, and type of seizures (i.e., focal vs. generalized) is important factors when deciding AED withdrawal. Studies are needed to determine the optimal practice of AED withdrawal after seizure cessation for acute brain injury.

Conclusions

There are numerous types of seizures encountered in critically ill patients, with the vast majority being nonconvulsive. NCS and NCSE are detectable only with cEEG monitoring, therefore this is an essential component to the management of seizures in critical care. What is less certain in the field of critical care seizure management is which medications should be used and in what order. In addition, there is a great deal of uncertainty regarding the urgency and aggressiveness of critical care seizure management.

It has been established that GCSE is a medical emergency with high morbidity and mortality, however, GCSE represents a minority of the seizure types encountered in the ICU. Due to the lack of available evidence, the treatment paradigm for NCS and NCSE (the types of seizures encountered most frequently in the ICU) reflects that of GCSE. But, recent evidence suggests that sedative medications often used to treat GCSE may not be necessarily appropriate. The concept of "appropriately aggressive treatment" has arisen from the notion that the aggressiveness of seizure treatment should reflect the degree of ongoing neuronal injury. More data is needed to understand the pathology and clinical implications of NCS and NCSE. In addition, more data is needed to determine ideal treatment for NCS and NCSE. Clinical trials are needed to advance the field of critical care seizure management.

References

1. Claassen J, Mayer SA, Kowalski RG, Emerson RG, Hirsch LJ. Detection of electrographic seizures with continuous EEG monitoring in critically ill patients. Neurology. 2004;62(10): 1743–8.
2. Treiman DM, Walker MC. Treatment of seizure emergencies: convulsive and non-convulsive status epilepticus. Epilepsy Res. 2006;68:77–82.
3. ARNAUTOVA EN, NESMEIANOVA TN. A proposed international classification of epileptic seizures. Epilepsia. 1964;5: 297–306.
4. Treatment of convulsive status epilepticus. Recommendations of the epilepsy foundation of America's working group on status epilepticus. JAMA. 1993;270:854–9.
5. Lowenstein DH, Alldredge BK. Status epilepticus. N Engl J Med. 1998;338(14):970–6.
6. Jenssen S, Gracely EJ, Sperling MR. How long do most seizures last? a systematic comparison of seizures recorded in the epilepsy monitoring unit. Epilepsia. 2006;47(9):1499–503.
7. Meldrum BS, Horton RW. Physiology of status epilepticus in primates. Arch Neurol. 1973;28(1):1–9.
8. Brophy GM, Bell R, Claassen J, Alldredge B, Bleck TP, Glauser T, et al. Guidelines for the evaluation and management of status epilepticus. Neurocrit Care. 2012;17:3–23.
9. Husain AM, Horn GJ, Jacobson MP. Non-convulsive status epilepticus: usefulness of clinical features in selecting patients for urgent EEG. J Neurol Neurosurg Psychiatry. 2003;74(2): 189–91.
10. Chong DJ, Hirsch LJ. Which EEG patterns warrant treatment in the critically ill? reviewing the evidence for treatment of periodic epileptiform discharges and related patterns. J Clin Neurophys. 2005;22(2):79–91.
11. Beniczky S, Hirsch LJ, Kaplan PW, Pressler R, Bauer G, Aurlien H, et al. Unified EEG terminology and criteria for nonconvulsive status epilepticus. Epilepsia. 2013;6(s6):28–9.
12. Husain AM. Treatment of recurrent electrographic nonconvulsive seizures (TRENdS) study. Epilepsia. 2013;6(s6):84–8.
13. Ferlisi M, Shorvon S. The outcome of therapies in refractory and super-refractory convulsive status epilepticus and recommendations for therapy. Brain. 2012;135(Pt 8):2314–28.
14. Shorvon S, Ferlisi M. The treatment of super-refractory status epilepticus: a critical review of available therapies and a clinical treatment protocol. Brain. 2011;134(Pt 10):2802–18.

15. Swisher CB, Shah D, Sinha SR, Husain AM. Baseline EEG pattern on continuous ICU EEG monitoring and incidence of seizures. J Clin Neurophys. 2015;32(2):147–51.

16. Oddo M, Carrera E, Claassen J, Mayer SA, Hirsch LJ. Continuous electroencephalography in the medical intensive care unit. Crit Care Med. 2009 Jun;37(6):2051–6.

17. Husain AM. Lacosamide in status epilepticus: Update on the TRENdS study. Epilepsy Behav. 2015;49:337–9.

18. Wasim M, Husain AM. Nonconvulsive seizure control in the intensive care unit. Curr Treat Options Neurol. 2015;17(3):340.

19. Abend NS, Dlugos DJ, Hahn CD, Hirsch LJ, Herman ST. Use of EEG Monitoring and Management of Non-Convulsive Seizures in Critically Ill Patients: A Survey of Neurologists. Neurocrit Care. 2010;12(3):382–9.

20. Kowalski RG, Ziai WC, Rees RN, Werner Jr JK, Kim G, Goodwin H, et al. Third-line antiepileptic therapy and outcome in status epilepticus. Crit Care Med. 2012;40(9):2677–84.

21. Hocker SE, Shorvon S. Anesthetic drugs in status epilepticus: risk or rescue? A 6-year cohort study. Neurology. 2014;83(9):866.

22. Fountain NB, Lothman EW. Pathophysiology of status epilepticus. J Clin Neurophys. 1995;12(4):326–42.

23. Rabinowicz AL, Correale JD, Bracht KA, Smith TD, DeGiorgio CM. Neuron-specific enolase is increased after nonconvulsive status epilepticus. Epilepsia. 1995;36(5):475–9.

24. Vespa PM, Miller C, McArthur D, Eliseo M, Etchepare M, Hirt D, et al. Nonconvulsive electrographic seizures after traumatic brain injury result in a delayed, prolonged increase in intracranial pressure and metabolic crisis. Crit Care Med. 2007 Dec;35(12):2830–6.

25. Treiman DM, Meyers PD, Walton NY, Collins JF, Colling C, Rowan AJ, et al. A comparison of four treatments for generalized convulsive status epilepticus. Veterans affairs status epilepticus cooperative study group. N Engl J Med. 1998;339(12):792–8.

26. Holtkamp M. Predictors and prognosis of refractory status epilepticus treated in a neurological intensive care unit. J Neurol Neurosurg Psychiatry. 2005;76(4):534–9.

27. Mayer SA, Claassen J, Lokin J, Mendelsohn F, Dennis LJ, Fitzsimmons B-F. Refractory Status Epilepticus. Arch Neurol. 2002;59(2):205–10.

28. Cock HR. ESETT group. Established status epilepticus treatment trial (ESETT). Epilepsia. 2011;8(s8):50–2.

29. Bleck T, Cock H, Chamberlain J, Cloyd J, Connor J, Elm J, et al. The established status epilepticus trial 2013. Epilepsia. 2013;6(s6): 89–92.

30. Sutter R, Marsch S, Fuhr P, Kaplan PW, Rüegg S. Anesthetic drugs in status epilepticus: risk or rescue? a 6-year cohort study. Neurology. 2014;82(8):656–64.

31. Suzette MM, LaRoche MD. Handbook of ICU EEG monitoring: Demos Medical Publishing; 2012. New York p. 1.

32. Alldredge BK, Gelb AM, Isaacs SM, Corry MD, Allen F, Ulrich S, et al. A comparison of lorazepam, diazepam, and placebo for the treatment of out-of-hospital status epilepticus. N Engl J Med. 2001;345(9):631–7.

33. Leppik IE, Derivan AT, Homan RW, Walker J, Ramsay RE, Patrick B. Double-blind study of lorazepam and diazepam in status epilepticus. JAMA. 1983;249(11):1452–4.

34. Appleton R, Macleod S, Martland T. Drug management for acute tonic-clonic convulsions including convulsive status epilepticus in children. Appleton R, (ed). Cochrane database system review (3) Chichester: John Wiley & Sons, Ltd; 2008: CD001905.

35. Abend NS, Gutierrez-Colina AM, Topjian AA, Zhao H, Guo R, Donnelly M, et al. Nonconvulsive seizures are common in critically ill children. Neurology. 2011;76(12):1071–7.

36. French JA, Gazzola DM. Antiepileptic drug treatment: new drugs and new strategies. Continuum. 2013;19(3):643–55.

37. Dirksen MS, Vree TB, Driessen JJ. Clinical pharmacokinetics of long-term infusion of midazolam in critically ill patients--preliminary results. Anaesth Intensive Care. 1987;15(4):440–4.

38. Silbergleit R, Durkalski V, Lowenstein D, Conwit R, Pancioli A, Palesch Y, et al. Intramuscular versus intravenous therapy for prehospital status epilepticus. N Engl J Med. 2012;366(7):591–600.

39. Silbergleit R, Lowenstein D, Durkalski V, Conwit R. NETT investigators. Lessons from the RAMPART study—and which is the best route of administration of benzodiazepines in status epilepticus. Epilepsia. 2013;6(s6):74–7.

40. Abernethy DR, Greenblatt DJ. Phenytoin disposition in obesity. Determination of loading dose. Arch Neurol. 1985 May;42(5):468–71.

41. Yasiry Z, Shorvon SD. The relative effectiveness of five antiepileptic drugs in treatment of benzodiazepine-resistant convulsive status epilepticus: a meta-analysis of published studies. Seizure. 2014;23(3):167–74.

42. Dreifuss FE, Santilli N, Langer DH, Sweeney KP, Moline KA, Menander KB. Valproic acid hepatic fatalities: a retrospective review. Neurology. 1987;37(3):379–85.

43. Sinha S, Naritoku DK. Intravenous valproate is well tolerated in unstable patients with status epilepticus. Neurology. 2000;55(5): 722–4.

44. Al-Mufti F, Claassen J. Neurocritical care: status epilepticus review. Crit Care Clin. 2014;30(4):751–64.

45. Crepeau AZ, Treiman DM. Levetiracetam: a comprehensive review. Expert Rev. Neurother. 2010;10(2):159–71.

46. Rossetti AO, Bromfield EB. Determinants of success in the use of oral levetiracetam in status epilepticus. Epilepsy Behav. 2006;8(3): 651–4.

47. Höfler J, Trinka E. Lacosamide as a new treatment option in status epilepticus. Epilepsia. 2013;54(3):393–404.

48. Moreno Morales EY, Fernandez Peleteiro M, Bondy Peña EC, Domínguez Lorenzo JM, Pardellas Santiago E, Fernández A. Observational study of intravenous lacosamide in patients with convulsive versus non-convulsive status epilepticus. Clin Drug Invest. 2015;35(7):463–9.

49. Gajraj NM. Pregabalin: its pharmacology and use in pain management. Anesth Analg. 2007;105(6):1805–15.

50. Ben-Menachem E. Pregabalin pharmacology and its relevance to clinical practice. Epilepsia. 2004;45(s6):13–8.

51. Swisher CB, Doreswamy M, Husain AM. Use of pregabalin for nonconvulsive seizures and nonconvulsive status epilepticus. Seizure. 2013;22(2):116–8.

52. Swisher CB, Doreswamy M, Gingrich KJ, Vredenburgh JJ, Kolls BJ. Phenytoin, levetiracetam, and pregabalin in the acute management of refractory status epilepticus in patients with brain tumors. Neurocrit Care. 2012;16(1):109–13.

53. Novy J, Rossetti AO. Oral pregabalin as an add-on treatment for status epilepticus. Epilepsia. 2010;51(10):2207–10.

54. Pandey CK, Singh N, Bose N, Sahay S. Gabapentin and propofol for treatment of status epilepticus in acute intermittent porphyria. J Postgrad Med. 2003;49(3):285.

55. Bhatia R, Vibha D, Srivastava MVP, Prasad K, Tripathi M, Bhushan SM. Use of propofol anesthesia and adjunctive treatment with levetiracetam and gabapentin in managing status epilepticus in a patient of acute intermittent porphyria. Epilepsia. 2008;49(5): 934–6.

56. Hottinger A, Sutter R, Marsch S, Rüegg S. Topiramate as an adjunctive treatment in patients with refractory status epilepticus: an observational cohort study. CNS Drugs. 2012;26(9):761–72.

57. Stojanova V, Rossetti AO. Oral topiramate as an add-on treatment for refractory status epilepticus. Acta Neurol. 2012;125(2): e7–e11.

58. Synowiec AS, Yandora KA, Yenugadhati V, Valeriano JP, Schramke CJ, Kelly KM. The efficacy of topiramate in adult refractory status epilepticus: experience of a tertiary care center. Epilepsy Res. 2012;98(2–3):232–7.

59. Towne AR, Garnett LK, Waterhouse EJ, Morton LD, DeLorenzo RJ. The use of topiramate in refractory status epilepticus. Neurology. 2003;60(2):332–4.

60. Takeoka M, Holmes GL, Thiele E, Bourgeois BF, Helmers SL, Duffy FH, et al. Topiramate and metabolic acidosis in pediatric epilepsy. Epilepsia. 2001;42(3):387–92.
61. Borland RG, Nicholson AN. Immediate effects on human performance of a 1,5-genzodiazepine (clobazam) compared with the 1,4-benzodiazepines, chlordiazepoxide hydrochloride and diazepam. Br J Clin Pharmacol. 1975;2(3):215–21.
62. Walzer M, Bekersky I, Blum RA, Tolbert D. Pharmacokinetic drug interactions between clobazam and drugs metabolized by cytochrome P450 isoenzymes. Pharmacotherapy. 2012;32(4):340–53.
63. Sivakumar S, Ibrahim M, Parker Jr D, Norris G, Shah A, Mohamed W. Clobazam: an effective add-on therapy in refractory status epilepticus. Epilepsia. 2015;56(6):e83–9.
64. Corman C, Guberman A, Benavente O. Clobazam in partial status epilepticus. Seizure. 1998;7(3):243–7.
65. Tinuper P, Aguglia U, Gastaut H. Use of clobazam in certain forms of status epilepticus and in startle-induced epileptic seizures. Epilepsia. 1986;27(1):S18–26.
66. Kellinghaus C, Berning S, Stögbauer F. Use of oxcarbazepine for treatment of refractory status epilepticus. Seizure. 2014;23(2):151–4.

Management of Status Epilepticus in the Intensive Care Unit

Panayiotis N. Varelas and Jan Claassen

Introduction

Based on a proposed operational definition of SE by Lowenstein, SE refers to at least 5 min of (a) continuous seizures or (b) two or more discrete seizures between which there is incomplete recovery of consciousness [1]. Status epilepticus (SE) is a true medical emergency that requires aggressive and prompt therapeutic intervention preferably in an ICU environment. The physician may encounter a patient with SE in the ICU, either because the patient was admitted for management of the SE or because the patient developed SE during the course of his admission for another medical reason. SE is particularly frequently seen with CNS infection/inflammation and brain hemorrhages, but may also be encountered in those patients with systemic inflammatory processes such as sepsis [2, 3]. In the Neuro-ICU additionally some patients, who are admitted for continuous electroencephalogram (EEG) monitoring after intracranial electrode placement, may develop frank SE (after the antiepileptic medications are withdrawn) and constitute a third category of "semi-intentional" iatrogenic SE.

The most important principle in the treatment of SE is that time to initiation of the first anti-seizure medication is likely the most important predictor of seizure control and outcome [4, 5]. Undertreatment of the seizures should be avoided as this may lead to more refractory seizures and some may even

go straight to continuous infusion of anesthetic drips if the first anticonvulsant fails to control the seizures [6]. Persistent convulsive or nonconvulsive seizure activity not responding to first-line treatment requires ICU admission and an aggressive treatment approach [7], as untreated SE has an overall poor prognosis. Most agree that NCSE should be treated just as CSE, but based on mostly retrospective case series some doubt has been raised about the use of anesthetic infusions as these are associated with medical complications and poor outcome [8]. Likely these associations are based on the fact that more aggressive interventions are given to sicker and more refractory patients. Diagnosis of the underlying etiology for SE is important as certain etiologies may only be successfully controlled if the precipitating offender is corrected. SE in the setting of hypoglycemia illustrates this well, as correction of the underlying metabolic abnormality is a prerequisite for successful seizure control. The seizure burden in SE of acute brain injury has been associated with a cumulative increase of worse functional and cognitive outcome for each additional time period spent seizing in both children and adults [9–11].

Pathophysiology

Physicians need to understand the underlying pathophysiology of SE because this is important in order to adjust the treatment of SE, as some treatments such as ketamine are aimed at the evolving, self-sustaining pathophysiologic changes seen with ongoing seizure activity. Most seizures are self-terminating phenomena lasting from few seconds to few minutes. A single seizure is followed by a refractory period characterized by higher seizure threshold that prevents seizure recurrence. However, under certain conditions the mechanisms responsible for seizure termination fail and seizures recur, i.e. SE ensues. This may lead to CNS damage either directly or indirectly and further seizures.

Direct mechanisms include abnormal release of excitatory aminoacids and decreased release of inhibitory ones at the

P.N. Varelas (✉)
Departments of Neurology and Neurosurgery, Henry Ford Hospital, 2799 West Grand Blvd, Detroit, MI 48202, USA

Department of Neurology, Wayne State University, Detroit, MI, USA
e-mail: varelas@neuro.hfh.edu

J. Claassen
Neurocritical Care, Columbia University College of Physicians and Surgeons, New York, NY, USA

Division of Critical Care and Hospitalist Neurology, Department of Neurology, Columbia

University Medical Center, New York Presbyterian Hospital, New York, NY, USA
e-mail: jc1439@columbia.edu

P.N. Varelas, J. Claassen (eds.), *Seizures in Critical Care*, Current Clinical Neurology, DOI 10.1007/978-3-319-49557-6_8

synapse [12]. There is increased glutamate release with repetitive presynaptic activation (called facilitation) eventually leading to excitotoxic damage through Ca++ influx to the neurons via NMDA and AMPA receptors. At the same time, release of GABA from the presynaptic storage sites is decreased when the presynaptic neuron is activated repetitively (referred to as fading of inhibition) [13]. Except for the transient synaptic effects, there are additional longer lasting ones affecting the expression of genes and leading to apoptosis of more vulnerable classes of cells, especially in the hippocampus. In addition, local epileptogenic processes, if repeated, can lead to dissemination of seizure propensity to other regions of the brain, a process named secondary epileptogenesis [14].

The effect that antiepileptic medications have in controlling SE may also vary with the duration of seizures and drug resistance may develop. As mentioned above, this drug resistance may be due to antiepileptic drug (AED) target alterations induced by SE, such as reduced membrane expression or increased trafficking of $GABA_A$ receptors [15], in addition to reduced GABA release. Apart from target alterations by receptor trafficking (i.e., from the synaptic membrane into endosomes, making them unavailable to the neurotransmitter), SE is known to increase the brain expression of drug efflux transporters such as P-glycoprotein (Pgp) at the blood-brain barrier, which might reduce concentrations of AEDs at their brain targets. In a study of two rat SE models, no increase of Pgp expression in brain capillary endothelial cells during SE was found, whereas significant overexpression was determined in both models 48h after SE. These data suggest that alterations in Pgp are not critically involved in refractory SE, at least in the first couple of days [16]. If SE occurs in the context of pre-existing epilepsy, increased Pgp expression may already be present at the time of status onset. In this case, drugs such as verapamil (a Pgp inhibitor) may reverse the resistance to AEDs, which are substrates to Pgp (phenytoin, phenobarbital), in long-lasting refractory SE [17].

Indirect CNS damage from SE is the result of systemic derangements that follow. The seminal animal studies by Meldrum have shed a light on this issue. After prolonged bicuculline-induced convulsive SE in baboons, neuronal damage and cell loss was evident in the neocortex, cerebellum, and hippocampus. When systemic factors were kept within normal physiological limits (paralyzed and artificially ventilated animals with adequate serum glucose levels), there was decreased but still present neocortical and hippocampal cell damage, but absent cerebellar cell injury [18, 19]. These experiments suggest that the seizure activity per se is responsible for the neuronal damage and the systemic derangements play an additional role.

These derangements are especially important for the ICU patient who is in SE, because they are amenable to ICU treatment. Table 8.1 presents the most common changes by system involved. Lothman divided the systemic changes after

Table 8.1 Systemic physiologic changes induced by prolonged generalized convulsions or generalized convulsive SE

CNS
Tissue hypoxia (decreased O_2 delivery and increased demand)
Cerebral edema (angiogenic and cytotoxic)
Increased CBF-CMRO$_2$
Increased intracranial pressure
CSF pleocytosis
Hemorrhage
Cerebral venous thrombosis
Cardiovascular
Hypertension followed by hypotension
Tachycardia
Myocardial ischemia
Arrhythmias
Cardiac arrest
Respiratory
Hypopnea/apnea
Hypoventilation
Aspiration
Pulmonary hypertension and edema
Pulmonary embolus
Metabolic
Acidosis (both metabolic and respiratory)
Dehydration
Electrolyte changes (hyponatremia, hyperkalemia)
Hypoglycemia
Hyperthermia
Skeletomuscular
Rhabdomyolysis
Dislocations
Fractures (bilateral humeral head, compression of the first four lumbar bodies)
Renal
Acute tubular necrosis
Gastrointestinal
Hepatic failure
Hematologic
Peripheral leukocytosis
Disseminated intravascular coagulopathy

Adapted from [44, 76]

convulsive SE into two phases [13]. During phase 1 (or early phase, within the first 30 min) the initial consequences of a prolonged seizure or SE are an increase in the cerebral blood flow (CBF) and a massive increase of plasma catecholamines, leading to increased blood pressure, heart rate, serum glucose, sweating, and body temperature. Cardiac arrhythmias are common. Acidosis is the result of increased serum lactate and CO_2 retention. Minute ventilation may be increased in this phase, but later, periods of hypopnea predominate and can be exacerbated with respiratory depressant antiepileptics, such as barbiturates and benzodiazepines. In a clinical study, the pH ranged between 6.28 and 7.5 in 70 spontaneously ventilating patients with SE: it was <7.35 in

59 and <7.0 in 23 patients. Thirteen patients had $PaCO_2 > 60$ mmHg and overall 30 patients had a respiratory component to the acidosis [20]. Acidosis is markedly attenuated with neuromuscular blockade, indicating anaerobic muscle metabolism as a major source of lactate [19]. Hypoxia, on the other hand, is usually modest. In primate models of SE, the mean PaO_2 was 58–68 mmHg and alone did not seem to induce cerebral injury [18, 21]. After approximately 30 min of seizing the patient enters the 2 phase (or late phase) of SE. The systemic and cerebral protective mechanisms progressively fail, leading to multi-organ compromise: Hypotension, cardiac failure with increased pulmonary capillary leaking (leading to neurogenic pulmonary edema), loss of cerebral autoregulation (resulting in a systemic pressure dependent CBF, which together with the increased intracranial pressure exacerbates the cerebral hypoperfusion), renal failure secondary to rhabdomyolysis or acute tubular necrosis, hypoglycemia and hepatic failure, severe electrolyte abnormalities (hyperkalemia which may reach life-threatening levels), and a disseminated coagulopathy. Cardiac arrhythmias are life-threatening in up to 60% of patients with prolonged SE [22]. Sinus tachycardia or supraventricular tachycardia is most common and can be complicated by the rapid infusion of antiepileptics such as phenytoin. Temperature elevation of 40° in seizing primates can be reached within 60–90 min after SE onset and, if persisting for >3 h, leads to neuropathic changes greater than those predicted from the seizure duration alone. When the baboons were paralyzed, the mean temperature increase was only 2.05°C over a 7-h observation. A similar dangerous temperature elevation has been observed in humans. Seventy out of 90 patients with SE had hyperthermia, with maximum temperature reaching 107°F. The duration of hyperthermia outlasted the duration of SE, with most patients remaining febrile at 12 h after the cessation of the convulsions, but only 3/27 were febrile at 48 h [20].

Patients that develop SE in the setting of acute brain injury may be particularly susceptible to acquire additional brain injury due to the brain being more susceptible to injury, as well as some of the stabilizing pathophysiologic processes being affected, such as loss of autoregulation leading to a delayed increase in regional cerebral blood flow to compensate for the increased metabolic demands of the seizing brain tissue [23].

Another important characteristic of late-phase status is an electromechanical dissociation that occurs and may lead to misinterpretation of the clinical situation: convulsions may decrease or evolve to minor twitching, although electrical cerebral seizure activity continues as NCSE [24]. Table 8.2 presents a scheme of these evolving stages. It is interesting to note that SE is a dynamic state, with different characteristics, depending on when the patient is examined [25]. Thus depending on the time of observation in the ICU, the patient

Table 8.2 Clinical and EEG seizure correlation during generalized SE

Time	Clinical activity	EEG activity
Onset	Discrete convulsions	Discrete seizure activity
	Continuous convulsions	Merging seizure activity
Minutes	Continuous convulsions	Continuous seizure activity
	Minimal twitching in face or distal extremities	Intermittent suppression between bursts of seizure activity
Hours	No muscular activity	Periodic epileptiform discharges on a flat background

Adapted from [25, 76, 225]

may have obvious grand-mal convulsions or only subtle twitching of the fingers, abdomen or face or nystagmoid jerks of the eyes or no clinical activity, but being in deep coma state. Although the chances in the ICU are that the intensivist will be notified early, because of vital sign monitoring and frequent examinations by the ICU staff, this may not be the case with a patient who was just admitted for ongoing status. This possibility must be kept in mind and all previously seizing patients, who do not regain consciousness soon, should be monitored with a continuous EEG to exclude ongoing NCSE.

Goals of ICU Management and Treatment Options for SE

Management of ICU seizures and SE should include (1) emergent medical management, (2) termination of seizures, (3) prevention of recurrence of seizures, (4) diagnosis and address of the underlying cause of seizures, and (4) prevention and treatment of complications. In a survey of 408 intensivists from the UK, it was shown that following failure of initial management of resistant SE, a benzodiazepine infusion (35%) or anesthetic induction agent (32%) was the preferred second-line treatments. The majority of respondents (57%) gave anesthetic induction agents within 60 min of the start of SE. Thiopentone was administered in 82% of these cases. Clinical assessment was used to monitor the response to the treatment in almost half the cases. However, in more specialized ICUs, such as pediatric or neurological or neurosurgical units the majority of responders used a cerebral function monitor in addition to the clinical examination, emphasizing the greater experience these physicians had [26]. In a more recent survey of international experts in the treatment of SE with a 50% response rate (60/120), there was consensus for using intravenous lorazepam for the emergent (first-line) therapy of SE in children and adults. For urgent (second-line) therapy, the most common agents chosen were phenytoin/fosphenytoin, valproate sodium, and levetiracetam; these choices varied by the patient age in the case scenarios. Physicians who care for adult patients chose cIV therapy for RSE, especially midazolam and propofol, rather than a standard AED sooner than those who care for children; and in children, there is a reluctance to choose propofol. Pentobarbital was chosen later in the therapy for all ages [27].

As a general principle, the time to initiate treatment and to not undertreat early after onset of SE is a more important factor in determining seizure control and outcome than the specific choice of antiepileptic agent [28, 29]. This is illustrated by evidence that early treatment initiation for SE has been shown to be effective [4, 5] and by the fact that while lorazepam was superior to other options in the treatment of SE, the difference was not tremendous (i.e., when compared to phenobarbital [30]), and second agent add-on therapy in the out of hospital setting was ineffective but higher than usual doses of benzodiazepine in the out of hospital setting were effective in controlling SE [28, 29]. A general treatment algorithm for convulsive SE is presented in Table 8.3. The treatment is divided in stages, based on the response to seizure cessation (clinical or electroencephalographic).

Emergent Medical Management

Prehospital Management

Management of SE must begin by the emergency medical services in a prehospital setting. Several studies have attempted to assess the possibility of aborting SE even prior to the hospital. In a randomized, double-blinded study, lorazepam was 4.8 and diazepam 2.3 times more effective than placebo in terminating SE on the arrival at the emergency department when given intravenously (IV) by paramedics [4]. In another prehospital study, midazolam at doses of 2 mg/kg for children or 10 mg for adults intranasally or intramuscularly (IM) was comparable or better than IV diazepam [31]. The RAMPART study was a double-blind, randomized, noninferiority trial comparing the efficacy of intramuscular (IM) midazolam (10 mg followed by placebo IV, $n = 448$) with that of IM placebo followed by intravenous lorazepam (4 mg, $n = 445$) for children and adults in SE treated by paramedics. At the time of arrival in the emergency department, seizures had ceased without rescue therapy in 73.4% and 63.4%, respectively, favoring midazolam by an absolute 10% (95% CI 4.0–16.1, $p <$ 0.001). Based on this data the authors concluded that midazolam IM is at least as safe and effective as lorazepam IV for prehospital seizure cessation [5].

If there is a history of diabetes mellitus or insulin use, an emergent glucose measurement should be done by paramedics and if an accucheck is not available, glucose in the form of orally administered juice or sugar or IV injection of DW 50% should be considered. As soon as measurement of glucose becomes available, glucose should be rechecked and thiamine administration also considered.

Oxygen should be administered in a convulsing patient in the ambulance and all prehospital measures to keep an open airway should also be taken.

In-Hospital Management in the Emergency Department or ICU

Management of the convulsing patient who arrived in the Emergency Department or was transferred to an ICU room comprises general medical supportive and diagnostic measures and at the same time specific treatment to terminate the seizures. It is unclear what type of ICU setting is a better fit to deal with SE and current data do not necessarily support admission to a specialized Neuro-ICU. In a single center, non-randomized study of 151 patients (with 168 episodes of SE), 46 (27%) were admitted to an NICU and 122 (73%) to an MICU based on bed availability. APACHE II scores were significant higher in the MICU group (17.5 vs 13.4, $p = 0.003$) and age in the NICU (58.3 vs 51.5 years, $p = 0.041$). More continuous EEGs were ordered in the NICU (85 vs 30 %, $p <$ 0.001), where fewer patients were intubated, but more eventually tracheostomized. The NICU had a higher rate of complex partial SE and more alert or somnolent patients, whereas the MICU had a higher rate of generalized SE and more stuporous or comatose patients. Admission diagnoses also differed, with the NICU having higher rates of strokes and the MICU higher rates of toxic metabolic etiologies (39 vs 12% and 11 vs 21 %, $p = 0.002$). After adjustment, no difference was found in mortality, the ICU or hospital length of stay and modified Rankin score at discharge [32], but discharge status is typically not a great outcome measure as the recovery process is potentially still ongoing and benefits of an intervention or treatment setting may be underappreciated.

General Medical Supportive and Diagnostic Measures for SE

Basic life support with maintenance of airway, breathing and circulation should be provided as soon as the diagnosis of SE is established [6]. Endotracheal intubation (ETI) is important in maintaining adequate oxygenation and preventing aspiration pneumonia. However, few patients with SE require intubation. In the RAMPART study, out of 1023 enrollments, 218 (21%) patients received ETI. Two hundred four (93.6%) of the ETIs were performed in the hospital and 14 (6.4%) in the prehospital setting. Intubated patients were older and men underwent ETI more often than women. Patients with ongoing seizures on ED arrival had a higher rate of ETI, as did those who received rescue anti-seizure medication. Most ETI (62%) occurred early on (prior to or within 30 min after ED arrival). Late ETI was associated with higher mortality (14%) compared to early ETI (3%) [33]. Adequate oxygen supply with a non-rebreather facial mask and airway patency with oral or nasopharyngeal devices may be enough measures for a patient who has had one or more seizures, but has stopped having convulsions.

Table 8.3 Treatment algorithm for SE

3A Prehospital measures
IM midazolam 10 mg or, if not available, lorazepam 4 mg IV, intranasal midazolam or clonazepam
Provide oxygen by nasal cannula or face mask
If a history of diabetes, check finger-stick blood glucose, if available. Administer 1 amp of DW 50% IV if <60 mg/100 dl
3B In-hospital measures
Stage 1: Emergent initial measures
Preserve airway and oxygenation by oxygen face mask or intubation, as needed
Establish IV access
Order EEG to be available during therapy
Measure finger-stick blood glucose. Administer 1 amp of DW 50% IV if <60 mg/100 dL and 100 mg Thiamine IV
Send to the Lab: antiepileptic drug(s) blood levels, electrolytes, basic metabolic panel, serum glucose, complete blood count, total and ionized calcium, magnesium, and arterial blood gases
At the same time with the above: Immediate benzodiazepines—IV lorazepam 0.07–0.1 mg/kg [4 mg IV with an additional 4 mg if no response, if no weight available] or diazepam 0.15–0.25 mg/kg IV. If no IV access, diazepam 20 mg per rectum or midazolam 10 mg IM, buccally or intranasally. Skip this step and go directly to Stage 2, if patient has already received prehospital treatment with benzodiazepines
Stage 2: Urgent Control
Give one of the following two agents
• Phenytoin loading dose 20 mg/kg IV at 50 mg/min or fosphenytoin 20 mg/kg PE (phenytoin equivalents) IV at 150 mg/min or IM or
• Valproate 25–40 mg/kg IV load at 1.5–3 mg/kg/min
• If seizures continue after this step maybe give additional phenytoin or fosphenytoin (load additional 5 mg/kg PE to 10 mg/kg PE; goal serum level 20 mg/dl to 25 mg/dl) or valproate (load additional 20 mg/kg IV)
• Alternatives if allergies or unavailability of the above prevent administration to consider: levetiracetam 30–70 mg/kg IV (500–mg/min) or Phenobarbital 20 mg/kg IV (rate 100 mg/min)
EEG connected and running
Stage 3: Refractory SE
Intubation and mechanical ventilation
Hemodynamic support by pressors and IV fluid boluses
AEDs for RSE:
• Midazolam 0.1–0.2 mg/kg IV bolus, which can be repeated every 5 min up to total 2 mg/kg, followed by infusion 0.1–2.0 mg/kg/h, suppress seizure activity for 24 h then start weaning
• If for any reason unable to give midazolam, give Propofol 2 mg/kg IV bolus and 150 μg/kg/min to 200 μg/kg/min infusion, suppress seizure activity for 24 h then start weaning
• If not used yet and in patients with DNR status may use valproate (dosing as above)
• Additional AED alternatives include levetiracetam, phenobarbital, or lacosamide
Need continuous EEG monitoring at this point. NCSE should be managed the same as CSE.
Stage 4: Super-refractory SE
Stage 4.1
AEDs for (consider one of the following)
• Pentobarbital 10 mg/kg IV load at up to 50 mg/min, can be repeated several times until EEG burst-suppression pattern with 20–30 s suppression goal is achieved. Start at the same time continuous infusion 1 mg/kg/h and titrate up to 10 mg/kg/h for same goal.
• Thiopental 2–3 mg/kg IV bolus and 0.3 mg/kg/min to 0.4 mg/kg/min infusion or
• Additional agents to consider especially if breakthrough or withdrawal seizures are recorded:
o Ketamine 0.5–4.5 mg/kg bolus IV and up to 5 mg/kg/hour infusion for 24–48 h
o Phenobarbital 15–20 mg/kg load
Stage 4.2
Can be used after 4.1 measures fail or in parallel with them (in order from the first to the last resort)
• Isoflurane or desflurane or gabapentin or levetiracetam (in acute intermittent porphyria)
• Topiramate 300–1600 mg/day per orogastric tube (if no increased stomach residuals)
• Magnesium 4 g bolus IV and 2–6 g/h infusion (keep serum levels <6 mEq/L)
• Pyridoxine 100–600 mg/day IV or via orogastric tube
• Methyl-prednisolone 1 g/day IV for 5 days, followed by prednisone 1 mg/kg/day for 1 week
• IVIG 0.4 g/kg/day IV for 5 days
• Plasmapheresis for 5 sessions
• Hypothermia 33–35°C for 24–48 h and rewarming by 0.1–0.2°C/h
• Ketogenic diet 4:1
• Neurosurgical resection of epileptogenic focus if any
• Electroconvulsive therapy
• Vagal nerve stimulation or deep brain stimulation or transcranial magnetic stimulation
Stage 4.3
If several weaning attempts have failed over a period of months, consider end-of-life discussion with family or surrogate decision maker and withdrawal of life support with subsequent autopsy (if no etiology has been found)

Modified from [35, 190, 226, 227]

On the other hand, most ICU physicians would intubate a patient in SE for airway protection and for anticipation of administration of respiratory depressant antiepileptics. The goal after intubation is adequate oxygenation (initially 100% FiO_2) and ventilation with a goal of normal pH: initial hyperventilation in a paralyzed patient with metabolic acidosis is acceptable, but frequent arterial blood gases are necessary to avoid subsequent respiratory alkalosis, which may further decrease seizure threshold [34].

Paralytics are almost always used for the intubation of a seizing patient, but short-acting agents such as IV rocuronium (0.6–1.2 mg/kg) or vecuronium (0.1 mg/kg) are preferable to succinylcholine, which can induce severe hyperkalemia in neurological patients. As for sedation, thiopental can be used at 3–5 mg/kg, a drug which can also help in seizure control. At least two large IV catheters should be inserted and carefully secured for fluid, drug administration, and withdrawal of blood samples. This is not easy in a convulsing patient: an alternative site such as external jugular catheterization or an alternative route such as intramuscular or rectal administration should be sought [5].

Continuous electrocardiogram, pulse oximetry, and temperature monitoring should be initiated. Non-invasive blood pressure measurements should be started, but the physician should be reluctant to treat elevated pressure during the convulsion phase, unless it is extreme (for example >230 mmHg systolic) or there is suspicion it is the primary cause of the seizures (see the Chapter on hypertension and ICU seizures). Usually, control of the seizures with the first-line AEDs would be enough to reduce the blood pressure. Continuous invasive monitoring of blood pressure should be initiated for all patients in SE as many of the AEDs of choice have strong hypotensive effect, especially barbiturates.

EEG recording should be used to assess the presence or absence of ongoing seizure activity and to direct treatment, but this should not delay initiation of the urgent treatment of SE (see above).

Blood of all patients should be sent for blood glucose, complete blood count, basic metabolic panel, calcium (total and ionized), magnesium, AED levels [35]. On a case-by-case basis work-up should also include a comprehensive urine and blood toxicology panel (focussing on toxins that frequently cause seizures such as isoniazid, tricyclic antidepressants, theophylline, cocaine, sympathomimetics, alcohol, organophosphates, and cyclosporine), liver function tests, serial troponins, coagulation studies, arterial blood gas, and tests to detect inborn errors of metabolism.

For those with diagnosed hypoglycemia (typically via a finger-stick-accucheck), 50 ml of 50% glucose solution should be given. Hyperglycemia may exacerbate neuronal damage caused by SE, therefore glucose should be only administered when lab results confirm hypoglycemia [36,

37]. In case of suspected or confirmed history of alcoholism or other suspected dietary deficiency, 100 mg of IV thiamine is given first along with glucose to avoid precipitating Wernicke's encephalopathy.

Lumbar puncture is indicated, if there are no signs of increased intracranial pressure or non-communicating hydrocephalus and an infectious process causing SE is suspected. Twenty percent of patients with SE may have "benign postictal pleocytosis" (up to 70 white blood cells/mm^3) [38]. This SE-induced pleocytosis is usually polymorphonucleocitic in the differential [20] and this may help differentiate from a primary viral encephalitis as the cause of SE (where the differential is mainly mononucleocytic [7]). This latter case may be resistant to treatment to the point that the term "malignant SE" has been coined [39]. Eight out of 54 (15%) patients with SE may have CSF protein elevation >50 mg/100 ml but in only one case the value exceeded 75 mg/100 ml [20].

Termination of Seizures During SE

Management of an isolated seizure is discussed in another chapter but prolonged or recurring seizures, such as those seen in SE, should be treated aggressively and without delay. The earlier the treatment is initiated, the easier the termination of seizures: 80% of patients had termination of SE when treated within 30 min of onset and <40% when treated after the first 2 h from onset [40]. Compared to the ED, where recurrent convulsive seizures are easily recognized as SE, in the ICU many seizures are nonconvulsive in nature, and are only discovered on EEG. In this situation most intensivists would try to break the convulsion or electrographic seizures by administering benzodiazepines IV (such as lorazepam) for the short-term control of the seizing patient (first-line treatment) and loading the patient with an IV antiepileptic, such as phenytoin or valproate for the long-term control (second-line treatments) (Table 8.3). Because at this point it may not be clear if the flurry of seizures heralds the entry of SE, a very low threshold should exist to intubate the patient in anticipation of more seizures and the need for airway control during the work-up.

If the seizures persist despite 2 AEDs, SE is considered *refractory* (RSE) and special measures are taken in the ICU (Stage 3, Table 8.3), including the administration of anesthetic doses of short-half-life anti-seizure medications (third-line treatment). In select cases additional dose of second-line AEDs (such as phenobarbital or lacosamide) may be considered but most would start continuous infusions of anesthetic IV drugs, such as midazolam or propofol at this point, which also current guidelines recommend [27, 35]. As mentioned above some question the benefits for anesthetic agents to treat RSE altogether [8], while others consider giving anesthetic agents even earlier in the management course potentially as a second-line agent [35]. If these measures fail, induced barbiturate coma with longer-half-life agents such as pentobarbital is performed which marks the transition to *super-refractory (SRSE)* (Stage 4). Barbiturate treatments can be used for a short period (24–48 h) with subsequent slow emergence of the patient from coma or, in case seizures recur, for a longer period (usually a week). Additional agents such as ketamine are used at this stage (Table 8.3, Stage 4.1) and additional measures should be considered with various reported success rates based on small case-series at best (Table 8.3, Stage 4.2). Throughout the management and particularly if seizures are difficult to control the underlying cause for SE should be kept in mind and constantly questioned as disease modifying interventions such as plasmapheresis or neurosurgical interventions may be successful in certain scenarios. Prolonged SE may have a very favorable outcome and particularly in young patients with an unclear underlying etiology. Such an example is an 18-year-old man with SRSE who remained in the ICU for 79 days, but subsequently recovered [41]. End-of-life discussions with the family should only be entertained if these extreme and unproven measures fail to control the seizures in the ICU and only after all possible etiologically treatable causes have been considered (Table 8.3, Stage 4.3).

It should be noted that as the intensivist moves down the list of treatment options, the data supporting these treatments become more and more thin and expert-opinion-based. In fact, some of them may be independently associated with worse outcomes. In a recent study, mentioned above, 171 patients were treated over 6 years for SE, of whom 37% were treated with IVADs. Mortality was 18%. Patients with anesthetic drugs had more infections during SE (43% vs 11%; $p < 0.0001$) and a 2.9-fold relative risk for death (2.88; 95% confidence interval 1.45–5.73), independent of possible confounders (i.e., duration and severity of SE, non-anesthetic third-line antiepileptic drugs, and critical medical conditions) and without significant effect modification by different grades of SE severity and etiologies [8].

The intensity of treatment with therapeutic coma has also been challenged. In another recent study, 50 out of 467 (10.7%) patients with incident SE were managed with therapeutic coma. Therapeutic coma was associated with poorer outcome in the whole cohort: these patients had higher relative risk ratio for new disability (6.86; 95% CI, 2.84–16.56) and higher for mortality (9.10; 95% CI, 3.17–26.16). This effect was more important in patients with complex partial compared with generalized convulsive or nonconvulsive SE in coma. Prevalence of infections was higher (odds ratio, 3.81; 95% CI, 1.66–8.75), and median hospital stay in patients discharged alive was longer (16 days [range, 2–240 days] vs 9 days [range, 1–57 days]; $p < 0.001$) in subjects managed with therapeutic coma [42].

The intensivist, however, has to remember the more refractory the status is the worst the outcome and these chal-lenging and unproven treatments may be the last resorts to save the life of the patient and stop the seizures. Of the general anesthetics, pentobarbital coma is probably the one treatment with the most challenges (see below in the specific section). However, it may be an efficacious and safe drug to use in super-refractory SE cases. In a recent study from Columbia Presbyterian Hospital in New York, 31 SRSE patients were treated with continuous pentobarbital infusion. Only 8 (26%) of them had a history of epilepsy and 23 (74%) presented with convulsive SE. Underlying etiology was acute symptomatic seizures in 16 (52%, 12/16 with encephalitis), remote seizures in 10 (30%), and unknown in 5 (16%). The mean duration of pentobarbital infusion was 6 days and it controlled seizures in 90% of patients. Seizures recurred in 48% while weaning the infusion, despite the fact that burst-suppression was attained in 90% of patients and persisted >72 h in 56% of them. Weaning was successful after adding phenobarbital in 12 out of 15 (80%) of patients with withdrawal seizures. Complications during or after pentobarbital infusion included pneumonia (32%), hypotension requiring pressors (29%), urinary tract infection (13%), and propylene glycol toxicity and cardiac arrest in one patient each. Interestingly, one third (35%) of patients had no identified new complication after starting the infusion. At one year after discharge, 74% of patients were dead or in a state of unresponsive wakefulness, 16% were severely disabled, and only 3 out of 31 (10%) had no or minimal disability. The authors concluded that pentobarbital-induced coma for SRSE leads to infrequent complications, effectively aborts seizures, and may be successful even after weaning if combined with phenobarbital [43].

All of these studies are observational case series and not randomized controlled trials and therefore the reported associations between treatment and outcome will always remain circumstantial at best. At the heart of it, the chicken-and-egg problem with underlying etiology and SE on the one side and SE treatment on the other side (all being related to each other and affecting the ultimate outcome to different degrees), will remain unresolved in an observational data set. Clearly patients with RSE will not spontaneously stop seizing and recover without intervention. In the following sections we will review the available medication options and the rationale for their use.

Rationale for Using Specific Antiepileptic Medications

Treatment of recurrent seizures and status epilepticus requires fast drug absorption and therefore parenteral administration is essential. Among the currently available standard antiepileptics, only phenytoin, phenobarbital, levetiracetam, lacosamide, and valproate are available in injectable preparations. In addition, benodiazepines such as diazepam, lorazepam and general anesthetics (such as pentobarbital, thiopental, midazolam, and propofol) are available in parenteral forms. In order to act rapidly, the drugs need to cross the blood-brain barrier readily. This is the case with most drugs that are effective in acute seizure management: they are highly lipid-soluble and thus cross in seconds to minutes. High lipid solubility also leads to redistribution from the central compartment (blood and extracellular fluid) to peripheral compartments (fat and organs). The redistribution leads to a drop in plasma concentrations. Therefore repeat infusions are necessary to maintain adequate plasma levels. Continuous administration increases the concentration of the drug in the central compartment and leads to saturation of the peripheral compartment to the degree that the drug no longer redistributes. If drug administration ceases, plasma levels will be maintained by diffusion from the peripheral to the central compartment, which may result in unfavorable side effects, such as prolonged obtundation or cardiorespiratory collapse. These effects are dangerous and account for some of the morbidity and mortality associated with SE [44]. When administered in an ICU setting with readily available central access for urgent administration of IV fluids and vasopressors to counteract any drug-induced hypotension, this side effect is not associated with worse outcome [45].

The rationale for using benzodiazepines as first-line drug was based on a number of randomized controlled trials. The first randomized, double-blind study was conducted by Leppik et al., who compared diazepam to lorazepam in patients with SE. Both drugs were highly efficacious at controlling the seizures (see below) [46]. Another randomized, non-blinded clinical trial compared a combination of diazepam and phenytoin to phenobarbital in 36 patients with generalized convulsive SE. The cumulative convulsion time had a strong trend to be shorter for the phenobarbital group than for the diazepam/phenytoin group (median 5 vs 9 min, $P <$ 0.06). The response latency (elapsed time from the initiation of therapy to the end of the last convulsion) had also a tendency for being shorter for the phenobarbital group (median 5.5 vs 15 min, $P < 0.10$). The frequencies of intubation, hypotension, and arrhythmias were similar in the two groups [47]. The results of his study, although not reaching statistical significance due to the small number of patients, provided evidence of the safety and efficacy of phenobarbital, but did not convince the majority of the medical community, who preferred shorter acting agents with a safer clinical profile.

Ten years later, the landmark study from the Veterans Affairs Status Epilepticus Cooperative Study Group was published [30]. It was a randomized, double-blind, multicenter trial from 16 VA medical centers of four IV regimens, either for overt SE or subtle SE: diazepam (0.15 mg/kg) followed by phenytoin (18 mg/kg), lorazepam (0.1 mg/kg), phenobarbital (15 mg/kg), and phenytoin alone (18 mg/kg). Interestingly, lorazepam followed by phenytoin, the most commonly used

combination today, was not included. If the first treatment had failed, an algorithm to follow with a second and third treatment regimen was also available. Treatment was considered successful when all motor and EEG seizure activity ceased within 20 min after the beginning of the drug infusion and when there was no return of seizure activity during the following 40 min. Five hundred seventy patients were enrolled. Three hundred eighty-four patients had verified overt convulsive SE and 134 subtle SE. An important finding was that SE has to be controlled with the first antiepileptic agent: the second agent was successful in only 7% of cases when the first one failed. In the convulsive SE group, lorazepam was successful in 64.9% of patients, phenobarbital in 58.2%, diazepam plus phenytoin in 55.8%, and phenytoin in 43.6% (P = 0.02, but in the intention-to-treat analysis only with a trend). Lorazepam was significantly superior to phenytoin in a pairwise comparison ($P = 0.002$). In the subtle SE group no significant differences among the treatments were detected (17.9%, 24.2%, 8.3%, and 7.7%, respectively, for the four regimens, $P = 0.18$, in the intention-to-treat analysis $P = 0.91$). There were no differences among the treatment groups with respect to recurrence during the 12-h study period, the incidence of adverse reactions (hypoventilation, hypotension, cardiac arrhythmias), or the outcome at 30 days. However, comparing the two types of SE, outcomes for subtle SE were significantly worse at 30 days (50.1% of patients with overt SE were discharged from the hospitals vs only 8.8% of those with subtle SE, $P < 0.001$). Similarly, hypotension requiring treatment occurred more often in patients with subtle SE ($p <$ 0.001). During the first 12 h after the end of the infusions, no patient with subtle SE regained consciousness, compared to 17% of patients with overt SE (but with no significant difference among the four treatment groups).

At 30 days, the outcome of patients who responded to the first-line drug in both the overt and subtle SE groups was better than those who did not respond in the Veterans Affairs Status Epilepticus Cooperative Study Group [30]. Mortality in the non-responders was twice as high as that in the responders. Based on these results, Treiman and colleagues concluded that lorazepam was more efficacious than phenytoin in overt SE treatment and overall easier to use than the other regimens. Also based on these results, various treatment algorithms have been proposed which combine treatment first with lorazepam and then with phenytoin within the first 30 min after SE onset [48].

Recently a small French study compared a single to an early double antiepileptic agent approach for the treatment of SE in the out of hospital setting (68 patients in each arm). This randomized, double-blind, placebo-controlled trial explored the efficacy of levetiracetam as add-on therapy to benzodiazepines (clonazepam 1 mg) for generalized CSE [29]. This study found no difference for the primary outcome measure defined as cessation of convulsions at 15 min after drug administration and also no difference in the predefined post-hoc analyses of secondary safety and efficacy endpoints. Impressively, 84% of patients in the control arm who only received 1 mg of clonazepam were seizure free, which is higher than the 59% and 65% for intravenous lorazepam (4 mg or 0.1 mg/kg) and 73% for intramuscular injection of midazolam (10 mg) [4, 5, 30]. Patients were allowed to get an extra dose of clonazepam and possibly the higher dosed benzodiazepine should be credited with the high response rate.

After these measures fail and if the patient is in the ICU, anesthesia with midazolam or propofol is suggested for treatment of RSE. Alternatively, phenobarbital is tried first for the next 30 min, before one proceeds to general anesthesia. The notion, however, is to individualize the treatment to the patient, than follow a strict, inflexible algorithm: for example, there are selected patients with good response to IV lorazepam, who may benefit from subsequent oral administration of the drug instead of an additional medication [49]. When the first-line drugs fail to control SE, the subsequent choices have markedly reduced efficacy [30], either due to intrinsic refractoriness or delay of treatment with reduced probability for response [50]. Until now we do not have a way to predict which patient will not respond to treatment and for whom the intensivist should, for example, skip treatment steps and go directly to general anesthesia. Mayer et al. examined the issue of predictive factors for refractory SE in a retrospective study of 74 patients with 83 episodes of SE. Refractory SE was defined as seizures occurring >60 min despite treatment with benzodiazepines and an adequate loading of a second standard IV antiepileptic. In 57 (69%)

episodes seizures occurred after benzodiazepine treatment and in 26 (31%) even after a second agent was administered (i.e., fulfilling the criteria for RSE). NCSE and focal motor seizures at onset were independent risk factors for RSE in the multivariate analysis (odds ratio 11.6, 95% CI 1.3–11.1, $P = 0.03$ and 3.1, 1.1–9.1, $P = 0.04$, respectively) [51].

However, there is no standardized management of RSE even among neurologists specializing in critical care. A survey among 63 (out of 91 participants who responded) experts in this field from Austria, Germany and Switzerland found that two thirds would apply another non-anesthetizing drug (such as phenobarbital) for both convulsive and complex partial SE after the failure of first-line drugs. A general anesthetic was more often used in convulsive than in complex partial SE as an alternative (35% vs 16%, $P = 0.02$). All participants would proceed to general anesthesia for ongoing seizures after these measures had failed, in case of CSE and, interestingly, 75% of them in case of NCSE. One third of participants would not use EEG, but only aim for clinical seizure termination. The vast majority (72%) responded that they would start weaning general anesthesia within 24–48 h [52]. The more recent international survey of critical care experts, however, suggested that for adult patients the preference was to choose continuous IV therapy for RSE, especially midazolam and propofol, rather than a standard AED, which may reflect a shift in the treatment paradigm [27].

In the following sections we will present the individual drugs used in the treatment of ICU seizures. Some of the most important data regarding pharmacokinetics, adverse effects,

Table 8.4 Doses, half-life and elimination route for antiepileptic medications used in the ICU for prolonged seizures or SE [48, 62, 76, 79, 142, 168, 228]

	IV Loading dose	Maximum Rate	Maintenance (po-IV)	T 1/2	Elimination
Diazepam	0.15–0.25 mg/kg	5 mg/min		24–57 h	Hepatic
Lorazepam	0.05–0.1 mg/kg	2 mg/min		8–25 h	Hepatic
Midazolam	0.1–0.3 mg/kg	4 mg/min	0.08–0.4 mg/kg/h	1.5–4 h	Hepatic
Clonazepam	1 mg (repeat × 4)	2 mg/min	10 mg/day	20–40 h	Hepatic
Phenytoin	15–20 mg/kg	50 mg/min	4–5 mg/kg/day	12–48 h	Hepatic
Fosphenytoin	15–20 mg PE/kg	150 mg PE/min	4–5 mg PE/kg/day	10–15 min	Hepatic, RBC, tissues
Lidocaine	1.5–2 mg/kg	50 mg/min	3–4 mg/kg/h	1.8 h	Hepatic
Lacosamide	100 mg	1–2 mg/min	50–400 mg/day	13 h	Renal
Levetiracetam	1500 mg (up to 3 g)	Within 15 min	1–3 g/day	7 h	Renal
Valproic acid	10–25 mg/kg	1.5–3 mg/kg/min	15–50 mg/kg/day	7–18 h	Hepatic
Thiopental	2–4 mg/kg	250 mg/min	3–5 mg/kg/h	14–34 h	Hepatic
Pentobarbital	6–12 mg/kg	50 mg/min	0.5–2 mg/kg/h	20 h	Hepatic
Phenobarbital	1520 mg/kg	100 mg/min	1–4 mg/kg/day	75–120 h	Hepatic, renal (25%)
Propofol	1–2 mg/kg	5 min	5–10 mg/kg/h initially, reduced to 1–3 mg/kg/h	0.5–1 h	Hepatic
Paraldeyde	5–10 ml rectally	Glass syringes	Repeated in 15–30 min	3 h	Hepatic, lungs
Isoflurane	0.8–2% inhaled	Anesthetic system	Titrate to burst-suppression		Lungs

PE phenytoin equivalents

and efficacy, based on published studies pertinent to the ICU, will be presented to the interested reader. Table 8.4 presents an overview of these medications. A more in-depth analysis can be found in standard Epilepsy and Pharmacology textbooks.

Medications Used to Control ICU Seizures and SE (Table 8.4)

Benzodiazepines

Introduction

Benzodiazepines have maintained a significant role as first-line IV treatment for acute seizures or SE since they were shown to be broad spectrum and potent anticonvulsant agents [53]. Their effect is at the synaptic level via the benzodiazepine $GABA_A$ receptor complex. They enhance the inhibitory GABA action by increasing the Cl-channel openings and hyperpolarizing the postsynaptic neuron [54, 55]. However, one must keep in mind that first-line anticonvulsants like benzodiazepines and phenytoin fail to terminate convulsive SE in 31–50% of cases [1, 4, 5, 30, 51]. Recent data suggests that possibly the dose of the benzodiazepine as much as the time lapse between seizure onset and medication administration predicts the rate of response, though this was not specifically tested in the trial [29].

Diazepam

Diazepam is a highly lipid-soluble benzodiazepine, which has been used extensively for the treatment of SE, but recently has at least in the USA lost some popularity to lorazepam. It is recommended that diazepam be administered by direct IV injection through a needle or a catheter rather than by infusion. Due to its solubility profile it rapidly enters the brain tissue. However, it redistributes to other parts of the body (fat stores and muscle) in approximately 15–20 min after it enters the brain. This results in loss of the clinical effect due to a fall in the brain drug levels. Its distribution half-life is 30–60 min and its elimination half-life 24–57 h [56]. Nonetheless, sedative adverse effects are persistent and cumulative in particular with repeated administration, since the drug remains in the fat stores. It has been shown that 5–10 mg/min of diazepam can terminate seizures in 5–10 min in 70–80% of patients. The recommended dose is 10–20 mg (0.15–0.25 mg/kg, at a rate of ≤5 mg/min) [46].

In cases that prolonged IV treatment is recommended for longer term management, the use of an alternative drug is advised. The injectable solution contains 5 mg/ml diazepam in a mixture containing 40% propylene glycol and 10% ethanol and can cause local tissue irritation, venous thrombosis or phlebitis, and pain at the site of injection. Careful monitoring of vital signs is recommended to prevent systemic adverse effects such as hypotension, respiratory depression, profound sedation and coma.

Co-administration of other sedatives such as barbiturates can increase the risk of serious systemic side effects [44, 57–59].

Diazepam can also be given by rectal administration. Two controlled clinical studies were conducted to demonstrate the effectiveness of rectal diazepam in treating seizure clusters. The trials were randomized, double-blind, placebo-controlled with the first dose administered at the onset of an identified episode. Seizure frequency was measured over the course of 12 h. Both trials showed that a significantly greater percentage of diazepam-treated patients that ranged from 55 to 62% were seizure free during the observation periods compared with placebo-treated patients. Somnolence was the most commonly reported adverse effect and in over 500 patients treated with rectal diazepam not a single episode of respiratory depression was reported [60, 61]. Despite this favorable drug profile, rectal diazepam administration in the ICU should be considered only in the very few patients without immediate IV access (for example those who, during their convulsions, lose their IV access, continue to seize, and have no obvious veins for cannulation). However, newer benzodiazepines, such as IM midazolam, may be better suited for those problematic administration route cases (see below).

Lorazepam

Lorazepam is closely related to diazepam in terms of efficacy and adverse effects. It has become the drug of choice in the acute management of seizures since the drug is less lipid-soluble than diazepam and subject to less rapid redistribution. Its distribution half-life is <10 min and its elimination half-life 8–25 h [56]. A single injection is highly effective and it has been associated with lower risk of cardiorespiratory depression and hypotension than diazepam. The anticonvulsant effect lasts approximately 6–12 h, making it preferable to diazepam (15–30 min) and particularly appropriate for the management of withdrawal seizures [62]. In a randomized, double-blind trial, lorazepam was compared with diazepam in the treatment of 81 episodes of SE. Patients received one or two doses of 10 mg of diazepam or 4 mg of lorazepam IV. The onset of action did not differ significantly (mean time to end the seizures was 2 min for diazepam and 3 for lorazepam). Seizures were controlled in 89% of the episodes treated with lorazepam and 76% treated with diazepam. Adverse effects, such as respiratory depression, occurred in 13% of the lorazepam-treated and in 12% of the diazepam-treated patients [46]. This slightly superior clinical profile of the drug was also confirmed in the pediatric population. The two drugs were compared in 102 children in a prospective, open, "odd and even dates" trial. Convulsions were controlled in 76% of patients treated with a single dose of lorazepam and in 51% of those treated with a single dose of diazepam. In this study, some patients received lorazepam rectally with 100% efficacy. Significantly fewer patients treated with lorazepam required additional anticonvulsants to terminate the seizures. Respiratory depression occurred in 3% of lorazepam-treated patients and 15% of diazepam-treated patients. Interestingly, no patient who received lorazepam required admission to an ICU [63].

In another retrospective study, efficacy, safety, and cost of lorazepam treatment in 90 episodes of SE was compared to diazepam. Fewer seizure recurrences followed lorazepam administration (given either as first, second, or third dose of benzodiazepine, $P = 0.0006$). There was no difference in adverse effects or cost. The authors recommended that lorazepam be the first-line therapy in preference to diazepam in adults with convulsive SE [64].

Most importantly, as discussed above, lorazepam was found to be the most efficacious and safe treatment for treatment of SE when compared to diazepam with phenytoin, phenytoin alone, and phenobarbital [30], and also shown to be safely administered in the out of hospital setting [4].

Due to the strong tendency for tolerance following lorazepam treatment, longer-term maintenance antiepileptic drugs must be given in addition. The recommended dose of lorazepam is 0.05–0.1 mg/kg (usually 4 mg), repeated after 10 min if necessary. The rate of injection should not exceed 2 mg/min.

Midazolam

Midazolam is a unique water-soluble compound, whose benzepine ring closes when in contact with serum and converts it into a highly lipophilic structure, crossing rapidly the blood-brain barrier. Its water solubility leads to rapid absorption by intramuscular injection or by intranasal or buccal administration. Midazolam is 96% protein-bound and is metabolized in the liver before renal excretion. It has an ultra-short distribution half-life of <5 min and a short elimination half-life of 1.5–4 h [56]. Thus, its action is very short and seizures may recur few minutes after they have stopped. However, in the ICU the volume of distribution may be expanded and the half-life may be prolonged, especially with liver dysfunction [65]. Acidosis can also reduce the lipid solubility of the drug by opening the benzepine ring structure and thus, decrease CNS entrance and seizure control. Despite these deficiencies, midazolam is probably the best benzodiazepine that can be used as a continuous infusion, because of its favorable kinetics and the lack of propylene glycol as a vehicle (which can cause cardiac arrhythmias). An IV bolus of 0.1–0.3 mg/kg at a rate not to exceed 4 mg/min can be repeated once after 15 min. The recommended rate for IV infusion is 0.08–2 mg/kg/h [35]. Higher rates may be associated with hypotension but when given in a critical care setting rates up to 2.9 mg/kg/h are likely safe [45]. The high water solubility of midazolam and rapid absorption makes it a better agent for IM injection than the other benzodiazepines, when IV administration route becomes a problem in the ICU [66]. The mean

half-life of IM midazolam (2 h) is slightly longer than the IV route. IM diazepam and lorazepam have a relatively slower absorption, induce local discomfort or can precipitate at the injection site and are not recommended for the treatment of SE [62]. However, IM midazolam has been successfully used to stop frequent seizures or SE within 5–10 min in children and adults [67–71]. In a prospective, randomized study in the emergency department IM midazolam was compared to IV diazepam in their ability to stop seizures. Eleven patients received diazepam (0.3 mg/kg, maximum 10 mg) and 13 midazolam (0.2 mg/kg, maximum 7 mg). Midazolam was administered faster, because of no need for starting an IV line (mean time from arrival to administration of the drug was 3.3 vs 7.8 min, $P = 0.001$) and resulted in faster cessation of seizures (mean time from arrival to cessation 7.8 vs 11.2 min, $P = 0.047$) [69]. The usual IM dose of midazolam is 5–10 mg (0.2 mg/kg).

More recently, Ulvi et al. prospectively evaluated midazolam infusion in 19 patients with refractory SE (not responding to initial IV administration of 0.3 mg/kg diazepam (three times at 5-min intervals), 20 mg/kg phenytoin, and 20 mg/kg phenobarbital. These patients were given an IV bolus of midazolam (200 mcg/kg) followed by a continuous infusion at 1 mcg/kg/min. The dose was increased by 1 mcg/kg/min every 15 min until seizures were controlled. In 18 (94.7%) patients, seizures were completely controlled in a mean time of 45 min, at a mean infusion rate of 8 mcg/kg/min. No significant changes in blood pressure, heart rate, oxygen saturation, or respiratory status were noticed. The mean time to full consciousness after stopping the infusion was 1.6 h and the mean infusion duration of midazolam was 14.5 h [72].

A recent randomized controlled trial demonstrated that intramuscular injections of midazolam as first-line treatments for convulsive SE were in the out of hospital setting at least as effective and safe as intravenous administration of lorazepam [5]. One of the advantages of this approach is that midazolam unlike lorazepam does not have to be refrigerated making it a more practical choice to use in the field for many emergency services.

Phenytoin and Fosphenytoin

Phenytoin is insoluble in water, and the parenteral formulation contains 40% propylene glycol, 10% alcohol, as well as sodium hydroxide to adjust the pH to 12. This solution is highly caustic to veins and it may cause necrosis to the surrounding tissues by extravasation. The rate of administration has been limited to a maximum of 50 mg/min, although in clinical practice it is given more slowly—over 25–45 min in the adult patient—to minimize the pain at the injection site and reduce the risk of cardiovascular toxicity from the propylene glycol diluent. It should be mixed only with normal saline and other drug administration through the same line should be avoided. As a lipid-soluble compound, phenytoin readily enters the brain (it reaches peak levels within 15 min) and its redistribution out of the CNS is slower than the benzodiazepines [73]. The drug is 96% protein bound and competes with other highly bound medications. With low albumin levels, one should consider measuring free instead of total phenytoin levels. Fast infusion of the drug carries the risk for hypotension and QT prolongation, therefore ECG and frequent blood pressure measurements are recommended. Pain, edema, and distal to the infusion site ischemia characterizes the "purple-glove" syndrome, which may occur in 9/152 (5.9%) patients who received phenytoin through a peripheral IV line [74]. There may be a delay of several hours between the infusion and the clinical presentation of the syndrome, which makes the recognition difficult. Nevertheless, phenytoin is a highly effective drug in treating SE [75].

Fosphenytoin sodium is a phosphate ester prodrug of phenytoin that was developed as a replacement for parenteral phenytoin and was approved in the US market in 1996. After administration, phenytoin is cleaved from the prodrug by phosphatases found in the liver, red blood cells, and many other tissues. The conversion rate is not affected by age, hepatic status or the presence of other drugs. Unlike phenytoin, fosphenytoin is freely soluble in aqueous solutions, including IV solutions. It is supplied as a ready-mixed solution of 50 mg/ml in water for injection and is buffered to a pH 8.6–9.0. This relatively lower pH of the vehicle for fosphenytoin is responsible for the lack of local adverse side effects at the injection site as opposed to the highly alkaline IV phenytoin solution. Fosphenytoin can be administered IV or IM and it is extensively bound (~95%) to plasma albumin. The dosage of the drug is expressed in phenytoin equivalents (PE). Seventy-five mg of fosphenytoin results in 50 mg of phenytoin in the serum after the enzymatic conversion; 75 mg of fosphenytoin is therefore labeled as 50 mg phenytoin equivalent (thus 15 mg PE of fosphenytoin is the same as 15 mg of phenytoin) [76]. The drug is administered IV or IM at doses corresponding to customary phenytoin sodium loading (15–20 mg PE/kg) and consistently produces therapeutic plasma phenytoin concentrations (total 10–20 μg/ml and free 1–2 μg/ml). A maintenance dose of 4–7 mg PE/kg can be given either IV or IM. Therapeutic phenytoin concentrations are attained in most patients within 10 min of rapid IV fosphenytoin infusion (up to 150 mg PE/min) and within 30 min of slower IV infusion (<100 mg/min) or IM injection. Maximal total plasma phenytoin concentration increases with increasing fosphenytoin dose, but is less affected by increasing the infusion rate at a given dose level. It is recommended, following fosphenytoin administration, that phenytoin concentrations not be monitored until complete conversion of fosphenytoin to phenytoin is established. Since the conversion half-life is approximately 10–15 min [77], conversion is completed within 1–1.5 h; serum phenytoin peaks at 30 min following the start of IV fosphenytoin infusion and at 3 h after IM injection.

Fosphenytoin has fewer local adverse side effects (pain, itching, or burning at the site of injection) when given IV or IM compared with IV phenytoin. The most common CNS side effect incidence, such as nystagmus, somnolence, ataxia, and headache does not differ between phenytoin and fosphenytoin [78]. Fosphenytoin has been associated with hypotension in 7.7% of patients, which rarely lead to an intervention and with higher pruritus than phenytoin [79]. Phenytoin administered at fosphenytoin rates can lead to cardiac arrest [80], therefore intensivists have to be very careful while prescribing the drug in the ICU during emergencies. Paresthesias of the lower abdomen, back, head, or neck have been reported with fosphenytoin in particular, when high doses and rapid infusion rate were used. They rapidly resolve without sequelae. A possible explanation is the competitive displacement of derived phenytoin from plasma protein binding sites by fosphenytoin. Earlier and higher unbound phenytoin plasma concentrations, and thus an increase in systemic adverse effects, may also occur following IV fosphenytoin loading doses in patients with a decreased ability to bind fosphenytoin and phenytoin (renal or hepatic disease, hypoalbuminemia, the elderly). Close vital sign monitoring and reduction in the infusion rate by 25–50% are recommended for these, frequently encountered, ICU patients [81].

Valproic Acid (VPA)

Valproate is an antiepileptic drug with broad spectrum activity against absence seizures [82], generalized tonic-clonic seizures [83], focal seizures [84, 85] and myoclonic seizures [86].

The drug has enjoyed increasing popularity in the ICU, especially after the introduction of the parenteral formulation. Although VPA is safe and generally well tolerated, there have been early reports of altered hepatic function and of several fatalities in patients taking VPA in combination with other antiepileptics [87]. Careful monitoring of hepatic function is required in patients being treated with VPA, but dose reduction alone may be effective in preventing hepatic complications. In order to provide information on which patients are at risk for VPA-induced hepatotoxicity, Dreifuss et al. conducted a retrospective review of all reports of fatal hepatic dysfunction received by Abbott laboratories between 1978–1984. Patients found to be at the greatest risk for developing fatal hepatotoxicity where children <2 years treated with multiple antiepileptics, and who had other medical conditions, congenital abnormalities, mental retardation, developmental delay, or other neurologic diseases [88]. From 1980 to 1986 the number of VPA-related hepatic fatalities had declined from eight to one, while the number of patients treated had increased nearly six-fold. Nevertheless, VPA is relatively contraindicated in cirrhosis or hepatic failure where it can accumulate and further promote liver damage (see below). Additional side effects include a dose-related thrombocytopenia, platelet dysfunction and coagulopathies (4% incidence in children [89]), pancreatitis, and elevated ammonia.

Valproate sodium injection (Depacon) is approved for use when clinical factors make oral administration difficult or impossible. The pharmacokinetics of the oral and parenteral forms are similar, but if fast therapeutic levels is the goal, like in many ICU situations, the IV form has significant advantages. It can be delivered at a more physiological pH, does not require organic solvents, and has a wider range of solution compatibility compared to phenytoin. In addition, it does not cause sedation or respiratory compromise like the barbiturates or benzodiazepines and has a safer hypotension profile compared to phenytoin and the barbiturates [90]. The drug has an elimination half-life between 7.2 and 17.7 h in studies given to healthy volunteers and this may be due to its 90–95% plasma protein binding [91–93]. Depacon was approved for infusions up to 10–15 mg/kg at 1.5–3 mg/kg/min in the absence of other antiepileptics and in patients valproate-naive. IM injection may produce muscle necrosis and should be avoided.

In a multicenter, open-label trial examining safety of IV VPA, 318 patients with previously treated epilepsy were enrolled; a need for parenteral VPA therapy for various reasons was documented. The median dose of IV VPA was 375 mg given over 1 h. Fifty-four (17%) patients experienced transient adverse effects, such as headache (2.4%), local reactions (2.2%), somnolence and nausea without vomiting (2.2%). The side effects led six patients to withdraw from the study [93]. However, these recommended doses generally result in sub-therapeutic levels of VPA, and they have been challenged in subsequent studies. In a small study by Venkataraman and Wheless, 24 infusions of IV valproate were carried out electively in 21 patients with epilepsy. The dose ranged from 21–28 mg/kg (mean 24.2 mg/kg) and was weight-adjusted. Target infusion rates were 3 or 6 mg/kg/min, i.e. over 4–8 min. No significant BP changes or EKG abnormalities were reported. Based on these results the authors suggested a rate of 6 mg/kg/min [94]. Doses up to 40 mg/kg [95] have been given without serious side effects including significant changes in blood pressure or electrographic abnormalities or respiratory depression. This is in contrast to other commonly used parenteral antiepileptics, such as lorazepam, phenobarbital, diazepam, and fosphenytoin, which have been variably associated with hypoventilation, cardiac arrhythmias, or hypotension [30, 96].

Of special concern in the ICU is co-administration of VPA with phenytoin, two highly albumin-bound AEDs. Two factors, hypoalbuminemia and VPA co-administration with phenytoin have been shown to increase free phenytoin fraction, and a combination of these two markedly increased free PHT fraction. In this case, free levels of both drugs should be measured in addition to total levels [97].

Intravenous VPA has not been approved for the management of status epilepticus (SE). However, the use of IV valproate in SE has been reported in the medical literature in both children and adults [98–102] and in a rat model of SE induced by intra-hippocampal application of 4-aminopyridine [103]. It has been used in both CSE and NCSE.

Price evaluated 24 neurosurgical patients with generalized CSE refractory to diazepam, treated with IV VPA, either as a bolus of 400 mg followed by infusion of 100 mg/h or 15 mg/kg load followed by 6 mg/kg/h infusion. Seizure control was achieved in 6/15 (40%) patients within 2 h in the first group and in 7/9 (78%) patients within 1 h in the second. Only one patient developed thrombocytopenia, without a clear cause-and-effect relationship ever established [104].

In one study conducted in Europe, the efficacy of IV sodium valproate was evaluated in 23 valproate-naïve adult patients with SE (8 with convulsive and 15 with nonconvulsive). A loading dose of 15 mg/kg followed by 1 mg/kg/h infusion led to VPA levels of 68.5 mg/l at 1 h, which was deemed satisfactory. Disappearance of SE in <20 min was considered successful, while in >30 min was considered a failure. Use of IV valproate resulted in the resolution of SE in 19 (83%) patients (7/8 with convulsive and 12/15 with NCSE). All four patients who failed to respond to VPA, as well as to other antiepileptics, had SE secondary to cerebral lesions. There were no relapses of SE within the first 24 h. All patients showed a slight reduction in systolic blood pressure and heart rate, but none required treatment for that. The serum concentrations varied most in four patients older than 80 years, but valproate was still well tolerated. Despite these promising results, the authors suggested that IV valproate be used cautiously in the elderly [101].

Another study assessed the safety and efficacy of IV valproate in 35 patients with SE. Twenty patients had failed treatment with benzodiazepines, and three patients had failed phenytoin treatment. SE was interrupted in 27/35 (77%) patients; the majority of them responded during the bolus infusion. Among the eight patients considered treatment failures, five patients were also refractory to other antiepileptic drugs, two patients responded to an increased valproate dose, and one patient responded to clonazepam. Two patients developed nausea and allergic skin rash after the VPA in these series [105].

In a small retrospective review of hospital records, 13 patients with SE and hypotension received IV VPA therapy. Mean age of patients was 74 and the mean loading dose of

VPA was 25 mg/kg (range 14.7–32.7), at a mean rate of 36.6 mg/min (range 6.3–100). There were no significant changes in blood pressure, pulse, or use of vasopressors, suggesting that VPA loading at these high rates is well tolerated, even in patients with cardiovascular instability. Seizures were controlled in 4 (31%) patients with IV VPA, but eventually all patients died as a consequence of their underlying illness (six were post-anoxic and 3 had stroke) [96]. The same group presented their results of using IV VPA in 30 patients on a later occasion. Control of seizures was achieved in 5/11 (45%) of patients with overt convulsive SE, 2/6 (33%) of patients with subtle SE, 4/8 (50%) patients with complex partial SE and all four (100%) patients with simple partial SE. Among patients with overt convulsive SE, the mean duration of SE prior to treatment in patients who responded was 2.6 h vs 36 h in those who did not respond [106].

Based on a review of the available literature until mid-2000, Hodges and Mazur suggested 3 clinical situations, where IV VPA could be considered as a third or fourth-line agent for the treatment of SE (Table 8.5). We also added a use in patients who have a well-documented allergic reaction to phenytoin or fosphenytoin.

This sequence of treatment options may be challenged by new data comparing phenytoin to VPA. In a retrospective study of 63 patients treated with IV VPA (average dose 31.5 mg/kg, range 10–78 mg/kg) because of allergy to phenytoin, myoclonus or refractoriness to the other AEDs, Limdi et al. reported 63.3% efficacy, which was increasing with the order that the drug was used (higher as a 4th AED than as a 1st AED). The rate of administration in this study reached 500 mg/min in the majority of patients, with minimal adverse events [107]. In a prospective study from India, Misra et al. evaluated 68 patients with CSE who were randomly assigned to two treatment groups, either VPA 30 mg/kg IV over 15 min or phenytoin 18 mg/kg IV at a rate of 50 mg/min. Interestingly, no benzodiazepines were used before VPA or phenytoin. If seizures failed to be controlled after this first-line treatment, the other agent was subsequently used. Seizures were aborted in 66% in the VPA group and 42% in the PHT group. As a second-line treatment in refractory

patients, VPA was effective in 79% and PHT was effective in 25%. The side effects in the two groups did not differ [108].

This study is the first to demonstrate superiority of VPA over phenytoin, but generalizability is questionable as skipping a first-line benzodiazepine clearly deviated from generally accepted standard of care. Further, these results were not replicated in a subsequent randomized study, which compared 50 patients treated with IV VPA with 50 age and sex-matched patients treated with phenytoin, but after administration of benzodiazepines without success. Intravenous VPA was successful in 88% and IV phenytoin in 84% of patients of SE (no significant difference), with a significantly better response in patients of SE <2 h. As in the study by Misra et al., the total number of adverse events did not differ significantly between the two treatment groups [109]. Lastly, in a prospective, quasi-randomized open-label study, Gilad et al. treated patients who presented in the emergency department with SE or acute repetitive seizures with either IV VPA 30 mg/kg or IV phenytoin 18 mg/kg over 20 min in a 2:1 ratio. No benzodiazepines were initially used and in case of failure of the first drug to control seizures, the other one followed. Seventy-four adult patients participated in the study, 49 in the VPA and 25 in the phenytoin arm. In 43 (87.8%) of the VPA patients, the seizures discontinued, and no rescue medication was needed. Similar results were found in the PHT group in which seizures of 22 (88%) patients were well controlled. Side effects were found in 12% of the PHT group, and in none of the VPA group [110]. In another prospective study from Norway, Olsen et al. treated 41 patients with SE or serial seizure attacks with 25 mg/kg of IV VPA loading dose over 30 min, followed by continuous infusion of 100 mg/h for at least 24 h. All patients had initially received diazepam as first-line unsuccessful treatment. In 76% of the cases (31 of 41), seizures stopped and anesthetic agents were not required [111].

Despite the small numbers and conflicting results, these small unblinded studies show better safety profile of VPA compared to phenytoin, at least equivalent efficacy, tolerability of higher infusion rates (up to 6 mg/kg/min) and may begin to challenge the current treatment algorithms. In fact recent European and US guidelines recommend IV VPA (20–40 mg/kg IV, allowing for additional 20 mg/kg if seizures continue) as an alternative to phenytoin second-line treatment for benzodiazepine resistant SE [6, 35]

Table 8.5 Indications for use of IV valproic acid in SE

1. As adjunctive agent, after benzodiazepines and phenytoin/fosphenytoin have been properly given and while preparations are being made for third-line agents (propofol, midazolam or barbiturates)
2. Once third-line agents have been given without complete cessation of SE
3. Instead of third-line agents in patients who do not wish to be mechanically ventilated
4. Patients allergic to one or more other antiepileptics
5. Absence SE or myoclonic SE as first or second-line agent

Adapted from [90]

Levetiracetam (LEV)

Levetiracetam (LEV) was approved as add-on therapy for refractory partial-onset seizures with or without secondarily generalization. The mechanism of action is poorly understood. It binds to the synaptic vesicle protein 2A (which regulates vesicular traffic and neurotransmitter release), inhibits the N-type high voltage-activated Ca^{++} channel currents, and suppresses the activity of negative allosteric modulators (such as zinc and beta carbolines) in the chloride influx via GABA and glycine-gated channels (therefore restoring chloride influx) [112–114]. It is metabolized by plasma hydrolysis and not through the cytochrome P450 system. LEV and its inactive metabolites are excreted 60–70% renally and the remaining 30% via the fecal route. Renal elimination is proportional to the renal clearance, and the half-life increases in renal insufficiency.

A significant advantage of the drug is that it virtually has no known interaction with the majority of ICU-used drugs, including other antiepileptics. This was explored in a retrospective study conducted in the NICU at the University of Cincinnati by Szaflarski et al. [115]. These authors analyzed the data of 379 critically ill patients and reported that phenytoin used prior to the NICU admission was frequently replaced with LEV monotherapy. Patients treated with LEV monotherapy when compared to other AEDs had lower complication rates and shorter NICU stays. Older patients and patients with brain tumors or strokes were preferentially treated with LEV for prevention and/or management of seizures.

LEV has been used in the treatment of SE because of its IV formulation advantage, although it has never been FDA-approved for this indication. Rossetti et al. retrospectively analyzed 23 patients with SE treated with enteral LEV [116]. The median daily dose of LEV was 2000 mg (range: 750–9000 mg). Ten patients (43%) responded. Initiation of treatment and dosage were significantly different between responders and non-responders: all responders had received LEV within 4 days after the beginning of their SE episode and were administered less than 3000 mg LEV/day. These authors concluded that LEV may be a useful alternative in SE if administered early, even in intubated patients, and that escalating the dosage beyond 3000 mg/day will unlikely provide additional benefit.

In another study from Jena, Germany, Rupprecht et al. compared 8 patients who received LEV as a second-line agent for NCSE with 11 patients treated with conventional IV medications for NCSE [117]. Those patients treated with LEV showed a marked clinical improvement with final cessation of ictal EEG-activity and clinical symptoms of NCSE within 3 days (mean 1.5 days). The response to conventional treatment was similarly effective but there were severe side effects whereas no relevant side effects in the LEV-treated group were noticed. The authors report no significant differences in hospitalization time, time in intensive care unit and outcome between the LEV group and the control group.

LEV has also been used in patients with refractory SE. Patel et al. published a small series of 6 patients with refractory SE (not responding to at least 2 antiepileptic medications), who eventually responded to enteral LEV (dose range 500–3000 mg/day) within 12–96 h [118].

LEV became also available in a parenteral form. Although it is considered bioequivalent to the enteral form and should be administered IV at a similar to the per os dose, it will build serum levels at a much faster rates (500–1500 mg can be given within 15 min), a potential advantage in case of SE. In fact, even higher infusion rates (up to 2500 mg IV over 5 min) were tolerated in healthy adults, with adverse effects (dizziness, 52.8%; somnolence, 33.3%; fatigue, 11.1%; headache, 8.3%) consistent with the established safety profile for the oral formulation [119]. Additionally, it may be considered an attractive alternative in critically ill patients in general, where the enteral administration may lead to delayed or erratic absorption or when swallowing or nasogastric tube placement is not deemed possible. Parenteral LEV has been used for treatment of SE in a study from Basel, Switzerland [120]. In this retrospective study, Ruegg et al. used IV LEV to treat 50 critically ill patients, 24 of which were in SE. These patients in SE received 20 mg/kg IV LEV within 15 min and in 16 (67%) of them (including 4, who received the drug as first-line treatment for simple partial or NCSE) SE ceased. Except for transient thrombocytopenia in 2/50 patients, no other serious or life-threatening side effects were reported by the authors. These results were replicated in the study by Knake et al., who reported their experience with the use of IV LEV for the treatment of 18 episodes of benzodiazepine refractory focal SE in 16 patients, including four patients with secondary generalized SE [121]. SE was controlled in all patients by the given combination of drugs. Additional antiepileptic medications after the IV LEV were necessary in two episodes.

Whether or not these retrospective data from small case series support the notion that LEV can be effectively used to treat SE remains to be seen. More recently, a randomized, double-blind, placebo-controlled study from France, for add-on therapy of LEV (2.5 g IV) or placebo to benzodiazepine (clonazepam 1 mg) in the prehospital setting was prematurely stopped after 3.5 years and after 107 patients were randomly assigned to receive placebo and 96 were assigned to receive levetiracetam. The interim analysis showed no evidence of a treatment difference in the modified intention-to-treat analysis [29].

Lacosamide

This novel agent was approved by FDA on 28 October 2008 for the adjunctive treatment of partial-onset seizures in patients 17 years of age and older with epilepsy. Despite the advantage conferred to ICU patients because of the IV formulation availability, lacosamide has not been FDA-approved for status epilepticus. The mode of action is unclear, but the drug binds to the collapsin response mediator protein 2 (CRMP-2), a phosphoprotein expressed mainly in the CNS and playing a role in neuronal differentiation and control of axonal outgrowth. This drug is renally eliminated [122].

Although a substrate for the CYP2C19, its metabolite is inactive. Reduction of the maximum daily dose up to 300 mg/day is recommended in patients with severe renal insufficiency and in those with mild to moderate hepatic insufficiency. After hemodialysis, an extra dose of 50% should be considered. It is available in oral and IV formulations (a potential advantage in ICU patients). In a double-blind, double-dummy, randomized inpatient trial, 60 patients with partial-onset epilepsy received either IV lacosamide plus oral placebo or IV placebo plus oral lacosamide. During treatment period, patients received twice-daily doses of lacosamide equivalent to their oral dose in an other open-label lacosamide trial (range 200–600 mg/day). Intravenous lacosamide showed a similar safety and tolerability profile to oral lacosamide when used as replacement therapy [123]. There is only one case report of its use in a patient with NCSE, who responded to its IV formulation (200 mg IV bolus within 3–5 min, followed by 100 mg po q12 h the next day) [124].

In an uncontrolled case series and systematic case series some efficacy of lacosamide was reported for patients with convulsive and nonconvulsive SE [125, 126], but not enough evidence exists at this point to recommend its routine use for benzodiazepine refractory SE [127].

Barbiturates

Barbiturates are potent antiepileptic medications and can be used either as additives to the antiepileptic regimen for better seizure control (such a s phenobarbital, infrequently as first or second-line drugs due to sedation risk in non-intubated patients) or as inducers of general anesthesia in case of refractory SE. A number of barbiturates are used as intravenous scheduled medications (i.e., phenobarbital) and continuous drips (i.e., thiopental and pentobarbital) to treat SE in the ICU. They are very potent but may be associated with serious side effects.

Issues with Barbiturate Infusions in the ICU

A number of side effects need to be taken into account when making the decision to use pentobarbital or thiopental infusions to treat SE. A major problem with barbiturate drips is the need for complete and prolonged support of vital organs when administered in high doses that challenges and exhausts many ICU resources. The neurological examination, an important assessment tool in all cases where an intracranial pathology is associated with SE (for example, hemorrhage, tumor, or trauma) is reduced to few brainstem reflexes (the last retained reflex with increasing depth of coma being the pupillary response) or complete disappearance of all indications of brain activity. This reduces our ability to differentiate between brain death and profound sedation and obviates the need for ancillary bedside tests including EEG and pos-

sibly tests to determine the presence of cerebral flow such as Transcranial Doppler or CT angiogram and CT perfusion. Respiratory depression with barbiturates obligates endotracheal intubation and mechanical ventilation. Frequent suctioning of respiratory secretions is necessary due to ciliary immobility and cough suppression. Hypotension due to both vasodilatation and myocardial depression is frequently encountered. Arterial blood pressure monitoring should be performed for all patients that undergo pentobarbital infusions, and on a case-by-case functional cardiac monitoring using pulse contour analysis or less often pulmonary wedge pressure (goal 12–14 mm Hg) monitoring may be helpful in case of prolonged administration of high dose pentobarbital or other barbiturates [128]. Most patients will need some kind of vasopressor or inotropic infusion (dopamine 10–20 mcg/kg/min or neosynephrine 1–8 mcg/kg/min). These measures will also keep adequate renal perfusion and urinary output that are usually decreased with barbiturate coma. With high dose barbiturate infusion, propylene glycol toxicity may ensue. It presents with hyperosmolarity and lactic acidosis, which may progress to develop refractory hypotension, arrhythmias, hemolysis, renal dysfunction, and multiorgan failure. An elevated osmolar gap may guide the intensivist to the correct diagnosis and early discontinuation of the barbiturate infusion to improvement [129]. With deep coma, poikilothermia ensues and special care should be taken to keep the temperature to the predefined range. On the other hand, all barbiturates are potent immunosuppressives [130] and special care should be taken to avoid nosocomial infections. All procedures should be performed under strict sterility, samples of potentially infected fluids (bronchial secretions, urine, blood) should be collected with even low suspicion level and all infections should be aggressively treated. Enteral nutrition through nasogastric or nasojejunal tubes, although feasible and preferable [131], can become problematic due to gastric and bowel hypomobility with high gastric residuals and risk of regurgitation-aspiration. Intestinal infarction can complicate ileus during high barbiturate dosage [132]. Therefore, in some cases total parenteral nutrition through a dedicated central line port becomes a viable alternative. Immobility leads to skin ulceration and deep venous thromboses, increasing the risk for pulmonary embolism. Frequent repositioning of the patient in bed and special inflatable or rotating mattresses decrease the incidence of the former. Sequential compression devices and low-molecular weight heparin administration are common measures taken in the ICU to avoid the latter.

Despite these myriad problems with barbiturate-induced coma, these are effective drugs in highly refractory SE cases. The intensivist should not forget that patients with CSE or NCSE may be in coma anyway with minimal neurological responses and if left untreated have few chances of survival or independent living. New data support this balance between risks-benefits of barbiturates. In a recent study from Columbia-Presbyterian Hospital in New York, 31 patients with SRSE were treated with pentobarbital infusion for an average of 6 days. Seizures were controlled in 90% of patients but recurred in 48% upon weaning the infusion and were eventually controlled with the addition of another barbiturate, phenobarbital, in 80% of previously un-weanable patients. Interestingly, complications did not occur in 11 (35%) patients and in the rest were pneumonia (32%), hypotension requiring pressors (29%), urinary tract infection (13%), and propylene glycol toxicity and cardiac arrest in one patient each. At one year after discharge, 74% of patients were dead or in a state of unresponsive wakefulness and another 16% severely disabled, but 10% had a good outcome [43].

Depth and Duration of Barbiturate Coma

Most authorities agree that ICU patients on barbiturate coma should be monitored with EEG, preferably in a continuous basis. However, there is no consensus regarding the depth of the EEG suppression that must be achieved. Some experts recommend a burst-suppression pattern of 5–10 s [128, 133], while others advocate for complete suppression or "flat record" [134]. In a retrospective study of 35 patients treated with pentobarbital for refractory SE, persistent seizure control was achieved in 6/12 (50%) patients reaching a burst-suppression level as the greatest depth of EEG suppression and in 17/20 (85%) patients reaching a "flat" record ($P = 0.049$). Three patients with neither pattern and just slow EEG had also persistent control. Survival was non-significantly better in the more suppressed group (25% vs 60%, $P = 0.08$). Isolated epileptiform discharges during the barbiturate infusion did not correlate with relapse of status. These results suggest that patients with deeper suppression appear to have fewer relapses and a better outcome, as well as that it is not necessary to suppress all epileptiform discharges [135]. However, these patients were not randomized to different treatments, the study was small and underpowered, and one needs to balance the benefits of the deeper suppression level with the adverse effects such a more aggressive treatment portends. A systematic review evaluated studies describing use of midazolam or propofol or pentobarbital for refractory SE. Compared with seizure suppression, titration of treatment to EEG background suppression level was associated with a lower frequency of breakthrough seizures (4 vs. 53%; $p < 0.001$), but also a higher frequency of hypotension (76 vs. 29%; $p < 0.001$). No difference in short-term mortality was found between these three anesthetic agents [136]. Another recent retrospective study of 127 episodes of SE (excluding post-anoxic cases), 49 of which were refractory to treatment, did not find any benefit regarding mortality in achieving burst suppression (via barbiturates or propofol or combination of anesthetic agents) [137]. The criticism of this study was that one third of patients were not monitored by continuous EEG and that no patient achieved complete and sustained burst suppression [138]. Acknowledging the lack of high quality data, current guidelines recommend cessation of electrographic seizures or achieving burst suppression as the titration goal for anesthetic infusion of antiepileptic medications (strong recommendation, very low quality) [35].

There is also no general agreement regarding the duration of the induced barbiturate coma [139]. Most authorities believe that 24–48 h are enough (weak recommendation, very low quality) [35], but some recommend up to 96 h [140]. Krishnamurthy and Drislane conducted a retrospective analysis of 40 patients with 44 refractory SE episodes on pentobarbital coma. Patients with more prolonged treatment (>96 h) and those receiving phenobarbital at the time of pentobarbital taper were less likely to relapse [141]. Treatment is gradually tapered and the patient is closely monitored clinically and electrographically for recurrence of seizures. If seizures return, the process is reversed and the patient re-anesthetized for progressively longer periods, as needed. Therapeutic levels of additional antiepileptics should be reached (for example, phenytoin level of 20–25 mcg/ml) before a new weaning trial. A load of phenobarbital sometimes is helpful. Mirski et al. described a patient with refractory generalized SE, who was treated with barbiturate-induced burst suppression coma for 53 days with good neurologic recovery [41]. Initially, pentobarbital was used, with serum pentobarbital levels necessary to control EEG seizure activity ranging from 40 to 95 mg/l (177 to 419 μmol/l). After the first 15 days, phenobarbital was introduced and kept at levels that reached 220–290 mg/l (947–1249 μmol/l) for seizure control. In addition, phenytoin with over-therapeutic levels of 25–35 mg/l (99–139 μmol/l; unbound phenytoin concentration 2.0–4.0 mg/l [7.9–15.9 μmol/l]) was used. Maintaining these concentrations required 2500–3000 mg/day of phenobarbital and 800–1200 mg/day of phenytoin. Overall, the patient spent 79 days in the ICU. This extreme case reveals the feasibility of an aggressive treatment approach. More recently, phenobarbital has been shown to support successful weaning from pentobarbital infusion in a case series of patients with SRSE [43].

Phenobarbital

Parenteral phenobarbital is available in preparations that are highly alkaline and may irritate the tissues. Phenobarbital's entry into the brain is more gradual than with more lipid-soluble compounds such as benzodiazepines. Therefore, peak concentrations in the brain may not occur for 15–20 min after the peak blood concentration is reached. This represents a limitation that makes phenobarbital not the best choice as a first-line drug. Phenobarbital is solely eliminated by the liver and has a prolonged half-life of 4 days (75–120 h). This pharmacokinetic property may be advantageous since it is associated with prolonged antiepileptic effect. However, if the dose is excessive, reversal of the effect will be slow. Phenobarbital can cause severe sedation and even coma, but in children paradoxical hyperkinetic reactions are not uncommon. Elderly with cerebral disease may also exhibit confusion and irritability rather than sedation. Sedation subsides with chronic therapy. Respiratory depression and hypotension can occur especially if it is given as a second or third-line drug to a patient previously treated with benzodiazepines or other barbiturates. In most cases, intubation and maintenance of ventilation are essential if phenobarbital is administered. The recommended loading dose is 10–20 mg/kg at a rate of 100 mg/min (usual adult dose 600–800 mg) followed by a maintenance dose of 1–4 mg/kg/day [48, 62, 76].

Thiopental

Thiopental is a highly effective anticonvulsant medication with some potential cerebral protective action. It has rapid onset of action and reduces the intracranial pressure, cerebral blood flow, and cerebral metabolism. Thiopental is the preferred drug for barbiturate-induced anesthesia for refractory SE in Europe [26]. A study from Finland reported the outcomes of 10 patients treated with high-dose thiopental for refractory SE in an ICU. The median time from seizure onset to burst-suppression EEG was 11.5 (6–12) hours and from ICU admission to starting thiopental anesthesia 113 (80–132) minutes. The median dose of thiopental to achieve burst-suppression was 19 (13–21) mg/kg and the median infusion rate to maintain the burst suppression 7 (5–8) mg/kg/h. The median duration of ventilation was 8.5 days and the median ICU length of stay 10 days. Eight patients developed atelectasis and nine received antibiotics based on clinical signs of infection [128]. This small study is indicative of the difficulties encountered in the ICU with such treatment. Sedation, hypotension, and respiratory depression that require intubation and mechanical ventilation usually occur. The drug has a strong tendency to accumulate, the elimination half-life may extend to 14–36 h [139] and a prolonged recovery time of days should be expected after the anesthetic doses used for the treatment of SE. Monitoring of the blood levels of the drug or its active metabolite pentobarbitone is advisable. Other less common adverse effects include spasm at the site of injection, hepatic dysfunction, pancreatitis and hypersensitivity reactions. Administration of thiopental requires full cardiorespiratory support with IV fluids, pressors and prolonged EEG monitoring to maintain a burst-suppression pattern. Hypotension below 90 mmHg is a sign that thiopental should be lowered. All these adverse effects make the drug less suitable for elderly patients or those with cardiac, hepatic, or renal disease [142]. The recommended dose is 2–4 mg/kg IV bolus given over 20 s followed by 3–5 mg/kg/h infusion in 0.9% sodium chloride solution. Thiopental should be slowly withdrawn 12 h after the last seizure has ceased and when optimal levels of antiepileptic drugs are documented.

Pentobarbital

Pentobarbital is an alternative to thiopental (and an active metabolite of the latter). It has a shorter elimination half-life than phenobarbital (approximately 24 h, range 15–60 h) [133]. Due to the short action of the drug, withdrawal results in a fairly prompt recovery of consciousness. However, seizures may also recur, as with all barbiturates, during the withdrawal period. In the retrospective study by Krishnamurthy and Drislane, 40 patients were treated for refractory SE with pentobarbital coma. Eight of 9 (89%) patients with relapse of seizures after the drug was discontinued died, compared to only 9/26 (35%) with persistently controlled seizures ($P < 0.005$). Etiology was the major determinant of relapse and survival, with 19/20 (95%) patients with chronic epilepsy, infections, or focal lesions having achieved good control as compared with 2/9 (22%) with multiple medical problems ($P < 0.001$). In this study, treatment delay did not predict a worsened outcome. Hypotension caused dose reduction, but never required treatment discontinuation [141].

Sedation, respiratory depression, and hypotension due to both vasodilatation and myocardial depression commonly occur. Decerebrate posturing and flaccid paralysis have been reported. Flaccid paresis may persist for weeks after withholding pentobarbital. Blood level monitoring is not very helpful, since there is inconsistent relationship between serum level and seizure control. Lactic acidosis due to 40% v/v propylene glycol content in pentobarbital infusion has been reported. An anion gap metabolic lactic acidosis, hyperosmolality with increased osmolal gap, refractory hypotension, renal and multi-organ failure, constitute alerts for propylene glycol toxicity syndrome that can be resolved after discontinuation of the drug [129, 143]. The recommended IV dose is 5–15 mg/kg over 1 h followed by infusion of 0.5–5.0 mg/kg/h or higher until burst-suppression EEG pattern is evident [35]. In a literature review until September 2001, Claassen et al. compared the efficacy of midazolam, propofol, and pentobarbital for the treatment of refractory SE [136]. No prospective, randomized trial was found. Overall 28 studies, mainly case series, with a total of 193 patients were included. Mortality was not different between the groups. Compared to the other two medications, pentobarbital was associated with a lower frequency of short-term treatment failure (8 vs. 23%; $P < 0.01$), breakthrough seizures (12 vs 42%; $P < 0.001$), and changes to a different continuously infused antiepileptic (3 vs 21%; $P < 0.001$). However, a higher frequency of hypotension was reported with pentobarbital (77 vs 34%; $P < 0.001$).

There are no large randomized controlled trials to guide the use of anesthetic drips for the treatment of status epilepticus except from one underpowered study by Rosetti and colleagues that compared RSE treated with infusion of propofol to those treated with pentobarbital. Medications were titrated towards EEG burst-suppression for 36–48 h and then progressively weaned. This study reported comparable efficacy of seizure control (RSE controlled after a first course of study medication in 43% in the propofol versus 22% in the barbiturates arm, $P = 0.40$), functional outcomes, and complications, except for longer days of mechanical ventilation in the pentobarbital arm. However, findings have to be interpreted with caution as the study was terminated early due to poor recruitment (enrolled 23 of 150 needed) [144].

Propofol

Propofol is a potent anticonvulsant non-barbiturate anesthetic, with barbiturate-like and benzodiazepine-like effects at the $GABA_A$ receptor [145]. It has rapid onset of action (within 3 min) and recovery (5–10 min after the drug has been stopped). It is metabolized in the liver and thus, affected by liver disease. Usage for SE management in anesthetic doses always requires assisted ventilation. Neuroexcitatory effects possibly through subcortical disinhibition result in muscle rigidity, opisthotonos, or myoclonic jerks [142]. These involuntary movements are usually not associated with EEG changes. However, not all experts agree with this thesis [146]: propofol has been shown to increase the frequency of spikes during electrocorticography and to activate neocortical foci [147, 148]. A systemic review of reports on seizure-like phenomena (SLP) associated with propofol was conducted by Walder et al. In 70 patients without epilepsy, SLP happened during induction in 24 (34%), during maintenance in two (3%), during emergence in 28 (40%), and were delayed in 16 (23%). Most frequent clinical presentations of SLP were generalized tonic-clonic seizures in 30 patients (43%), increased tone with twitching and rhythmic movements not perceived as generalized tonic-clonic seizures in 20 (36%), and involuntary movements in 11 (16%). EEG was performed in 24 patients, in all after the SLP had stopped. Two patients had generalized spikes and three general slowing. Out of 11 patients with epilepsy, seven (64%) had generalized tonic-clonic seizures during emergence. Only two patients had an EEG that showed generalized spikes and slowing in one patient and focal temporal spikes in the other. The time point of the SLP occurrence according to this study suggests that a change in cerebral concentration of propofol may be causative, because it is quite rare to witness these phenomena during the maintenance phase of anesthesia [146].

The recommended dose is 2 mg/kg bolus followed by continuous infusion of 5–15 mg/kg/h initially, reducing to 1–3 mg/kg/h. When seizures have been controlled for at least 12 h the drug should be slowly tapered over 12 h. To prevent rebound seizures, a decremental rate of 5% of the maintenance infusion per hour (i.e., over approximately 24 h [142]) or 1 mg/kg or less every 2 h has been recommended. Propofol infusion may cause hypotension that can be prevented by adequate use of vasopressors and IV fluids. Bradycardia including asystole has also been reported [149]. Metabolic acidosis, increased incidence of infection, rhabdomyolysis [149] and lipidemia may occur after prolonged use, but the use of 2% formulation of propofol has reduced the incidence of the latter. A propofol-infusion syndrome has been described in children and adults [150, 151]. Cremer et al. reported 7 adult cases with head injury in a neurosurgical ICU. Five of them died due to progressive myocardial failure and arrhythmias, rhabdomyolysis, metabolic acidosis, and hyperkalemia. All patients received propofol at rates >5 mg/kg/h for >58 h. Interestingly, the incidence was higher after the introduction of 2% propofol (5% before vs 17% after), although it did not reach statistical significance. The authors discouraged these high doses of propofol for long periods [152]. An association between propofol and catecholamine infusions (to support low blood pressure) in patients with traumatic head injury has also been reported [153]. Although it is unclear if the same risk is present in patients with SE, the intensivist treating these patients with high dose propofol should be cognizant of this possibility. A small retrospective study comparing propofol to midazolam for the treatment of refractory SE found that the two agents did not differ in clinical or electrographic seizure control. Propofol-treated patients with Acute Physiology and Chronic Health Evaluation (APACHE) II score of ≥20 had higher mortality ($P = 0.05$) [154].

A more recent, prospective study—mentioned above—of 10 patients with refractory SE showed that propofol had to be titrated at high doses (median rate 9.5 mg/kg/h) to induce burst-suppression pattern for at least 12 h. Three patients had recurrence of their seizures after the propofol was tapered [155]. These preliminary data suggest that midazolam may be tried before propofol, especially if used for several days and propofol before pentobarbital, because of shorter mechanical ventilation risk, as per the aforementioned randomized-controlled trial's results [144].

Ketamine

Animal data suggest that during SE there is an initial response to GABAergic agonists, which is lost later in the course, at about the same time that NMDA receptor-mediated transmission becomes enhanced [156]. NMDA antagonism at this late state, when SE becomes refractory (i.e., not responding to benzodiazepines, propofol or barbiturates) seems a logical next step [157]. Ketamine is an NMDA antagonist, which has been used in refractory SE in both animal models [158] and humans [159]. In a report, for example, a 22-year-old woman with mitochondriopathy and pre-existing epilepsy developed SE not responding to benzodiazepines, phenytoin, thiopental, and propofol. SE was terminated within days after supplemental administration of continuous ketamine infusion to midazolam. The authors suggested that ketamine should be incorporated into therapeutic regimens for difficult-to-treat SE [160].

In a multicenter case-series of 60 patients with RSE, permanent seizure control was achieved in 57% of patients and in 32% of these ketamine contributed to permanent control in the judgement of the investigators. No likely responses were observed when infusion rates were lower than 0.9 mg/kg/h, when ketamine was introduced at least 8 days after SE onset, or after failure of seven or more drugs. The study observed a 43% mortality rate but ketamine was discontinued due to side effects in only five patients (only one with propofol-related infusion syndrome) [161]. In a case report of subtle SE, ketamine controlled the seizures, but 3 months later diffuse cerebellar and worsened cerebral atrophy, raising the possibility of NMDA antagonist-mediated neurotoxicity was found [162], but these observations are difficult to differentiate from the underlying cause of status. Based on these data the intensivist should consider ketamine as a treatment of SRSE not as the last resort, but earlier than before.

Other Less Commonly Used Medications for SE

In support of these options are mostly anecdotal reports or at most single case series. Isoflurane, which produces electrographic suppression and has no reported organ toxicity is the most commonly used volatile anesthetic for treating refractory SE not responding to IV agents [163]. It has minimal hepatic or renal metabolism (thus, no toxicity to the organs) and most is exhaled unchanged. Compared to other volatile anesthetics it also has less cardiac and blood pressure effects. Its major limitation for more widespread use is the lack of scavenging apparatus in most ICUs. In addition the experience with the agent has been limited: only small case series of its use have been reported. Kofke et al. have administered isoflurane for 1–55 h, in 9 patients with 11 episodes of SE. Seizures stopped in all patients and burst-suppression patterns on EEGs were achieved. Hypotension was recorded in all patients. Seizures resumed upon discontinuation of isoflurane on eight of 11 occasions. Six of the nine patients died and the three survivors sustained cognitive deficits. This small series suggest that isoflurane is an effective, rapidly titratable anticonvulsant, but with potential seizure recurrence after its discontinuation [164]. In another retrospective study, Mirsattari et al. reported seven patients treated with an average of ten AEDs in addition to isoflurane (one patient also received desflurane for 19 days). Regardless of seizure type, isoflurane and desflurane consistently stopped epileptic discharges with adequate, sustained EEG burst suppression within minutes of initiation of the inhalation therapy. Four patients had good outcomes and three died. Complications during the inhalation therapy included hypotension (7/7), atelectasis (7/7), infections (5/7), paralytic ileus (3/7), and deep venous thrombosis (2/7) [165]. Isoflurane has also been suggested as an antiepileptic agent in patients with acute intermittent porphyria [79]. Its dose is titrated for end-tidal concentration of 0.8–2% and burst-suppression on the EEG.

Lidocaine can be tried as a second-line drug for the treatment of early SE [166]. The drug has a cell membrane stabilizing effect that reduces ion exchange and depolarization. Its action is not prolonged and with repeated doses there is significant risk for toxicity and even exacerbation of seizures (see Chapter of Drugs Used for the Critically Ill and Critical Care Seizures). Based on a study which showed efficacy in 31/42 episodes of SE after the first bolus of the drug, lidocaine is administered as a bolus of 1.5–2 mg/kg IV over 2 min, which can be repeated only once (total dose up to 200 mg). A continuous IV infusion of 3–4 mg/kg/h should not extend for >12 h [167].

Paraldeyde is a cyclic polymer of acetaldehyde with foul odor that has to be administered through a glass syringe (plastic tubing systems or syringes should be avoided). It has been used in the past extensively for treating SE, but during the last decades has lost popularity with the advent of newer antiepileptics. It has to be taken from fresh preparations kept in dark containers, because, if decomposed, it can induce toxicity or thrombosis of veins and microembolism if given IV. The preferred route is per rectum. It is rapidly absorbed and its antiepileptic effect is evident within few minutes and is usually long lasting. Most of the metabolism occurs in the liver, but 20–30% of the dose is exhaled through the lungs. Sedation, cardiorespiratory depression, and metabolic acidosis with increased lactate are the major adverse effects. The drug is diluted by the same volume of water (5–10 ml for adults) and given rectally in a dose of 5–10 g.

Clomethiazole is given as an IV bolus followed by a continuous infusion, but its popularity has declined because of the risk for accumulation with prolonged use. However, the drug has rapid onset of action and can be titrated to desired effect. Cardiorespiratory arrest is a real risk with higher infusion rates or prolonged use and the patient should be continuously monitored. Other adverse effects include sedation, vomiting, phlebitis, fluid overload, and electrolyte disturbances. It is administered as a bolus of 320–800 mg (40–100 ml) at a rate of 5–15 ml/min, followed by an infusion of 1–4 ml/min and titration to response [168].

Verapamil, a Ca^{++} channel antagonist with inhibitory effects on the P-glycoprotein (an efflux transporter for several AEDs, the overexpression of which is thought to convey resistance to AEDs during prolonged SE—see above in Pathophysiology), has been successfully administered IV (0.034 mg/min) to terminate SE after 37 days in an 11-year-old boy [17].

Other Potential Treatment Options for SRSE (Table 8.3, Stage 4.2)

Hypothermia

Hypothermia decreases the oxygen consumption and metabolic rate of the brain. There has been growing evidence of its beneficial effects in stroke and head trauma. Even in earlier studies, hypothermia has been recognized as a useful measure to decrease seizure activity [169]. There are animal data showing that hypothermia ameliorates and hyperthermia aggravates brain damage from seizures or SE [170]. In a rat model of kainic acid-induced seizures and SE, ictal discharges were decreased by 50% with mild hypothermia (28°C) and nearly abolished when body temperature was further lowered to 23°C. There was no hippocampal cell loss in hypothermic rats, whereas gross cell loss in the hippocampus was observed at normal body temperature. Hyperthermia (42°C), on the other hand, markedly aggravated the seizures and hippocampal damage induced by kainic acid in all rats; all animals died of tonic seizures within 2 h [171, 172]. In a more recent animal study, rats with SE induced by lithium and pilocarpine and refractory to midazolam were exposed to deep hypothermia (20°C for 30 min). A reduced EEG power over 50-fold was observed, SE was stopped within 12 min, and hypothermia reduced EEG spikes by 87% [173].

In addition, hypothermia may have a synergistic effect on thiopental-induced burst-suppression EEG pattern. Kim et al. compared normothermic to hypothermic (33.3°C) patients undergoing cerebral aneurysm clipping with EEG monitoring after a thiopental bolus was given: the onset time for suppression was shortened and the duration of suppression and of isoelectric EEG was prolonged in the group with mild hypothermia [174]. Moderate hypothermia (30–31°C) in addition to thiopental-induced coma has been used in three children with refractory SE. The seizures were controlled and 48 h to 5 days later the patients were rewarmed at a rate of 1°C every 3–4 h [175].

Corry et al. treated four patients with refractory SE with hypothermia (goal 31–33°C) via an endovascular cooling system [176]. These patients also received midazolam or pentobarbital infusions for rapid seizure control and were maintained hypothermic for 24 h. If no seizures recurred, they were rewarmed at a rate of 0.5°C every 4 h. Therapeutic hypothermia was successful in aborting seizure activity in all four patients, allowing midazolam infusions to be discontin-

ued. In 3 patients a burst-suppression EEG was reached. After rewarming, two patients remained seizure-free, and all four demonstrated a marked reduction in seizure frequency. Thus, although there are no randomized clinical studies evaluating the effect of hypothermia on SE, we prefer to keep our ICU patients with SE normothermic or slightly hypothermic.

More recently, a systematic review of studies utilizing hypothermia in the treatment of RSE has been published. Overall, 13 studies were identified, with 10 manuscripts and 3 meeting abstracts. A total of 40 patients were treated until May 2014. The common target temperature was 33° Celsius and was sustained for a median 48 h. Patients displayed a 62.5%, 15%, and 22.5% rate of seizure cessation, seizure reduction, and failure of treatment, respectively. External cooling was utilized in the majority of cases. Deep venous thrombosis, coagulopathy, and infections were the commonly reported complications. Based on this data, the authors conclude that Oxford level 4, GRADE D evidence exists to support the use of therapeutic hypothermia to control seizures in RSE [177]. Because several recent trials showing harm in the hypothermia arm of patients treated with traumatic brain injury [178] or meningitis [179] warrant caution as to its unrestricted application.

Resective Surgery

This strategy is usually reserved for cases of partial refractory SE, with an identifiable epileptic focus. This approach has been reported in a child with complex partial SE or in patients who fail to respond to three courses of cerebral suppressant therapy for at least 2 weeks [180, 181]. Duane et al. reported a 7-year-old boy with left hemiparesis secondary to right hemispheric cortical dysplasia. Burst-suppression pattern during pentobarbital coma was not successful and he seemingly had generalized spike and waves on the EEG and scattered areas of regional hypometabolism bilaterally on the [18F]fluorodeoxyglucose positron emission tomography. When the EEG was reviewed with increased time resolution, however, spikes suggested a right hemisphere origin. The patient underwent bilateral intracarotid amobarbital spike-suppression test that showed only minimal suppression of epileptiform discharges with injection of the left carotid, but complete suppression of spike activity after right-sided carotid injection. A right hemispherectomy was performed with complete cessation of status epilepticus [182].

In 10 children, who all failed high-dose suppressive therapy for at least 2 weeks and all had neuroimaging abnormalities, resective therapy acutely terminated SE in all of them with no mortality and no substantial morbidity. At median follow-up of 7 months, 7 (70%) of 10 patients were seizure free, and 3 (30%) of 10 had significant improvement in their epilepsy [183]. In a study, Ng et al.

reported a total of five children who presented with refractory SE, including complex partial SE, epilepsia partialis continua, and "status gelasticus." Multiple medical therapies had failed to control their seizures, and focal resection was performed. Seizures were fully controlled in four patients, and in one patient seizure frequency was reduced by more than 90% [184].

A case of neuro-sarcoidosis admitted to an NICU with refractory complex partial SE, with occasional generalization, who failed barbiturate coma treatment has been reported. This patient had an epileptic focus identified through intracranial electrode placement, surgical resection and successful outcome [185]. Despite these case reports or small case series, safety and effectiveness of resective surgery has yet to be proved in a controlled study. The approach appears most promising if a single, identifiable focus can be seen on imaging (including ictal SPECT/PET).

Brain Stimulation

Refractory SE has been reported to respond to various methods of brain stimulation, including low frequency cortical stimulation via subdural electrodes (0.5 Hz stimulations to the ictal onset zones in 30 min trains daily for 7 consecutive days). This 26 year-old woman, who was on two anesthetics plus high doses of 2–4 enteral AEDs responded after 1 day of stimulation and one anesthetic agent was successfully discontinued. Seizures only returned by the 4th day when the second anesthetic had been reduced by 60%. Upon returning, seizures arose from only one of the five original ictal onset zones [186].

Vagal nerve stimulation has also become one of the treatment options in epilepsy. A 30-year-old man with refractory SE was placed on pentobarbital coma in another case report. He underwent left vagal nerve stimulator placement after nearly 9 days of barbiturate coma, with stimulation initiated in the operating room. On the following day, EEG revealed resolution of previously observed periodic lateral epileptiform discharges and the patient was free of seizures [187].

Thalamic stimulation has been proposed and showed a good electrographic result but clinical improvement was lacking in a 27-year-old man with encephalopathy of unknown origin, post cardiac arrest and with EEG showing generalized periodic epileptiform discharges [188].

Electroconvulsive therapy (ECT) has been reported in a number of case series of RSE but has not been systematically evaluated [189, 190]. In one case report, ECT (3 sessions/week, 6 total) was administered in a patient who was in refractory SE, not responding to pentobarbital coma for 40 days. After the 2nd session the barbiturate was removed and eventually the patient recovered within 1 month [191].

Immunosuppressive Therapy

The decision to start blindly immunotherapy for suspected autoimmune SRSE is difficult. One should remember that these cases are treatment-resistant and no randomized trials have been published. When no other etiology has been found, such an approach should be considered after a paraneoplastic antibody panel has been collected (serum or CSF), even in the waiting period before the results are back. Higher clinical suspicion for autoimmune SE should be present when no longstanding history of epilepsy is reported, when prominent memory loss and psychiatric symptomatology is quickly evolving, when a known malignancy is present and other neurological signs, such as ataxia or autonomic dysfunction, coexist [192]. If on CT or PET of the entire body a tumor is discovered, then resection of the mass may improve seizure control. The AEDs are the same as those used against SRSE. Many patients in SE already host infections and immunosuppressive treatments should be initiated only after the infection is under control. In parallel with the AEDs, high dose corticosteroids (1 g methylprednisolone IV for 5 days, followed by 1 mg/kg prednisone/day) with or without intravenous immunoglobulin (2 g/kg over 5 days) [193, 194] or plasmapheresis (5 sessions) [195] are treatments that can be used based on expert opinions and anecdotal experience. Second-line treatments include cyclophosphamide or rituximab [196] and, for maintenance or recurrences, mycophenolate mofetil or azathioprine. Surgical resection of an epileptogenic focus or for Rassmussen's encephalitis should also be considered [192].

Management of Focal SE

Although single or multiple focal involuntary movements are not uncommonly encountered in the ICU, the intensivist should be familiar with the remote possibility that sensory complaints, changes of mental status or speech or visual disturbances represent seizures. Focal SE encompasses a wide range of clinical manifestations lasting for >30 min, including epilepsia partialis continua (EPC or Kojewnikoff's epilepsy, defined as continuous focal jerking of a body part, usually distal limb, over hours, days or years) [197], opercular myoclonic SE (OMASE, characterized by fluctuating cortical dysarthria without true aphasia associated with epileptic myoclonus involving bilaterally the glossopharyngeal musculature) [198], sensory SE [199], aphasic SE [200], or occipital lobe SE (presenting as visual loss, mimicking migraine) [201]. These unusual clinical presentations generate a lot of questions in the ICU, regarding their nature as epileptic phenomena, their need for treatment and their outcome, because staff is more familiar with the clinical presentation and treatment of generalized tonic-clonic SE. However, until a more diffuse process is excluded (for example, hypoglycemia), their very presence indicates focal cerebral pathology that should alert the clinician. Common causes include vascular or traumatic lesions, epilepsy (benign epilepsy of childhood with rolandic spikes), tumors or Russian spring-summer or Rasmussen's encephalitis (see in the Chapter on Presentation and Pathophysiology of Seizures in the Critical Care Environment). More diffuse processes are much less common, with non-ketotic hyperglycemic diabetes mellitus [202] and hyponatremia, mitochondrial encephalopathies (MELAS-MERRF), paraneoplastic syndromes [203] or antibiotics (penicillin, azlocillin-cefotaxime [204]) the most prominent [205]. Rasmussen's encephalitis was the most common cause of EPC in patients younger than 16 and cerebrovascular disease in older patients in a British series of 36 cases [197]. Acute disease was also found in most of the 41 patients described by Drislane et al., vascular disease being present in over half of them [206]. Inflammatory or autoimmune EPC has also been reported. In a case from Turkey, a patient diagnosed with neuro-Behcet disease developed EPC resistant to treatment [207]. In another case report from the same country, a 37-year-old woman presented with migrating focal motor SE. She was found to have autoimmune thyroiditis and was treated successfully with IV steroids. The authors recommended anti-thyroid antibody screening for multifocal motor status epilepticus cases of unspecified cause [208]. In another case report, a 19-year-old Japanese man presented with EPC. Clobazam improved the EPC, but action myoclonus developed, which responded to oral tandospirone (30 mg/day, since 5-hydroxyindole acetic acid was markedly decreased in the CSF). In this patient, the MR structural images were unremarkable, but cerebral SPECT showed decreased uptake in the left thalamus and bilateral frontal lobes. Antibodies against glutamate receptor subunit $\varepsilon 2$ was positive in the CSF [209].

Focal SE except for the etiologic implications is also important because it may precede or follow generalized clinical seizures or SE [206]. An EEG may be ordered when there is suspicion of secondary generalization or when a new focal neurologic deficit cannot be explained by neuroimaging alone. Subdural hematomas in particular are lesions in which it is important to consider the possibility of focal SE as the reason of worsening symptoms or mental status changes [206].

Although EPC is notoriously resistant to antiepileptics, in up to one third of cases there may be improvement or complete resolution with treatment [197]. Focal SE usually necessitates polypharmacy, which, in our experience as well as in others, must include phenytoin or phenobarbital, although there are no randomized studies comparing these medications to the newer antiepileptics or placebo. The same guidelines presented in Tables 8.6, 8.7, and 8.8 can be used, but most physicians would be reluctant to reach general anesthesia to control focal seizures. In non-motor simple partial SE there is no evidence that secondary brain damage ensues. On the other hand, the outcome of focal SE with motor symptoms is more strongly related to the underlying condition. As an example, tight glucose control in a case of non-ketotic hyperglycemia resolved the EPC in two separate episodes [202]. EPC following Rasmussen's has worse prognosis, because of the progressive nature of the disease [206, 210]. It should be kept in mind that the longer acting antiepileptics appear more helpful and that the response to the drugs may be quite delayed in focal SE (up to 48 h in one series [206]). Intravenous nimodipine, a calcium channel blocker, has been used to successfully treat two patients with EPC [211], but no controlled trials exist. In another study, all four patients with simple partial SE treated with IV valproate (mean loading dose of 22.9 ± 7.9 mg/kg) achieved seizure control with mean levels of 92.2 ± 50.1 mg/l [106]. Repetitive transcranial magnetic stimulation (rTMS) has also been used in several reports. Seven patients with EPC of mixed etiologies were treated with rTMS applied over the seizure. rTMS was delivered in high-frequency (20–100 Hz) bursts or as prolonged low-frequency (1 Hz) trains and resulted in a brief (20–30 min) pause in seizures in 3/7 patients and a lasting (>or=1 day) pause in 2/7. These authors also conducted a literature search, which identified six additional reports of EPC treated with rTMS where seizures were suppressed in 3/6. Seizures were not exacerbated by rTMS in any patient. Generally mild side effects included transient head and limb pain, and limb stiffening during high-frequency rTMS trains [212].

Prevention and treatment of complications

Complications of generalized tonic-clonic seizures can be divided into acute systemic complications due to the sympathetic overdrive and the stress of extreme motor activity and to persistent neurological complications that occur at a later stage [213]. Most of these complications have been already presented under the section pathophysiology of SE.

One of the most common complications encountered with SE is hyperthermia: it is usually due to excessive muscle activity rather than infection [20], but there are few cases where a CNS infection is the cause of SE. Therefore, the intensivist should be vigilant and order the appropriate work-up in atypical cases. Hyperthermia can spontaneously resolve following seizure control. However active cooling is recommended if body temperature exceeds 40°C. Because of the aforementioned beneficial results of hypothermia from experimental animal models [171], we believe more aggressive and earlier treatment of fever should be instituted in the ICU. Pilot data of hypothermia use in SE in humans suggests some efficacy (see above).

Extreme muscle activity also leads to lactic acidosis [21]. Catecholamine excess can cause hyperglycemia, which can further exacerbate acidosis through anaerobic metabolism. Lactic acidosis has also been reported with high-dose propofol and pentobarbital use (see above). Acidosis, induced by

Table 8.6 Effects of common ICU medications on anti-epileptics

	Phenytoin	Carbamazepine	Valproate
ADDED DRUG			
Salicylates	↑		↑
Ibuprofen	↑		
Erythromycin		↑↑	↑
Chloramphenicol	↑		
Trimethoprim	↑		
Isoniazid	↑	↑	↑
Fluconazole, ketoconazole	↑↑	↑	
Propoxyphene	↑	↑↑	
Amiodarone	↑	↑	
Diltiazem, verapamil		↑	
Cimetidine	↑↑	↑	
Omeprazole	↑		
Chlorpromazine			↑
Ethanol	↓		
Folic acid	↓		
Rifampicin	↓		
Digitoxin	↓		
Cyclosporine	↓		
Warfarin	↓		
Theophylline	↓		
Glucocorticosteroids	↓		

Adapted from [229–232]
↓ = decrease, ↑ = increase

Table 8.7 Effects of anti-epileptics on common ICU medications

	Phenytoin	Carbamazepine	Phenobarbital
ICU MEDICATION			
Warfarin	↓	↓↓	↓↓
Theophylline	↓↓	↓↓	↓↓
Corticosteroids	↓↓	↓↓	↓↓
Haloperidol		↓	↓
Lithium		↑	
Tricyclics	↓	↓	↓
Cyclosporine	↓↓	↓↓	↓↓
Nimodipine	↓	↓	↓
Non-depolarizing paralytics	↓	↓	

↓ = decrease, ↑ = increase
Adapted from [229–232]

hypercarbic ventilation attenuates neuronal injury in a rat model of SE [214].

Hyperglycemia, on the other hand, may have detrimental effects in several types of brain injury (for example, ischemia), but its effects are less clear in SE. Regional brain glucose utilization during seizures is increased in the brain, especially the hippocampus [215]. In a rat model of L-allylglycine-induced SE, Swan et al. studied the lactate and glucose content of hippocampal cells at increasing plasma glucose concentrations. Although brain lactate concentration was elevated in SE and maximal in the high-glucose group, it did not reach ischemia levels thought to induce cell death nor did it correlate with neuropathologic damage [216]. The intracellular pH, however, decreased in hyperglycemic rabbits with pentylenetetrazole induced SE [37]. Therefore, although hyperglycemia should be avoided in the management of several underlying cerebral injurious processes, which may lead to SE, this may not be the case when seizures or SE ensue. Our personal preference is to start all our ICU non-hypoglycemic patients in SE on finger-stick checks q6 h for the first 24 h and treat glucose readings >130 mg/dl with subcutaneous insulin based on a "non-aggressive" sliding scale (part of a tight glucose control protocol that is used in all patients admitted to our Neuro-ICU).

Table 8.8 Interaction between anti-epileptic medications

	PHT	PB	CBZ	OXC	VPA	TB	LTG	ZNS	BDZ
Added drug									
PHT		~	↓	↓	↓	↓	↓	↓	
PB	↑, then ↓		~	↓	↓	↓	↓		↓
CBZ	~	~	↓	↓	↓	↓	↓	↓	↓
OXC			↑ **			↓			
VPA	↓ *	↑	~ or ↑ **				↑		↑
ZNS			↑ **						
BDZ	↓	~			~				

Adapted from [232]

PHT phenytoin, *PB* phenobarbital, *CBZ* carbamazepine, *VPA* valproate, *TB* tiagabine, *OXC* oxcarbazepine, *ZNS* zonisamide, *BDZ* benzodiazepines

↓ = decrease, ↑ = increase, ~ = variable, * = ↑ free DPH level, ** = epoxide

Another common complication is rhabdomyolysis, which may cause acute tubular necrosis and renal failure if left untreated. Patients should be screened for myoglobinuria and serum creatinine level should be measured. If myoglobinuria is detected or creatinine levels are highly elevated, serum potassium monitoring, urinary alkalinization and forced diuresis should be considered. Special attention to rhabdomyolysis after high-dose, prolonged propofol infusions (as part of the propofol infusion syndrome) should be paid in the Neuro-ICU, especially if catecholamine infusions are used to support the blood pressure [153].

Cardiorespiratory complications include arrhythmias, hypotension, respiratory depression, neurogenic pulmonary edema, central apnea, and pulmonary aspiration (see above). Mean arterial pressure is elevated due to elevated total peripheral resistance, which can lead to decreased cardiac output. Patients with atherosclerotic cardiovascular risk factors may have a gradual deterioration in hemodynamic parameters, whereas other patients decline acutely [22, 217–219]

Management of Seizures and SE with Antiepileptics in ICU Patients with Organ Dysfunction

Hepatic Failure

Because of their renal clearance, low protein binding and metabolism, gabapentin, levetiracetam, vigabatrin, pregabalin seem excellent choices. However, there are not many data regarding these newer antiepileptic drugs. Vigabatrin may normalize plasma alanine aminotransferase levels, making impossible to use it as an index of the hepatic dysfunction [220].

Phenytoin can accumulate and its plasma protein binding capacity is reduced. Reduction of the dose and frequent determinations of free levels are required in order to continue using the drug. Phenobarbital is metabolized in the liver, but is also partially excreted unchanged in the urine (20–25% of the dose). Biliary excretion is minimal and cholestasis is not a reason to adjust the dosage. Therefore, it can be used po or IV, but one should remember that its half-life in hepatic failure may be prolonged up to 130 h. Measuring serum levels of the drug and close monitoring for respiratory depression is recommended. The same is true for the benzodiazepines: oxazepam is a short-acting drug without oxidative metabolism, but is not available in IV form. All benzodiazepine dosing, except for oxazepam, should be reduced with liver failure. Lack of active metabolites makes lorazepam a better choice than diazepam, which should be avoided. The short acting barbiturates, such as pentobarbital and thiopental are completely metabolized in the liver and should not be used because of poor elimination. In addition to hepatotoxicity, which is idiosyncratic and mainly encountered in young children (see above), and pancreatitis, valproic acid can induce elevations of ammonia. In epileptic patients without hepatic disease, this adverse effect does not require treatment, unless symptomatic [221]. However, it can lead to confusion when treating patients with hepatic dysfunction and baseline hyperammonemia, who may clinically worsen; therefore, VPA is generally contraindicated in hepatic failure. If absolutely necessary to be used, the dosage should be reduced, because the half-life of the drug is increased up to 18 ± 5 h. Although large, randomized controlled trials of levocarnitine treatment in valproic-acid-induced hyperammonemic encephalopathy are lacking, levocarnitine has been shown to be generally safe and effective in retrospective trials and case reports. Overall, there is more literature supporting the use of levocarnitine in encephalopathy associated with acute overdose than with short- or long-term treatment with usual dosages of valproic acid [222]. If this translates to supplementation with L-carnitine, when using valproic acid to treat SE in a patient with liver failure, is unknown.

Renal failure

Drugs hepatically metabolized should be used instead of those with renal elimination, but there are several details that are important to remember. Phenytoin has decreased half-life and the unbound fraction is increased. Free levels should be followed and doses should be smaller and more frequent (q8 h). Only the free fraction is dialyzable, therefore, there is usually no need for extra dosing post dialysis. A significant amount of phenobarbital, on the other hand, is dialyzable and has to be supplemented post dialysis with careful monitoring of the levels. Because of the potential for accumulation, the dosage of the drug should be reduced. Valproic acid is barely affected by renal failure, since it is mainly hepatically metabolized. As with phenytoin, the decreased protein binding in uremia may lead to elevated free levels, which should be followed. Dialysis does not affect its levels. An increased risk for valproic-induced pancreatitis has been reported in uremic patients [223] and amylase should be measured in case of unexplained abdominal pain. Benzodiazepines do not seem to be affected by uremia or dialysis and, generally, their dose does not need adjustment. Because diazepam's active metabolite and oxazepam are renally excreted, caution is advised with their use in severe uremia.

Among the enterally administered antiepileptic drugs, carbamazepine is together with valproic acid a good option, since its levels are barely affected in uremia and there is no need for post dialysis supplementation. However, rare instances of idiosyncratic renal damage have been reported with this drug [224]. Tiagabine, a hepatically metabolized antiepileptic can also be used without any dosage adjustment in uremia, but if the patient is in status, it should probably be avoided (see above). With gabapentin a sliding scale dosage based on creatinine clearance has been recommended:

- 60 ml/min, 400 mg tid
- 30–60 ml/min, 300 mg bid
- 15–30 ml/min, 300 mg qd
- <15 ml/min, 300 mg every other day

Because the drug is highly dialyzable, an extra dose of 200–300 mg should be also given after each dialysis session.

If levetiracetam is used in renal failure, the following dosing schedule is recommended based on creatinine clearance:

- >80 ml/min, 500–1000 mg bid
- 50–80 ml/min, 500–1000 mg bid
- 30–50 ml/min, 250–750 bid
- <30 ml/min, 250–500 mg bid
- End stage renal disease—hemodialysis, 500–1000 mg/day

Following dialysis, 250–500 mg extra IV or po levetiracetam can be administered.

Topiramate and zonisamide induce formation of renal calculi and should be probably avoided in case of single kidney, history of renal stones and after kidney transplantation.

Hemato-Poetic Dysfunction

Immunosuppressed or post chemotherapy ICU patients have special needs regarding the antiepileptic drug use. Phenytoin can lead to megaloblastic anemia, responding to folate supplementation. An idiosyncratic pseudolymphoma syndrome, with diffuse lymphadenopathy, fever and skin rash, different than the more common hydantoin lupus-like rash, can be misdiagnosed as true lymphoma and lead to unnecessary diagnostic work-up. Thrombocytopenia is much less common with phenytoin, but is a dose-related adverse effect of valproic acid. Usually only purpura or petechiae occur and only rarely organ bleeding. However, in the ICU, in pre- or postoperative patients or those with active bleeding or coagulopathy, any drop in the platelet count should lead to a decrease of the dose of the drug or substitution with an alternative agent. Neutropenia is less common with valproic acid, but a well-known adverse effect of carbamazepine (10%, usually during the first few months of use). The drug should be stopped only in case of white cell count <2500 or absolute neutropenia (<1000 polymorphonuclear cells). Carbamazepine can also induce aplastic anemia. Phenobarbital when chronically administered can induce folate-deficient megaloblastic anemia, but this is rarely a problem in the ICU. The benzodiazepines have no significant hematologic adverse effects.

Drug interaction in the ICU

Several of the interactions between antiepileptics and common medications used in the ICU have been mentioned in the other chapters of this book. The physician treating ICU seizures or SE should be familiar with the most important of them, before he assumes treatment failure or is surprised by obvious signs of toxicity. Table 8.6 presents the effects of these drugs on antiepileptic medication levels. Aluminium hydroxide, magnesium hydroxide, and calcium antiacids can decrease the absorption of enterally administered phenytoin, lowering its level. Conversely, antiepileptic medications can affect the metabolism of numerous ICU drugs and few of these interactions are presented in Table 8.7. Finally, antiepileptic medications interact with each other (Table 8.8) and the intensivist using polypharmacy in the management of epileptic seizures should consider potential changes in the free or total levels of individual medications.

References

1. Lowenstein DH. Status epilepticus: an overview of the clinical problem. Epilepsia. 1999;40(Suppl 1):S3–8. discussion S21-22
2. Claassen J, Albers D, Schmidt JM, et al. Nonconvulsive seizures in subarachnoid hemorrhage link inflammation and outcome. Ann Neurol. 2014;75:771–81.
3. Gilmore EJ, Gaspard N, Choi HA, et al. Acute brain failure in severe sepsis: a prospective study in the medical intensive care unit utilizing continuous EEG monitoring. Intensive Care Med. 2015;41:686–94.

4. Alldredge BK, Gelb AM, Isaacs SM, et al. A comparison of loraz-epam, diazepam, and placebo for the treatment of out-of-hospital status epilepticus. N Engl J Med. 2001;345:631–7.

5. Silbergleit R, Durkalski V, Lowenstein D, et al. Intramuscular versus intravenous therapy for prehospital status epilepticus. N Engl J Med. 2012;366:591–600.

6. Claassen J, Riviello Jr JJ, Silbergleit R. Emergency Neurological Life Support: Status Epilepticus. Neurocrit Care. 2015;23(Suppl 2):136–42.

7. Holtkamp M. The anaesthetic and intensive care of status epilepticus. Curr Opin Neurol. 2007;20:188–93.

8. Sutter R, Marsch S, Fuhr P, Kaplan PW, Ruegg S. Anesthetic drugs in status epilepticus: risk or rescue? a 6-year cohort study. Neurology. 2014;82:656–64.

9. Payne ET, Hahn CD. Reply: the circular dilemma of seizure-induced brain injury. Brain. 2014;137:e306.

10. Payne ET, Zhao XY, Frndova H, et al. Seizure burden is independently associated with short term outcome in critically ill children. Brain. 2014;137:1429–38.

11. De Marchis GM, Pugin D, Meyers E, et al. Seizure burden in sub-arachnoid hemorrhage associated with functional and cognitive outcome. Neurology. 2015;86(3):253–60.

12. Chen JW, Wasterlain CG. Status epilepticus: pathophysiology and management in adults. Lancet Neurol. 2006;5:246–56.

13. Lothman EW. Biological consequences of repeated seizures. In: Engel J, Pedley TA, editors. Epilepsy: a comprehensive textbook. Philadelphia-New York: Lippincott-Raven; 1998. p. 481–97.

14. Betjemann JP, Lowenstein DH. Status epilepticus in adults. Lancet Neurol. 2015;14:615–24.

15. Loscher W. Mechanisms of drug resistance in status epilepticus. Epilepsia. 2007;48(Suppl 8):74–7.

16. Bankstahl JP, Loscher W. Resistance to antiepileptic drugs and expression of P-glycoprotein in two rat models of status epilepticus. Epilepsy Res. 2008;82(1):70–85.

17. Iannetti P, Spalice A, Parisi P. Calcium-channel blocker verapamil administration in prolonged and refractory status epilepticus. Epilepsia. 2005;46:967–9.

18. Meldrum BS, Brierley JB. Prolonged epileptic seizures in primates. Ischemic cell change and its relation to ictal physiological events. Arch Neurol. 1973;28:10–7.

19. Meldrum BS, Vigouroux RA, Brierley JB. Systemic factors and epileptic brain damage. Prolonged seizures in paralyzed, artificially ventilated baboons. Arch Neurol. 1973;29:82–7.

20. Aminoff MJ, Simon RP. Status epilepticus. Causes, clinical features and consequences in 98 patients. Am J Med. 1980;69:657–66.

21. Meldrum BS, Horton RW. Physiology of status epilepticus in primates. Arch Neurol. 1973;28:1–9.

22. Boggs JG, Painter JA, DeLorenzo RJ. Analysis of electrocardiographic changes in status epilepticus. Epilepsy Res. 1993;14:87–94.

23. Claassen J, Perotte A, Albers D, et al. Nonconvulsive seizures after subarachnoid hemorrhage: Multimodal detection and outcomes. Ann Neurol. 2013;74:53–64.

24. DeLorenzo RJ, Waterhouse EJ, Towne AR, et al. Persistent nonconvulsive status epilepticus after the control of convulsive status epilepticus. Epilepsia. 1998;39:833–40.

25. Treiman DM. Electroclinical features of status epilepticus. J Clin Neurophysiol. 1995;12:343–62.

26. Walker MC, Smith SJ, Shorvon SD. The intensive care treatment of convulsive status epilepticus in the UK. Results of a national survey and recommendations. Anaesthesia. 1995;50:130–5.

27. Riviello Jr JJ, Claassen J, LaRoche SM, et al. Treatment of status epilepticus: an international survey of experts. Neurocrit Care. 2013;18:193–200.

28. Claassen J. Dr No: double drug fails to eliminate status epilepticus. Lancet Neurol. 2016;15:23–4.

29. Navarro V, Dagron C, Elie C, et al. Prehospital treatment with levetiracetam plus clonazepam or placebo plus clonazepam in status epilepticus (SAMUKeppra): a randomised, double-blind, phase 3 trial. Lancet Neurol. 2015.

30. Treiman DM, Meyers PD, Walton NY, et al. A comparison of four treatments for generalized convulsive status epilepticus. Veterans affairs status epilepticus cooperative study group. N Engl J Med. 1998;339:792–8.

31. Millikan D, Rice B, Silbergleit R. Emergency treatment of status epilepticus: current thinking. Emerg Med Clin North Am. 2009;27:101–13. ix

32. Varelas PN, Corry J, Rehman M, et al. Management of status epilepticus in neurological versus medical intensive care unit: does it matter? Neurocrit Care. 2013;19:4–9.

33. Vohra TT, Miller JB, Nicholas KS, et al. Endotracheal Intubation in Patients Treated for Prehospital Status Epilepticus. Neurocrit Care. 2015;23:33–43.

34. Guaranha MS, Garzon E, Buchpiguel CA, Tazima S, Yacubian EM, Sakamoto AC. Hyperventilation revisited: physiological effects and efficacy on focal seizure activation in the era of video-EEG monitoring. Epilepsia. 2005;46:69–75.

35. Brophy GM, Bell R, Claassen J, et al. Guidelines for the evaluation and management of status epilepticus. Neurocrit Care. 2012;17:3–23.

36. Pulsinelli WA, Levy DE, Sigsbee B, Scherer P, Plum F. Increased damage after ischemic stroke in patients with hyperglycemia with or without established diabetes mellitus. Am J Med. 1983;74:540–4.

37. Tomlinson FH, Anderson RE, Meyer FB. Effect of arterial blood pressure and serum glucose on brain intracellular pH, cerebral and cortical blood flow during status epilepticus in the white New Zealand rabbit. Epilepsy Res. 1993;14:123–37.

38. Simon RP. Physiologic consequences of status epilepticus. Epilepsia. 1985;26(Suppl 1):S58–66.

39. Holtkamp M, Othman J, Buchheim K, Masuhr F, Schielke E, Meierkord H. A "malignant" variant of status epilepticus. Arch Neurol. 2005;62:1428–31.

40. Lowenstein DH, Alldredge BK. Status epilepticus at an urban public hospital in the 1980s. Neurology. 1993;43:483–8.

41. Mirski MA, Williams MA, Hanley DF. Prolonged pentobarbital and phenobarbital coma for refractory generalized status epilepticus. Crit Care Med. 1995;23:400–4.

42. Marchi NA, Novy J, Faouzi M, Stahli C, Burnand B, Rossetti AO. Status epilepticus: impact of therapeutic coma on outcome. Crit Care Med. 2015;43:1003–9.

43. Pugin D, Foreman B, De Marchis GM, et al. Is pentobarbital safe and efficacious in the treatment of super-refractory status epilepticus: a cohort study. Crit Care. 2014;18:R103.

44. Shorvon S. Emergency treatment of epilepsy. In: Shorvon S, editor. Handbook of epilepsy treatment. Malden: Blackwell; 2000. p. 173–94.

45. Fernandez A, Lantigua H, Lesch C, et al. High-dose midazolam infusion for refractory status epilepticus. Neurology. 2014;82:359–65.

46. Leppik IE, Derivan AT, Homan RW, Walker J, Ramsay RE, Patrick B. Double-blind study of lorazepam and diazepam in status epilepticus. JAMA. 1983;249:1452–4.

47. Shaner DM, McCurdy SA, Herring MO, Gabor AJ. Treatment of status epilepticus: a prospective comparison of diazepam and phenytoin versus phenobarbital and optional phenytoin. Neurology. 1988;38:202–7.

48. Lowenstein DH, Alldredge BK. Status epilepticus. N Engl J Med. 1998;338:970–6.

49. Lowenstein DH. Treatment options for status epilepticus. Curr Opin Pharmacol. 2003;3:6–11.

50. Bleck TP. Refractory status epilepticus in 2001. Arch Neurol. 2002;59:188–9.

51. Mayer SA, Claassen J, Lokin J, Mendelsohn F, Dennis LJ, Fitzsimmons BF. Refractory status epilepticus: frequency, risk factors, and impact on outcome. Arch Neurol. 2002;59:205–10.

52. Holtkamp M, Masuhr F, Harms L, Einhaupl KM, Meierkord H, Buchheim K. The management of refractory generalised convulsive and complex partial status epilepticus in three European countries: a survey among epileptologists and critical care neurologists. J Neurol Neurosurg Psychiatry. 2003;74:1095–9.

53. Zbinden G, Randall LO. Pharmacology of benzodiazepines: laboratory and clinical correlations. Adv Pharmacol. 1967;5:213–91.

54. Meldrum BS, Chapman AG. Benzodiazepine receptors and their relationship to the treatment of epilepsy. Epilepsia. 1986;27(Suppl 1):S3–13.

55. Amrein R, Hetzel W. Pharmacology of drugs frequently used in ICUs: midazolam and flumazenil. Intensive Care Med. 1991;17(Suppl 1):S1–10.

56. Reves JG, Fragen RJ, Vinik HR, Greenblatt DJ. Midazolam: pharmacology and uses. Anesthesiology. 1985;62:310–24.

57. Bell DS. Dangers of treatment of status epilepticus with diazepam. Br Med J. 1969;1:159–61.

58. Parry T, Hirsch N. Psychogenic seizures after general anaesthesia. Anaesthesia. 1992;47:534.

59. Shorvon S. Antiepileptic drugs. In: Shorvon S, editor. Handbook of epilepsy treatment. Oxford: Blackwell; 2000. p. 85–172.

60. Cereghino JJ, Mitchell WG, Murphy J, Kriel RL, Rosenfeld WE, Trevathan E. Treating repetitive seizures with a rectal diazepam formulation: a randomized study. The North American Diastat Study Group. Neurology. 1998;51:1274–82.

61. Dreifuss FE, Rosman NP, Cloyd JC, et al. A comparison of rectal diazepam gel and placebo for acute repetitive seizures. N Engl J Med. 1998;338:1869–75.

62. Treatment of convulsive status epilepticus. Recommendations of the epilepsy foundation of America's working group on status epilepticus. JAMA. 1993;270:854–9.

63. Appleton R, Sweeney A, Choonara I, Robson J, Molyneux E. Lorazepam versus diazepam in the acute treatment of epileptic seizures and status epilepticus. Dev Med Child Neurol. 1995;37:682–8.

64. Cock HR, Schapira AH. A comparison of lorazepam and diazepam as initial therapy in convulsive status epilepticus. QJM. 2002;95:225–31.

65. Dirksen MS, Vree TB, Driessen JJ. Clinical pharmacokinetics of long-term infusion of midazolam in critically ill patients—preliminary results. Anaesth Intensive Care. 1987;15:440–4.

66. Towne AR, DeLorenzo RJ. Use of intramuscular midazolam for status epilepticus. J Emerg Med. 1999;17:323–8.

67. Wroblewski BA, Joseph AB. The use of intramuscular midazolam for acute seizure cessation or behavioral emergencies in patients with traumatic brain injury. Clin Neuropharmacol. 1992;15:44–9.

68. Galdames D, Aguilera M, Fabres L. Midazolam in the treatment of status epilepticus and frequent seizures in adults. Epilepsia. 1997;38:12.

69. Chamberlain JM, Altieri MA, Futterman C, Young GM, Ochsenschlager DW, Waisman Y. A prospective, randomized study comparing intramuscular midazolam with intravenous diazepam for the treatment of seizures in children. Pediatr Emerg Care. 1997;13:92–4.

70. Mayhue FE. IM midazolam for status epilepticus in the emergency department. Ann Emerg Med. 1988;17:643–5.

71. McDonagh TJ, Jelinek GA, Galvin GM. Intramuscular midazolam rapidly terminates seizures in children and adults. Emerg Med. 1992;4:77–81.

72. Ulvi H, Yoldas T, Mungen B, Yigiter R. Continuous infusion of midazolam in the treatment of refractory generalized convulsive status epilepticus. Neurol Sci. 2002;23:177–82.

73. Treiman DM. Pharmacokinetics and clinical use of benzodiazepines in the management of status epilepticus. Epilepsia. 1989;30(Suppl 2):S4–10.

74. Jamerson BD, Dukes GE, Brouwer KL, Donn KH, Messenheimer JA, Powell JR. Venous irritation related to intravenous administration of phenytoin versus fosphenytoin. Pharmacotherapy. 1994;14:47–52.

75. Jones GL, Wimbish GH, McIntosh WE. Phenytoin: basic and clinical pharmacology. Med Res Rev. 1983;3:383–434.

76. Chapman MG, Smith M, Hirsch NP. Status epilepticus. Anaesthesia. 2001;56:648–59.

77. Browne TR, Kugler AR, Eldon MA. Pharmacology and pharmacokinetics of fosphenytoin. Neurology. 1996;46:S3–7.

78. Boucher BA. Fosphenytoin: a novel phenytoin prodrug. Pharmacotherapy. 1996;16:777–91.

79. Payne TA, Bleck TP. Status epilepticus. Crit Care Clin. 1997;13:17–38.

80. DeToledo JC, Lowe MR, Rabinstein A, Villaviza N. Cardiac arrest after fast intravenous infusion of phenytoin mistaken for fosphenytoin. Epilepsia. 2001;42:288.

81. Fischer JH, Patel TV, Fischer PA. Fosphenytoin: clinical pharmacokinetics and comparative advantages in the acute treatment of seizures. Clin Pharmacokinet. 2003;42:33–58.

82. Villarreal HJ, Wilder BJ, Willmore LJ, Bauman AW, Hammond EJ, Bruni J. Effect of valproic acid on spike and wave discharges in patients with absence seizures. Neurology. 1978;28:886–91.

83. Wilder BJ, Ramsay RE, Murphy JV, Karas BJ, Marquardt K, Hammond EJ. Comparison of valproic acid and phenytoin in newly diagnosed tonic-clonic seizures. Neurology. 1983;33:1474–6.

84. Beydoun A, Sackellares JC, Shu V. Safety and efficacy of divalproex sodium monotherapy in partial epilepsy: a double-blind, concentration-response design clinical trial. Depakote Monotherapy for Partial Seizures Study Group. Neurology. 1997;48:182–8.

85. Penry JK, Dean JC. Valproate monotherapy in partial seizures. Am J Med. 1988;84:14–6.

86. Bourgeois BFD. Valproic: clinical use. In: Levy RH, Mattson RH, Meldrum BS, editors. Antiepileptic drugs. New York: Raven Press; 1995.

87. Willmore LJ, Wilder BJ, Bruni J, Villarreal HJ. Effect of valproic acid on hepatic function. Neurology. 1978;28:961–4.

88. Dreifuss FE, Santilli N, Langer DH, Sweeney KP, Moline KA, Menander KB. Valproic acid hepatic fatalities: a retrospective review. Neurology. 1987;37:379–85.

89. Gerstner T, Teich M, Bell N, et al. Valproate-associated coagulopathies are frequent and variable in children. Epilepsia. 2006;47:1136–43.

90. Hodges BM, Mazur JE. Intravenous valproate in status epilepticus. Ann Pharmacother. 2001;35:1465–70.

91. Zaccara G, Messori A, Moroni F. Clinical pharmacokinetics of valproic acid—1988. Clin Pharmacokinet. 1988;15:367–89.

92. Ramsay RE, Uthman B, Leppik IE, et al. The tolerability and safety of valproate sodium injection given as an intravenous infusion. J Epilepsy. 1997;10:187–93.

93. Devinsky O, Leppik I, Willmore LJ, et al. Safety of intravenous valproate. Ann Neurol. 1995;38:670–4.

94. Venkataraman V, Wheless JW. Safety of rapid intravenous infusion of valproate loading doses in epilepsy patients. Epilepsy Res. 1999;35:147–53.

95. Uberall MA, Trollmann R, Wunsiedler U, Wenzel D. Intravenous valproate in pediatric epilepsy patients with refractory status epilepticus. Neurology. 2000;54:2188–9.

96. Sinha S, Naritoku DK. Intravenous valproate is well tolerated in unstable patients with status epilepticus. Neurology. 2000;55:722–4.

97. Mamiya K, Yukawa E, Matsumoto T, Aita C, Goto S. Synergistic effect of valproate coadministration and hypoalbuminemia on

the serum-free phenytoin concentration in patients with severe motor and intellectual disabilities. Clin Neuropharmacol. 2002;25:230–3.

98. Kaplan PW. Intravenous valproate treatment of generalized nonconvulsive status epilepticus. Clin Electroencephalogr. 1999;30:1–4.

99. Chez MG, Hammer MS, Loeffel M, Nowinski C, Bagan BT. Clinical experience of three pediatric and one adult case of spike-and-wave status epilepticus treated with injectable valproic acid. J Child Neurol. 1999;14:239–42.

100. Alehan FK, Morton LD, Pellock JM. Treatment of absence status with intravenous valproate. Neurology. 1999;52:889–90.

101. Giroud M, Gras D, Escousse A. Use of injectable valproic in status epilepticus. Drug Invest. 1993;5:154–9.

102. Yu KT, Mills S, Thompson N, Cunanan C. Safety and efficacy of intravenous valproate in pediatric status epilepticus and acute repetitive seizures. Epilepsia. 2003;44:724–6.

103. Martin ED, Pozo MA. Valproate suppresses status epilepticus induced by 4-aminopyridine in CA1 hippocampus region. Epilepsia. 2003;44:1375–9.

104. Price DJ. Intravenous valproate: experience in neurosurgery. In: Chadwick D, editor. Royal society of medicine service international congress and symposium series. London: Royal Society of Medicine Services Limited; 1989. p. 197–203.

105. Peters CN, Pohlmann-Eden B. Efficacy and safety of intravenous valproate in status epilepticus. Epilepsia. 1999;40:149–50.

106. Naritoku DK, Sinha S. Outcome of status epilepticus treated with intravenous valproate. Neurology. 2001;56:A235.

107. Limdi NA, Shimpi AV, Faught E, Gomez CR, Burneo JG. Efficacy of rapid IV administration of valproic acid for status epilepticus. Neurology. 2005;64:353–5.

108. Misra UK, Kalita J, Patel R. Sodium valproate vs phenytoin in status epilepticus: a pilot study. Neurology. 2006;67:340–2.

109. Agarwal P, Kumar N, Chandra R, Gupta G, Antony AR, Garg N. Randomized study of intravenous valproate and phenytoin in status epilepticus. Seizure. 2007;16:527–32.

110. Gilad R, Izkovitz N, Dabby R, et al. Treatment of status epilepticus and acute repetitive seizures with i.v. valproic acid vs phenytoin. Acta Neurol Scand 2008;118(5):296–300.

111. Olsen KB, Tauboll E, Gjerstad L. Valproate is an effective, well-tolerated drug for treatment of status epilepticus/serial attacks in adults. Acta Neurol Scand Suppl. 2007;187:51–4.

112. Lynch BA, Lambeng N, Nocka K, et al. The synaptic vesicle protein SV2A is the binding site for the antiepileptic drug levetiracetam. Proc Natl Acad Sci U S A. 2004;101:9861–6.

113. Niespodziany I, Klitgaard H, Margineanu DG. Levetiracetam inhibits the high-voltage-activated Ca(2+) current in pyramidal neurones of rat hippocampal slices. Neurosci Lett. 2001;306:5–8.

114. Rigo JM, Hans G, Nguyen L, et al. The anti-epileptic drug levetiracetam reverses the inhibition by negative allosteric modulators of neuronal GABA- and glycine-gated currents. Br J Pharmacol. 2002;136:659–72.

115. Szaflarski JP, Meckler JM, Szaflarski M, Shutter LA, Privitera MD, Yates SL. Levetiracetam use in critically ill patients. Neurocrit Care. 2007;7:140–7.

116. Rossetti AO, Bromfield EB. Determinants of success in the use of oral levetiracetam in status epilepticus. Epilepsy Behav. 2006;8:651–4.

117. Rupprecht S, Franke K, Fitzek S, Witte OW, Hagemann G. Levetiracetam as a treatment option in non-convulsive status epilepticus. Epilepsy Res. 2007;73:238–44.

118. Patel NC, Landan IR, Levin J, Szaflarski J, Wilner AN. The use of levetiracetam in refractory status epilepticus. Seizure. 2006;15:137–41.

119. Ramael S, Daoust A, Otoul C, et al. Levetiracetam intravenous infusion: a randomized, placebo-controlled safety and pharmacokinetic study. Epilepsia. 2006;47:1128–35.

120. Ruegg S, Naegelin Y, Hardmeier M, Winkler DT, Marsch S, Fuhr P. Intravenous levetiracetam: treatment experience with the first 50 critically ill patients. Epilepsy Behav. 2008;12:477–80.

121. Knake S, Gruener J, Hattemer K, et al. Intravenous levetiracetam in the treatment of benzodiazepine refractory status epilepticus. J Neurol Neurosurg Psychiatry. 2008;79:588–9.

122. Doty P, Rudd GD, Stoehr T, Thomas D. Lacosamide. Neurotherapeutics. 2007;4:145–8.

123. Biton V, Rosenfeld WE, Whitesides J, Fountain NB, Vaiciene N, Rudd GD. Intravenous lacosamide as replacement for oral lacosamide in patients with partial-onset seizures. Epilepsia. 2008;49:418–24.

124. Kellinghaus C, Berning S, Besselmann M. Intravenous lacosamide as successful treatment for nonconvulsive status epilepticus after failure of first-line therapy. Epilepsy Behav. 2009 ;14(2):429–31.

125. Moreno Morales EY, Fernandez Peleteiro M, Bondy Pena EC, Dominguez Lorenzo JM, Pardellas Santiago E, Fernandez A. Observational study of intravenous lacosamide in patients with convulsive versus non-convulsive status epilepticus. Clin Drug Investig. 2015;35:463–9.

126. Paquette V, Culley C, Greanya ED, Ensom MH. Lacosamide as adjunctive therapy in refractory epilepsy in adults: a systematic review. Seizure. 2015;25:1–17.

127. Yasiry Z, Shorvon SD. The relative effectiveness of five antiepileptic drugs in treatment of benzodiazepine-resistant convulsive status epilepticus: a meta-analysis of published studies. Seizure. 2014;23:167–74.

128. Parviainen I, Uusaro A, Kalviainen R, Kaukanen E, Mervaala E, Ruokonen E. High-dose thiopental in the treatment of refractory status epilepticus in intensive care unit. Neurology. 2002;59:1249–51.

129. Bledsoe KA, Kramer AH. Propylene glycol toxicity complicating use of barbiturate coma. Neurocrit Care. 2008;9:122–4.

130. Devlin EG, Clarke RS, Mirakhur RK, McNeill TA. Effect of four i.v. induction agents on T-lymphocyte proliferations to PHA in vitro. Br J Anaesth. 1994;73:315–7.

131. Magnuson B, Hatton J, Williams S, Loan T. Tolerance and efficacy of enteral nutrition for neurosurgical patients on pentobarbital coma. Nutr Clin Pract. 1999;14:131–4.

132. Olson KR, Pond SM, Verrier ED, Federle M. Intestinal infarction complicating phenobarbital overdose. Arch Intern Med. 1984;144:407–8.

133. Rashkin MC, Youngs C, Penovich P. Pentobarbital treatment of refractory status epilepticus. Neurology. 1987;37:500–3.

134. Ramsay RE. Treatment of status epilepticus. Epilepsia. 1993;34:S71–81.

135. Krishnamurthy KB, Drislane FW. Depth of EEG suppression and outcome in barbiturate anesthetic treatment for refractory status epilepticus. Epilepsia. 1999;40:759–62.

136. Claassen J, Hirsch LJ, Emerson RG, Mayer SA. Treatment of refractory status epilepticus with pentobarbital, propofol, or midazolam: a systematic review. Epilepsia. 2002;43:146–53.

137. Rossetti AO, Logroscino G, Bromfield EB. Refractory status epilepticus: effect of treatment aggressiveness on prognosis. Arch Neurol. 2005;62:1698–702.

138. Bergey GK. Refractory status epilepticus: is EEG burst suppression an appropriate treatment target during drug-induced coma? What is the Holy Grail? Epilepsy Curr. 2006;6:119–20.

139. Rossetti AO. Which anesthetic should be used in the treatment of refractory status epilepticus? Epilepsia. 2007;48(Suppl 8):52–5.

140. Treiman DM. Convulsive status epilepticus. Curr Treat Options Neurol. 1999;1:359–69.

141. Krishnamurthy KB, Drislane FW. Relapse and survival after barbiturate anesthetic treatment of refractory status epilepticus. Epilepsia. 1996;37:863–7.

142. Walker MC. Status epilepticus on the intensive care unit. J Neurol. 2003;250:401–6.

143. Miller MA, Forni A, Yogaratnam D. Propylene glycol-induced lactic acidosis in a patient receiving continuous infusion pentobarbital. Ann Pharmacother. 2008;42:1502–6.

144. Rossetti AO, Milligan TA, Vulliemoz S, Michaelides C, Bertschi M, Lee JW. A randomized trial for the treatment of refractory status epilepticus. Neurocrit Care. 2011;14:4–10.

145. Stecker MM, Kramer TH, Raps EC, O'Meeghan R, Dulaney E, Skaar DJ. Treatment of refractory status epilepticus with propofol: clinical and pharmacokinetic findings. Epilepsia. 1998;39:18–26.

146. Walder B, Tramer MR, Seeck M. Seizure-like phenomena and propofol: a systematic review. Neurology. 2002;58:1327–32.

147. Hodkinson BP, Frith RW, Mee EW. Propofol and the electroencephalogram. Lancet. 1987;2:1518.

148. Hufnagel A, Elger CE, Nadstawek J, Stoeckel H, Bocker DK. Specific response of the epileptic focus to anesthesia with propofol. J Epilepsy. 1990;3:37–45.

149. Hanna JP, Ramundo ML. Rhabdomyolysis and hypoxia associated with prolonged propofol infusion in children. Neurology. 1998;50:301–3.

150. Strickland RA, Murray MJ. Fatal metabolic acidosis in a pediatric patient receiving an infusion of propofol in the intensive care unit: is there a relationship? Crit Care Med. 1995;23:405–9.

151. Perrier ND, Baerga-Varela Y, Murray MJ. Death related to propofol use in an adult patient. Crit Care Med. 2000;28:3071–4.

152. Cremer OL, Moons KG, Bouman EA, Kruijswijk JE, de Smet AM, Kalkman CJ. Long-term propofol infusion and cardiac failure in adult head-injured patients. Lancet. 2001;357:117–8.

153. Smith H, Sinson G. Varelas P. Neurocrit Care: Vasopressors and propofol infusion syndrome in severe head trauma; 2008.

154. Prasad A, Worrall BB, Bertram EH, Bleck TP. Propofol and midazolam in the treatment of refractory status epilepticus. Epilepsia. 2001;42:380–6.

155. Parviainen I, Uusaro A, Kalviainen R, Mervaala E, Ruokonen E. Propofol in the treatment of refractory status epilepticus. Intensive Care Med. 2006;32:1075–9.

156. Walton NY, Treiman DM. Motor and electroencephalographic response of refractory experimental status epilepticus in rats to treatment with MK-801, diazepam, or MK-801 plus diazepam. Brain Res. 1991;553:97–104.

157. Rice AC, DeLorenzo RJ. N-methyl-D-aspartate receptor activation regulates refractoriness of status epilepticus to diazepam. Neuroscience. 1999;93:117–23.

158. Borris DJ, Bertram EH, Kapur J. Ketamine controls prolonged status epilepticus. Epilepsy Res. 2000;42:117–22.

159. Sheth RD, Gidal BE. Refractory status epilepticus: response to ketamine. Neurology. 1998;51:1765–6.

160. Pruss H, Holtkamp M. Ketamine successfully terminates malignant status epilepticus. Epilepsy Res. 2008;82(2–3):219–22.

161. Gaspard N, Foreman B, Judd LM, et al. Intravenous ketamine for the treatment of refractory status epilepticus: a retrospective multicenter study. Epilepsia. 2013;54:1498–503.

162. Ubogu EE, Sagar SM, Lerner AJ, Maddux BN, Suarez JI, Werz MA. Ketamine for refractory status epilepticus: a case of possible ketamine-induced neurotoxicity. Epilepsy Behav. 2003;4:70–5.

163. Kofke WA, Bloom MJ, Van Cott A, Brenner RP. Electrographic tachyphylaxis to etomidate and ketamine used for refractory status epilepticus controlled with isoflurane. J Neurosurg Anesthesiol. 1997;9:269–72.

164. Kofke WA, Young RS, Davis P, et al. Isoflurane for refractory status epilepticus: a clinical series. Anesthesiology. 1989;71:653–9.

165. Mirsattari SM, Sharpe MD, Young GB. Treatment of refractory status epilepticus with inhalational anesthetic agents isoflurane and desflurane. Arch Neurol. 2004;61:1254–9.

166. Aggarwal P, Wali JP. Lidocaine in refractory status epilepticus: a forgotten drug in the emergency department. Am J Emerg Med. 1993;11:243–4.

167. Pascual J, Ciudad J, Berciano J. Role of lidocaine (lignocaine) in managing status epilepticus. J Neurol Neurosurg Psychiatry. 1992;55:49–51.

168. Shorvon S. The management of status epilepticus. J Neurol Neurosurg Psychiatry. 2001;70:ii22–7.

169. Vastola EF, Homan R, Rosen A. Inhibition of focal seizures by moderate hypothermia. A clinical and experimental study. Arch Neurol. 1969;20:430–9.

170. Lundgren J, Smith ML, Blennow G, Siesjo BK. Hyperthermia aggravates and hypothermia ameliorates epileptic brain damage. Exp Brain Res. 1994;99:43–55.

171. Liu Z, Gatt A, Mikati M, Holmes GL. Effect of temperature on kainic acid-induced seizures. Brain Res. 1993;631:51–8.

172. Maeda T, Hashizume K, Tanaka T. Effect of hypothermia on kainic acid-induced limbic seizures: an electroencephalographic and 14C-deoxyglucose autoradiographic study. Brain Res. 1999;818:228–35.

173. Niquet J, Baldwin R, Gezalian M, Wasterlain CG. Deep hypothermia for the treatment of refractory status epilepticus. Epilepsy Behav. 2015;49:313–7.

174. Kim JH, Kim SH, Yoo SK, Kim JY, Nam YT. The effects of mild hypothermia on thiopental-induced electroencephalogram burst suppression. J Neurosurg Anesthesiol. 1998;10:137–41.

175. Orlowski JP, Erenberg G, Lueders H, Cruse RP. Hypothermia and barbiturate coma for refractory status epilepticus. Crit Care Med. 1984;12:367–72.

176. Corry JJ, Dhar R, Murphy T, Diringer MN. Hypothermia for refractory status epilepticus. Neurocrit Care. 2008;9:189–97.

177. Zeiler FA, Zeiler KJ, Teitelbaum J, Gillman LM, West M. Therapeutic hypothermia for refractory status epilepticus. Can J Neurol. 2015;42:221–9.

178. Andrews PJ, Sinclair HL, Rodriguez A, et al. Hypothermia for intracranial hypertension after traumatic brain injury. N Engl J Med. 2015;373:2403–12.

179. Mourvillier B, Tubach F, van de Beek D, et al. Induced hypothermia in severe bacterial meningitis: a randomized clinical trial. JAMA. 2013;310:2174–83.

180. Ma X, Liporace J, O'Connor MJ, Sperling MR. Neurosurgical treatment of medically intractable status epilepticus. Epilepsy Res. 2001;46:33–8.

181. Ng YT, Kim HL, Wheless JW. Successful neurosurgical treatment of childhood complex partial status epilepticus with focal resection. Epilepsia. 2003;44:468–71.

182. Duane DC, Ng YT, Rekate HL, Chung S, Bodensteiner JB, Kerrigan JF. Treatment of refractory status epilepticus with hemispherectomy. Epilepsia. 2004;45:1001–4.

183. Alexopoulos A, Lachhwani DK, Gupta A, et al. Resective surgery to treat refractory status epilepticus in children with focal epileptogenesis. Neurology. 2005;64:567–70.

184. Ng YT, Kerrigan JF, Rekate HL. Neurosurgical treatment of status epilepticus. J Neurosurg. 2006;105:378–81.

185. Varelas PN. How I treat status epilepticus in the Neuro-ICU. Neurocrit Care. 2008;9:153–7.

186. Schrader LM, Stern JM, Wilson CL, et al. Low frequency electrical stimulation through subdural electrodes in a case of refractory status epilepticus. Clin Neurophysiol. 2006;117:781–8.

187. Patwardhan RV, Dellabadia Jr J, Rashidi M, Grier L, Nanda A. Control of refractory status epilepticus precipitated by anticonvulsant withdrawal using left vagal nerve stimulation: a case report. Surg Neurol. 2005;64:170–3.

188. Valentin A, Nguyen HQ, Skupenova AM, et al. Centromedian thalamic nuclei deep brain stimulation in refractory status epilepticus. Brain Stimul. 2012;5:594–8.

189. Rossetti AO, Lowenstein DH. Management of refractory status epilepticus in adults: still more questions than answers. Lancet Neurol. 2011;10:922–30.

190. Cuero MR, Varelas PN. Super-refractory status epilepticus. Curr Neurol Neurosci Rep. 2015;15:74.
191. Carrasco Gonzalez MD, Palomar M, Rovira R. Electroconvulsive therapy for status epilepticus. Ann Intern Med. 1997;127:247–8.
192. Lopinto-Khoury C, Sperling MR. Autoimmune status epilepticus. Curr Treat Options Neurol. 2013;15:545–56.
193. Wilder-Smith EP, Lim EC, Teoh HL, et al. The NORSE (new-onset refractory status epilepticus) syndrome: defining a disease entity. Ann Acad Med Singap. 2005;34:417–20.
194. Gall CR, Jumma O, Mohanraj R. Five cases of new onset refractory status epilepticus (NORSE) syndrome: outcomes with early immunotherapy. Seizure. 2013;22:217–20.
195. Li J, Saldivar C, Maganti RK. Plasma exchange in cryptogenic new onset refractory status epilepticus. Seizure. 2013;22:70–3.
196. Kadoya M, Onoue H, Kadoya A, Ikewaki K, Kaida K. Refractory status epilepticus caused by anti-NMDA receptor encephalitis that markedly improved following combination therapy with rituximab and cyclophosphamide. Intern Med. 2015;54:209–13.
197. Cockerell OC, Rothwell J, Thompson PD, Marsden CD, Shorvon SD. Clinical and physiological features of epilepsia partialis continua. Cases ascertained in the UK. Brain. 1996;119(Pt 2):393–407.
198. Thomas P, Borg M, Suisse G, Chatel M. Opercular myoclonic-anarthric status epilepticus. Epilepsia. 1995;36:281–9.
199. Manford M, Shorvon SD. Prolonged sensory or visceral symptoms: an under-diagnosed form of non-convulsive focal (simple partial) status epilepticus. J Neurol Neurosurg Psychiatry. 1992;55:714–6.
200. Wells CR, Labar DR, Solomon GE. Aphasia as the sole manifestation of simple partial status epilepticus. Epilepsia. 1992;33:84–7.
201. Walker MC, Smith SJ, Sisodiya SM, Shorvon SD. Case of simple partial status epilepticus in occipital lobe epilepsy misdiagnosed as migraine: clinical, electrophysiological, and magnetic resonance imaging characteristics. Epilepsia. 1995;36:1233–6.
202. Huang CW, Hsieh YJ, Pai MC, Tsai JJ, Huang CC. Nonketotic hyperglycemia-related epilepsia partialis continua with ictal unilateral parietal hyperperfusion. Epilepsia. 2005;46:1843–4.
203. Mut M, Schiff D, Dalmau J. Paraneoplastic recurrent multifocal encephalitis presenting with epilepsia partialis continua. J Neuro-Oncol. 2005;72:63–6.
204. Wroe SJ, Ellershaw JE, Whittaker JA, Richens A. Focal motor status epilepticus following treatment with azlocillin and cefotaxime. Med Toxicol. 1987;2:233–4.
205. Schomer DL. Focal status epilepticus and epilepsia partialis continua in adults and children. Epilepsia. 1993;34(Suppl 1):S29–36.
206. Drislane FW, Blum AS, Schomer DL. Focal status epilepticus: clinical features and significance of different EEG patterns. Epilepsia. 1999;40:1254–60.
207. Aktekin B, Dogan EA, Oguz Y, Karaali K. Epilepsia partialis continua in a patient with Behcet's disease. Clin Neurol Neurosurg. 2006;108:392–5.
208. Aydin-Ozemir Z, Tuzun E, Baykan B, et al. Autoimmune thyroid encephalopathy presenting with epilepsia partialis continua. Clin EEG Neurosci. 2006;37:204–9.
209. Kato Y, Nakazato Y, Tamura N, Tomioka R, Takahashi Y, Shimazu K. Autoimmune encephalitis with anti-glutamate receptor antibody presenting as epilepsia partialis continua and action myoclonus: a case report. Rinsho Shinkeigaku. 2007;47:429–33.
210. Scholtes FB, Renier WO, Meinardi H. Simple partial status epilepticus: causes, treatment, and outcome in 47 patients. J Neurol Neurosurg Psychiatry. 1996;61:90–2.
211. Brandt L, Saveland H, Ljunggren B, Andersson KE. Control of epilepsy partialis continuans with intravenous nimodipine: report of two cases. J Neurosurg. 1988;69:949–50.
212. Rotenberg A, Bae EH, Takeoka M, Tormos JM, Schachter SC, Pascual-Leone A. Repetitive transcranial magnetic stimulation in the treatment of epilepsia partialis continua. Epilepsy Behav. 2009;14:253–7.
213. Fountain NB. Status epilepticus: risk factors and complications. Epilepsia. 2000;41(Suppl 2):S23–30.
214. Sasahira M, Lowry T, Simon RP. Neuronal injury in experimental status epilepticus in the rat: role of acidosis. Neurosci Lett. 1997;224:177–80.
215. Evans MC, Meldrum BS. Regional brain glucose metabolism in chemically-induced seizures in the rat. Brain Res. 1984;297:235–45.
216. Swan JH, Meldrum BS, Simon RP. Hyperglycemia does not augment neuronal damage in experimental status epilepticus. Neurology. 1986;36:1351–4.
217. Kreisman NR, Gauthier-Lewis ML, Conklin SG, Voss NF, Barbee RW. Cardiac output and regional hemodynamics during recurrent seizures in rats. Brain Res. 1993;626:295–302.
218. Darnell JC, Jay SJ. Recurrent postictal pulmonary edema: a case report and review of the literature. Epilepsia. 1982;23:71–83.
219. Terrence CF, Rao GR, Perper JA. Neurogenic pulmonary edema in unexpected, unexplained death of epileptic patients. Ann Neurol. 1981;9:458–64.
220. Williams A, Sekaninova S, Coakley J. Suppression of elevated alanine aminotransferase activity in liver disease by vigabatrin. J Paediatr Child Health. 1998;34:395–7.
221. Zaret BS, Beckner RR, Marini AM, Wagle W, Passarelli C. Sodium valproate-induced hyperammonemia without clinical hepatic dysfunction. Neurology. 1982;32:206–8.
222. Mock CM, Schwetschenau KH. Levocarnitine for valproic-acid-induced hyperammonemic encephalopathy. Am J Health Syst Pharm. 2012;69:35–9.
223. Moreiras Plaza M, Rodriguez Goyanes G, Cuina L, Alonso R. On the toxicity of valproic-acid. Clin Nephrol. 1999;51:187–9.
224. Hogg RJ, Sawyer M, Hecox K, Eigenbrodt E. Carbamazepine-induced acute tubulointerstitial nephritis. J Pediatr. 1981;98:830–2.
225. Treiman DM, Walton NY, Kendrick C. A progressive sequence of electroencephalographic changes during generalized convulsive status epilepticus. Epilepsy Res. 1990;5:49–60.
226. Varelas PN, Spanaki MV, Mirski MA. Status epilepticus: an update. Curr Neurol Neurosci Rep. 2013;13:357.
227. Ferlisi M, Shorvon S. The outcome of therapies in refractory and super-refractory convulsive status epilepticus and recommendations for therapy. Brain. 2012;135:2314–28.
228. Walker MC, Howard RS, Smith SJ, Miller DH, Shorvon SD, Hirsch NP. Diagnosis and treatment of status epilepticus on a neurological intensive care unit. QJM. 1996;89:913–20.
229. Roberts C, French JA. Anticonvulsants in acute medical illness. In: Delanty N, editor. Seizures medical causes and management. Totowa, NJ: Humana Press, Inc; 2002. p. 333–56.
230. Shorvon S. The drug treatment of epilepsy. In: Hopkins A, Shorvon S, Cascino G, editors. Epilepsy. 2nd ed. London: Chapman and Hall; 1993. p. 178.
231. Leppik IE, Wolff DL. Antiepileptic medication interactions. Neurol Clin. 1993;11:905–21.
232. Varelas PN, Mirski MA. Seizures in the adult intensive care unit. J Neurosurg Anesthesiol. 2001;13:163–75.

Ischemic Stroke, Hyperperfusion Syndrome, Cerebral Sinus Thrombosis, and Critical Care Seizures

9

Panayiotis N. Varelas and Lotfi Hacein-Bey

Introduction

Seizures following stroke have been reported since the 19th century. Hughlings Jackson in 1864 reported convulsions in the paralyzed side after a middle cerebral artery (MCA) embolism [1] and few years later William Gowers, in 1885, introduced the term "post-hemiplegic epilepsy" [2].

Seizures can occur early following a stroke (within the first 2 weeks) or start at later stages. They can occur >24 h before clinical evidence of stroke ("antecedent" seizures) or within the 24 h period before or after the initial neurologic deficit ("at onset" or "acute phase" seizures) [3, 4]. Early seizures may be seen during the index admission in the ICU for stroke, or may occur later in the course of the event, justifying admission or re-admission to the Unit. Three major questions arise in the ICU when a patient with stroke develops one or more seizures: (1) how do the seizures impact on the stroke (2) are the seizures, especially the early ones, a mode of entrance into epilepsy, and (3) when and for how long is anti-epileptic treatment appropriate. While trying to address the importance of the problem, one may encounter several difficulties reviewing the literature: many studies are older, from the pre-computed tomography (CT) era, retrospective, based on small numbers of patients, not including all types of stroke, not considering the timing (not

differentiating between early or late seizures). It is important, however, to differentiate between early and late post-stroke seizures because there are several clinical, etiological, and prognostic differences, justifying a separate analysis [5]. Moreover, in several studies, the time between stroke onset and admission is unclear, making uncertain whether seizures occurred before a health care personnel encountered the patient, an important detail since many seizures occur during the very first minutes or hours after the onset of a stroke. Finally, many studies do not control effectively for the presence of anti-epileptic medications when the seizures occur, potentially underestimating the natural history of post-stroke seizures.

Seizures After Ischemic Stroke

Clinical Studies

The reported incidence of post-stroke seizures varies between 4.4% and 13.8% depending on the design of the study, the patient selection included in the analysis, the methods used to evaluate the stroke, the neurophysiological type of monitoring, and the follow-up period [5–14]. A male preponderance has been reported in two studies [5, 15]. Early seizures (definition varying from the first 24 h to the first 4 weeks post stroke) usually occur at the stroke onset in 1.8–33% of patients and constitute the majority of post-stroke seizures [5, 6, 8, 9, 11, 12, 16–20]. The majority of early seizures occur immediately post-stroke and the most of those are inaugural of stroke [12]. In a study of 10,261 patients in the Canadian Stroke network Registry, seizures at ischemic stroke presentation occurred in 1.53% and seizures during hospitalization post-ischemic stroke in 2.03% of patients [21]. Late post-stroke seizure occurrence also depends on the definition and the duration of follow-up, with a reported incidence of 2.5–67% of cases [6, 10, 12, 20, 22–25]. Recurrent seizures (epilepsy) after stroke can occur in 4–9% of patients [26, 27]. Although some studies have reported that early

P.N. Varelas (✉)
Departments of Neurology and Neurosurgery, Henry Ford Hospital, 2799 West Grand Blvd, Detroit, MI 48202, USA

Department of Neurology, Wayne State University, Detroit, MI, USA
e-mail: pvarela1@hfhs.org

L. Hacein-Bey
Sutter Imaging Division, Interventional and Diagnostic Neuroradiology, Sutter Medical Group, 1500 Expo Parkway, Sacramento, CA 95815, USA

Radiology Department, UC Davis School of Medicine, Sacramento, CA 95817, USA
e-mail: lhaceinbey@yahoo.com

© Springer International Publishing AG 2017
P.N. Varelas, J. Claassen (eds.), *Seizures in Critical Care*, Current Clinical Neurology, DOI 10.1007/978-3-319-49557-6_9

seizures did not lead to the development of late seizures [28, 29], the cumulative risk for epilepsy may reach 19% by 6 years, a figure 22 times higher than the expected age-specific incidence of epilepsy in the general population [17]. Loiseau et al., in a large epidemiological study from southwestern France, found that cerebrovascular disease was the most frequently recognized etiology of seizures in the aging population: it was the underlying cause in 36.6% of patients with spontaneous seizures and in 53.9% of the patients with confirmed epilepsy [15]. Therefore, although only 5% of epilepsy is due to cerebrovascular disease (pre-CT data from Rochester, Minnesota) [17], because stroke incidence is high in the elderly, stroke may account for 25–50% of new epilepsy cases in this population segment [15, 30–34].

Most of the seizures after stroke have a focal onset and are of the simple partial type [9–11, 35, 36]. Almost half of them show secondary generalization, making it difficult in the ICU to differentiate between the two types, unless the onset was witnessed or there is continuous video-EEG monitoring. Complex partial seizures are less frequent, although in one retrospective study their incidence reached 24% of all post-stroke seizures [36]. The incidence of primary generalized seizure lies between the two, although this may be an overestimate since most authorities agree that most of them are secondary generalized [37].

There have been very few studies conducted in a Stroke Unit or other ICU, since the majority of stroke patients are managed in an acute floor setting and get admitted to an ICU environment only if they have significant co-morbidities or they deteriorate. In this chapter, we provide a review of all currently available data, so that the reader may form his own opinion.

Several studies were conducted in the pre-CT era, the most notable being that by Louis and McDowell, who reviewed the records of 1000 patients with presumed thrombotic infarction based on clinical criteria [10]. The incidence of seizures was 7.7%. Early seizures were reported in 55% and late in 45% of 60 patients with seizures. Epilepsy developed in 3% of patients with early seizures and 81% of patients with late seizures during an average follow-up period of 27 months.

Another early report of a large stroke population admitted to an Acute Stroke Unit in Toronto found 83/827 (10%) patients to have seizures during the first admission or during the 2- to 5-year follow-up [38]. Seizures occurred only in patients with hemispheric lesions and were equally represented in those with infarcts and hemorrhages. Early seizures (within 1 week) occurred in 57% of those patients (39% within the first day). By the first year 88% of those 83 patients had seizures. Mortality during the first week was not different in those patients with and without seizures.

In a retrospective analysis of 90 patients with post-ischemic stroke seizures, immediate seizures (defined as occurring within 24 h) were observed in 30% and early seizures (within 2 weeks) in 33% [35]. Overall, 98% of the initial post-stroke seizures were observed within 2 years. The authors could identify precipitating factors for initial seizures in four patients (one with hypoglycemia, one with hyponatremia, and two with fever due to pneumonia). Early seizures were more likely partial and late seizures generalized. Recurrent seizures occurred in 35/90 (39%) patients with a mean follow-up of 30 months. Eighty six percent of patients with recurrent seizures had identifiable precipitating factors, the major being non-compliance with the antiepileptic medications. There was no difference in the recurrence rate between those patients with early (40%) and late seizures (38%).

In a retrospective analysis of medical records from Taiwan, approximately 2000 patients were admitted with presumed cerebral infarction and 118 of them had seizures [36]. A bimodal distribution of post-thrombotic stroke seizures was found, with an early peak within 2 weeks (early seizures) and a late one between 6 months and 1 year [36]. Early seizures were reported in 13/118 (11%) patients with seizures and late seizures in 66/118 (66%). However, this study has several limitations, including 42/118 patients with unknown interval between seizure and stroke onset. Twenty three out of 118 patients (19.5%) with a first seizure had silent infarcts proven by CT of the head and no history of previous stroke. In those patients with a single infarct (excluding lacunes and border zone infarcts), the frontal and the temporal lobes were the most commonly involved lobes, either solely or partially (58% each), followed by the parietal lobe (43%) and the occipital lobe (20%). Most of the seizures were simple partial (58%) or complex partial (24%) with or without secondary generalization. Status epilepticus (SE) occurred in 15% of the patients. For patients with ischemic stroke, epilepsy developed in 35% of patients after early seizures and in 90% of patients with late seizures.

In another hospital-based study from Buenos Aires, Argentina, 22 (10%) of 230 patients with stroke developed seizures, including 7.1% of those with ischemic stroke and 25% of those with ICH [6]. The risk for seizures was higher in those patients with ICH, cortical involvement and large stroke (defined as a lesion involving more than one lobe). Early onset seizures (within the first month) occurred in 54.5% and seizure recurrence in 6/22 (27%) of patients with seizures. There was no difference in the type, location, and size of stroke between those patients with early and late seizures.

In a prospective study conducted in Birmingham, UK, 230 patients were followed for at least 27 months after acute stroke [11]. Early seizures at the onset of stroke (defined as within a 24 h period before or after the initial neurological deficit onset) occurred in 13 (5.7%) of patients, all with strokes in the internal carotid artery distribution. In the ischemic stroke subgroup the percentage was 4.3%, in the ICH 10.7% and the SAH

11.1%. Mortality in patients with seizures was significantly higher than the whole stroke group only during the first 48 h after admission. This study has several limitations. Only 86% of patients were admitted to the hospital within the first 48 h of stroke onset, and only 20% had confirmation of the stroke type by CT, angiogram, or necropsy. Six out of 13 patients with seizures had epilepsy or were taking anti-epileptic medications before the onset of the stroke. None of the remaining patients with post-stroke seizures, who survived their stroke (5/7) had further seizures during a minimum follow-up of 30 months. The authors concluded that anti-epileptics failed to control seizures in these patients.

A large prospective study was conducted in Australia, following 1000 patients admitted for stroke [9]. The incidence of early seizures (within 2 weeks) was 4.4% (44 patients) and in 43/44 (97%) occurred within the first 48 h. Four patients had SE (0.4%) and 18 (1.8%) multiple seizures. All patients that received anti-epileptic treatment (77%) had readily controlled seizures. The highest incidence of early seizures (15.4%) was found in patients with supratentorial lobar or extensive (lobar and deep) ICH, followed by 8.5% in patients with SAH, 6.5% in patients with carotid territory infarcts, and 3.7% in patients with hemispheric TIAs. No early seizures were found in any patients with subcortical, lacunar, or vertebrobasilar distribution infarcts or deep cerebral or infratentorial ICHs. There was no difference in the incidence of seizures after cardioembolic infarct compared to large vessel extracranial disease. As a follow-up to the previous study from Australia, the same authors reported the incidence of late seizures (defined as seizures occurring after discharge) in 31/44 patients with early seizures without TIA, who survived [39]. Late seizures occurred in 32% of these patients, compared to 10% of age, sex, and type of stroke matched patients without early seizures from the same cohort. In patients with ischemic stroke, late seizures occurred in 26% and 0%, respectively, and in patients with ICH in 62.5% and 25%, respectively. The mean time from early to late seizure was 12 months (3 months to 2.5 years) and the type of seizure was not associated with seizure recurrence. Twenty one patients were on anti-epileptic treatment at discharge, but the authors could not conclude about their usefulness to prevent late seizures due to the small numbers.

Early seizures (within 2 weeks) occurred in 2.5% of 1200 patients admitted for acute stroke in a large, retrospective study from China [16]. The incidence of early seizures was 2.3% in infarction, 2.8% in ICH, and 2.7% in SAH. There was no association between the stroke subtype and early seizure occurrence. Carotid artery territory cortical infarctions had tenfold increased incidence of seizures compared to non-cortical infarctions and lobar ICH 20-fold increased incidence compared to nonlobar ICH ($p < 0.001$). Two thirds of early seizures were partial, 24% generalized, and 10% SE.

Another large retrospective hospital-based study was conducted in Marseille, France [12]. Seventy eight patients out of 2016 (3.9%) developed seizures after acute stroke and were followed for an average of 30.2 months. The authors observed a biphasic chronological distribution of seizures: early seizures (within the 1st month) were observed in 28/78 (36%) of patients with seizures and late seizures (after the 3rd month) in 64%. Among those with early seizures, two thirds occurred within the first 24 h (23% of all seizures) and among the late ones, two thirds occurred between the 3rd and 12th months (42% of all seizures). Compared to ischemic strokes, ICH was followed more frequently by early seizures ($p = 0.05$). The proportion of seizures following cardioembolic stroke was analogous to that from other causes. Simple partial seizures (with or without secondary generalization) were observed in 64%, primary generalized in 32%, and complex partial in 4% of patients. SE presenting as first seizure occurred in 14% of cases. EEG was performed in 97% of patients with seizures and showed focal slowing abnormalities in 63% and focal irritative abnormalities in 37% of cases. The earlier it was performed after stroke (within the first 48 h or not), the higher the percentage of irritative abnormalities found. Recurrent seizures occurred in 51% of 70 patients with seizures that survived the stroke and no difference was found between those with early or late seizure onset.

In a retrospective, hospital-based study from Palermo, Italy, 217 out of 4425 (4.7%) patients with acute stroke had one or more seizures [40]. Seizures after ischemic stroke occurred in 4.7% of patients and after ICH in 5.7%. In the ischemic group, seizures heralded the stroke in 10.7% of patients with seizures, were early (within 2 weeks) in 44.3% and late in 44.9% of patients with seizures. The location of ischemic stroke was cortical in 45.5% of cases, subcortical in 32.6%, and mixed in 21.9%.

In a prospective hospital-based registry of 1099 patients with stroke conducted in Barcelona, Spain, 27 (2.5%) had early (within the first 48 h) seizures [18]. Younger age, confusional syndrome, hemorrhagic stroke, large lesion size, involvement of parietal and temporal lobes were more frequently found in patients who developed early seizures. There was no increased frequency of early seizures in those patients with TIAs, embolic infarcts, and lacunar strokes. Patients with seizures had 33.3% mortality (vs 14.2% for those without seizures, $p = 0.02$). Presence of early seizures after stroke was an independent predictor of in-hospital mortality (odds, 95% CI 6.17, 2.13–17.93). In a subsequent article, with one more year of data included, the authors reported similar findings, regarding early seizures: in the multivariate analysis only cortical involvement (6, 2.5–14) and acute agitated confusional state (4.4, 1.4–13.8) were independent predictors for early post-stroke seizures [41].

In a prospective multicenter international study (Seizures after Stroke Study Group, SASS), 1897 patients with acute stroke were admitted to teaching hospitals [7]. Seizures were present in 8.6% of patients with ischemic stroke and 10.6% of patients with ICH. Early onset seizures (within 2 weeks) occurred in 4.8% of patients with ischemic stroke. Forty percent of all seizures (3.4% of patients with ischemic stroke) occurred within the first 24 h. Recurrent seizures (epilepsy) occurred in 2.5% of all patients (28% of patients who had seizures) or 2.1% of patients with ischemic stroke (55% of patients with late-onset seizures). Partial seizures accounted for 52% of all seizures. The 1 year actuarial risk for seizures was 20% for patients with ICH and 14% for patients with ischemic stroke. Using a Cox proportional hazards model, late-onset seizures conveyed in the total cohort an almost 24-fold increased risk for epilepsy. In the ischemic stroke group, cortical involvement and stroke disability (as measured by the modified Canadian Neurological score) were independent factors for development of seizures and late-onset seizures for the development of epilepsy (12-fold increased risk).

In a retrospective study from Hong Kong, 34/994 patients (3.4%) with stroke developed post-stroke seizures. No patient with subarachnoid hemorrhage or posterior circulation infarct developed seizures. Male sex and cortical stroke location were the only independent factors associated with seizures (odds ratios 3.2, 95% CI 1.45–7.08 and 3.83, 1.05–14, respectively). Early seizures (within 30 days from onset of stroke) occurred in 1.6% (47% of patients with post-stroke seizures) and epilepsy in 0.7% [42].

In a prospective study from Norway, 484 patients were followed for 7–8 years after ischemic stroke. Post-stroke epilepsy (defined as ≥2 seizures ≥1 week after the stroke) developed in 5.7% of patients and in all of them it was partial epilepsy. Scandinavian Stroke Scale (SSS) score <30 on admission was a significant independent predictor for developing post-stroke epilepsy (odds ratio 4.9) [43].

In a large study from Turkey, 1428 patients admitted to a stroke unit were followed for a mean period of 5.5 years. Although details regarding the timing of seizure presentation are not provided, 3.6% of patients developed epilepsy (2.7% with ischemic and 12.8% with hemorrhagic stroke and 26.6% with venous infarction). Using TOAST classification criteria [44], the authors reported post-stroke epilepsy in 2.7% of patients with atherothrombotic, in 2.6% with cardioembolic, and in 1.3% with lacunar strokes [45].

Another retrospective study from Turkey evaluated 1880 patients with stroke and found 200 (10.6%) of them having seizures. These patients with seizures were compared with 400 control patients, but there was no matching between the groups. Instead, the controls were matched to the rest of the patients without seizures (i.e., they were a good random sample). This study is unique because it reported similar incidence of seizures between ischemic (10.6%) and hemorrhagic (10.7%) strokes. Early seizures (within 2 weeks) occurred in 38.5% of patients with seizures and late seizures in 61.5% [46].

In a large retrospective study from Croatia, 3542 patients with stroke and seizures, defined as convulsions immediately before or within 24 h from the onset of neurological deficits, were evaluated. Seizures were observed in 1.43% of patients with ischemic stroke and in 3.76% of patients with hemorrhagic stroke. Total inpatient mortality was 21.4% in the group without seizures, and significantly more (30.8%) in the group with seizures [47].

In a prospective study of 638 patients with first-ever stroke (543 ischemic and 95 hemorrhagic) admitted to a Stroke Unit in Perugia, Italy, early seizures were observed in 4.8%. Seizures were significantly more common in patients with cortical involvement, severe and large stroke, and in patients with cortical hemorrhagic transformation of ischemic stroke. Hemorrhagic transformation was the only independent predictor for early seizures. There was no association between these seizures and worse outcome [48].

In a prospective study of 400 patients treated with t-PA in Calgary, Canada, seizures occurred in 4% (62.5% of those presented within a week and the rest later). Atrial fibrillation was associated with seizures and their presence with higher mortality. There was no adjustment for co-variates in this study [49].

In the Registry of the Canadian Stroke Network, 10,261 patients were evaluated for post-stroke seizures. Compared to stroke patients without seizures, post-stroke patients with presentation or during hospitalization seizures were younger, had more severe strokes, a higher admission rate to the ICU, higher morbidity, and higher mortality. Presentation seizure was associated with female sex and less limb weakness, while hospitalization seizure with pneumonia and the presence of hemineglect [21].

The only prospective hospital-based study conducted in the ICU examining the incidence of post-stroke seizures was conducted at UCLA, Los Angeles, CA, using CEEG monitoring [50]. None of the ischemic stroke patients received prophylactic anti-epileptic treatment. All patients with ICH were covered with such a regimen. Despite the prophylaxis difference, seizures occurred in 18/63 (28%) of patients with ICH and 3/46 (6%) patients with ischemic stroke (odds ratio 5.7, 95% CI 1.4–26.5, $p < 0.004$). Most seizures (89%) occurred within the first 72 h after the insult and most of them (76%) were non-convulsive (unresponsive patients with absence of overt convulsions).

In a retrospective study from Taiwan, 143 patients with first-time ischemic stroke were followed for a minimum of 6 years. Seizures occurred in 13 (9.1%) of them. Acute symptomatic seizures developed in two (1.4%) and unprovoked seizures in the other 11 (7.7%) patients [51].

In a large prospective hospital-based Stroke registry in Germany, 58,874 patients with TIA, ischemic stroke, or ICH were included. Acute post-stroke seizures were identified in 0.7% of patients with TIA, 2.2% of patients with ischemic stroke and in 5.1% of patients with ICH. Lower age, higher stroke severity, acute nonneurologic infection, history of diabetes mellitus, and history of preceding TIA were independent predictors of acute post-stroke seizures in patients with ischemic stroke, whereas younger age, acute infection, and a history of TIA were predictors after ICH [52].

In a more recent prospective study of 2053 patients admitted to a Stroke Unit, 58 (2.8%) with ischemic stroke presented with early seizures (first week) [53]. The severity of strokes in patients with early seizures was greater than in those without (NIHSS >14 in 50 vs. 25%), as well as the 30-day mortality (29 vs. 14%). Independent seizure predictors were: total anterior circulation infarct, hemorrhagic transformation, hyperglycemia, and the interaction term diabetes x hyperglycemia.

Most of the aforementioned studies are hospital-based studies, introducing a potential bias for more severe stroke admissions. Such bias can be avoided by studying population-based cohorts. These studies give information for both acute onset seizures after stroke (usually hospitalized patients) and for the long-term risk (and thus influence the decision about prophylactic anti-epileptic management).

The oldest population-based study was conducted in Rochester, Minnesota and included 535 patients with first ischemic stroke [54]. Onset seizures (within 24 h) occurred in 4.8% of these patients and early seizures (within 1 week) in 6%. The cumulative probability of developing late seizures (after the 1st week) within the 1st year was 3% (a risk 23-fold higher than for the general population), by 5 years 7.4% and by 10 years 8.9%. In the multivariate analysis, anterior hemisphere location of the infarct was a strong predictor of early seizures (odds ratio 4, 95% CI 1.2–13.7). Early seizures and stroke recurrence were independent predictors for late seizures and recurrent seizures (epilepsy). A criticism of these results may be based on the fact that several patients had their first stroke in the sixties, when computed tomography was not available and might have had hemorrhagic instead of ischemic strokes.

Another large prospective population-based study was performed in France between 1985–1992 [5]. Using the Stroke Registry of Dijon, the authors reported 90 (5.4%) patients with early seizures (within the first 15 days) out of 1640 patients with acute stroke, with an understudy population of 150,000. All patients had CT of the head and all patients with seizures an EEG evaluation. Patients with cerebral infarct due to atheroma had seizures in 4.4%, those with cardiogenic embolus in 16.6%, those with lacunes in 1%, and those with TIAs in 1.9%. An interesting observation in this study is the high incidence of seizures with infarcts of the occipital lobe (11.3%). There were no seizures in patients with brainstem, thalamic, cerebellar, or retinal infarcts. The authors reported higher incidence of seizures after cardioembolic infarction (20.8%) compared to infarction from atheroma (5%, $p = 0.01$) in the anterior circulation distribution. There was no such difference in the vertebrobasilar distribution. This study is also interesting because it reports male predominance as an independent factor for early seizures after stroke and also EEG findings. All patients with seizures had abnormal EEGs: nonspecific focal slow waves in 43 patients, bilateral slow waves in 18, periodic lateralized epileptiform discharges (PLEDS) in 15, paroxysmal features in ten and electrical partial SE in four.

A second large, prospective, population-based study was conducted in Besancon, France [24]. Out of 3205 patients with first-time ischemic or hemorrhagic stroke, 159 (5%) had first-time seizures. Early onset seizures occurred in 57 (1.8%) patients and late ones in 102 (3.2%) patients. During a mean follow-up period of 47 months, 68/135 (50%) patients with a first post-stroke seizure had seizure recurrence. A second seizure occurred more often in patients with late as opposed to early seizures ($p < 0.01$). Occipital involvement and late-onset first seizure were independent predictors of multiple seizure recurrences.

A large European population study was conducted in the Oxfordshire community, UK [8]. Over 4 years, 675 patients with first stroke were registered from a study population of about 105,000. Onset seizures (within the first 24 h) occurred in 14 (2%) of acute stroke patients and were generalized in seven, simple partial in six and complex partial in one. The risk for onset seizures was higher in patients with SAH (6%) and ICH (3%) than in patients with ischemic stroke (2%). Onset seizures conveyed a 7.5 times higher risk (95% CI 2.5–23) for subsequent seizures in comparison to patients with acute stroke but no onset seizures. In the actuarial analysis, the cumulative risk for seizures after ischemic stroke was 4.2% (2.2–6.2%) within the first year and 9.7% (3.7–15.7%) within 5 years. The risks for seizures from ICH were 19.9% (1.5–38.3%) and 26.1% (0–54.8%) and from SAH 22% (2.6–41.8%) and 34.3% (0–100%), respectively. Survivors of total anterior circulation infarction had a 34% (12–57%) risk for post-stroke seizures within 2 years, a risk much higher than in those with other stroke subtypes. On the other hand, the lowest risk for seizures was found in those patients with lacunar strokes (only 3% developed seizures) and in those who were independent at 1 month post stroke (actuarial risk at 5 years 4.2% (0.1–8.3%). Compared to the general population, ischemic stroke conveyed a 29-fold increased risk for seizures within the 1st year and a 21-fold increased risk within the 2nd year. This difference was accentuated in the age group <65 years, where the risk for seizures within the 1st year was 76-fold increased compared to the general population without stroke. Interestingly, in this age group and during the second year, the risk for seizures, although still higher than for the general population, was lower than for the other age groups (17.2-fold increase versus 18.5–23.2-fold increase in patients >65 years old). Thus, younger patients were noted to have a dramatically increased risk for seizures during the 1st year after stroke, which dropped during the second year.

Another population-based study was conducted in Copenhagen, where 1195 patients with acute stroke out of a population of 240,000 inhabitants were followed for 3 years [19]. Early seizures (within the first 14 days after stroke) occurred in 4.2% of patients, most within the first 72 h (86%). Early seizures were only related to the severity of stroke, as estimated by the Scandinavian Stroke Scale (SSS). For each ten point increase in the SSS the risk for early seizures increased by a factor of 1.65 (95% CI 1.4–1.9). This study did not include patients with SAH. Although ICH was more frequent in patients with early seizures than without (17% vs 7%), in the multivariate analysis it dropped as a predictor of seizures. Mortality in patients with early seizures was 50% compared to 20% in patients without seizures, but seizures did not stand as an independent predictor of mortality in the multivariate analysis (only stroke severity predicted mortality). Indeed, in survivors, this study found that early seizures were associated with a better outcome. The authors explained this finding by suggesting that seizures were emanating from a larger ischemic penumbra, which represents salvageable brain tissue. Interestingly, in a subsequent analysis of this cohort, followed for 7 years, the authors reported that 3.2% of patients developed post-stroke epilepsy, which was independently associated with younger age, higher onset stroke severity, larger lesion size, intracerebral hemorrhage, or presence of early seizures [55].

In another population-based study (Northern Manhattan Stroke Study—NOMASS), seizures within the first 7 days of the stroke onset occurred in 4.1% of all 904 patients enrolled and in 3.1% of 704 patients with ischemic strokes [56]. The most common type of seizures was complex partial seizures (48.7%), followed by primary generalized (24.3%), simple partial (10.8%), and undetermined (16.2%) seizures. Compared to ischemic infarcts, seizures post ICH conferred a 2.4 times increased risk for subsequent seizures (95% CI, 1.2–5.2). Compared to deep infarcts, lobar infarcts conferred an 11 times increased risk for seizures (95% CI 2.6–47.6). Deep and lobar ICH, as well as SAH also correlated with a significantly higher risk for seizures than deep ischemic infarcts (7.9, 1.4–43.6, 25.3, 5.1–125.2 and 13.2, 2.7–86.4, respectively). In a subgroup with recorded NIHSS scores, seizures were more commonly associated with NIHSS > 15 on admission. Early seizures post-ischemic stroke were not independently predictive of 30-day case fatality, a finding which was in conflict with earlier studies [18].

A large prospective study from Lausanne, Switzerland, using the Lausanne Stroke Registry reported 43/3628 (1.2%) patients with seizures [57]. Those patients with seizures were age, sex, and location-type of lesion-matched with two controls without seizures from the same cohort. Early seizures (within the first 24 h) occurred in 23/3270 (0.7%) patients with ischemic stroke and 14/352 (3.97%) patients with ICH. Patients with infarcts were statistically fewer than those with ICH to develop seizures. Hemorrhagic infarcts were associated with seizures, but embolic infarcts were not. All lesions in patients with seizures involved the cortex, except for three (one deep posterior circulation infarct and two striatocapsular ICH). In the multivariate analysis, a high blood cholesterol level was an independent predictor for decreased risk for early seizures (odds ratio 0.18, 95% CI 0.06–0.54).

A large population-based study from Cincinnati, Ohio, evaluated 6044 patients with acute stroke and reported 190 (3.1%) of them having acute onset seizures (within the first 24 h). No difference was found between first-ever versus recurrent strokes on the incidence of seizures. Ischemic strokes and TIAs had an overall 2.4% incidence of these early seizures, in contrast with 7.9% for ICH and 10.1% for SAH. Of the patients with ischemic stroke, there was higher incidence of seizures in cardioembolic (3%) versus small or large vessel ischemic strokes (1.7%). Independent risk factors for seizure development included hemorrhagic stroke, younger age, and pre-stroke Rankin score of ≥ 1 [58].

In a large recent meta-analysis of 102,008 patients from 34 longitudinal cohort studies, the pooled incidence rate of post-stroke (ischemic and hemorrhagic) seizures was found to be 0.07 (95% confidence interval, 0.05–0.09), while the rate of post-stroke epilepsy was 0.05, 0.04–0.06. The incidence of post-stroke seizures in hemorrhagic stroke (0.10, 0.08–0.13) was much higher than in ischemic stroke (0.06, 0.04–0.08) and when the cortical region was involved (0.15, 0.10–0.21) [14].

In summary, many studies suffer from retrospective design, mixed ischemic and hemorrhagic stroke populations and various definitions and follow-up periods. The best estimates from prospective studies place the incidence of early seizures after ischemic stroke in the 0.7–6.5% range, of late seizures in the 2.03–6.8% range, total seizures in the 1.02–8.6% range (with up to 16.6% for cardioembolic strokes) and of epilepsy in the 2.1–2.7%. Table 9.1 summarizes the aforementioned studies of stroke and seizures, as well as percentages of early, late, recurrent (epilepsy), or total seizures.

Status Epilepticus

SE may be an additional risk factor for increased mortality and morbidity after stroke, through systemic metabolic changes, increased risk for herniation secondary to elevated intracranial pressure, cardiac arrhythmias leading to sudden death or increased risk of aspiration pneumonia [56]. Thus SE is an unquestionable reason for ICU admission.

Table 9.1 Studies with reported seizure incidence after a stroke

Study	Type of study	No of patients	Type of stroke	Total seizures	Early seizures	Late seizures	Epilepsy
Louis and McDowell [10]	R	1000	Isc	7.7%	3.3%	2.7%	3% early, 81% late
Black et al. [38]	R	827	Isc, hem	10%	57%[a]	43%[a]	
Gupta et al. [35]	R	90	Isc		33%[a]	1 year 40%[a] 2 years 24%[a]	39%[a]
Sung et al. [36]	R	118	Isc	5.9%	11%8	66%[a]	35% early[a] 90% late[a]
Lancman et al. (6)	R	230	Isc, ICH	10%	5.4%	2.7%	
Shinton et al. [11]	P	230	Isc, ICH, SAH		5.7%		
Kilpatrick et al. [9]	P	1000	Isc, ICH, SAH		4.4%	32% early[a] 10% without early[a]	
Lo et al. [16]	R	1200	Isc, ICH, SAH		2.5%		
Milandre et al. [12]	R	2016	Isc, ICH	3.9%	1.4%	2.5%	1.7%
Daniele et al. [40]	R	4425	Isc, ICH	Isc 4.7% ICH 5.7%	Isc 2.6% ICH 3.6%	Isc 2.1% ICH 2.1%	
Arboix et al. [41]	P	1099	Isc, ICH, SAH		2.5%		
Bladin et al. [7]	P	1897	Isc, ICH	Isc 8.6% ICH 10.6%	Isc 4.8% ICH 7.9%	Isc 3.8% ICH 2.6%	Isc 2.1% ICH 2.6%
Vespa et al. [50]	P	109	Isc, ICH	Isc 6% ICH 28%			
So et al. [54]	R	535	Isc		6%	1 year 3% 5 year 7.4% 10 year 8.9%	
Giroud et al. [5]	P	1640	Isc, ICH, SAH	Ath 4% Card 16.6% Lac 1% TIA 1.7%	5.4%		
Berges et al. [24]	P	3205	Isc, hem	5%	1.8%	3.2%	50%[b]
Burn et al. [8]	P	675	Isc, ICH, SAH	Isc 4.2%/9.7% ICH 19.9%/26.1% SAH 22%/34.3%	2%		
Reith et al. [19, 55]	P	1195	Isc, ICH	4.1%	Isc 3% ICH 8%		3.2%
Labovitz et al. [56]	P	904	Isc, ICH, SAH		Isc 3.1% ICH 7.3% SAH 8%		
Devuyst et al. [57]	P	3628	Isc, ICH	1.02%	Isc 0.7%[c] ICH 3.97%[c]		
Neau et al. [113][e]	R	65	Isc	10.8%			
Lamy et al. [22][f]	P	581	Isc		2.4%	1 year 3.1% 3 years 5.5%	2.3%
Cheung et al. [42]	R	994	Isc, ICH, SAH	3.4%	Isc 3.3% ICH 4.1% SAH 0%		0.7%
Cordonnier et al. [116]	P	202	Isc, ICH		5.4% Isc 4.5% ICH 12%	6.9% Isc 6.8% ICH 8%	
Lossius et al. [43]	P	484	ICH				5.7%
Benbir et al. [45]	P	1428	Isc, ICH, CVT	3.6%			Isc 2.7% ICH 12.8% CVT 26.6%

(continued)

Table 9.1 (continued)

Study	Type of study	No of patients	Type of stroke	Total seizures	Early seizures	Late seizures	Epilepsy
Misirli et al., [46]	R	1880	Isc, ICH	10.6%	4.1%	6.5%	
Szaflarski et al. [58]	P	6044	Isc, ICH, SAH	3.1%	3.1% Isc 2.4% ICH 7.9% SAH 10.1%		
Basic-Baronica et al. [47]	R	3542	Isc, ICH	1.8%	Isc 1.43% ICH 3.76%		
Alberti et al. [48]	P	638	Isc, ICH		4.9% Isc 4.8% ICH 16.3%		
Chiang et al. [51]	R	143	Isc	9.1%			
Strzelczyk et al. [136]	P	264	Isc, ICH	10.9%	4.5%	6.4%	3.8%
Denier et al. [87]	P	328	Isc		4.3%		
Krakow et al. [52]	P	58,874	Isc, TIA, ICH	Isc 2.2% TIA 0.7% ICH 5.1%			
Mecarelli et al. [99]	P	232	Isc, ICH		6.5%		
Procaccianti et al. [53]	P	2053	Isc, ICH		3.2%		
Couillard et al. [49]	R	400	Isc	4%	2.5%	1.5%[d]	
Pezzini et al. [88]	P	516	Isc, ICH		3.9%		
Huang et al. [21]	P	10,261	Isc	3.6%	1.53%	2.03%[e]	
Zou et al. [14]	M	102,008	Isc, ICH	6.93% Isc 6% ICH 10%			5%

P prospective, *R* retrospective, *M* meta-analysis, *Isc* ischemic, *ICH* intracerebral hemorrhage, *SAH* subarachnoid hemorrhage, *hem* hemorrhage, *Ath* atheroma, *Card* cardioembolic, *CVT* cerebral venous thrombosis, *Lac* lacunar, *TIA* transient ischemic attack
[a]Patients with seizures
[b]Survivors with first seizure
[c]Excluding 6 pts with prodromal seizures
[d]After 1 week
[e]During hospitalization
[f]Age group 15–45 years
[g]Age group 18–55 years

Acute stroke is the third most common cause for SE [59], accounting for approximately 20% of all SE cases [60–62]. In a retrospective study, 8% of all initial post-stroke seizures presented as SE (6% focal and 2% generalized) [35]. SE was more common with early (14%) than late (5%) onset seizures, but did not occur as recurrent seizures. This was demonstrated in the largest pre-CT retrospective study of seizures following non-embolic cerebral infarction, that found the majority of SE attacks to occur in the acute post-stroke phase [10]. In another retrospective study, SE occurred in 13% of 118 patients with thrombotic stroke and was generalized tonic-clonic in 60%. This latter study reported only one patient with SE as the initial stroke manifestation and another three with SE in the acute stroke phase: 60% of patients had SE as late seizure manifestation post infarction [36]. Milandre et al. found that 14% of their patients with initial post-stroke seizures were in SE [12] and Lo et al. that 10% of early seizure patients were in SE [16]. Within the first 7 days following an ischemic stroke, SE occurs in 0.9% of patients in the NOMASS-population-based study, and represents 18.9–27% of first-time or early seizures after stroke, respectively [56, 63].

A large, prospective, population-based study was conducted in Besançon, France [63]. Out of 3205 patients with first-time strokes, 159 (5%) had first-time seizures. SE occurred in 31/159 (19%) patients with post-stroke seizures. Partial SE occurred in 12 patients, NCSE in ten, generalized in six, and unclassifiable in three patients. SE occurred in 22/2742 (0.8%) patients with ischemic stroke and 22/116 (19%) patients with ischemic stroke who had post-stroke seizures. SE occurred in 9/463 (1.9%) patients with ICH and 9/43 (21%) patients with ICH and post-stroke seizures. There was no significant difference between the two etiologies of stroke (ischemic stroke or ICH) regarding the occurrence of post-stroke SE. In 4/3205 (0.12%) patients stroke initially manifested as SE and in 17/159 (11%) SE occurred as the first post-stroke epileptic symptom. In patients with SE, it manifested as the first epileptic syndrome in 17/31 (55%) patients (in 7 as "early" SE—within the first 2 weeks—and in 10 as "late" SE) and in 14 patients it followed another seizure after the stroke (in two patients it was "early" SE and in 12 patients it was "late" SE). In an average 47-month follow-up of the 16/17 surviving patients with SE as the first epileptic symptom, only 3 (19%) developed additional episodes of SE and

50% were SE or seizure-free. By contrast, all 14 patients with SE after one or more seizures had recurrences: five with SE (36%) and 9 (64%) with only seizures. Thus, SE as the first epileptic symptom was associated with a lower risk for subsequent seizures ($p < 0.01$). Such favorable association was not noted with early or late occurrence of SE. Fifteen out of 31 (48%) patients with post-stroke SE died. In five of them (16%, all with infarction) SE was considered the direct cause of death. There was no significant difference in mortality for patients with post-stroke seizures and post-stroke SE. Permanent neurologic deterioration after SE occurred in two patients only and transient deterioration in 13 patients. However, there was no radiological change in these 15 patients. In another large, multicenter study of 346 patients with generalized convulsive SE, mortality reached 11% in those patients with stroke as the precipitating cause [60].

Another large, retrospective hospital-based study was reported from Turkey [64]. Out of 1174 patients with first-time stroke, 180 (15.3%) developed post-stroke seizures, of which 17 (9% or 1.45% of the whole cohort) developed SE. Twelve patients manifested SE after ischemic stroke and five after ICH. There was no difference between the group with SE and the group with post-stroke seizures regarding sex, age, stroke risk factors, seizure types, EEG findings, stroke type (ischemic or hemorrhagic), topography or cortical involvement or size of the lesion. However, SE occurred more frequently among more disabled patients (Rankin scale > 3, $p = 0.002$). Early onset (within the first week) SE was found in 7/17 patients, of whom SE occurred as the first epileptic symptom in six (stroke begun as SE in two patients) and as SE after at least one seizure in one patient. Late-onset SE was found in 10/17 patients, of whom SE occurred as the first epileptic symptom in three. Five of seven patients with early onset SE compared to none of those patients with late-onset SE experienced recurrence of SE ($p = 0.003$). Mortality was not different among patients with SE (53%) compared to those with post-stroke seizures (50%). However, it was higher in those patients with early onset SE, than in those with late-onset seizures ($p = 0.049$). Death was the direct consequence of SE in two patients (12%). Poor functional disability was the only independent clinical factor for developing post-stroke SE and age for mortality after post-stroke SE.

In the large prospective study from Lausanne, Switzerland, SE was reported in 3/37 (8%) patients with early seizures after stroke, but in only 0.08% of all patients with ischemic infarction or ICH in this cohort [57].

In a prospective study from Turkey that evaluated 121 patients with SE, 30 (24.8%) were associated with stroke. This study does not report incidence of post-stroke SE. All stroke types were evenly distributed within the early onset group (within 2 weeks), whereas only ischemic stroke was found in the late-onset group (after 2 weeks). Posterior cerebral artery (PCA) infarcts were significantly more common

within the late-onset group. NCSE was more frequent than convulsive SE in the early onset group [65].

In a retrospective study from Taiwan, 143 patients with first-time ischemic stroke were followed for a minimum of 6 years. One (0.07%) developed SE during hospitalization [51]

In a prospective study of 2053 patients admitted to a Stroke Unit, 58 (2.8%) with ischemic stroke presented with early seizures and 13 (0.6%) with SE [53].

In summary, the same methodological problems (see end of subsect. 2.1) are true for studies that report SE after stroke. From prospective studies, the best estimate is that SE occurs in 0.08–0.9% of patients after ischemic stroke.

Table 9.2 is a summary of the aforementioned studies reporting SE incidence after stroke.

Pathophysiology

Seizures Before Stroke: Chicken or Egg First?

Although the vast majority of seizures follow stroke, they can also precede it. Many studies excluded epileptic patients from the analysis if they suffered a stroke and had concurrent seizures. Others, however, reported the outcomes in these patients with "vascular precursor epilepsy" [10, 36]. In one particular study from UK, 46% of patients who developed seizures after acute stroke were epileptics, raising the possibility that epileptic patients may have more frequent seizures after a stroke than non-epileptic patients [11]. This could be explained either through recurrent or continuous focal ischemia capable of inducing an epileptogenic cortical focus or the activation of epileptiform discharges by regional hypoxia in patients with partial or primary generalized epilepsy, a mechanism not yet demonstrated in non-epileptic patients [3]. In another study from Taiwan, four patients had seizures preceding the thrombotic stroke onset from a few hours to 2–3 days [36]. In the Oxfordshire study 2% of patients had a seizure in the year before the stroke, a threefold increase compared to the general population [8]. Another case-control study of 230 patients showed an eightfold increased risk of epilepsy before stroke [66]. A more recent, population-based study from the UK matched 4709 patients who had seizures beginning at or after the age of 60 with controls and followed them for 5–7 years. In the seizures group, 10% of patients developed strokes and in the control only 4.4%. In a Cox model, the estimated relative hazard of stroke at any point for patients with seizures compared with the control group was 2.89 [67]. In addition, the previously cited large prospective study from Switzerland reported 6/3628 (0.16%) patients with seizures within the week preceding the stroke onset [57]. Three patients had infarcts and three ICH. The authors suggest that these pre-stroke seizures are caused by an initially pre-clinical lesion, which because of rebleeding,

Table 9.2 Studies with reported status epilepticus (SE) incidence after a stroke

Study	Type of study	No of pts	SE	Comments
Sung et al. [36]	R	118	15%	0.8% initial stroke manifestation
Kilpatrick et al. [9]	P	1000	0.4%	Pts with early seizures
Lo et al. [16]	R	1200	0.25%	Pts with early seizures
Milandre et al. [12]	R	2016	0.5%	
Gupta et al. [35]	R	90	8%	14% of pts with early seizures 5% of pts with late seizures
Labovitz et al. [56]	P	904	0.9%	
Rumbach et al. [63]	P	3205	Isc 0.9% ICH 1.9%	0.12% initial stroke manifestation 19% pts with SE had recurrent SE, when 1st epileptic symptom 36% pts with SE had recurrent SE, when SE followed seizures
Velioglu et al. [64]	R	1174	1.45% Isc 1% ICH 0.45%	0.17% initial stroke manifestation 71% pts with SE had recurrence, when early onset SE 0% pts with SE had recurrence, when late-onset SE
Devuyst et al. [57]	P	3628	0.08%	Excluding 6 pts with prodromal seizures
Lamy et al. [22]	P	581	0.34%	age group 18–55 years
Chiang et al. [51]	R	143	0.07%	
Procaccianti et al. [53]	P	2053	Isc, ICH 0.6%	

P prospective, *R* retrospective, *Isc* ischemic, *ICH* intracerebral hemorrhage

developing edema or extension or dysfunction of adjacent or remote structures (diaschisis) evolves into a clinical stroke syndrome. Because up to 11% of patients with first clinical strokes have asymptomatic cerebral infarctions on computed tomography (half of which involve the cortex) [68], it is conceivable that the preceding seizures arise from these asymptomatic lesions [36]. Two studies support this theory: in the first study, 15/132 (11.4%) patients with late age onset seizures and no history of stroke had infarcts on CT of the head versus two of age- and sex-matched controls ($p = 0.003$). However, 60% of these infarcts were lacunes [69]. In another study, 75/387 (19%) of patients older than 50 years with new-onset seizures had ischemic lesions on CT of the head, making cerebral vascular disease the most frequently identified cause of late-in-life-onset epilepsy [34].

Ischemic Changes in Time and Development of Seizures

The interplay between the depth and duration of ischemia and the development of epileptic epiphenomena is still unknown, but new developments have shed a light. Post-stroke seizures are associated with more severe brain ischemia as shown by positron emission tomography [70]. Seizures associated with migraine may be warning signs of an underlying cerebral infarction [71]. A causal relationship between TIAs and seizures has been difficult to establish. Repetitive involuntary movements in association with TIAs have been reported. EEG in these patients did not show epileptiform activity and the movements did not respond to phenytoin [3, 72].

Onset seizures after acute stroke have common features with acute seizures after traumatic brain injury and imply a common pathogenesis [7, 8]. In animal models, however, there may be differences. In rats, for example, non-convulsive seizures occur more acutely and intensely after permanent middle cerebral artery occlusion than penetrating ballistic-like brain injury [73].

Since there may be a free time interval between the development of late seizures after early post-stroke seizures, the pathophysiologic mechanisms may differ between early and late seizures or be evolving in time [12]. Early seizures are thought to emanate from electrically irritable tissue in the penumbra of the lesion [74, 75], due to regional metabolic dysfunction and excitotoxic neurotransmitter release, such as glutamate [76]. Dysfunction of inhibitory GABAergic circuits is another possibility. Accumulation of Ca^{++} and Na^+ inside the cell results in depolarization of the cellular membrane and the activation of several intracellular cascades. This has been shown in animal models of stroke [77], where cortical neurons in the neocortex and hippocampus had altered membrane potentials and increased excitability [78, 79], as well as in vitro models of hippocampal neuron cultures, where a single 30 min 5 mcM glutamate exposure produced dead cells or cells manifesting recurrent epileptiform discharges and with increased intracellular calcium levels [76].

In a rat model, Nedergaard and Hansen showed that the penumbral depolarization after MCA occlusion is either spreading depression waves (from K+ or glutamate release from the core of the infarct) or ischemic depolarizations (due to blood flow fluctuations around the threshold of anoxic membrane failure) [80]. These derangements do not remain stationary, but constitute an evolving process. In a rat model of forebrain ischemia, there was a differential seizure threshold to infused pro-epileptic agents, that was changing over time

[81]. Thus, it is suggested that after an initial critical period, estimated around 3 h, the progression of the penumbra tissue towards necrosis leads to lessened epileptogenic activity, which accounts for the decrease in seizure frequency between 3 and 24 h after stroke [57]. These findings are supported by another neurophysiological study using transcranial magnetic stimulation, where six out 84 patients with stroke showed a decrease in duration of the silent period in either the arm or leg of the affected side compared to the unaffected limb [82]. Five of these six patients had early or late post-stroke focal seizures and no interictal epileptiform activity on the EEG. The authors suggested that this finding was due to decreased cortical inhibitory activity related to functional or structural impairment of GABAergic interneurons.

The potential role that hypoxemia may play, in addition to the presence of a penumbra is exemplified in a large retrospective study from Belgium. Two hundred thirty seven patients with post-stroke seizures were compared with 939 stroke patients without seizures. The interesting finding from this study was that the only independent factors associated with post-stroke seizures were partial anterior circulation syndrome/infarct and presence of chronic obstructive pulmonary disease (COPD). The authors suggested that nocturnal desaturations in patients with COPD playing an additional role to stroke [83].

How much do seizures affect the evolution of the triggering stroke? The effect of seizures on the infarcted area, through hypoxia, lactic acidosis, ionic changes, and a higher metabolic demand of the brain, is thought to lead to persistent worsening of the neurologic deficits [18, 84]. In one particular study, persistent partial motor post-stroke seizures led to persistent worsening of the prior neurologic deficit in 10/48 patients, without new CT or MRI findings [84]. In a rat model of permanent occlusion of the middle cerebral artery, levetiracetam was given immediately before the surgery in one group and its vehicle to the controls. Both in drug-treated and in control rats, EEG activity was suppressed after the MCA occlusion. In control but not in drug-treated rats, EEG activity reappeared approximately 30–45 min after the occlusion and initially consisted in single spikes and, then, evolved into spike-and-wave and polyspike-and-wave discharges. In rats sacrificed 24 or 72 h after the occlusion, the ischemic lesion was approximately 50% smaller in drug-treated than in control rats, implying a neuroprotective effect of levetiracetam potentially through seizure-like phenomena suppression [85]. However, several other studies have failed to demonstrate worsening of prognosis after post-stroke seizures [9, 11, 19, 56].

Late seizures probably are due to gliosis and the development of meningocerebral cicatrix, leading to persistent hypoperfusion and anoxia, dendritic deformation and hypersensitivity or denervation supersensitivity [3, 35, 75].

Another interesting recent finding was the association of post-stroke seizures with subsequent development of dementia. In the Lille, France, large prospective stroke/dementia cohort, cognitive function before and after a stroke was evaluated longitudinally with a battery of tests. Early post-stroke seizures (within 1 week from stroke onset) were independently predicting new-onset dementia within 3 years (hazard ratio 3.81, 95% CI 1.13–12.8). The authors suggested that seizures were a marker of an underlying condition associated with an increased risk for dementia, such as more severe vascular pathology, an underlying pre-clinical degenerative disease such as Alzheimer's or post-stroke complications [86].

A summary of possible mechanisms for seizures in varying temporal relationships to stroke can be found in the article of Armon et al. [3] and Solverman et al. [75].

Localization and Etiology of Ischemic Stroke and Seizures

The importance of cerebral cortical involvement and specific cortical areas in the generation of post-stroke seizures is exemplified in a large prospective study of 661 patients admitted to a Stroke Unit. In this study, 328 patients had MRI-confirmed cerebral infarcts (with cortical involvement in 178 of them). Early onset seizures (defined as seizures within 14 days) were all initially partial seizures and occurred in 4.3% and at stroke onset in 1.5% of patients. These seizures occurred exclusively in patients with cortical involvement. With infarcts involving the cerebral cortex, there was a higher risk of early seizures in watershed infarctions than in territorial strokes (23.1% vs 5.3%). Logistic regression analysis showed an almost four fold increased risk of early seizures in patients with watershed infarctions compared with other cortical infarcts (odds ratio, 95% CI, 4.7, 1.5–15.4). Interestingly in this study, age, sex, diabetes mellitus, hypertension, smoking, NIHSS score, and cardioembolic origin were not significant predictors for early seizures [87]. Cortical distribution of the ischemic infarction was also independently associated with seizures (odds ratio, 95% CI 5.5, 1.53–20.2) in a retrospective study from Taiwan with a long follow-up period (minimum 6 years) [51]. In a prospective study from Perugia, Italy, cortical involvement, severe and large stroke size and cortical hemorrhagic transformation were predictors for early post-stroke seizures in the univariate analysis, but only hemorrhagic transformation was an independent predictor in the multivariate [48].

In addition, neurological complications within the first week of an acute stroke may influence the risk of early seizures. In the Brescia Stroke Registry in Italy, 3.9% of 516 patients with acute stroke developed early seizures. Patients with early seizures had a higher burden of complications compared with those without (30 vs. 4.2%, for patients with >6 complications). The odds ratio and 95% CI were 1.57, 1.21–2.01 for any increase of 1 in the number of complications [88].

Although the involvement of the cerebral cortex after ischemic stroke is thought to be necessary for the occurrence of seizures, there have been several reports of seizures associated with lesions involving subcortical structures. In mice exposed to permanent occlusion of the right common carotid artery and then systemic hypoxia, generalized motor seizures were observed within 72 h. These seizures occurred nearly exclusively in animals with extensive brain injury in the hemisphere ipsilateral to the carotid occlusion, but their generation was not associated with electroencephalographic discharges in bilateral hippocampal and neocortical recordings, suggesting origin from deep subcortical structures [89]. In humans, lacunar infarcts have been implicated in the development of seizures, either through more widespread cerebrovascular disease and involvement of adjacent cortex not apparent on the CT of the head or because subcortical lesions, such as those in the caudate head, may induce seizures [5, 29]. Four out of 13 patients with seizures after acute stroke had subcortical lesions in a prospective study from Birmingham, UK [11]. Only 3 out of 273 (1%) patients with lacunar infarcts had seizures in the previously quoted large prospective study from Dijon, France [5]. In the same population, the authors reported in a different study that 11/13 (85%) patients with seizures and CT-proven lenticulostriate strokes had an associated ipsilateral posterofrontal or anterotemporal cortical ischemic lesion demonstrated by MRI. On SPECT, 13/13 (100%) patients had decreased CBF in the ipsilateral frontal area. Also, in patients with a lenticulostriate stroke, a larger size of both the subcortical and ipsilateral cortical ischemic lesions were predictive of seizures [90]. Five patients (3%) in the Oxfordshire study with lacunes had seizures [8] and another five patients with lacunes and grand mal seizures have been reported in a case series from Israel [91]. In the multicenter, prospective SASS study, 2.6% of patients with lacunes developed seizures, but 7/8 had also other identifiable reasons [7]. In a prospective hospital-based registry, 113 patients with non-lacunar subcortical infarcts were studied. Seizures occurred in 4 (3.5%) of these patients, all with striatocapsular infarcts: two within the first 24 h, one within the first month and one within the first year. Cardioembolic strokes were more common in patients with seizures [92]. In the Hong Kong study, 1.5% of patients with lacunar strokes developed seizures, contrasting with the 8.8% of those with total anterior circulation infarcts and 7% of those with partial anterior circulation infarcts [42]. In the recent Turkish study, epilepsy developed in 1.3% of patients with lacunar strokes [45]. Other large studies have not found an association between lacunes and seizures [9].

Other subcortical or white matter changes have been implicated in post-stroke seizures. Ten percent of patients with CADASIL have seizures, usually related to ischemic stroke development [93]. In a case report, a patient with new-onset focal epilepsy showed on MRI FLAIR sequence white matter hyperintensities on both hemispheres with confluent lesions at the right parieto-occipital junction, with juxtacortical components. The authors suggested that these white matter lesions closer to the cortex may be the cause of seizures, like in multiple sclerosis [94].

Seizures associated with embolic infarcts may be due to commonly seen hemorrhagic conversion, since iron deposition in rat brain tissue is known to be epileptogenic [95]. The same way, iron deposition may play a significant role in seizure development after ICH, although this mechanism does not adequately explain the early onset frequently seen. In addition, thrombin is thought to play a significant role in seizures after ICH [96].

EEG Findings

In the ICU, EEG allows evaluation of post-stroke neurological symptoms [75], such as focal weakness (Todd's paralysis) or coma (due to NCSE) [97], which may be due to seizures rather than be permanent deficits from stroke and may be treatable. Normal EEG after post-stroke seizures has been reported in 4–15% of cases [9, 12, 16, 35]. As with ICH [50], the use of CEEG monitoring in the ICU has revolutionized the detection of seizures post-ischemic stroke, many of which are subclinical. [50]. In a study from Switzerland, which evaluated 100 patients admitted to a stroke unit with acute stroke (ischemic in 91 and hemorrhagic in nine patients), CEEG was performed for a mean duration of 17 h 34 min. Epileptic activity occurred in 17 patients and consisted of repetitive focal sharp waves in seven, repetitive focal spikes in seven, and PLEDs in three. Although clinical seizures occurred in three patients before CEEG (only one had repetitive focal spikes on CEEG), electrical seizures were only recorded in two patients without clinical seizures. On multivariate analysis, stroke severity (higher NIHSS) was the only independent predictor [98].

Abnormalities on the EEG may have a differential predictive value regarding the development of seizures after cerebral infarction. Holmes found that 98% of post-stroke patients with sharp waves, spikes and PLEDs on the EEG developed seizures, but did not correlate these findings with seizure recurrence [13]. Twenty six percent of patients who developed post-stroke seizures had PLEDs in this study compared to only 2% of those who never had one. The prognostic significance of post-stroke PLEDs has also been emphasized in another retrospective study, which noted that all four patients with PLEDs on the initial EEG had recurrent seizures [35]. Conversely, in patients with post-stroke seizures, focal irritative abnormalities (electrographic seizures, epileptiform abnormalities, PLEDs) can be found on the average in one fourth of cases and focal slowing in two thirds [12, 16, 35]. Epileptiform abnormalities on EEG performed within the first 24 h ("unless the patient was critically ill") were found in 14% of patients with peri-stroke seizures in a large recent prospective study [57]. In another study of 232 patients with stroke (177 with ischemic stroke) with EEG performed within 24 h after stroke onset, sporadic epileptiform focal abnormalities were found in 10% and PLEDs in 6%. SE was recorded in 71.4% of patients with PLEDs. At the multivariate analysis, only early epileptic manifestations were independently associated with PLEDs. These specific patterns, such as PLEDs, that are closely related to early seizures, could be detected with EEG monitoring only [99]. The specificity of the test is poor, since similar findings are not uncommon in patients with stroke without seizures [12]. The frequency of irritative abnormalities can be influenced by the timing and the repetition rate of the test. This may explain why in a prospective study from Denmark, epileptiform abnormalities were reported in only 2/77 (2.6%) patients with supratentorial strokes [26]. EEGs were obtained in all patients within the 1st week after the stroke and repeated at 3 and 6 months. All seven patients who developed epilepsy in this series had focal delta and theta activity on the EEG. One patient had epileptiform activity at 3 months post-stroke, before he developed epilepsy and another on the first EEG recorded 6 days after stroke and 5 days after the first seizure. The authors conclude that EEG was not helpful in determining the risk for developing epilepsy.

Figure 9.1 shows a patient who was in status epilepticus after an old ischemic stroke.

Figure 9.2 shows another patient who developed a stroke, followed by seizures while driving.

Neuroimaging

Diffusion-weighted MRI (DWI) and apparent diffusion coefficient (ADC) changes have been well described during acute ischemic stroke. In the acute phase, because of energy substrate depletion and Na+/K+—ATPase pump failure, ionic changes lead to cytotoxic edema and decreased diffusion of water. On DWI ischemic brain appears brighter (high signal) than normal brain, while it is darker on ADC maps (low ADC = decreased signal). Later, when the cells die and cellular membranes are disrupted these changes reverse (decreased DWI signal and increased ADC signal).

However, neuroimaging changes have also been reported after repetitive seizures or SE or NCSE [100], making interpretation more difficult when these conditions co-exist. Senn et al. reported a patient with partial status that had high DWI and ADC signal in the affected areas at the onset of seizures. Seven days later, DWI signal had regressed and ADC had further increased and 10 days later there was marked regression of all signals and signs of focal atrophy [101]. These findings contrast with those of Lansberg et al., who reported three patients with complex partial status epilepticus and decrease in ADC on the first day [102]. These differences may be due to timing of the MRI during SE. Low density changes on CT and high signals on T2-weighted MRI (that do not respect vascular territories), leptomeningeal contrast enhancement (indicative of alteration of the blood-brain barrier and vasogenic edema), local hyperperfusion on MRA and cerebral activation on functional MRI, all reversible, have been well associated with partial epilepsy and could help differentiate between ischemic stroke and seizure activity [101, 102]. Therefore, combining DWI and perfusion sequences may give more interpretable results than ADC and help distinguish the effect of seizures from that of oligemia or ischemia due to stroke. MRI shows hyperperfusion in seizing brain using gadolinium based or arterial spin labeling (ASL) sequences [103, 104]. DWI will display restricted diffusion despite increased perfusion during seizures [105]. In two patients who had partial status epilepticus associated with an old infarction and two episodes each of left hemiparesis and hemisensory disturbance without convulsion, DWI showed a hyperintense lesion in the cortex around the old infarction lesion mimicking current infarction. Although EEG failed to reveal ictal discharges or interictal paroxysmal activities in three of four episodes, perfusion images with ASL clearly demonstrated ictal hyperperfusion in the area corresponding to the cortical hyperintense lesion on DWI. The clinical deficits disappeared after appropriate anti-epileptic treatment [106]. Recent evidence suggests that DWI restriction adjacent to ongoing seizure activity may result from local cortical metabolic disturbances and more widespread cortico-cortical and cortico-thalamic synchronization abnormalities [107].

The long-term significance of these acute imaging findings is not entirely clear. DWI changes are largely reversible, but if prolonged seizures are present, may be associated with laminar necrosis and irreversible deficits [108]. One study of 26 patients with acutely seizures related MRI changes reported residual gliosis or focal atrophy in 42% of their cohort, while the remainder had reversible findings. Partial simple and complex seizures were associated with hippocampal involvement, but status epilepticus with incomplete reversibility of MRI abnormalities [109].

Seizures Post Stroke in the Young and the Elderly

Non-hemorrhagic stroke in young patients (before 45) accounts for 3–10% of all infarctions and has low mortality (1.5–8%) [110–112]. Only few studies have examined the incidence of post-stroke seizures in this younger population.

In a retrospective analysis of 65 young patients (aged 15–45) with stroke, followed for an average 32 months

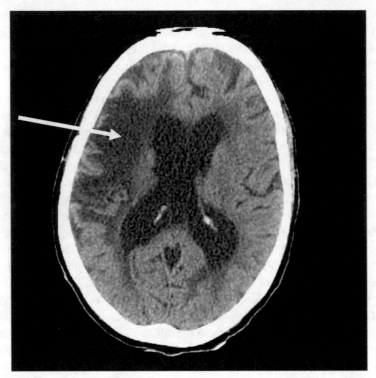

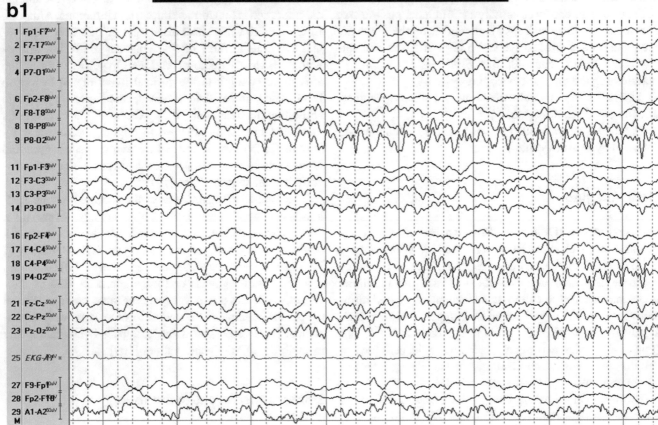

Fig. 9.1 81-year-old AA woman with history of old stroke and *left side* residual hemiplegia was admitted to the Neuro-ICU for altered mental status. Continuous EEG exhibited 162 electrographic seizures during the first day of recording, emanating from the right hemisphere. She was treated with IV valproic acid and IV phenytoin. Two days later the EEG showed only interictal activity and after an additional 2 days only

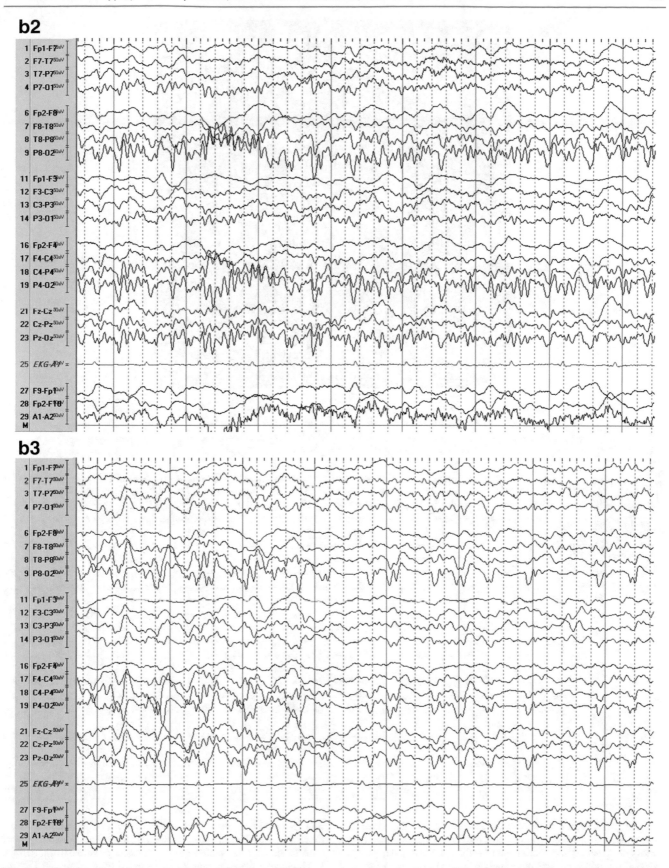

Fig. 9.1 (Continued) mild to moderate encephalopathy, while her mental status was improving. CT of the head showing an encephalomalacic area on the right fronto-parietal area from the old ischemic stroke (*white arrow*). Continuous EEG showing the beginning (B.1), evolution (B.2), and end (B.3) of a single electrographic seizure (without clinical correlate other than diminished mental status). The rhythmic, high amplitude theta/delta activity starts over P4, P8, and O2, but later spreads to the whole right hemisphere

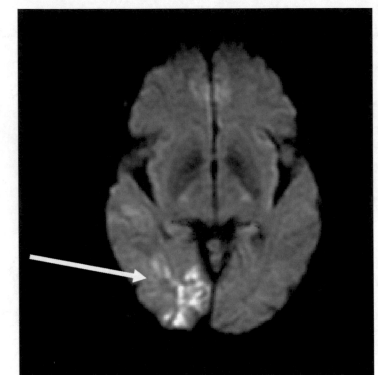

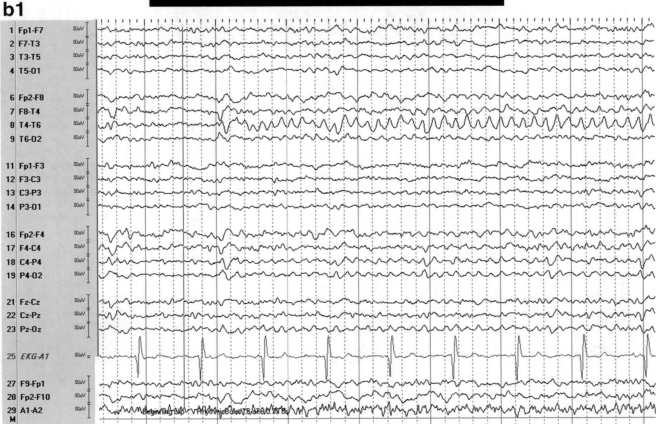

Fig. 9.2 An 84 AA diabetic woman was admitted to the Neuro-ICU after a motor vehicle accident (she was the driver) without head trauma or loss of consciousness. During her transfer she was found hypoglycemic and developed generalized tonic-clonic seizures. An MRI showed a right occipital stroke and an EEG several seizures emanating from the right temporal-occipital areas. She was loaded with phenytoin and levetiracetam IV and the seizures stopped. Diffusion-weighted imaging of the MRI showing the R inferior temporo -occipital stroke (*white arrow*). EEG showing the beginning from T4 to T6 of a seizure (B.1). This seizure evolved over the entire right hemisphere (B.2)

b2

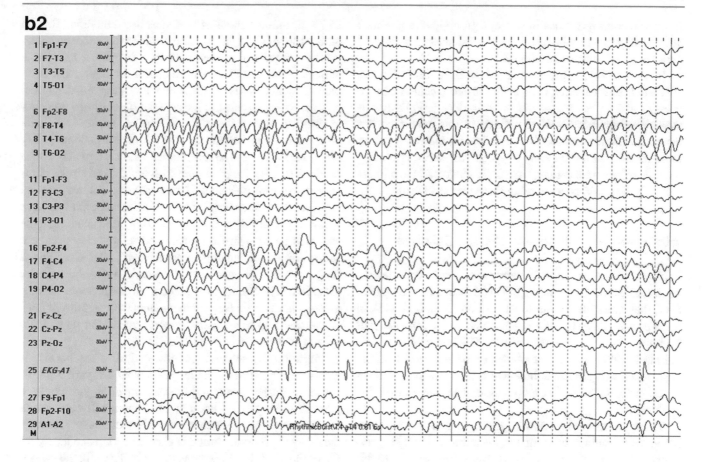

(range 12–59), the incidence of seizures was 10.8% and all occurred in patients with carotid artery territory infarction [113].

In a prospective, multicenter, European study (the PFO-ASA study), 581 patients with cryptogenic ischemic stroke, aged 18–55 years, were followed for seizures for an average of 38 months [22]. None of the six deaths was related to the occurrence of a seizure. Early seizures (within 1 week post-stroke) occurred in 14/581 (2.4%) of patients, 71% of them within the first 24 h. Two patients developed SE, one as an inaugural event. Rankin scale ≥ 3 (odds ratio, 95% CI, 3.9, 1.2–12.7) and cortical involvement (7.7, 1–61.1) were the only clinical and radiologic independent variables associated with early seizures. Late seizures occurred in 20/581 (3.4%) with a mean delay of 12.9 months post-stroke. Six of these patients had early seizures and 4/6 were on anti-epileptic treatment when the first late seizure occurred. Early seizures (5.1, 1.8–14.8), cortical signs (4.5, 1.6–13.1), and size of infarct larger than one-half hemisphere (9.7, 3.1–30.8) were independent predictors for late seizure development. Recurrent, unprovoked late seizures were found in 11/20 (55%) patients with late seizures and the risk for epilepsy was 2.3% within 3 years in this patient population.

In the large Canadian Stroke Network registry, seizures on stroke presentation or during hospitalization were more frequent in younger patients compared to patients with stroke without seizures. In addition to more severe strokes, older age, non-alert status on admission and higher Carlson index, seizures during hospitalization independently predicted overall mortality [21].

The incidence of seizures in the elderly is close to that in the first decade of life. With increasing age, more patients have an identifiable cause for their seizures and thus more seizures may have a focal onset [114]. Luhdorf et al. followed all patients within a definite area who developed seizures after the age of 60. The dominant cause of seizures was previous stroke in 32% of cases [32]. In a retrospective population-based study from Saskatchewan, Canada, 46/84 (55%) of patients 60 years and older with new-onset seizures had acute or remote cause identified (symptomatic). Of those, 22/46 (48% or 26% of all patients with new seizures) were due to acute or old stroke. All patients with non-life-threatening strokes had excellent prognosis, with seizures resolving in all but one patient. No information is provided about the number of elderly patients admitted to an ICU in these studies [115].

Similar findings were noted in a large, prospective, epidemiological study conducted in Southwest France [15]. The annual incidence of seizures in patients older than 60 years was 127/100,000. Cerebrovascular disease was the most frequently recognized cause in this age group and represented 36.6% of patients with spontaneous seizures and 54% of patients with confirmed epilepsy.

More recently, a prospective study from Lille, France, evaluated 202 patients with acute stroke (median age 76 years) for the presence of pre-existing dementia. Early seizures developed in 5.4% of patients in this cohort. Stroke patients with pre-existing dementia had an increased risk of late seizures, but not for early seizures. Any factor increasing the risk of seizures (drugs, metabolic changes), the authors concluded, should be avoided in these patients [116].

Treatment of Post-Ischemic Stroke Seizures

Seizures at the onset of an ischemic stroke were considered a contraindication for IV t-PA [117] and, based on prospective data, they were the reason for not administering IV t-PA in 0.9% of candidates [118]. Conversely, if stroke is treated, but eventually is not proven (usually by DWI on MRI), the initial stroke-like signs are attributed to *stroke mimics*. In the past, there was stricter adherence to this seizure exclusion criterion for IV t-PA, but more recent data undermined this exclusion.

There are more data now regarding the incidence, treatment, and complications of stroke mimics, including seizures. For example, stroke mimics were diagnosed in 13.4% of patients presenting to the Emergency department. Seizures were the second most common stroke mimic (19.5%). None of these patients received t-PA, mostly because of being outside the time window or because of minor deficits in the NIHSS before starting the infusion [119]. DWI MRI sequence in the setting of a new focal neurological deficit can be used to differentiate between these two conditions and was able to identify stroke mimics from ischemic stroke in another study, where seizures comprised 11.5% of former group [120]. Similarly, using MRI to exclude stroke in patients who received t-PA, seizures were diagnosed in 3.1% of 648 suspected ischemic stroke patients and comprised 47.6% of all stroke mimics. None of the stroke mimic patients deteriorated clinically post t-PA, but one developed orolingual angioedema [121]. The safety of administering fibrinolysis in patients who potentially may not have a stroke, but need to be treated emergently due to the narrow window, has been evaluated in few studies. In a retrospective study of 250 patients who received IV t-PA, 2.8% had stroke mimics (of which 71% were seizures, mostly with focal onset). There was a trend for lower NIHSS scores in mimics. Global aphasia without hemiparesis was the presenting symptom in 3 (42.9%) mimics versus 8 (3.3%) strokes. Orolingual angioedema (1.2%), symptomatic intracranial hemorrhage (5.3%), and asymptomatic intracranial hemorrhage (12.3%) complicated strokes, but were absent in mimics. After 3 months,

85.7% of mimics and 35.4% strokes had a modified Rankin Scale score of 0–1 [122]. In another large retrospective analysis of 539 patients treated with IV t-PA, 10.4% had stroke mimics. Seizures (19.6%) were one of the three most common final diagnoses at discharge for these misdiagnosed patients. No symptomatic intracranial hemorrhage was documented in any of these stroke mimics, suggesting a safe profile for administering IV t-PA in these patients [123]. More recently, in a single center study of patients who received IV t-PA for presumed stroke, 12% had stroke mimics (31.6% were seizures). None of these patients had an intracerebral hemorrhage after the fibrinolysis, but two have systemic hemorrhages [124]. Reflecting these changes in the approach towards stroke mimics and seizures at onset, is a survey of stroke clinicians from eight NIH Specialized Programs of Translational Research in Acute Stroke (SPOTRIAS). Ninety-one percent of responders recommended fibrinolytic therapy in patients with significant deficits attributable to an acute ischemic stroke but with also a seizure at symptom onset [125].

Interestingly, seizures occurring during the period of thrombolysis with IV t-PA may represent a sign of reperfusion or hyperperfusion and may enhance the thrombolytic process [126–128]. Although in these small case series these seizures were associated with a dramatic recovery, they may also herald hemorrhagic conversion and an urgent CT of the head should be considered if clinically the patient deteriorates. In a more recent case report, cortical myoclonus during the IV thrombolysis for a right middle cerebral artery stroke was recorded using back-average EEG analysis with time-locked electromyogram of the affected contralateral limb. There was no improvement in the deficit. Interestingly this patient had additional acute renal failure [129]. An alternative mechanism of seizures during IV fibrinolysis is a direct effect of the drug on seizure generation. For example, t-PA is an endogenous serine protease associated with neuronal activity and synaptic plasticity in the brain, its expression is enhanced after seizures, and is involved in seizure propagation throughout the brain. Although mice with neuronal over-expression of t-PA are more seizure-prone than wild-type, no significant differences were found in a study that compared patients who received t-PA and those who did not in early or late seizures or in the development of epilepsy [130].

The most recent guidelines from the Stroke Council of the American Stroke Association include seizures as a relative exclusion criterion for administration of fibrinolytics. After careful consideration of risk-benefit patients may receive fibrinolysis in this situation [131]. CT angiography may be a useful modality in differentiating Todd's paralysis from early seizure and ischemia by detection of intracranial occlusion and may contribute to decision-making for thrombolysis [132].

The same recent guidelines from the Stroke Council of the American Stroke Association mention that there are no studies to date showing a benefit of prophylactic anti-epileptic treatment after ischemic stroke and prophylactic treatment is not recommended (Class III, Level of Evidence C). Their recommendation is to treat recurrent seizures in a manner similar to other acute neurological conditions. The anti-epileptic drugs to be used should be selected by specific patient characteristics (Class I, Level of Evidence B). They also mention that little information exists on indications for the long-term use of anticonvulsant drugs after a seizure [131]. Reiterating these Guidelines, the Neurocritical Care Society Pharmacy Section issued a review of evidence-based support for seizure prophylaxis in Neurocritical Care. In this most recent special article, no additional data or recommendations beyond the aforementioned from the ASA are included for post-stroke seizures [133]. In the following paragraphs we will try to summarize the data available and have an in-depth look at the problem an intensivist faces.

As mentioned before, there are no randomized controlled trials evaluating specific treatment options in post-stroke seizures. Bladin et al. argue that such a trial would pose extensive logistic challenges and would likely be unethical [7]. Prophylactic treatment for seizures after ischemic stroke is controversial. The duration of treatment is also unknown. Should these patients be admitted to an ICU when they present with a seizure in the context of an acute or subacute stroke? Armon et al. have summarized the rationales for treating seizures at the onset of a stroke, as follows: (a) control of persistent or recurrent seizures (SE) (b) prevention of seizures within the first day of stroke (c) prevention within the first 2 weeks post stroke, and (d) prevention of recurrence of seizures after the first 2 weeks or the appearance of late seizures [3]. We suggest adapting the same rationale to the ICU setting by tailoring it to the following issues: (a) whether to treat or not a seizure that accompanies a stroke (b) whether to treat recurrent seizures or SE (c) whether to treat preventively post-stroke seizures (d) whether to prevent late seizures from occurring after an early seizure (e) whether to prevent epilepsy from developing after early or late seizures.

The current consensus in ischemic stroke management is to not treat patients unless they present with a first seizure or they are known as pre-existing epileptics [134]. If a patient had pre-stroke seizures, the rationale for covering with anti-epileptics is based on the prevention of pre-existing epilepsy to manifest in its usual form post stroke or as SE [3]. However, even before the occurrence of the first seizure, some subgroups of non-epileptic patients may be at higher risk for seizure development. Large infarct size, cortical involvement, watershed distribution, hemorrhagic stroke transformation, severe stroke and PLEDs on the EEG within 24 h from admission [5–7, 16, 19, 22, 35, 39, 41, 48, 53, 54, 56, 87, 99, 135] are typical situations where a physician could consider covering the patient with anti-epileptic treatment to prevent early seizures, especially if other co-morbidities make a seizure manifestation an unacceptably high risk for complications.

The occurrence of one or more seizures may trigger the decision to use anti-epileptics although that decision may also depend on the type and location of stroke. Because of the risk of progression to SE, further damage to the ischemic penumbra leading to deterioration of the stroke or aspirating oral secretions or vomitus, we believe these patients should be admitted and treated in an NICU or a stroke Unit. Are there any data that support this approach? In the series of Milandre et al., 51% of patients with seizures developed recurrent seizures, multiple in two thirds of them [12]. In the series by Gupta et al., 39% of patients had recurrent seizures, multiple in 57% of them [35]. In neither study was there any difference in the recurrence rate, whether the seizures occurred early or late post stroke. In the Oxfordshire study, 3% of patients with cerebral infarction developed a single post-stroke seizure and another 3% recurrent seizures, which overall occurred infrequently. The percentages for those with total anterior circulation infarction were 5% and 11% and in those with lacunes 2% and 1%, respectively. However, 40% of patients with seizures within the first 24 h post-ischemic stroke and 50% post ICH developed later seizures, although the numbers are very small [8]. Patients with lobar ICH or SAH had 14% and 8% incidence of early seizures in the Manhattan population study and the authors suggested prophylaxis for these subgroups for the first 24 h only, since almost 90% of seizures occurred within that time frame [56].

Usually late post-stroke seizures are not encountered in the ICU, unless one is dealing with SE. Occasionally, however, a patient who is admitted for another medical reason to the ICU develops seizures, that cannot be related to a drug or a metabolic derangement. Or the patient may develop seizures in the context of a recurrent stroke and it may be difficult (if there is no clear focality in the seizure onset or in the EEG) to associate the seizure with the new or the old stroke. As with early seizures, there are data supporting the use of anti-epileptic coverage for these late seizures. From the SASS study, although late-onset seizures (after the first 2 weeks) occurred in only 3.8% of all patients with ischemic stroke, they led to epilepsy in 55% of these patients and their presence was the only independent predictor for the development of epilepsy [7]. This has been also noted in other studies [36, 54] or younger patient populations [22]. However, it cannot be generalized. In a prospective study from Germany, including 264 patients with stroke, ten patients developed post-stroke epilepsy over a follow-up period of 1 year. Early onset seizures (within 2 weeks post stroke) occurred in 12 patients, seven of who developed epilepsy. Late-onset seizures were observed in 17 patients. Seven out of 13 patients with ischemic stroke who suffered from late seizures did not proceed to epilepsy during the 1 year follow-up and without anti-epileptic medications. This study is interesting because his authors attempted to create a post-stroke epilepsy risk scale (PoSERS). They included a 10-point scale (with variables such as supratentorial localization, ICH involving cortical areas, ischemia involving cortical or cortical-subcortical areas, ischemia plus evolving neurological deficit, large stroke, early or late seizure), which with score >5 was able to predict epilepsy with 100% sensitivity and negative predictive value and 96.9% specificity, but with only moderate positive predictive value (55.6%). Adding EEG evaluation in a subgroup of patients did not add value in the scale [136].

The role played by anti-epileptic medications in preventing early or late post-stroke seizures is also unclear [9, 11]. In a retrospective study, 88% of patients with post infarction seizures were controlled with monotherapy, mostly phenytoin, whereas another smaller percentage was initially started on multi-drug regimen [35]. An Israeli group retrospectively compared 35 patients with post-ischemic stroke treated immediately with anti-epileptic medications for 2 years after their first early seizure, with 26 patients who were untreated until they developed a second seizure [137]. The assignment was made based on the admission service that had accepted the patients. The mean time for the development of a first seizure post-stroke was 5.7 days and for the second 15.2 months. During the initial 2-year post event period the group that was treated immediately had lower relapse (14.3% vs 38.5%, $p = 0.03$) and higher seizure-free rates (85% vs 61%, $p = 0.042$). However, the treated group after discontinuing the anti-epileptic treatment had the same seizure risk than the untreated group during the period between the first and the second seizure (4.8% vs 6.2%, $p = 0.6$). This protective role of anti-epileptic medications was not confirmed in other larger studies. In a recent, multicenter, prospective European study of younger patients (<55 years old) with cryptogenic ischemic stroke, anti-epileptic treatment did not prevent late seizures in patients with early seizures [22].

Which anti-epileptic agents are most effective in preventing post-stroke seizures is also unknown. Overall, post-stroke seizures seem easily controlled and monotherapy usually suffices. For example, in a retrospective study from Taiwan, 143 patients with first-time ischemic stroke were followed for a minimum of 6 years. Seizures occurred in 13 (9.1%) of them. Regarding seizure control after discharge, 12 patients were seizure-free with or without anti-epileptic drugs and one had 1–3 seizures per year. [51].

Because the majority of seizures have a focal onset, first line drugs in the ICU were older parenteral agents, such as phenytoin or fosphenytoin [75]. However, if the patient's mental status and swallowing ability allows oral administration of other agents, such as carbamazepine or oxcarbamazepine, those should be considered.

The potential effect that anti-epileptic medications may have on ischemia or rehabilitation should also be considered.

Some anti-epileptics, such as carbamazepine, topiramate or sodium valproate, have additional neuroprotective properties against cerebral ischemia [138, 139]. On the other hand, other studies also suggest that phenytoin, barbiturates, and benzodiazepines may have a negative effect on recovery from stroke [140]. These older agents also have interactions with common drugs used for treatment or secondary prevention of stroke, such as warfarin or salicylic acid [134].

Because of more favorable side-effect profile and tolerability, newer agents such as lamotrigine should be also considered as monotherapy. Other oral agents that are approved only for primary or adjunctive treatment and are commonly used as monotherapy such as topiramate, levetiracetam, and zonisamide could also be used in individual cases. Age may also be another important factor for a decision which agent to use, since most stroke patients are elderly [134]. The International League Against Epilepsy has concluded that only lamotrigine and gabapentin have level A evidence to allow recommendation as first-line monotherapy for elderly adults with partial-onset seizures [141]. Gabapentin has been used as monotherapy in 71 patients with late post-stroke seizures in an uncontrolled study from Barcelona, Spain [142]. The initial dose of gabapentin was established based on weight: 900 mg/d for patients weighing under 75 kg and 1200 mg/d for patients weighing over 75 kg. If seizures recurred, the dose was increased by 300 mg/d. Seizures were observed in 18.2% of patients during an average follow-up period of 30 months. Overall, these patients achieved better control than patients with newly diagnosed nonvascular partial epilepsy [143]. Another monotherapy used in 25 elderly patients with late post-stroke seizures was levetiracetam. After 6 months, 76% of patients were still receiving the drug (at a median dose of 1052 mg/day (range 1–2 g/day) and 89.5% of them were seizure-free [144]. In another prospective study of 34 elderly patients with late post-stroke seizures, levetiracetam monotherapy (1000–2000 mg/day) conveyed 82.4% seizure freedom in a follow-up period of 18 months. Seven patients had side-effects, with only one discontinuing the drug. Two patients switched to another anti-epileptic drug because of uncontrolled seizures [145]. In a subsequent open-label prospective study of 35 patients with late post-stroke seizures (occurring at least 2 weeks after the stroke onset), levetiracetam in doses 1500–2000 mg/day achieved 1 year seizure freedom in 77.1%. Four patients discontinued the drug, three due to aggressive behavior, and one due to drowsiness and gait disturbance [146]. Compared to carbamazepine use, levetiracetam did not convey any significantly better proportion of seizure freedom in a multicenter, randomized, open-label study of 128 patients with late (2 weeks to 3 years) post-stroke seizures. The group treated with levetiracetam, however, had significantly lower side-effects [147].

The duration of the anti-epileptic treatment is also unknown. Most experts use the EEG together with the clinical picture and stroke type to decide about the length of treatment. Armon et al. suggested for cortical ICH and seizures a 12-month seizure-free interval and an EEG without epileptiform activity to consider withdrawing the treatment. For non-hemorrhagic stroke and one or more generalized tonic-clonic seizures (at the onset or early on) they suggested a 1- to 2-week course with phenytoin, then tapering if the EEG does not show an epileptogenic focus. If such a focus is present, they suggested a longer treatment. The same approach was used for epilepsia partialis continua, with the objective of minimizing the likelihood of secondary generalization [3].

Non-anti-epileptic drugs can also have impact on post-stroke seizures. For example, in a recent study of 1832 patients with stroke and no history of seizures before, 63 (3.4%) of who had early onset seizures and 91 (5%) had epilepsy. Statin use was associated with a lower risk of post-stroke early onset seizures (odds ratio, 95% CI 0.35, 0.20–0.60), but not with post stroke epilepsy. In those patients who presented with early onset seizures, statin use was associated with reduced risk of post-stroke epilepsy (0.34, 0.13–0.88). This reduced risk was seen mainly in patients who used a statin only in the acute phase [148].

Table 9.3 represents a suggested algorithm for the treatment of post-stroke seizures.

Reperfusion–Hyperperfusion Syndrome

First described by Sundt et al. [149], the reperfusion syndrome is an uncommon constellation of symptoms usually encountered following carotid endarterectomy (0.4–2% of cases [150, 151]) or other revascularization procedures, such as percutaneous transluminal angioplasty (PTA) [152, 153], carotid artery stenting (1–5% [154–156]), extracranial–intracranial

Table 9.3 Treatment with anti-epileptic medications after ischemic stroke

1. Infarct and pre-existing seizures: continue or restart anti-epileptic regimen, keep therapeutic levels.
2. Infarct and no seizures:
Observe
Consider Rx if large, cortical infarct, with hemorrhagic component or significant co-morbidities (lung, heart, presence of aneurysm, etc.) for at least 2 weeks
3. Infarct and early 1st seizure:
Start monotherapy. If subcortical or lacune, continue for 2 weeks. If anterior circulation cortical infarct, continue for 1–2 years (seizure-free interval). Assess with EEG before discontinuation?
4. Infarct and SE:
Treat according to SE protocol in the NICU. Continue Rx for at least 4 years (seizure-free interval), if SE was the first epileptic symptom. Assess with EEG before discontinuation and individualize. Treat indefinitely, if SE followed early or late seizures
5. Infarct and late 1st seizure:
Treat with monotherapy for at least 2 years (seizure-free interval). Assess with EEG before discontinuation and individualize.

arterial bypass [157], intracranial artery stenting [158, 159], innominate endarterectomy [160] or left ventricular device implantation for end-stage heart failure [161]. It comprises transient focal seizures (always emanating from the vascular territory ipsilateral to the treated artery), ipsilateral headache with atypical migrainous features and intracerebral hemorrhage or brain edema, usually a few days to up to 3 weeks after revascularization [162]. The syndrome should not be related to thromboembolism and no new infarct should be demonstrated on neuroimaging [163]. Occasionally, SE ensues [75]. Severe ICA stenosis with preoperative ICA/CCA pressure ratio <0.7 leads to significant increase of CBF in both hemispheres after CEA, more pronounced ipsilaterally [164]. In many centers these patients are monitored in the ICU for the first few postoperative days [165]. Symptoms post carotid angioplasty-stenting typically present within 36 h after the procedure, contrasting with those after CEA, which usually present later (4–7th postoperative day) [166].

Seizures are thought to result from cerebral embolization from the operative site (although some authors require a stricter definition of the syndrome and exclude thromboembolism [163]), hemorrhage secondary to the lack of autoregulation or simply to the reperfusion syndrome effect. If they occur during or early after surgery, they are more likely caused by intraoperative or immediate postoperative embolization or inadequate perfusion during clamping of the carotid. The predisposing role of preoperative strokes towards seizures in symptomatic patients is unclear. If seizures occur late during the postoperative course, especially when there is severe carotid stenosis and if preceded by headache, they are most likely caused by the hyperperfusion syndrome [162]. The syndrome is thought to be due to impaired cerebral autoregulation, as a result of chronic cerebral hypoperfusion distal to high grade carotid stenosis [167]. The intracranial distal arterioles are maximally and chronically dilated and do not respond to the flush of blood by vasoconstriction after correction of the stenosis, leading to cerebral edema and, if cortical, to seizures [168]. Carotid baroreceptor insensitivity and the secondary hypertensive response after CEA are additional factors [152], as most patients have uncontrolled hypertensive blood pressure levels both before and after surgery [162]. Pathological findings in the hyperperfusion syndrome resemble the findings in hypertensive encephalopathy and the reperfusion syndrome after cerebral AVM resection [162].

Sundt et al. reported a 11/1145 (0.9%) incidence of seizures after CEA [149]. A total of 20 (1.8%) patients in their series displayed the characteristic constellation of symptoms, that were given the name of hyperperfusion syndrome. Seizures presented between the 5th and 7th postoperative day. Five patients had a history of preoperative strokes and two developed postoperative ICH. Riegel et al. reported the lowest incidence of seizures so far in their large series from the Mayo Clinic (10/2439, 0.4%), which included some patients from Sundt's series [169]. Four patients had a history of preoperative strokes and seven had a Xenon CBF study during surgery, which demonstrated an increase in CBF ipsilaterally to the CEA. Nine of ten patients had initial focal onset of seizures, which then generalized. Although all patients had PLEDs on EEG, all had complete resolution of their neurologic deficits. The authors suggested that patients with preoperative hypertension and high grade bilateral carotid stenoses were at the greatest risk for developing seizures post CEA. They recommended caution with anticoagulant or antiplatelet agents in these patients and prompt treatment of blood pressure and seizures.

Kieburtz et al. described eight patients with focal and generalized seizures following 650 CEAs (1.2%) [170]. Six patients had pre-CEA TIAs, while two were asymptomatic. Seizures occurred with a mean of 7.6 (range 6 to 13) days after CEA. All patients initially had focal motor seizures contralateral to the side of the CEA, but six patients had seizures that became generalized. All patients had post-ictal hemiparesis. Lorazepam given initially and phenytoin/phenobarbital sodium for maintenance resulted in control of the seizures. CT showed old strokes in two patients (one ipsilateral to the CEA and the other contralaterally), diffuse cerebral edema ipsilateral to the CEA in another two, ICH in one and no abnormalities in three patients. Five patients without CT evidence of stroke were normal at follow-up and had no further seizures. The other three patients had mild deficits. One developed a chronic seizure disorder.

Reversible cerebral edema was reported in 5/184 (2.7%) patients with severe carotid stenosis or occlusion who underwent CEA or bypass [162]. Headache, focal neurologic deficits, and white matter edema on CT developed after discharge from the hospital. Focal seizures occurred in four and generalized seizures in three of these patients and the EEG showed PLEDs in two and ipsilateral slowing in another two of them. The authors suggested that hyperperfusion syndrome has been underreported and that many cases of cerebral edema, especially in older series, were misinterpreted as cerebral infarction.

In a large prospective study from the U.K., Naylor et al. identified 8/949 (0.8%) patients who developed seizures after CEA [171]. Seven were treated hypertensives but 4 patients had labile BP preoperatively. Five had severe bilateral carotid disease and four had vertebral/subclavian stenoses. Five required treatment for postoperative hypertension. Two suffered seizures <36 h of CEA, the remainder at 3–8 days. All eight had significantly elevated blood pressure at onset of seizures. CT scanning/autopsy showed normal scans in three, white matter edema in four, and petechial or diffuse ICH in 2 patients. Seven developed a post-ictal neurological deficit (stroke in five, TIA in two). In this case series, post-CEA seizure was associated with adverse outcomes (one patient died, one had a disabling stroke and four had non-

fatal strokes). Interestingly, the authors report that clinicians treating these patients in acute medical units were generally unaware of the "post-CEA hyperperfusion syndrome" and tended to treat the hypertension less aggressively.

In a retrospective study of CEAs from Brooklyn, NY, 9/404 (2%) patients developed hyperperfusion syndrome and three of them seizures [150]. One of these patients had intraoperative mean ICA volume flow by carotid artery duplex scanning of 178 ml/min, which during seizures 1 week postoperatively increased to 632 ml/min and subsequently decreased to 141 ml/min after symptoms subsided. This study suggested that contralateral CEA within 3 months from the index CEA may be a predictive factor for hyperperfusion syndrome.

In a retrospective study from India, 6/87 (7%) patients developed hyperperfusion syndrome after stenting (47 cases) or CEA (40 cases) [165]. Two patients were the presenting symptom in two patients and occurred 5 h and 1 day after the intervention. Both patients had either high degree stenosis in one side or occlusion and occlusion on the opposite side. Although only the second patient had an ICH, they both died.

In another large retrospective study from Los Angeles, CA, 6/1602 (0.4%) developed hyperperfusion syndrome and only one seizures 8 days after the surgery [151]. This patient was treated for 3 months with phenytoin, without recurrence.

In a prospective study from Boston, MA, 841 CEAs were performed over 2 years and hyperperfusion syndrome occurred in 14 (1.7%) patients. Seizures occurred in 5 (0.6%) patients and ICH in 4 (0.5%). In this study, non-elective CEA was the only independent factor associated with hyperperfusion syndrome [172].

Percutaneous transluminal angioplasty (PTA) and stenting is gaining acceptance as a safe alternative to CEA in some patient subgroups. Two patients who developed seizures secondary to hyperperfusion syndrome have also been reported by Schoser et al., 16 h and 3 days after PTA and stenting of the ICA [152, 153]. Although the management of seizures is not discussed in the article, marked increase of CBFVs was demonstrated by TCD. Two patients reported by Ho et al., with high grade bilateral ICA stenoses and preexisting hypertension developed recurrent seizures with focal onset and secondary generalization 7 h and 14 days, respectively, after successful endovascular treatment [153]. Seizures were controlled by intravenous diazepam and phenytoin, and by lowering the blood pressure during the events. CT of the head did not reveal new infarcts and follow-up angiograms showed widely patent ICAs. In a retrospective study from Canada, 129 patients underwent reperfusion procedures [163]. Hyperperfusion syndrome developed in 4/129 (3.1%) patients with CEA and 3/44 (6.8%) patients with ICA stenting. Two patients developed delayed seizures. In a large retrospective study from the Cleveland Clinic, OH, 5/450 (1.1%) patients post carotid artery stenting developed hyperperfusion syndrome within a median of 10 h (range 6 h to 4 days) [173]. One patient developed a seizure on the 5th postoperative day. The authors concluded that similarly to patients after CEA, patients after ICA stenting may be at higher risk for hyperperfusion syndrome, if they have a critical ICA stenosis of ≥90%, severe contralateral ICA disease, poor collateral flow, hypertension, and recent stroke or ischemia.

Except for extracranial carotid stenting, intracranial intervention may also lead to hyperperfusion syndrome. A recent case report exemplifies that. A patient, who underwent left supraclinoid internal carotid artery stenting (after a right internal carotid artery stenting at the neck origin; both for >90% stenosis), developed post-stenting right focal seizures with secondary generalization and eventually epilepsia partialis continua. Patient was treated successfully with IV antiepileptics and BP control (which was initially 200/120 mm Hg). He underwent neuroimaging which did show left frontoparietal vasogenic edema without a hemorrhage or infarct. He gradually improved over 1 month. This study provides a nice review of hyperperfusion syndrome after intracranial angioplasty or stenting [159].

Seizures induced by cerebral reperfusion after thrombolytic therapy for acute ischemic stroke is a rare phenomenon. Hafeez et al. report a case where a patient who received IV rt-PA within 3 h of stroke symptom onset developed the new-onset symptom of continuous, primary motor seizure activity within 20 min of drug administration. These epileptic seizures originated in the same area as the acute brain ischemia and occurred during the anticipated period of cerebral reperfusion [127].

A more recent study of 69 patients who underwent left ventricular assist device (LVAD) implantation for end-stage heart failure in a single center over a period of 47 months found 19 patients who developed neurological dysfunction (27.5%) including encephalopathy (16%), coma (4.3%), and seizures (4.3%). Only in 1/3 of these patients with seizures an infarct was found in neuroimaging. The multivariate analysis showed that an increase in cardiac index from the preoperative baseline value and a previous coronary bypass operation were the only independent predictors of neurologic dysfunction. Reduction of left ventricular assist device flow in 16 of the 19 symptomatic patients led to improvement of symptoms in 14 (87%) patients with clinical improvement or resolution by 48 h and without negative consequences [161].

TCD can be used in the ICU to evaluate patients with a suspicion of hyperperfusion syndrome. Thirty six high grade stenosis patients (>90% stenosis of ICA) were evaluated with TCD before and after IV infusion of 1 g acetazolamide [174]. Thirty three patients showed increased MCA CBFVs after the challenge (preserved reserve capacity) and three decreased (loss of reserve capacity). After CEA, those three patients developed unilateral headache and an increase of mean MCA CBFVs, while the other 33 patients showed little difference. None of these patients developed seizures, suggesting a mild hyperperfusion syndrome.

In a landmark paper, Jorgensen and Schroeder evaluated 95 patients with TCD before and after symptomatic CEA [167]. Hyperperfusion syndrome developed in 18/95 (19%) and two separate groups were identified: in nine patients symptoms lasted for a mean of 3 h and in the other nine for a mean of 12 days. The longer the duration of the symptoms of hyperperfusion, the more likely the preoperative finding of increased mean blood pressure gradient across the stenosis, the lower the CO_2 reactivity index on both sides of the brain and the absence of decrease of the pulsatility index during CO_2 inhalation. Following surgery in patients with symptoms of hyperperfusion, MCA CBFVs were shown to decrease significantly with labetalol from a mean high of 104 to 68 cm/s on the side of CEA, a reaction not seen on the contralateral side. This asymmetric response diminished overtime as the episodes of hyperperfusion subsided. At discharge, cerebral CO_2 reactivity improved bilaterally in these patients, a change not seen in patients without hyperperfusion syndrome. Interestingly, 2/9 (22%) patients with longer lasting hyperperfusion symptoms developed seizures on the 5–6th postoperative day. MCA CBFVs on the side of the CEA in these two patients during seizures were 104 and 120 cm/sec with MAP 130 and 120 mmHg, respectively. After labetalol was administered, MAP dropped to 100 and 67 mmHg and CBFVs to 38 and 60 cm/s, respectively, and the seizures stopped. In both patients MCA CBFVs contralateral to the CEA remained unchanged, implying a defective cerebral autoregulation only present on the side ipsilateral to the CEA. Both patients who developed seizures had contralateral ICA occlusions, consistent with previous observations [165, 169]. None had postoperative infarcts on CT of the head, although they demonstrated patchy edema. These results prompted the authors to suggest that post-CEA patients should have their blood pressure meticulously controlled and that TCD may help identify patients at high risk for developing the hyperperfusion syndrome and seizures. If anticipated, a baseline study before or another immediately after surgery may be helpful [162, 167, 175].

Another monitor used in Neuro-ICUs is transcranial near-infrared spectroscopy. Using this method to monitor regional cerebral oxygen saturation (rSO_2), Ogasawara examined 50 patients with CEA [176]. Post-CEA hyperperfusion (CBF increase of ≥100%, compared with preoperative values) was observed for six patients, one of which developed hyperperfusion syndrome with seizures on the sixth postoperative day.

All this strongly suggests that high risk patients (history of hypertension, bilateral high grade stenoses, low CBFVs or CO2 reactivity by TCD, previous contralateral CEA within 3 months) should be monitored in the ICU for symptoms of hyperperfusion syndrome after revascularization of the cerebral vessels [165]. The blood pressure should be tightly controlled with aggressive titration of blood pressure to a systolic value of <120–140 mm Hg [158] and if symptoms develop, the first step of treatment should include further lowering of

BP (to a level of equalization of ipsilateral and contralateral CBFVs [167]). Agents with pure vasodilatory properties, such as sodium nitroprusside, should be avoided [158]. The ICU staff should be alerted to the possibility of seizures, and initiation of an anticonvulsant regimen in the setting of seizures (prophylactic use is not indicated) should be undertaken for few days [158, 168]. Neuroimaging to exclude a new ICH or infarct should be considered if there is new change in the neurological exam. If a new cortical hemorrhage is found, prophylactic seizure treatment with fosphenytoin or levetiracetam for 7 days could be entertained [168].

Table 9.4 represents a suggested algorithm for the treatment of reperfusion–hyperperfusion syndrome-related seizures.

Cerebral Vein and Dural Sinus Thrombosis

Clinical Studies

Several medical or surgical complications have been associated with the development of cerebral venous thrombosis (CVT). Also CVT is not infrequently encountered in ICU patients with the following conditions: various infectious processes (local or systemic), hematologic disorders (genetic prothrombotic conditions [like antithrombin III or protein C or S deficiencies, hyperhomocysteinemia, Factor V Leiden mutation, prothrombin gene mutation, Factor VIII excess], leukemia, thrombocytemia, paroxysmal nocturnal hemoglobinuria), cancer, non-infectious inflammatory disease, Behçet disease, nephrotic syndrome, dehydration and congestive heart failure, complications of pregnancy and the puerperium and mechanical causes, such as lumbar puncture (LP) alone or associated with the diagnosis of multiple sclerosis and high dose corticosteroids [177–182]. Patients with cerebral venous thrombosis

Table 9.4 Treatment with anti-epileptic medications after revascularization

1. Revascularization and pre-existing seizures: continue Rx
2. Revascularization and prophylactic seizure treatment: not indicated
3. Revascularization with cortical hemorrhage: prophylactic seizure treatment for 7 days may be undertaken
4. Revascularization and immediate or early (<day 5) seizure:
Neuroimaging to rule out ICH or artery to artery embolization
Treat seizures as after stroke, strict SBP control to 120–140 mm Hg range
5. Revascularization and late seizure (5th day-3rd week), with focal onset contralateral to procedure side:
Neuroimaging to rule out ICH
If pre-existing high grade stenosis and history of severe hypertension plus headache now: treat hyperperfusion syndrome with lorazepam and phenytoin or phenobarbital or valproic acid IV and hypertension with IV labetalol or enalapril or clonidine to reduce SBP to a level where CBFVs by TCD are symmetrical. Continue Rx for at least 3 weeks and discontinue if neuroimaging negative

(CVT) are frequently also admitted to the ICU for cerebral edema, signs of increased intracranial pressure (headache, papilledema), focal neurologic deficits or seizures.

Outcomes after CVT in recent years have improved, with mortality in the 5–10% range and independent life in almost 80–86% of patients [183–187]. Seizures occur frequently after CVT and in several cases they are the presenting sign. Indeed, seizures were present in the first clinical description of CVT in 1825 by Ribes [188]. In the angiographically proven cases reported by Bousser et al., Jacksonian or grand mal seizures occurred in 11/38 (29%) patients, and were the 4th most common symptom, following headache (74%), papilledema (45%), and hemiplegia (34%) [189]. In more recent studies, however, seizures have been recorded as one of the two most common signs of CVT [183, 186, 190].

It is interesting to note that several of the causative factors for CVT can also independently cause seizures (head trauma, intracranial surgery, CNS infection, primary or secondary brain tumors, vasculitis), although no attempt has been made to differentiate the relative roles of each [189, 191]. Other common etiologies for CVT include the aforementioned conditions, but in up to a quarter of cases the etiology remains unknown. Since lumbar punctures are commonly performed in the ICUs, the reported association between CVT and LP is of special interest to the intensivist. All five patients reported by Wilder-Smith et al. developed a characteristic pattern of headache (initially postural, then continuous) and seizures after LP or complicated peridural anesthesia and were found to have CVT [179]. Three out of four tested had Factor V Leiden deficiency. Other similar cases of CVT after LP complicated by seizure onset have also been reported [192–194].

Several studies report on the incidence of early or late seizures.

In a retrospective study of 78 patients with CVT, generalized seizures occurred in 24 (31%) patients and were the presenting symptom in 13 (17%, seven with partial motor and six with generalized seizures) [195]. Seizures were associated with a poor outcome in the univariate analysis and were included in a prognostic scale (0–11 points) developed by the authors, with 0.98 positive prognostic value for good and 0.96 positive prognostic value for poor prognosis.

In another retrospective study from the Bronx, NY, seizures were observed in 35/112 (31%) patients with acute CVT. Only 5% of patients had epilepsy after a mean follow-up period of 77.8 months [185]. Among those patients with early seizures and follow-up records, 4/28 (14%) had epilepsy, all with focal signs in the acute stage of CVT. Those seizures manifested in three of four patients during the first year and in one patient 2 years after CVT. The authors concluded that because of the low risk of recurrent seizures and of late recurrences, anti-epileptic treatment seems appropriate only for one-year post CVT, after which it can be tapered off gradually, unless seizures recur.

In a retrospective multicenter study from Italy, focal deficits and/or seizures were recorded in 19/35 (54.3%) patients with cortical and 4/13 (30.8%) patients with deep CVT [190]. EEG was performed in 18 patients and in two thirds revealed diffuse abnormalities. Only 2/18 (11%) of EEGs showed epileptic focal abnormalities. All patients with seizures, but one, were treated with AEDs.

In a more recent retrospective study from India, 90 patients with CVT were included over a 16-year period. Seizures occurred at presentation in 42/90 (47%) of patients (focal in 11, focal with secondary generalized in 19, and generalized tonic-clonic in 16). SE occurred in 10 (11.1%). Only four patients had early seizures (within 14 days from onset of CVT) and none had late seizures. On multivariate analysis, only supratentorial parenchymal lesion on MRI (odds ratio 4.67, 95% CI 1.51–15.08) was independently associated with higher risk of presenting seizure. Seizures were not associated with death nor with 6 month functional outcome in this study [196].

In the prospective, randomized, placebo-controlled Dutch-European Cerebral Sinus Thrombosis Trial, low molecular weight heparin (nadroparin 180 anti-factor Xa units/kg/day for 3 weeks, followed by oral anticoagulation with a target INR 2.5–3.5 for 10 weeks) was compared to placebo [197]. Seizures were reported in 28/59 (47%) patients, 41% in the placebo, and 53% in the treatment arm, but the study did not comment on their relationship with outcomes at 12 weeks [184].

In a prospective French study from Lille, seizures were the most common symptom overall, occurred in 28/55 (50.9%) patients with CVT and were the presenting symptom in one (1.8%) patient [183]. There is no mention of anti-epileptic treatment in this series. With a median follow-up of 36 months, recurrent seizures developed in 7/28 (25%) patients with seizures in the acute stage (i.e., 14.5% of all 3-year survivors from CVT). Focal or generalized seizures were not associated with outcome as measured with the modified Rankin disability score.

In another prospective study from Portugal (VENOPORT study), data were collected retrospectively for 51 patients and prospectively in another 91 patients (who were followed for an average of 1 year) with CVT [191, 198]. Early seizures (within the first 2 weeks after the diagnosis) were observed in 31/91 (34%) patients. In 29 (31.9%) patients early seizures were the presenting feature of CVT (in one patient seizures evolved to grand mal SE). The frequency of seizures was the same whether the superior sagittal sinus (33%) or the lateral/sigmoid sinus (25%) was thrombosed, but no seizures were observed in the seven patients with involvement of the deep venous system. Early seizures were independently predicted by sensory deficits (odds ratio 7.8, 95% CI 0.8–74.8) and the presence of a parenchymal lesion on admission, including focal edema, ischemic infarct, or

hemorrhage (3.7, 1.4–9.4). Late seizures were found in 6/43 (14%) of survivors in the retrospective arm of the study [198] and in 8/84 (9.5%) of survivors in the prospective arm [191], who were followed up to 10 months from the onset of the CVT. Epilepsy developed in 4/84 (4.8%) patients. Seven out of 8 (87.5%) patients with late seizures were on anti-epileptic treatment when the seizures occurred. Late seizures were generalized in almost two thirds of patients and were independently predicted by the presence of hemorrhage on the neuroimaging study performed upon admission. In the multivariate analysis early or late seizures were not independent predictors of increased mortality or dependency, although early seizures directly contributed to death in two patients (intractable SE and cardiorespiratory arrest after grand mal seizure). The authors concluded that prophylactic AEDs during the 1st year after CVT is justified only in those patients with hemorrhage on CT/MRI or early symptomatic seizures, but could probably be avoided in patients without such high risk factors.

Another small prospective study from Lyon, France reported a high percentage of pro-thrombotic states in patients with CVT admitted in a stroke Unit [199]. Seizures were observed in 8/16 (50%), five of whom had an hemorrhagic infarct. A pro-thrombotic state was detected in 6/8 (75%, a high factor VIII level in four patients), the same percentage as in patients without seizures.

In a prospective study (with a retrospective arm) from Germany, 79 patients with CVT were followed for an average of 52 months [187]. Twenty-two patients required NICU admission and mechanical ventilation. Thirty-one (39.2%) patients developed seizures and all were treated with AEDs (phenytoin IV in 20, barbiturates IV in 4, and oral AEDs in seven patients). More than two seizures despite anti-epileptic treatment was among other factors (age, the NIHSS on admission, venous infarct, and hemorrhagic transformation of the venous infarct) significantly related to acute death (15% of patients). Epilepsy developed in 9/58 (16%) of surviving patients during the long-term follow-up and was associated with more than two seizures despite anti-epileptic treatment during hospitalization.

Another large prospective study from Turkey included 1428 patients with stroke, among which 15 had CVT. Four of these patients developed seizures (26.6%), a significantly higher percentage than ICH (12.7%) or ischemic stroke (2.7%) [45].

In a large prospective study from Germany, 194 patients with CVT were admitted in two hospitals over 28 years [200]. Early seizures (within the first 14 days) occurred in 86 (44.3%) patients, the majority of which had focal onset and subsequent Todd's paralysis. SE occurred in 11 (12.8%) patients. Patients with early seizures were more likely to be admitted to the NICU than patients without seizures. Amongst patients with seizures, mortality was three times higher in those with SE than in those without SE (36.4% and 12%, respectively). Motor deficit (odds ratio 5.8, 95% CI 2.98–11.42), ICH (2.8, 1.46–5.56), and cortical vein thrombosis (2.9, 1.43–5.96) were independent predictors of early seizures. The authors concluded that prophylactic anti-epileptic treatment may be an option for patients with these predictor variables.

One of the largest studies is the International Study on Cerebral Vein and Dural Sinus Thrombosis (ISCVT) [186, 201]. This prospective, multicenter study included 624 patients. Most patients were treated with heparin (83%) and only 13.4% had a poor outcome (death or dependency). Prognostic factors for poor outcome were age >37 years, male sex, coma, mental status disorder, hemorrhage on admission CT scan, thrombosis of the deep cerebral venous system, central nervous system infection, and cancer. Presenting seizures occurred in 245 (39.3%, the second most common symptom after headache) and early seizures (within 2 weeks) in 43 (6.9%) patients with CVT. Sixty percent of early seizures were in reality recurrent, because they occurred in patients with presenting seizures. Supratentorial lesion (4.05, 2.74–5.95), cortical vein thrombosis (2.31, 1.44–3.73), sagittal sinus thrombosis (2.18, 1.50–3.18), and puerperal CVT (2.06, 1.19–3.55) were associated with presenting seizures, whereas supratentorial lesion (3.09, 1.56–9.62) and presenting seizures (1.74, 0.90–3.37) predicted early seizures.

More recently a five-year prospective study from Iran has reported that 32/94 (34%) patients experienced at least one seizure after CVT. Epilepsy, defined as more than one remote (after the first 2 weeks) seizures after discharge, occurred in 4 (6.3%) patients. Seizure in the acute phase (within the first 2 weeks) was the strongest predictor of remote seizure in the bivariate analysis. However, in the logistic regression analysis no factor predicted acute or remote seizure development [202].

In summary, seizures may be the most common or second most common sign after CVT and they occur in 26.6–50.9% of patients in prospective studies. Early seizures occur in 6.9–34%, late seizures in 9.5%, and epilepsy in 4.8–25% (especially when associated with hemorrhage).

Treatment of Seizures Related to CVT

The treatment of seizures that follow CVT obeys to the same principles as the treatment of seizures not related to this condition. If onset or presenting seizures occur, they should be treated with AEDs, because presenting seizures are predictive of early seizures based on the ISCVT results [201]. In this large study, the risk of early seizures in patients with supratentorial lesions and presenting seizures was significantly lower when AED prophylaxis was used (one patient

with seizures out of 148 patients with AEDs vs 25 out of 47 patients without AEDs, OR 0.006, 95% CI 0.001–0.05).

Should every patient with CVT be treated prophylactically with AEDs? In a recent Cochrane Review, Kwan et al. did not find any randomized and quasi-randomized controlled trial for treatment of seizures after CVT. Based on that, the authors concluded that there is no evidence to support or refute the use of anti-epileptic drugs for the primary or secondary prevention of seizures related to CVT [203]. However, other studies have reported factors associated with seizure incidence, such as supratentorial lesions, motor or sensory deficits, ICH or isolated cortical vein thrombosis [191, 200, 201]. These patients should probably be started on AEDs, because early seizures can lead to neurologic or systemic deterioration, SE, or death [201]. In the ISCVT study, however, seizures were not an independent predictor of death and/or dependency [186]. Moreover, the duration of treatment is unclear. Prolonged treatment for 1 year should be considered in patients with CVT who developed early seizures and ICH, because late seizures may occur within the first 12 months [183, 185, 191, 200]. Despite the fact that all patients with acute seizures were treated with anti-epileptic drugs during hospitalization and after discharge, no association was found in the Iranian study between remote seizures and anti-epileptics prescription [202].

In 2010, the European Federation of Neurological Societies published guidelines on treatment of cerebral venous and sinus thrombosis in adults. These guidelines state that prophylactic treatment may be a therapeutic option in patients with focal neurological deficits or supratentorial lesions on admission CT/MRI. This recommendation recognizes that there is lack of evidence, but also that there was a clear consensus among the Task Force members. They also state that the optimal treatment duration in patients with seizures is unclear [204].

How does treatment, which is aimed at recanalizing the thrombosed venous channel using various available options, affect the incidence or severity of seizures? Few data are currently available to help answer that question. In the Dutch-European prospective study, seizures occurred in 16/30 (53%) patients on the nadroparin arm and in 12/29 (41%) patients on the controls arm ($p > 0.05$). In the most recent prospective Dutch study, 20 patients with severe CVT (i.e., selected for thrombolysis if they had an altered mental status, coma, straight sinus thrombosis, or large space-occupying lesions) were treated with Urokinase infused into the sinuses [205]. Some patients received thrombosuction with a rheolytic catheter, combined with thrombectomy via a Fogarty catheter. Six patients died in these case series by transtentorial herniation. Interestingly, seizures occurred less frequently in the fatal cases (1/6) than in the surviving patients (10/14). Even the single patient with SE had an excellent outcome. Although no specific mention about AEDs was found in this study, the explanation provided for the better outcomes in patients with seizures was that some of these patients might be enrolled in the study with decreased mental status or coma due to seizures (and not due to severe infarcts or ICHs) and quickly recovered with anti-epileptic treatment.

Are seizures in patients with CVT treated with IV heparin more likely to lead to fatal complications? One retrospective study from Freiburg, Germany, analyzed 79 patients with CVT [206]. All patients received a 5000 IU IV bolus of heparin and a subsequent infusion with target aPTT of 80–90 s. There was no difference in fatal compared to non-fatal outcome in those patients with seizures (58% of all patients) or those patients with series of seizures or status (28% of patients with seizures).

Other studies evaluating novel treatments for CVT usually do not report data regarding seizures, either because the numbers are too small to draw meaningful conclusions or because they have a different focus. Niwa et al. reported treating a woman in her 10th month of pregnancy and superior sagittal sinus thrombosis with direct t-PA instillation [207]. The patient presented with generalized seizure and tetraparesis, but was discharged without neurologic deficit. Another interesting and informative case was reported by Gerszten et al., who treated an 18-year-old man with deep cerebral venous system thrombosis secondary to antithrombin III deficiency [208]. The patient, who presented with a focal motor seizure, was started on anti-epileptics and became comatose with fixed pupils before he received the endovascular treatment. He was treated with Urokinase delivered in the straight sinus and the vein of Galen 27 h after the onset and despite the presence of edema in both basal ganglia and thalami bilaterally, and a hemorrhage in the left thalamus. The procedure resulted in deep system recanalization and subsequently continuous infusion of heparin was given. The patient remained in the ICU on pentobarbital coma for 20 days for ICP control, but eventually improved to the point of independent living and was able to graduate from high school on time.

Table 9.5 represents a suggested algorithm for the treatment of CVT-related seizures.

Table 9.5 Treatment with anti-epileptic medications after CVT

1. CVT and no seizures:
Observe
Consider Rx if there are supratentorial lesions or parenchymal lesion (focal edema, infarct, or hemorrhage), focal motor or sensory deficits or cortical vein thrombosis on the admission CT/ MRI. Continue Rx for at least 1 year (seizure-free interval). Assess with EEG before discontinuation?
2. CVT and onset or early seizures:
Treat with monotherapy first for 1 year (seizure-free interval). Assess with EEG before discontinuation?

References

1. Jackson J. On the scientific and empirical investigation of epilepsies. In: Taylor J, editor. Selected writtings of John Hughlings Jackson. London: Hodder and Stoughton; 1931. p. 233.
2. Gowers W. Epilepsy and other chronic convulsive disorders. New York: Dover; 1964. p. 106.
3. Armon C, Radtke RA, Massey EW. Therapy of seizures associated with stroke. Clin Neuropharmacol. 1991;14(1):17–27.
4. Barolin GS. The cerebrovascular epilepsies. Electroencephalogr Clin Neurophysiol Suppl. 1982;35:287–95.
5. Giroud M, Gras P, Fayolle H, Andre N, Soichot P, Dumas R. Early seizures after acute stroke: a study of 1,640 cases. Epilepsia. 1994;35(5):959–64.
6. Lancman ME, Golimstok A, Norscini J, Granillo R. Risk factors for developing seizures after a stroke. Epilepsia. 1993;34(1):141–3.
7. Bladin CF, Alexandrov AV, Bellavance A, Bornstein N, Chambers B, Cote R, et al. Seizures after stroke: a prospective multicenter study. Arch Neurol. 2000;57(11):1617–22.
8. Burn J, Dennis M, Bamford J, Sandercock P, Wade D, Warlow C. Epileptic seizures after a first stroke: the oxfordshire community stroke project. BMJ. 1997;315(7122):1582–7.
9. Kilpatrick CJ, Davis SM, Tress BM, Rossiter SC, Hopper JL, Vandendriesen ML. Epileptic seizures in acute stroke. Arch Neurol. 1990;47(2):157–60.
10. Louis S, McDowell F. Epileptic seizures in nonembolic cerebral infarction. Arch Neurol. 1967;17(4):414–8.
11. Shinton RA, Gill JS, Melnick SC, Gupta AK, Beevers DG. The frequency, characteristics and prognosis of epileptic seizures at the onset of stroke. J Neurol Neurosurg Psychiatry. 1988;51(2):273–6.
12. Milandre L, Broca P, Sambuc R, Khalil R. Epileptic crisis during and after cerebrovascular diseases. A clinical analysis of 78 cases. Rev Neurol. 1992;148(12):767–72.
13. Holmes GL. The electroencephalogram as a predictor of seizures following cerebral infarction. Clin Electroencephalogr. 1980;11(2):83–6.
14. Zou S, Wu X, Zhu B, Yu J, Yang B, Shi J. The pooled incidence of post-stroke seizure in 102 008 patients. Top Stroke Rehabil. 2015;22:460–7.
15. Loiseau J, Loiseau P, Duche B, Guyot M, Dartigues JF, Aublet B. A survey of epileptic disorders in southwest France: seizures in elderly patients. Ann Neurol. 1990;27(3):232–7.
16. Lo YK, Yiu CH, Hu HH, Su MS, Laeuchli SC. Frequency and characteristics of early seizures in Chinese acute stroke. Acta Neurol Scand. 1994;90(2):83–5.
17. Hauser WA, Kurland LT. The epidemiology of epilepsy in Rochester, Minnesota, 1935 through 1967. Epilepsia. 1975;16(1):1–66.
18. Arboix A, Comes E, Massons J, Garcia L, Oliveres M. Relevance of early seizures for in-hospital mortality in acute cerebrovascular disease. Neurology. 1996;47(6):1429–35.
19. Reith J, Jorgensen HS, Nakayama H, Raaschou HO, Olsen TS. Seizures in acute stroke: predictors and prognostic significance The Copenhagen Stroke Study. Stroke. 1997;28(8):1585–9.
20. Camilo O, Goldstein LB. Seizures and epilepsy after ischemic stroke. Stroke. 2004;35(7):1769–75.
21. Huang CW, Saposnik G, Fang J, Steven DA, Burneo JG. Influence of seizures on stroke outcomes: a large multicenter study. Neurology. 2014;82(9):768–76.
22. Lamy C, Domigo V, Semah F, Arquizan C, Trystram D, Coste J, et al. Early and late seizures after cryptogenic ischemic stroke in young adults. Neurology. 2003;60(3):400–4.
23. Paolucci S, Silvestri G, Lubich S, Pratesi L, Traballesi M, Gigli GL. Poststroke late seizures and their role in rehabilitation of inpatients. Epilepsia. 1997;38(3):266–70.

24. Berges S, Moulin T, Berger E, Tatu L, Sablot D, Challier B, et al. Seizures and epilepsy following strokes: recurrence factors. Eur Neurol. 2000;43(1):3–8.

25. De Carolis P, D'Alessandro R, Ferrara R, Andreoli A, Sacquegna T, Lugaresi E. Late seizures in patients with internal carotid and middle cerebral artery occlusive disease following ischaemic events. J Neurol Neurosurg Psychiatry. 1984;47(12):1345–7.

26. Olsen TS, Hogenhaven H, Thage O. Epilepsy after stroke. Neurology. 1987;37(7):1209–11.

27. Viitanen M, Eriksson S, Asplund K. Risk of recurrent stroke, myocardial infarction and epilepsy during long-term follow-up after stroke. Eur Neurol. 1988;28(4):227–31.

28. Fish DR, Miller DH, Roberts RC, Blackie JD, Gilliatt RW. The natural history of late-onset epilepsy secondary to vascular disease. Acta Neurol Scand. 1989;80(6):524–6.

29. Faught E, Peters D, Bartolucci A, Moore L, Miller PC. Seizures after primary intracerebral hemorrhage. Neurology. 1989;39(8):1089–93.

30. Sundaram MB. Etiology and patterns of seizures in the elderly. Neuroepidemiology. 1989;8(5):234–8.

31. Mahler ME. Seizures: common causes and treatment in the elderly. Geriatrics. 1987;42(7):73–8.

32. Luhdorf K, Jensen LK, Plesner AM. Etiology of seizures in the elderly. Epilepsia. 1986;27(4):458–63.

33. Dam AM, Fuglsang-Frederiksen A, Svarre-Olsen U, Dam M. Late-onset epilepsy: etiologies, types of seizure, and value of clinical investigation, EEG, and computerized tomography scan. Epilepsia. 1985;26(3):227–31.

34. de la Sayette V, Cosgrove R, Melanson D, Ethier R. CT findings in late-onset epilepsy. Can J Neurol Sci. 1987;14(3):286–9.

35. Gupta SR, Naheedy MH, Elias D, Rubino FA. Postinfarction seizures. A clinical study. Stroke. 1988;19(12):1477–81.

36. Sung CY, Chu NS. Epileptic seizures in thrombotic stroke. J Neurol. 1990;237(3):166–70.

37. Pohlman-Eden B, Hoch D, Cochius J, Hennerici M. Stroke and epilepsy: critical review of the literature. Cerebrovasc Dis. 1996;6:332–8.

38. Black SE, Norris JW, Hachinski V. Post-stroke seizures. Stroke. 1983;14(1):134.

39. Kilpatrick CJ, Davis SM, Hopper JL, Rossiter SC. Early seizures after acute stroke. Risk of late seizures. Arch Neurol. 1992;49(5):509–11.

40. Daniele O, Caravaglios G, Ferraro G, Mattaliano A, Tassinari C, Natale E. Stroke-related seizures and the role of cortical and subcortical structures. J Epilepsy. 1996;9:184–8.

41. Arboix A, Garcia-Eroles L, Massons JB, Oliveres M, Comes E. Predictive factors of early seizures after acute cerebrovascular disease. Stroke. 1997;28(8):1590–4.

42. Cheung CM, Tsoi TH, Au-Yeung M, Tang AS. Epileptic seizure after stroke in Chinese patients. J Neurol. 2003;250(7):839–43.

43. Lossius MI, Ronning OM, Slapo GD, Mowinckel P, Gjerstad L. Poststroke epilepsy: occurrence and predictors—a long-term prospective controlled study (Akershus Stroke Study). Epilepsia. 2005;46(8):1246–51.

44. Adams Jr HP, Woolson RF, Biller J, Clarke W. Studies of Org 10172 in patients with acute ischemic stroke TOAST Study Group. Haemostasis. 1992;22(2):99–103.

45. Benbir G, Ince B, Bozluolcay M. The epidemiology of poststroke epilepsy according to stroke subtypes. Acta Neurol Scand. 2006;114(1):8–12.

46. Misirli H, Ozge A, Somay G, Erdogan N, Erkal H, Erenoglu NY. Seizure development after stroke. Int J Clin Pract. 2006;60(12):1536–41.

47. Basic Baronica K, Sruk A, Planjar-Prvan M, Bielen I. Epilepticki napadaji u perakutnoj fazi mozdanog udara: incidencija i utjecaj na unutarbolnicki letalitet [Seizures in the peracute stage of stroke:

incidence and effect on inpatient mortality]. Acta Med Croatica. 2008;62(1):29–32.

48. Alberti A, Paciaroni M, Caso V, Venti M, Palmerini F, Agnelli G. Early seizures in patients with acute stroke: frequency, predictive factors, and effect on clinical outcome. Vasc Health Risk Manag. 2008;4(3):715–20.

49. Couillard P, Almekhlafi MA, Irvine A, Jette N, Pow J, St Germaine-Smith C, et al. Subacute seizure incidence in thrombolysis-treated ischemic stroke patients. Neurocrit Care. 2012;16(2):241–5.

50. Vespa PM, O'Phelan K, Shah M, Mirabelli J, Starkman S, Kidwell C, et al. Acute seizures after intracerebral hemorrhage: A factor in progressive midline shift and outcome. Neurology. 2003;60(9):1441–6. PubMed PMID: 12743228

51. Chiang IH, Chang WN, Lin WC, Chuang YC, Chang KC, Tsai NW, et al. Risk factors for seizures after first-time ischemic stroke by magnetic resonance imaging. Acta Neurol Taiwanica. 2010;19(1):26–32.

52. Krakow K, Sitzer M, Rosenow F, Steinmetz H, Foerch C; Arbeitsgruppe Schlaganfall Hessen. Predictors of acute poststroke seizures. Cerebrovasc Dis 2010;30(6):584–589.

53. Procaccianti G, Zaniboni A, Rondelli F, Crisci M, Sacquegna T. Seizures in acute stroke: incidence, risk factors and prognosis. Neuroepidemiology. 2012;39(1):45–50.

54. So EL, Annegers JF, Hauser WA, O'Brien PC, Whisnant JP. Population-based study of seizure disorders after cerebral infarction. Neurology. 1996;46(2):350–5.

55. Kammersgaard LP, Olsen TS. Poststroke epilepsy in the Copenhagen stroke study: incidence and predictors. J Stroke Cerebrovasc Dis. 2005;14(5):210–4.

56. Labovitz DL, Hauser WA, Sacco RL. Prevalence and predictors of early seizure and status epilepticus after first stroke. Neurology. 2001;57(2):200–6.

57. Devuyst G, Karapanayiotides T, Hottinger I, Van Melle G, Bogousslavsky J. Prodromal and early epileptic seizures in acute stroke: Does higher serum cholesterol protect? Neurology. 2003;61(2):249–52.

58. Szaflarski JP, Rackley AY, Kleindorfer DO, Khoury J, Woo D, Miller R, et al. Incidence of seizures in the acute phase of stroke: a population-based study. Epilepsia. 2008;30

59. DeLorenzo RJ, Hauser WA, Towne AR, Boggs JG, Pellock JM, Penberthy L, et al. A prospective, population-based epidemiologic study of status epilepticus in Richmond Virginia. Neurology. 1996;46(4):1029–35.

60. Scholtes FB, Renier WO, Meinardi H. Generalized convulsive status epilepticus: causes, therapy, and outcome in 346 patients. Epilepsia. 1994;35(5):1104–12.

61. Towne AR, Pellock JM, Ko D, DeLorenzo RJ. Determinants of mortality in status epilepticus. Epilepsia. 1994;35(1):27–34.

62. Barry E, Hauser WA. Status epilepticus: the interaction of epilepsy and acute brain disease. Neurology. 1993;43(8):1473–8.

63. Rumbach L, Sablot D, Berger E, Tatu L, Vuillier F, Moulin T. Status epilepticus in stroke: report on a hospital-based stroke cohort. Neurology. 2000;54(2):350–4.

64. Velioglu SK, Ozmenoglu M, Boz C, Alioglu Z. Status epilepticus after stroke. Stroke. 2001;32(5):1169–72.

65. Afsar N, Kaya D, Aktan S, Sykut-Bingol C. Stroke and status epilepticus: stroke type, type of status epilepticus, and prognosis. Seizure. 2003;12(1):23–7.

66. Shinton RA, Gill JS, Zezulka AV, Beevers DG. The frequency of epilepsy preceding stroke. Case-control study in 230 patients. Lancet. 1987;1(8523):11–3.

67. Cleary P, Shorvon S, Tallis R. Late-onset seizures as a predictor of subsequent stroke. Lancet. 2004;363(9416):1184–6.

68. Kase CS, Wolf PA, Chodosh EH, Zacker HB, Kelly-Hayes M, Kannel WB, et al. Prevalence of silent stroke in patients

presenting with initial stroke: the framingham study. Stroke. 1989;20(7):850–2.

69. Roberts RC, Shorvon SD, Cox TC, Gilliatt RW. Clinically unsuspected cerebral infarction revealed by computed tomography scanning in late onset epilepsy. Epilepsia. 1988;29(2):190–4.

70. De Reuck J, Decoo D, Algoed L, et al. Epileptic seizures after thromboembolic cerebral infarcts: a positron emission tomographic study. Cerebrovasc Dis. 1995;5:328–33.

71. Shuaib A, Lee MA. Seizures in migraine: warning of an underlying cerebral infarction? Headache. 1987;27(9):500–2.

72. Yanagihara T, Piepgras DG, Klass DW. Repetitive involuntary movement associated with episodic cerebral ischemia. Ann Neurol. 1985;18(2):244–50.

73. Lu XC, Mountney A, Chen Z, Wei G, Cao Y, Leung LY, et al. Similarities and differences of acute nonconvulsive seizures and other epileptic activities following penetrating and ischemic brain injuries in rats. J Neurotrauma. 2013;30(7):580–90.

74. Heiss WD, Huber M, Fink GR, Herholz K, Pietrzyk U, Wagner R, et al. Progressive derangement of periinfarct viable tissue in ischemic stroke. J Cereb Blood Flow Metab. 1992;12(2):193–203.

75. Silverman IE, Restrepo L, Mathews GC. Poststroke seizures. Arch Neurol. 2002;59(2):195–201.

76. DeLorenzo RJ, Sun DA, Blair RE, Sombati S. An in vitro model of stroke-induced epilepsy: elucidation of the roles of glutamate and calcium in the induction and maintenance of stroke-induced epileptogenesis. Int Rev Neurobiol. 2007;81:59–84.

77. Comi AM, Weisz CJ, Highet BH, Johnston MV, Wilson MA. A new model of stroke and ischemic seizures in the immature mouse. Pediatr Neurol. 2004;31(4):254–7.

78. Buchkremer-Ratzmann I, August M, Hagemann G, Witte OW. Epileptiform discharges to extracellular stimuli in rat neocortical slices after photothrombotic infarction. J Neurol Sci. 1998;156(2):133–7.

79. Congar P, Gaiarsa JL, Popovici T, Ben-Ari Y, Crepel V. Permanent reduction of seizure threshold in post-ischemic CA3 pyramidal neurons. J Neurophysiol. 2000;83(4):2040–6.

80. Nedergaard M, Hansen AJ. Characterization of cortical depolarizations evoked in focal cerebral ischemia. J Cereb Blood Flow Metab. 1993;13(4):568–74.

81. Kim DC, Todd MM. Forebrain ischemia: effect on pharmacologically induced seizure thresholds in the rat. Brain Res. 1999;831(1–2):131–9.

82. Kessler KR, Schnitzler A, Classen J, Benecke R. Reduced inhibition within primary motor cortex in patients with poststroke focal motor seizures. Neurology. 2002;59(7):1028–33.

83. De Reuck J, Proot P, Van Maele G. Chronic obstructive pulmonary disease as a risk factor for stroke-related seizures. Eur J Neurol. 2007;14(9):989–92.

84. Bogousslavsky J, Martin R, Regli F, Despland PA, Bolyn S. Persistent worsening of stroke sequelae after delayed seizures. Arch Neurol. 1992;49(4):385–8.

85. Cuomo O, Rispoli V, Leo A, Politi GB, Vinciguerra A, di Renzo G, et al. The antiepileptic drug levetiracetam suppresses nonconvulsive seizure activity and reduces ischemic brain damage in rats subjected to permanent middle cerebral artery occlusion. PLoS One. 2013;8(11):e80852.

86. Cordonnier C, Henon H, Derambure P, Pasquier F, Leys D. Early epileptic seizures after stroke are associated with increased risk of new-onset dementia. J Neurol Neurosurg Psychiatry. 2007;78(5):514–6.

87. Denier C, Masnou P, Mapoure Y, Souillard-Scemama R, Guedj T, Theaudin M, et al. Watershed infarctions are more prone than other cortical infarcts to cause early-onset seizures. Arch Neurol. 2010;67(10):1219–23.

88. Pezzini A, Grassi M, Del Zotto E, Giossi A, Volonghi I, Costa P, et al. Complications of acute stroke and the occurrence of early seizures. Cerebrovasc Dis. 2013;35(5):444–50.

89. El-Hayek YH, Wu C, Chen R, Al-Sharif AR, Huang S, Patel N, et al. Acute postischemic seizures are associated with increased mortality and brain damage in adult mice. Cereb Cortex. 2011;21(12):2863–75.

90. Giroud M, Dumas R. Role of associated cortical lesions in motor partial seizures and lenticulostriate infarcts. Epilepsia. 1995;36(5):465–70.

91. Avrahami E, Drory VE, Rabey MJ, Cohn DF. Generalized epileptic seizures as the presenting symptom of lacunar infarction in the brain. J Neurol. 1988;235(8):472–4.

92. Bentes C, Pimentel J, Ferro JM. Epileptic seizures following subcortical infarcts. Cerebrovasc Dis. 2001;12(4):331–4.

93. Dichgans M, Mayer M, Uttner I, Bruning R, Muller-Hocker J, Rungger G, et al. The phenotypic spectrum of CADASIL: clinical findings in 102 cases. Ann Neurol. 1998;44(5):731–9.

94. Velizarova R, Mourand I, Serafini A, Crespel A, Gelisse P. Focal epilepsy as first symptom in CADASIL. Seizure. 2011;20(6):502–4.

95. Willmore LJ, Sypert GW, Munson JB. Recurrent seizures induced by cortical iron injection: a model of posttraumatic epilepsy. Ann Neurol. 1978;4(4):329–36.

96. Lee KR, Drury I, Vitarbo E, Hoff JT. Seizures induced by intracerebral injection of thrombin: a model of intracerebral hemorrhage. J Neurosurg. 1997;87(1):73–8.

97. Jordan KG. Continuous EEG monitoring in the neuroscience intensive care unit and emergency department. J Clin Neurophysiol. 1999;16(1):14–39.

98. Carrera E, Michel P, Despland PA, Maeder-Ingvar M, Ruffieux C, Debatisse D, et al. Continuous assessment of electrical epileptic activity in acute stroke. Neurology. 2006;67(1):99–104.

99. Mecarelli O, Pro S, Randi F, Dispenza S, Correnti A, Pulitano P, et al. EEG patterns and epileptic seizures in acute phase stroke. Cerebrovasc Dis. 2011;31(2):191–8.

100. Chu K, Kang DW, Kim JY, Chang KH, Lee SK. Diffusion-weighted magnetic resonance imaging in nonconvulsive status epilepticus. Arch Neurol. 2001;58(6):993–8.

101. Senn P, Lovblad KO, Zutter D, Bassetti C, Zeller O, Donati F, et al. Changes on diffusion-weighted MRI with focal motor status epilepticus: case report. Neuroradiology. 2003;45(4):246–9.

102. Lansberg MG, O'Brien MW, Norbash AM, Moseley ME, Morrell M, Albers GW. MRI abnormalities associated with partial status epilepticus. Neurology. 1999;52(5):1021–7.

103. Warach S, Levin JM, Schomer DL, Holman BL, Edelman RR. Hyperperfusion of ictal seizure focus demonstrated by MR perfusion imaging. AJNR Am J Neuroradiol. 1994;15(5):965–8.

104. Nguyen D, Kapina V, Seeck M, Viallon M, Fedespiel A, Lovblad KO. Ictal hyperperfusion demonstrated by arterial spin-labeling MRI in status epilepticus. J Neuroradiol. 2010;37(4):250–1.

105. Szabo K, Poepel A, Pohlmann-Eden B, Hirsch J, Back T, Sedlaczek O, et al. Diffusion-weighted and perfusion MRI demonstrates parenchymal changes in complex partial status epilepticus. Brain. 2005;128(Pt 6):1369–76.

106. Kanazawa Y, Morioka T, Arakawa S, Furuta Y, Nakanishi A, Kitazono T. Nonconvulsive partial status epilepticus mimicking recurrent infarction revealed by diffusion-weighted and arterial spin labeling perfusion magnetic resonance images. J Stroke Cerebrovasc Dis. 2015;24(4):731–8.

107. Rennebaum F, Kassubek J, Pinkhardt E, Hubers A, Ludolph AC, Schocke M, et al. Status epilepticus: Clinical characteristics and EEG patterns associated with and without MRI diffusion restriction in 69 patients. Epilepsy Res. 2016;120:55–64.

108. Donaire A, Carreno M, Gomez B, Fossas P, Bargallo N, Agudo R, et al. Cortical laminar necrosis related to prolonged focal status epilepticus. J Neurol Neurosurg Psychiatry. 2006;77(1):104–6.

109. Cianfoni A, Caulo M, Cerase A, Della Marca G, Falcone C, Di Lella GM, et al. Seizure-induced brain lesions: a wide spectrum of variably reversible MRI abnormalities. Eur J Radiol. 2013;82(11):1964–72.

110. Kappelle LJ, Adams Jr HP, Heffner ML, Torner JC, Gomez F, Biller J. Prognosis of young adults with ischemic stroke. A long-term follow-up study assessing recurrent vascular events and functional outcome in the Iowa registry of stroke in young adults. Stroke. 1994;25(7):1360–5.

111. Kristensen B, Malm J, Carlberg B, Stegmayr B, Backman C, Fagerlund M, et al. Epidemiology and etiology of ischemic stroke in young adults aged 18 to 44 years in northern Sweden. Stroke. 1997;28(9):1702–9.

112. Rozenthul-Sorokin N, Ronen R, Tamir A, Geva H, Eldar R. Stroke in the young in Israel. Incidence and outcomes. Stroke. 1996;27(5):838–41.

113. Neau JP, Ingrand P, Mouille-Brachet C, Rosier MP, Couderq C, Alvarez A, et al. Functional recovery and social outcome after cerebral infarction in young adults. Cerebrovasc Dis. 1998;8(5):296–302.

114. Hauser WA. Seizure disorders: the changes with age. Epilepsia. 1992;33(Suppl 4):S6–14.

115. Holt-Seitz A, Wirrell EC, Sundaram MB. Seizures in the elderly: etiology and prognosis. Can J Neurol Sci. 1999;26(2):110–4.

116. Cordonnier C, Henon H, Derambure P, Pasquier F, Leys D. Influence of pre-existing dementia on the risk of post-stroke epileptic seizures. J Neurol Neurosurg Psychiatry. 2005;76(12):1649–53.

117. The national institute of neurological disorders and stroke rt-PA stroke study group. N Engl J Med. 1995;333(24):1581–7.

118. Barber PA, Zhang J, Demchuk AM, Hill MD, Buchan AM. Why are stroke patients excluded from TPA therapy? An analysis of patient eligibility. Neurology. 2001;56(8):1015–20.

119. Brunser AM, Illanes S, Lavados PM, Munoz P, Carcamo D, Hoppe A, et al. Exclusion criteria for intravenous thrombolysis in stroke mimics: an observational study. J Stroke Cerebrovasc Dis. 2013;22(7):1140–5.

120. Eichel R, Hur TB, Gomori JM, Cohen JE, Leker RR. Use of DWI-only MR protocol for screening stroke mimics. J Neurol Sci. 2013;328(1–2):37–40.

121. Forster A, Griebe M, Wolf ME, Szabo K, Hennerici MG, Kern R. How to identify stroke mimics in patients eligible for intravenous thrombolysis? J Neurol. 2012;259(7):1347–53.

122. Winkler DT, Fluri F, Fuhr P, Wetzel SG, Lyrer PA, Ruegg S, et al. Thrombolysis in stroke mimics: frequency, clinical characteristics, and outcome. Stroke. 2009;40(4):1522–5.

123. Tsivgoulis G, Alexandrov AV, Chang J, Sharma VK, Hoover SL, Lao AY, et al. Safety and outcomes of intravenous thrombolysis in stroke mimics: a 6-year, single-care center study and a pooled analysis of reported series. Stroke. 2011;42(6):1771–4.

124. Lewandowski C, Mays-Wilson K, Miller J, Penstone P, Miller DJ, Bakoulas K, et al. Safety and outcomes in stroke mimics after intravenous tissue plasminogen activator administration: a single-center experience. J Stroke Cerebrovasc Dis. 2015;24(1):48–52.

125. De Los RF, Kleindorfer DO, Guzik A, Ortega-Gutierrez S, Sangha N, Kumar G, et al. Intravenous fibrinolysis eligibility: a survey of stroke clinicians' practice patterns and review of the literature. J Stroke Cerebrovasc Dis. 2014;23(8):2130–8.

126. Rodan LH, Aviv RI, Sahlas DJ, Murray BJ, Gladstone JP, Gladstone DJ. Seizures during stroke thrombolysis heralding dramatic neurologic recovery. Neurology. 2006;67(11):2048–9.

127. Hafeez F, Razzaq MA, Levine RL, Ramirez MA. Reperfusion seizures: a manifestation of cerebral reperfusion injury after administration of recombinant tissue plasminogen activator for acute ischemic stroke. J Stroke Cerebrovasc Dis. 2007;16(6):273–7.

128. Seeck M, Vulliemoz S. Seizures during stroke thrombolysis heralding dramatic neurologic recovery. Neurology. 2007;69(4):409–10.

129. Bentes C, Peralta R, Viana P, Morgado C, Melo TP, Ferro JM. Cortical myoclonus during IV thrombolysis for ischemic stroke. Epilepsy Behav Case Rep. 2014;2:186–8.

130. Tan ML, Ng A, Pandher PS, Sashindranath M, Hamilton JA, Davis SM, et al. Tissue plasminogen activator does not alter development of acquired epilepsy. Epilepsia. 2012;53(11):1998–2004.

131. Jauch EC, Saver JL, Adams Jr HP, Bruno A, Connors JJ, Demaerschalk BM, et al. Guidelines for the early management of patients with acute ischemic stroke: a guideline for healthcare professionals from the American Heart Association/American Stroke Association. Stroke. 2013;44(3):870–947.

132. Sylaja PN, Dzialowski I, Krol A, Roy J, Federico P, Demchuk AM. Role of CT angiography in thrombolysis decision-making for patients with presumed seizure at stroke onset. Stroke. 2006;37(3):915–7.

133. Rowe AS, Goodwin H, Brophy GM, Bushwitz J, Castle A, Deen D, et al. Seizure prophylaxis in neurocritical care: a review of evidence-based support. Pharmacotherapy. 2014;34(4):396–409.

134. Ryvlin P, Montavont A, Nighoghossian N. Optimizing therapy of seizures in stroke patients. Neurology. 2006;67(12 Suppl 4):S3–9.

135. Davalos A, Cendra E, Genis D, Lopez-Pousa S. The frequency, characteristics and prognosis of epileptic seizures at the onset of stroke. J Neurol Neurosurg Psychiatry. 1988;51(11):1464.

136. Strzelczyk A, Haag A, Raupach H, Herrendorf G, Hamer HM, Rosenow F. Prospective evaluation of a post-stroke epilepsy risk scale. J Neurol. 2010;257(8):1322–6.

137. Gilad R, Lampl Y, Eschel Y, Sadeh M. Antiepileptic treatment in patients with early postischemic stroke seizures: a retrospective study. Cerebrovasc Dis. 2001;12(1):39–43.

138. Leker RR, Neufeld MY. Anti-epileptic drugs as possible neuroprotectants in cerebral ischemia. Brain Res Brain Res Rev. 2003;42(3):187–203.

139. Costa C, Martella G, Picconi B, Prosperetti C, Pisani A, Di Filippo M, et al. Multiple mechanisms underlying the neuroprotective effects of antiepileptic drugs against in vitro ischemia. Stroke. 2006;37(5):1319–26.

140. Goldstein LB. Potential effects of common drugs on stroke recovery. Arch Neurol. 1998;55(4):454–6.

141. Glauser T, Ben-Menachem E, Bourgeois B, Cnaan A, Chadwick D, Guerreiro C, et al. ILAE treatment guidelines: evidence-based analysis of antiepileptic drug efficacy and effectiveness as initial monotherapy for epileptic seizures and syndromes. Epilepsia. 2006;47(7):1094–120.

142. Alvarez-Sabin J, Montaner J, Padro L, Molina CA, Rovira R, Codina A, et al. Gabapentin in late-onset poststroke seizures. Neurology. 2002;59(12):1991–3.

143. Chadwick DW, Anhut H, Greiner MJ, Alexander J, Murray GH, Garofalo EA, et al. A double-blind trial of gabapentin monotherapy for newly diagnosed partial seizures. International gabapentin monotherapy study group 945–77. Neurology. 1998;51(5):1282–8.

144. Garcia-Escriva A, Lopez-Hernandez N. Uso del levetiracetam en monoterapia en crisis postictus de la poblacion anciana [The use of levetiracetam in monotherapy in post-stroke seizures in the elderly population]. Rev Neurol. 2007;45(9):523–5.

145. Kutlu G, Gomceli YB, Unal Y, Inan LE. Levetiracetam monotherapy for late poststroke seizures in the elderly. Epilepsy Behav. 2008;13(3):542–4.

146. Belcastro V, Costa C, Galletti F, Autuori A, Pierguidi L, Pisani F, et al. Levetiracetam in newly diagnosed late-onset post-stroke seizures: a prospective observational study. Epilepsy Res. 2008;82(2–3):223–6.

147. Consoli D, Bosco D, Postorino P, Galati F, Plastino M, Perticoni GF, et al. Levetiracetam versus carbamazepine in patients with late poststroke seizures: a multicenter prospective randomized open-label study (EpIC Project). Cerebrovasc Dis. 2012;34(4):282–9.

148. Guo J, Guo J, Li J, Zhou M, Qin F, Zhang S, et al. Statin treatment reduces the risk of poststroke seizures. Neurology. 2015;85(8):701–7.

149. Sundt Jr TM, Sharbrough FW, Piepgras DG, Kearns TP, Messick Jr JM, O'Fallon WM. Correlation of cerebral blood flow and electroencephalographic changes during carotid endarterectomy: with results of surgery and hemodynamics of cerebral ischemia. Mayo Clin Proc. 1981;56(9):533–43.

150. Ascher E, Markevich N, Schutzer RW, Kallakuri S, Jacob T, Hingorani AP. Cerebral hyperperfusion syndrome after carotid endarterectomy: predictive factors and hemodynamic changes. J Vasc Surg. 2003;37(4):769–77.

151. Wagner WH, Cossman DV, Farber A, Levin PM, Cohen JL. Hyperperfusion syndrome after carotid endarterectomy. Ann Vasc Surg. 2005;19(4):479–86.

152. Schoser BG, Heesen C, Eckert B, Thie A. Cerebral hyperperfusion injury after percutaneous transluminal angioplasty of extracranial arteries. J Neurol. 1997;244(2):101–4.

153. Ho DS, Wang Y, Chui M, Ho SL, Cheung RT. Epileptic seizures attributed to cerebral hyperperfusion after percutaneous transluminal angioplasty and stenting of the internal carotid artery. Cerebrovasc Dis. 2000;10(5):374–9.

154. Abou-Chebl A, Reginelli J, Bajzer CT, Yadav JS. Intensive treatment of hypertension decreases the risk of hyperperfusion and intracerebral hemorrhage following carotid artery stenting. Catheter Cardiovasc Interv. 2007;69(5):690–6.

155. Morrish W, Grahovac S, Douen A, Cheung G, Hu W, Farb R, et al. Intracranial hemorrhage after stenting and angioplasty of extracranial carotid stenosis. AJNR Am J Neuroradiol. 2000;21(10):1911–6.

156. Ogasawara K, Sakai N, Kuroiwa T, Hosoda K, Iihara K, Toyoda K, et al. Intracranial hemorrhage associated with cerebral hyperperfusion syndrome following carotid endarterectomy and carotid artery stenting: retrospective review of 4494 patients. J Neurosurg. 2007;107(6):1130–6.

157. Stiver SI, Ogilvy CS. Acute hyperperfusion syndrome complicating EC-IC bypass. J Neurol Neurosurg Psychiatry. 2002;73(1):88–9.

158. Medel R, Crowley RW, Dumont AS. Hyperperfusion syndrome following endovascular cerebral revascularization. Neurosurg Focus. 2009;26(3):E4.

159. Mondel PK, Udare AS, Anand SV, Saraf RS, Limaye US. Recurrent cerebral hyperperfusion syndrome after intracranial angioplasty and stenting: case report with review of literature. Cardiovasc Intervent Radiol. 2014;37(4):1087–92.

160. MacGillivray DC, Valentine RJ, Rob CG. Reperfusion seizures after innominate endarterectomy. J Vasc Surg. 1987;6(5):521–3.

161. Lietz K, Brown K, Ali SS, Colvin-Adams M, Boyle AJ, Anderson D, et al. The role of cerebral hyperperfusion in postoperative neurologic dysfunction after left ventricular assist device implantation for end-stage heart failure. J Thorac Cardiovasc Surg. 2009;137(4):1012–9.

162. Breen JC, Caplan LR, DeWitt LD, Belkin M, Mackey WC, O'Donnell TP. Brain edema after carotid surgery. Neurology. 1996;46(1):175–81.

163. Coutts SB, Hill MD, Hu WY. Hyperperfusion syndrome: toward a stricter definition. Neurosurgery. 2003;53(5):1053–8. discussion 8–60

164. Schroeder T, Sillesen H, Sorensen O, Engell HC. Cerebral hyperperfusion following carotid endarterectomy. J Neurosurg. 1987;66(6):824–9.

165. Gupta AK, Purkayastha S, Unnikrishnan M, Vattoth S, Krishnamoorthy T, Kesavadas C. Hyperperfusion syndrome after supraaortic vessel interventions and bypass surgery. J Neuroradiol. 2005;32(5):352–8.

166. Lieb M, Shah U, Hines GL. Cerebral hyperperfusion syndrome after carotid intervention: a review. Cardiovasc Intervent Radiol. 2014;37:1087–92.

167. Jorgensen LG, Schroeder TV. Defective cerebrovascular autoregulation after carotid endarterectomy. Eur J Vasc Surg. 1993;7(4):370–9.

168. Badruddin A, Taqi MA, Abraham MG, Dani D, Zaidat OO. Neurocritical care of a reperfused brain. Curr Neurol Neurosci Rep. 2011;11(1):104–10.

169. Reigel MM, Hollier LH, Sundt Jr TM, Piepgras DG, Sharbrough FW, Cherry KJ. Cerebral hyperperfusion syndrome: a cause of neurologic dysfunction after carotid endarterectomy. J Vasc Surg. 1987;5(4):628–34.

170. Kieburtz K, Ricotta JJ, Moxley RT, 3rd. Seizures following carotid endarterectomy. Arch Neurol 1990;47(5):568–570.

171. Naylor AR, Evans J, Thompson MM, London NJ, Abbott RJ, Cherryman G, et al. Seizures after carotid endarterectomy: hyperperfusion, dysautoregulation or hypertensive encephalopathy? Eur J Vasc Endovasc Surg. 2003;26(1):39–44.

172. Maas MB, Kwolek CJ, Hirsch JA, Jaff MR, Rordorf GA. Clinical risk predictors for cerebral hyperperfusion syndrome after carotid endarterectomy. J Neurol Neurosurg Psychiatry. 2013;84(5):569–72.

173. Abou-Chebl A, Yadav JS, Reginelli JP, Bajzer C, Bhatt D, Krieger DW. Intracranial hemorrhage and hyperperfusion syndrome following carotid artery stenting: risk factors, prevention, and treatment. J Am Coll Cardiol. 2004;43(9):1596–601.

174. Sbarigia E, Speziale F, Giannoni MF, Colonna M, Panico MA, Fiorani P. Post-carotid endarterectomy hyperperfusion syndrome: preliminary observations for identifying at risk patients by transcranial Doppler sonography and the acetazolamide test. Eur J Vasc Surg. 1993;7(3):252–6.

175. Powers AD, Smith RR. Hyperperfusion syndrome after carotid endarterectomy: a transcranial doppler evaluation. Neurosurgery. 1990;26(1):56–9. discussion 9–60

176. Ogasawara K, Konno H, Yukawa H, Endo H, Inoue T, Ogawa A. Transcranial regional cerebral oxygen saturation monitoring during carotid endarterectomy as a predictor of postoperative hyperperfusion. Neurosurgery. 2003;53(2):309–14. discussion 14–5

177. Aidi S, Chaunu MP, Biousse V, Bousser MG. Changing pattern of headache pointing to cerebral venous thrombosis after lumbar puncture and intravenous high-dose corticosteroids. Headache. 1999;39(8):559–64.

178. Stam J. Cerebral venous and sinus thrombosis: incidence and causes. Adv Neurol. 2003;92:225–32.

179. Wilder-Smith E, Kothbauer-Margreiter I, Lammle B, Sturzenegger M, Ozdoba C, Hauser SP. Dural puncture and activated protein C resistance: risk factors for cerebral venous sinus thrombosis. J Neurol Neurosurg Psychiatry. 1997;63(3):351–6.

180. Ehtisham A, Stern BJ. Cerebral venous thrombosis: a review. Neurologist. 2006;12(1):32–8.

181. Ferro JM, Canhao P. Acute treatment of cerebral venous and dural sinus thrombosis. Curr Treat Options Neurol. 2008;10(2):126–37.

182. Kurkowska-Jastrzebska I, Wicha W, Dowzenko A, Vertun-Baranowska B, Pytlewski A, Boguslawska R, et al. Concomitant heterozygous factor V Leiden mutation and homozygous prothrombin gene variant (G20210A) in patient with cerebral venous thrombosis. Med Sci Monit. 2003;9(5):CS41–5.

183. Breteau G, Mounier-Vehier F, Godefroy O, Gauvrit JY, Mackowiak-Cordoliani MA, Girot M, et al. Cerebral venous

thrombosis 3-year clinical outcome in 55 consecutive patients. J Neurol. 2003;250(1):29–35.

184. de Bruijn SF, de Haan RJ, Stam J. Clinical features and prognostic factors of cerebral venous sinus thrombosis in a prospective series of 59 patients. For the cerebral venous sinus thrombosis study group. J Neurol Neurosurg Psychiatry. 2001;70(1):105–8.

185. Preter M, Tzourio C, Ameri A, Bousser MG. Long-term prognosis in cerebral venous thrombosis. Follow-up of 77 patients. Stroke. 1996;27(2):243–6.

186. Ferro JM, Canhao P, Stam J, Bousser MG, Barinagarrementeria F. Prognosis of cerebral vein and dural sinus thrombosis: results of the International Study on Cerebral Vein and Dural Sinus Thrombosis (ISCVT). Stroke. 2004;35(3):664–70.

187. Stolz E, Rahimi A, Gerriets T, Kraus J, Kaps M. Cerebral venous thrombosis: an all or nothing disease? Prognostic factors and long-term outcome. Clin Neurol Neurosurg. 2005;107(2):99–107.

188. Ribes M. Des recherches faites sur la phlebite. Revue Medicale Francaise et Etrangere et Journal de clinique de l' Hotel-Dieu et de la Charite de Paris. 1825;3:5–41.

189. Bousser MG, Chiras J, Bories J, Castaigne P. Cerebral venous thrombosis—a review of 38 cases. Stroke. 1985;16(2):199–213.

190. Terazzi E, Mittino D, Ruda R, Cerrato P, Monaco F, Sciolla R, et al. Cerebral venous thrombosis: a retrospective multicentre study of 48 patients. Neurol Sci. 2005;25(6):311–5.

191. Ferro JM, Correia M, Rosas MJ, Pinto AN, Neves G. Seizures in cerebral vein and dural sinus thrombosis. Cerebrovasc Dis. 2003;15(1–2):78–83.

192. Hubbert CH. Dural puncture headache suspected, cortical vein thrombosis diagnosed. Anesth Analg. 1987;66(3):285.

193. Ravindran RS, Zandstra GC, Viegas OJ. Postpartum headache following regional analgesia; a symptom of cerebral venous thrombosis. Can J Anaesth. 1989;36(6):705–7.

194. Schou J, Scherb M. Postoperative sagittal sinus thrombosis after spinal anesthesia. Anesth Analg. 1986;65(5):541–2.

195. Barinagarrementeria F, Cantu C, Arredondo H. Aseptic cerebral venous thrombosis: proposed prognostic scale. J Stroke Cerebrovasc Dis. 1992;2:34–9.

196. Kalita J, Chandra S, Misra UK. Significance of seizure in cerebral venous sinus thrombosis. Seizure. 2012;21(8):639–42.

197. de Bruijn SF, Stam J. Randomized, placebo-controlled trial of anticoagulant treatment with low-molecular-weight heparin for cerebral sinus thrombosis. Stroke. 1999;30(3):484–8.

198. Ferro JM, Lopes MG, Rosas MJ, Ferro MA, Fontes J. Long-term prognosis of cerebral vein and dural sinus thrombosis. results of the VENOPORT study. Cerebrovasc Dis. 2002;13(4):272–8.

199. Cakmak S, Derex L, Berruyer M, Nighoghossian N, Philippeau F, Adeleine P, et al. Cerebral venous thrombosis: clinical outcome and systematic screening of prothrombotic factors. Neurology. 2003;60(7):1175–8.

200. Masuhr F, Busch M, Amberger N, Ortwein H, Weih M, Neumann K, et al. Risk and predictors of early epileptic seizures in acute cerebral venous and sinus thrombosis. Eur J Neurol. 2006;13(8):852–6.

201. Ferro JM, Canhao P, Bousser MG, Stam J, Barinagarrementeria F. Early seizures in cerebral vein and dural sinus thrombosis: risk factors and role of antiepileptics. Stroke. 2008;39(4):1152–8.

202. Davoudi V, Keyhanian K, Saadatnia M. Risk factors for remote seizure development in patients with cerebral vein and dural sinus thrombosis. Seizure. 2014;23(2):135–9.

203. Kwan J, Guenther A. Antiepileptic drugs for the primary and secondary prevention of seizures after intracranial venous thrombosis. Cochrane Database Syst Rev. 2006;3:CD005501.

204. Einhaupl K, Stam J, Bousser MG, De Bruijn SF, Ferro JM, Martinelli I, et al. EFNS guideline on the treatment of cerebral venous and sinus thrombosis in adult patients. Eur J Neurol. 2010;17(10):1229–35.

205. Stam J, Majoie CB, van Delden OM, van Lienden KP, Reekers JA. Endovascular thrombectomy and thrombolysis for severe cerebral sinus thrombosis: a prospective study. Stroke. 2008;39(5):1487–90.

206. Mehraein S, Schmidtke K, Villringer A, Valdueza JM, Masuhr F. Heparin treatment in cerebral sinus and venous thrombosis: patients at risk of fatal outcome. Cerebrovasc Dis. 2003;15(1–2):17–21.

207. Niwa J, Ohyama H, Matumura S, Maeda Y, Shimizu T. Treatment of acute superior sagittal sinus thrombosis by t-PA infusion via venography—direct thrombolytic therapy in the acute phase. Surg Neurol. 1998;49(4):425–9.

208. Gerszten PC, Welch WC, Spearman MP, Jungreis CA, Redner RL. Isolated deep cerebral venous thrombosis treated by direct endovascular thrombolysis. Surg Neurol. 1997;48(3):261–6.

Hemorrhagic Stroke and Critical Care Seizures

Ali Mahta and Jan Claassen

Introduction

Seizures are a common complication of hemorrhagic stroke, which itself constitutes a wide variety of pathologies. The incidence of seizures after hemorrhagic stroke has been estimated to be higher than in ischemic strokes (Table 10.1) [1–3], but due to the heterogeneity of hemorrhagic strokes and lack of large observational or interventional trials many questions remain unanswered. Specifically, it is unclear how the pathophysiology of hemorrhages interplays with that of seizure activity and how treatment of either affects the overall outcome. Recent developments in continuous video EEG monitoring techniques particularly in the critical care settings suggest that electrographic seizures and status epilepticus are far more common than previously thought. Anti-epileptic prophylaxis as well as short- and long-term treatment of seizures following hemorrhagic strokes is controversial. The main focus of this chapter is to discuss clinical and in particular intensive care aspects of seizures in various types of hemorrhagic strokes in clinical practice.

A. Mahta
Division of Neurological Intensive Care, Department of Neurology, Columbia University College of Physicians and Surgeon, New York, NY 10032, USA
e-mail: am4370@cumc.columbia.edu

J. Claassen (✉)
Neurocritical Care, Columbia University College of Physicians and Surgeons, New York, NY, USA

Division of Critical Care and Hospitalist Neurology, Department of Neurology, Columbia

University Medical Center, New York Presbyterian Hospital, New York, NY, USA
e-mail: jc1439@columbia.edu

Subarachnoid Hemorrhage

Aneurysmal subarachnoid hemorrhage (SAH) accounts for about 3% of all strokes but it is associated with a high mortality and morbidity, typically affecting patients in the midst of their productivity. Approximately 10–15% of patients with aneurysmal SAH die within the first minutes or hours after hemorrhage, even before reaching a medical center [4]. Outcomes of aneurysmal SAH are better for patients that are treated at high volume medical facilities that have both neurosurgical and endovascular techniques available and treated more than 100 patients per year [5]. Case-fatality rates have been trending down over the past decade as a result of early securing of the aneurysm, better detection of complications including early treatment of hydrocephalus and delayed cerebral ischemia, and neurocritical care management in general [6]. For instance, Hop JW et al. demonstrated an 8% decline in case-fatality rate of aneurysmal SAH per decade between 1960 and 1992 [7]. Similar observation was made by Vergouwen MD et al. in a recent study which showed ninety-day case fatality in 2009–2012 compared to 1999–2002 period [8]. This also supports the value of neurointensive care in improvement of outcome of these patients.

Seizures are a well-known complication of SAH. The incidence of early and late convulsive seizures after SAH has been, respectively, reported to be 1.1–16% [9, 10] and 5.1–25% of patients [11, 12] in literature depending on the definition used. Seizures may occur at different stages of the disease, including at the time of initial presentation typically prior to hospital admission, within 2 weeks of ictus during the ICU or hospital stay, and in a delayed fashion up to years post-SAH [13]. Less frequently, seizure may be seen due to unruptured cerebral aneurysms. Kamali AW et al. reported five patients with complex partial seizures that were found to have cerebral aneurysms arising from middle cerebral or internal carotid arteries adjacent to the presumed epileptogenic area. The mechanisms implicated were calcification of the aneurysmal wall with compression or ischemia in the

P.N. Varelas, J. Claassen (eds.), *Seizures in Critical Care*, Current Clinical Neurology, DOI 10.1007/978-3-319-49557-6_10

Table 10.1 Different subtypes of hemorrhagic stroke and estimated risk of seizures

Hemorrhagic stroke subtype	Estimated risk of seizure (%)
Cerebral venous thrombosis	47–50
Cavernous malformation	23–79
Arteriovenous malformation	16–53
Subarachnoid hemorrhage	1.1–25
Hemorrhagic conversion of ischemic stroke	12
Intracerebral hemorrhage	8

adjacent tissue or distal emboli originating from the aneurysm itself [14].

Convulsive seizures after SAH have been associated with worse admission neurological function expressed as a higher aneurysm grade based on the Hunt Hess or World Federation of Neurosurgical Societies Scale [or lower Glasgow Coma Scale (GCS)], larger amount of subarachnoid blood on head CT scan, rebleeding of the aneurysm, and overall poor outcome [15, 16]. Seizures can also occur following the treatment of aneurysms. In the International Subarachnoid Aneurysm Trial (ISAT) trial, it has been showed that the risk of seizure is higher in patients who undergo surgical clipping than those patients who get endovascular coiling [17].

In two studies with aneurysmal SAH, the highest incidence of seizure was in anterior cerebral or communicating artery aneurysms, followed by middle cerebral artery aneurysms [18, 19]. In addition to the direct effect of SAH on seizure incidence as the result of cortical irritation from blood products, surgical or less likely endovascular treatment of an aneurysm may also contribute to early post-procedure seizures or epilepsy. Chang TR et al. conducted a prospective study of 1134 patients with aneurysmal SAH. Overall, 16% of 182 patients developed seizures, which were more frequently seen in younger patients (<40 years old), those with poor clinical grade, that also had intracerebral hemorrhage, MCA location of the aneurysm, and cocaine use [20].

Hyponatremia, which is a common electrolyte abnormality in patients with SAH, as a result of either cerebral salt wasting or SIADH, may lower seizure threshold after SAH. In a retrospective study of 316 patients with SAH, Sherlock M et al. showed that 179 patients (56.6%) developed hyponatremia (defined as serum sodium less than 135 mmol/L), which was due to SIADH in most of the patients (69%). Seizures developed in 14.5% of 62 patients with serum sodium less than 130 mmol/L, but in this study there was no significant difference in the incidence of seizures between patients with severe hyponatremia or plasma sodium less than 125 mmol/L (3/18) and patients with mild hyponatremia or plasma sodium between 125 and 130 mmol/L (6/44). Overall, hyponatremia was associated with longer hospital course, but it did not independently affect mortality [21].

Continuous EEG monitoring may detect non-convulsive status epilepticus (NCSE) as a cause of unexplained alteration of mental status or coma in SAH patients. Based on multiple studies, the rate of non-convulsive seizures and NCSE in patients with aneurysmal SAH has been estimated to be 7–18% and 3–13%, respectively (Kondziella, Claassen, Claassen) [22–24]. In poor grade SAH patients non-convulsive seizures may be particularly difficult to detect clinically. Dennis et al. found that almost every third patient with poor grade SAH and unexplained alteration of consciousness who underwent continuous video EEG monitoring was in NCSE. All of these patients received prophylactic anti-epileptics at the time of admission. Four patients were persistently comatose and four revealed deterioration to stupor or coma; only one demonstrated overt generalized tonic-clonic seizure before entering to coma; two patients had subtle eye blinking and facial twitching. NCSE was successfully treated for five patients (63%), but only one experienced clinical improvement, which was transient. In this small study, the mortality rate was 100% in all patients after a period of prolonged coma [25]. NCSE in SAH patients has been associated with older age (mean age 68 years) and high mortality (82–100%) [22]. The following risk factors for NCSE were identified in another study done by Claassen et al.: poor Hunt and Hess grade (IV or V), older age, ventricular drainage, and cerebral edema on CT [26]. In addition to seizures recorded on the surface recent studies indicate that focal seizures may be even more frequently recorded on invasive brain monitoring comatose SAH patients using depth electrodes [26].

EEG monitoring, initially used primarily to detect electrographic seizures, is now routinely applied for many SAH patients and has revealed a number of additional EEG patterns. Some of these, such as periodic discharges, while associated with poor outcome, are of uncertain significance and what is not clear is that their aggressive treatment affects outcome. In a prospective study of 756 patients with SAH, certain EEG findings on continuous video EEG monitoring during the time of hospitalization were associated with poor outcome. These EEG findings include the absence of sleep architecture, the presence of periodic lateralized epileptiform discharges (PLEDs), bilateral independent lateralized epileptiform discharges (BiPLEDs), and NCSE [24]. Interestingly, aside from seizure detection, continuous video EEG monitoring in patients with poor grade SAH can provide a diagnostic tool for detection of cerebral ischemia due to vasospasm as predictable EEG changes are observed with decreasing brain perfusion [23, 27, 28].

In the recent guidelines for the management of patients with SAH published by American Heart Association, it is recommended to use anti-epileptics for seizure prophylaxis for 3–7 days following the bleed (Class IIb; Level of Evidence B) [6]. The main reason for prophylactic use of anti-epileptics after SAH in the ICU setting is to decrease the likelihood of catastrophic events such as aneurysm re-rupture and ICP crisis which are usually associated with high mortality and morbidity. In addition, seizures may cause increasing cerebral metabolism in an already stressed brain after acute injury, which may precipitate additional brain injury. Following acute brain injury such as subarachnoid hemorrhage, increased metabolism and blood flow have been demonstrated with the onset of non-convulsive seizures. Interestingly, brain oxygen may drop, intracranial pressure may rise rapidly, but regional cerebral blood flow may increase only minutes and not seconds after the onset of the seizure [26, 29]. One possible explanation for these observations may be that seizures cause more damage in acutely brain injured patients than in those with epilepsy, damaging intrinsic defense mechanisms such as vasoreactivity.

Most series exploring the benefits of seizure prophylaxis after SAH studied the effects of phenytoin, which was associated with worse functional and cognitive outcomes in non-controlled case series [30, 31]. Phenytoin, metabolized by the hepatic cytochrome P450-3A4 system, increases the metabolism of the calcium channel antagonist nimodipine, therefore decreasing its bioavailability [32]. This is problematic since nimodipine is recommended based on clinical trials (Class I; Level of Evidence A) as a treatment to decreased morbidity from delayed cerebral ischemia [6]. With more favorable safety profiles, newer AEDs, such as levetiracetam, are increasingly used for seizure prophylaxis following SAH. In a recent survey from 25 centers in the USA, levetiracetam was used in 94% as the anti-epileptic agent of choice for seizure prophylaxis in SAH [33].

Early identification and treatment of seizures or status epilepticus (SE) is of paramount importance and should be achieved as soon as possible to avoid refractory or super-refractory status epilepticus. The first line agents in standard protocol for treatment of SE are parenteral lorazepam or midazolam. The second line treatment includes intravenous fosphenytoin or phenytoin, valproate, levetiracetam, or lacosamide based on comorbidities, availability of medications, and preference. In case of failure of first and second line agents, the third line therapy should be initiated promptly in conjunction with video EEG monitoring in an intensive care unit. At this point, patients need to be intubated for airway protection. The third line treatment includes phenobarbital, another second line agent or intravenous anesthetics such as midazolam, propofol, pentobarbital, or ketamine [34].

Intracerebral Hemorrhage

Spontaneous intracerebral hemorrhage (ICH) or intraparenchymal hemorrhage constitutes about 15% of all strokes and is associated with high mortality and morbidity. The most common causes of spontaneous ICH include hypertension, amyloid angiopathy, hemorrhagic conversion of ischemic stroke, arteriovenous malformation (AVM), cavernous malformation, other vascular abnormalities, and hemorrhagic complications of primary or metastatic brain tumors [35]. Aggressive management of secondary complications has been associated with improved outcomes after ICH.

Seizures are common following ICH with an estimated 30-day risk of 8% [36]. Most seizures (90%) occur in first 72 h of admission but delayed seizures and later development of epilepsy are also seen [37]. Neshige S et al. most recently performed a retrospective study of 1920 patients with ICH over a period of 8 years [38]. These researchers observed that the rate of seizures was 6.6% (127/1920) and more specifically 4.3% for early seizures (defined as seizures within one week of ICH onset) and 2.3% for late seizures (those occurring after the first week from ICH onset). Use of continuous video EEG monitoring in neuro-ICUs has played a major role in detecting and appropriately treating subclinical non-convulsive seizures in ICH, which are estimated at 18 to 28% [39–41].

A number of characteristics increase the risk of convulsive seizures in ICH including lobar hemorrhage (particularly non-occipital and juxtacortical locations), hematoma size, low GCS, focal neurologic deficit, presence of hydrocephalus, and midline shift on CT head (Bladin CF, 2000; De Reuck J, 2007; Weisberg LA, 1991). In multivariate analyses, the following were significantly associated with the development of both convulsive and non-convulsive seizures following ICH: cortical location of the ICH (odds ratio 7.37, 95% CI 4.77–11.45); non-hypertensive etiology (1.63, 1.02–2.56); high NIH stroke scale at the time of admission (1.04, 1.02–1.05), and younger age (0.97, 0.96–0.98). Interestingly, hematoma volume was the only independent factor associated with recurrence of seizures (1.02, 1.001–1.023) [38].

The association between ICH-related early seizures and prognosis or functional outcome has been recently studied. Brüning et al. in a retrospective study of 484 patients with spontaneous non-traumatic ICH from a single institution showed that there was no statistically significant association between early seizures and functional outcome measured by modified Rankin Scale (mRS) [42]. De Herdt et al. in a prospective study of 562 patients with spontaneous ICH found that early seizures did not affect functional outcome at 6 months [43]. Electrographic seizures, on the other hand, were associated with poor overall 3 months outcome and hematoma expansion [40] and increasing midline shift [43].

The underlying pathophysiology of seizures after ICH depends on the time that seizures are first recorded. Early onset seizures which occur within 2 weeks of ICH are primarily caused by anatomical destruction due to mass effects of hematoma and also biochemical disruption at the cellular level [3]. Delayed seizures that occur after 2 weeks of ICH onset are thought to be related to gliosis and chemico-cellular repair processes creating an epileptogenic focus [3, 40].

The role of seizure prophylaxis, choice of anti-epileptic agent, and its duration are controversial in the absence of randomized clinical trials. In the past, prophylactic AEDs were recommended for 30 days after lobar ICH [44, 45]; however, this is not generally accepted by many authorities any more. Based on the most recent American Heart Association guidelines regarding the management of ICH, prophylactic AEDs are not recommended (Class III, level of evidence B) [46]. Naidech AM et al. in a prospective study of 98 patients with ICH showed that prophylactic use of phenytoin was associated with poor functional outcome defined as mRS of 3–6 [47]. Gilad R et al. in a small randomized clinical trial of 72 patients with ICH showed that 7 patients of the treatment group (total 36) and 8 patients of the placebo group (total 36) developed seizures within a 1 year follow-up period, a non-significant difference. They concluded that prophylactic treatment with valproic acid for 1 month following ICH did not prevent seizures in 1 year follow-up [48]. Sheth KN et al. performed a prospective cohort study of 744 ICH patients. AEDs, mainly levetiracetam (89%), were prescribed for seizure prophylaxis in 289 (39%) patients. The authors found that use of prophylactic AEDs was associated with poor outcome in an unadjusted model (O.R 1.4; 95% CI 1.04–1.88); however, after adjusting for clinical data including age, hematoma volume, GCS, IVH presence, and lobar hemorrhage in multivariate logistic regression, no significant association was found (1.11, 0.74–1.65) [49].

Continuous video EEG monitoring is recommended in ICH patients with unexplained alteration of level of consciousness or any suspicion for subclinical seizures (Class IIa; level of evidence C) [46]. Brain hemorrhages themselves may cause alterations of EEG rhythms depending on their location, Delta activity may be observed over the affected hemisphere in deep capsular/basal ganglia hemorrhages, at times arising in rhythmic runs of moderate amplitude [50, 51]. Thalamic hemorrhages may be associated with ipsilateral delta activity, a reduction or enhancement of the alpha rhythm depending on the precise location within the thalamus, and absence of sleep spindles [50, 52]. Bleeds located in the mesencephalic area may cause diffuse theta activity [50]. Hemorrhages in the mid-lower brainstem can lead to diffuse attenuation or a lack of reactivity [50, 53].

Arteriovenous Malformations

Arteriovenous malformations (AVM) present frequently before age 40 and they are almost equally distributed between men and women. The most common indication for ICU admission for AVMs is ICH, which is seen in 30–82% of patients. The most common clinical presentations of cerebral AVMs include ICH, seizures, headache, and focal neurologic deficits [54]. The rate of seizure as initial manifestation of AVMs has been estimated to be about 16–53%. Seizures associated with the presence of an AVM can occur as a result of: (1) secondary ICH; (2) unruptured AVMs causing epileptogenesis in the surrounding brain tissue; (3) treatment, including post-surgical resection, post-endovascular coiling or even stereotactic radiosurgery [55–60]. In a prospective study of 229 patients with AVM, Josephson et al. found that the risk of developing epilepsy within 5 years after a first ever seizure was 58% (95% CI 40–76%). The risk of a first ever unprovoked seizure in 5 years was higher in patients with AVM and ICH or AVM with focal neurologic deficit compared to asymptomatic AVMs who were found incidentally (23%, 9–37% vs 8%0–20%) [61].

There are several factors that increase the risk for postoperative seizures in patients with AVMs. In a retrospective study, Hoh et al., a multidisciplinary neurovascular team, treated 424 patients with cerebral AVMs. One hundred forty-one (33%) of those had seizures before treatment. Follow-up data was available in 110 (78%) of these patients for a mean period of 2.9 years after treatment. Based on Engel Seizure Outcome Scale, there were 73 (66%) Class I (free of disabling seizures), 11 (10%) Class II (rare disabling seizures), 1 (0.9%) Class III (worthwhile improvement), and 22 (20%) Class IV (no worthwhile improvement) outcomes. Sixteen (5.7%) patients experienced new-onset seizures after treatment. A limited seizure history (<5 seizures before treatment), association of seizures with intracranial hemorrhage, generalized tonic-clonic seizure type, deep and posterior fossa AVM locations, surgical resection, and complete AVM obliteration were statistically associated with Class I outcomes. In the entire cohort, surgery resulted in seizure elimination in 81%, radiosurgery in 43%, and embolization in 50% of patients treated. When only completely obliterated AVMs were considered, no statistically significant differences between surgery, radiosurgery, and embolization were observed [62].

Other factors increasing the post-operative risk for seizures include age less than 30 years at seizure onset, preoperative seizure duration greater than 12 months, AVM size greater than 3 cm, location in the medial temporal or peri-Rolandic cortex, and previous hemorrhage or hemosiderin deposition [63–66].

Treatment for AVM-related seizures is controversial. In a recent meta-analysis, Josephson et al. concluded that it is still unclear whether invasive treatment for AVM-related seizures is superior to AEDs or not. Interestingly, there is still no randomized clinical trial to compare invasive treatment versus medical management for AVM-related seizures, probably because the focus of the treatment is to obliterate the AVM and decrease the risk for bleeding instead of treating seizures [67].

Cavernous Malformations

Cerebral cavernous malformation (CCM) consists of a tangle of blood vessels which lack elastic and muscular layers without intervening brain tissue. In addition, the endothelial cells are not connected together via tight junctions causing them susceptible to hemorrhage (Al-Shahi Salman R, 2012). CCMs can occur sporadically or be familial with an autosomal dominance inheritance pattern with incomplete penetrance and variable clinical presentations. Their overall incidence has been reported to be around 0.5% in the general population. The most common clinical presentation of CCMs is seizures, which occur in 23–79% of patients [68–70]. ICH is another frequent complication of CCMs, particularly in Hispanic patients, and this may also lead to seizures [71]. Of those patients who present with seizures, 40% develop medically refractory epilepsy for which surgical resection is the treatment of choice [72]. The exact mechanism of epileptogenesis in CCM is still unclear. It has been hypothesized that chronic microhemorrhages from the CCM causes deposition of hemosiderin, a blood degradation product, in the adjacent brain tissue. Hemosiderin can irritate the brain parenchyma by generating free radicals and lipid peroxides causing excitotoxicity on the adjacent neuronal tissues [73, 74]. Based on a recent meta-analysis, total surgical resection of CCMs including complete removal of the hemosiderin ring is associated with better seizure control compared to surgical resection without excision of the hemosiderin ring [75].

Ischemic Stroke with Hemorrhagic Conversion

Ischemic stroke and seizures in critical care is extensively discussed in a separate chapter. In this section we present data about seizures associated with hemorrhagic conversion of an ischemic stroke. Hemorrhagic transformation of an ischemic stroke can range from subtle asymptomatic petechial hemorrhages found on neuroimaging to large clinically significant (symptomatic) hematomas extending within or beyond the infarcted area [76]. In a prospective cohort study of 714 patients with stroke, Beghi et al. have reported that compared to cerebral infarction, primary ICH carried the highest risk (OR 7.2, 95% CI 3.5–14.9) for symptomatic seizures within 7 days of stroke onset followed by cerebral infarction with hemorrhagic stroke transformation (2.7, 0.8–9.6) [77]. In another prospective study of 2053 patients with stroke (both ischemic and hemorrhagic) over a period of four years, Procaccianti et al. found that 64 patients presented with seizures within the first week from stroke onset. They described the following factors as independent seizure predictors in patients with stroke: total anterior circulation infarcts, hemorrhagic transformation, cortical location of the lesion, and hyperglycemia in patients without diabetes [78]. Zhang et al. performed a meta-analysis to evaluate risk factors for seizures in patients with stroke. The following risk factors were significantly associated with the development of early seizures in all stroke patients: intracerebral hemorrhage (OR = 1.88, 95% CI 1.43–2.47), cerebral infarction with hemorrhagic transformation (3.28, 2.09–5.16), stroke severity (3.10, 2.00–4.81), and alcoholism (1.70, 1.23–2.34). On the other hand, cortical involvement (2.50, 1.93–3.23) and stroke severity (5.72, 4.23–7.22) were significantly associated with late onset seizures. Interestingly, there was no significant difference in the probability of single late onset seizure episode between patients with ICH and ischemic stroke (1.20, 0.92–1.55) [79].

Lastly, the treatment modality of ischemic stroke and its hemorrhagic complications may affect the development of seizures. In a prospective study of 805 patients with stroke treated endovascularly, 44 (5.5%) patients had seizures between stroke onset and 3-month follow-up (26 patients had early and 18 had late seizures). Early seizures (within the first 24 h from stroke onset) were independently predicted by asymptomatic ICH (OR 2.763, 95% CI, 1.185–6.442). Early seizures were also independently associated with unfavorable outcome (4.7, 0.376–3.914), similarly to symptomatic ICH (4.749, 0.376–3.914) [80]. It is unknown whether there is any potential benefit from prophylactic anticonvulsive treatment in patients receiving endovascular therapy for acute stroke, particularly for those with hemorrhagic conversion.

Conclusion

In summary, both convulsive and non-convulsive electrographic seizures are common complications of various types of hemorrhagic strokes. The risk of both early and late development of clinical or electrographic seizures mainly depends on the mechanism of hemorrhagic stroke and also its anatomical location. Early identification of electrographic seizures and status epilepticus using video EEG monitoring mostly in neurocritical care units has been associated with more aggressive treatment and in general better outcomes in most cases.

References

1. Giroud M, Gras P, Fayolle H, Andre N, Soichot P, Dumas R. Early seizures after acute stroke: a study of 1,640 cases. Epilepsia. 1994;35:959–64.
2. Lancman ME, Golimstok A, Norscini J, Granillo R. Risk factors for developing seizures after a stroke. Epilepsia. 1993;34:141–3.

3. Bladin CF, Alexandrov AV, Bellavance A, Bornstein N, Chambers B, Cote R, et al. Seizures after stroke: a prospective multicenter study. Arch Neurol. 2000;57:1617–22.
4. Huang J, Van Gelder JM. The probability of sudden death from rupture of intracranial aneurysms: a meta-analysis. Neurosurgery. 2002;51:1101–7.
5. Rinkel GJ. Management of patients with aneurysmal subarachnoid haemorrhage. Curr Opin Neurol 2016 Feb;29(1):37–41.
6. Connolly Jr ES, Rabinstein AA, Carhuapoma JR, et al. Guidelines for the management of aneurysmal subarachnoid hemorrhage: a guideline for healthcare professionals from the American Heart Association/American Stroke Association. Stroke. 2012;43(6):1711.
7. Hop JW, Rinkel GJ, Algra A, van Gijn J. Case-fatality rates and functional outcome after subarachnoid hemorrhage: a systematic review. Stroke. 1997;28(3):660–4.
8. Vergouwen MD, Jong-Tjien-Fa AV, Algra A, Rinkel GJ. Time trends in causes of death after aneurysmal subarachnoid hemorrhage: a hospital-based study. Neurology. 2016;86(1):59–63.
9. Byrne JV, Boardman P, Ioannidis I, Adcock J, Traill Z. Seizures after aneurysmal subarachnoid hemorrhage treated with coil embolization. Neurosurgery. 2003;52:545–52.
10. Pinto AN, Canhao P, Ferro JM. Seizures at the onset of subarachnoid haemorrhage. J Neurol. 1996;243:161–4.
11. Olafsson E, Gudmundsson G, Hauser WA. Risk of epilepsy in long-term survivors of surgery for aneurysmal subarachnoid hemorrhage: a population-based study in Iceland. Epilepsia. 2000;41:1201–5.
12. Keranen T, Tapaninaho A, Hernesniemi J, Vapalahti M. Late epilepsy after aneurysm operations. Neurosurgery. 1985;17:897–900.
13. Marigold R, Günther A, Tiwari D, Kwan J. Antiepileptic drugs for the primary and secondary prevention of seizures after subarachnoid haemorrhage. Cochrane Database Syst Rev. 2013;6:CD008710.
14. Kamali AW, Cockerell OC, Butlar P. Aneurysms and epilepsy: an increasingly recognised cause. Seizure. 2004;13:40–4.
15. Raper DM, Starke RM, Komotar RJ, Allan R, Connolly Jr ES. Seizures after aneurysmal subarachnoid hemorrhage: a systematic review of outcomes. World Neurosurg. 2013;79(5–6):682–90.
16. Butzkueven H, Evans AH, Pitman A, Leopold C, Jolley DJ, Kaye AH, et al. Onset seizures independently predict poor outcome after subarachnoid hemorrhage. Neurology. 2000;55:1315–20.
17. Molyneux AJ, Kerr RS, Yu LM, Clarke M, Sneade M, Yarnold JA. International subarachnoid aneurysm trial (ISAT) of neurosurgical clipping vs. endovascular coiling in 2143 patients with ruptured intracranial aneurysms: a randomised comparison of effects on survival, dependency, seizures, rebleeding, subgroups, and aneurysm occlusion. Lancet. 2005;366:809–17.
18. Hasan D, Schonck RS, Avezaat CJ, Tanghe HL, van Gijn J, van der Lugt PJ. Epileptic seizures after subarachnoid hemorrhage. Ann Neurol. 1993;33:286–91.
19. Rhoney DH, Tipps LB, Murry KR, Basham MC, Michael DB, Coplin WM. Anticonvulsant prophylaxis and timing of seizures after aneurysmal subarachnoid hemorrhage. Neurology. 2000;55:258–65.
20. Chang TR, Kowalski RG, Carhuapoma JR, Tamargo RJ, Naval NS. Cocaine use as an independent predictor of seizures after aneurysmal subarachnoid hemorrhage. J Neurosurg. 2016 Mar;124(3):730–5.
21. Sherlock M, O'Sullivan E, Agha A, Behan LA, Rawluk D, Brennan P, et al. The incidence and pathophysiology of hyponatraemia after subarachnoid haemorrhage. Clin Endocrinol. 2006;64:250–4.
22. Kondziella D, Friberg CK, Wellwood I, Reiffurth C, Fabricius M, Dreier JP. Continuous EEG monitoring in aneurysmal subarachnoid hemorrhage: a systematic review. Neurocrit Care. 2015;22(3):450–61.
23. Claassen J, Mayer SA, Kowalski RG, et al. Detection of electrographic seizures with continuous EEG monitoring in critically ill patients. Neurology. 2004;62:1743–8.
24. Claassen J, Hirsch LJ, Frontera JA, Fernandez A, Schmidt M, et al. Prognostic significance of continuous EEG monitoring in patients with poor grade subarachnoid hemorrhage. Neurocrit Care. 2006;4(2):103–12.
25. Dennis LJ, Claassen J, Hirsch LJ, Emerson RG, Connolly ES, Mayer SA. Nonconvulsive status epilepticus after subarachnoid hemorrhage. Neurosurgery. 2002;51:1136–43. discussion 1144
26. Claassen J, Perotte A, Albers D, et al. Nonconvulsive seizures after subarachnoid hemorrhage: multimodal detection and outcomes. Ann Neurol. 2013;74:53–64.
27. Vespa PM, Nuwer MR, Juhász C, et al. Early detection of vasospasm after acute subarachnoid hemorrhage using continuous EEG ICU monitoring. Electroencephalogr Clin Neurophysiol. 1997;103(6):607–15.
28. Rots ML, van Putten MJ, Hoedemaekers CW, Horn J. Continuous EEG monitoring for early detection of delayed cerebral ischemia in subarachnoid hemorrhage: a pilot study. Neurocrit Care. 2016 Apr;24(2):207–16.
29. Kishore S, Ko N, Soares BP, Higashi da RT, et al. Perfusion-CT assessment of blood-brain barrier permeability in patients with aneurysmal subarachnoid hemorrhage. J Neuroradiol. 2012;39(5):317–25.
30. Naidech AM, Kreiter KT, Janjua N, Ostapkovich N, Parra A, Commichau C, Connolly ES, Mayer SA, Fitzsimmons BF. Phenytoin exposure is associated with functional and cognitive disability after subarachnoid hemorrhage. Stroke. 2005;36:583–7.
31. Rosengart AJ, Huo JD, Tolentino J, et al. Outcome in patients with subarachnoid hemorrhage treated with antiepileptic drugs. J Neurosurg. 2007;107(2):253–60.
32. Wong GK, Poon WS. Use of phenytoin and other anticonvulsant prophylaxis in patients with aneurysmal subarachnoid hemorrhage. Stroke. 2005;36:2532. author reply 2532
33. Dewan MC, Mocco J. Current practice regarding seizure prophylaxis in aneurysmal subarachnoid hemorrhage across academic centers. J Neurointerv Surg. 2015;7(2):146–9.
34. Brophy GM, Bell R, Claassen J, et al. Guidelines for the evaluation and management of status epilepticus. Neurocrit Care. 2012;17(1):3–23.
35. Fiorella D, Zuckerman SL, Khan IS, Ganesh NK, Mocco J. Intracerebral hemorrhage: a common and devastating disease in need of better treatment. World Neurosurg. 2015;84(4):1136–41.
36. Passero S, Rocchi R, Rossi S, Ulivelli M, Vatti G. Seizures after spontaneous supratentorial intracerebral hemorrhage. Epilepsia. 2002;43:1175–80.
37. Balami JS, Buchan AM. Complications of intracerebral haemorrhage. Lancet Neurol. 2012;11(1):101–18.
38. Neshige S, Kuriyama M, Yoshimoto T, et al. Seizures after intracerebral hemorrhage; risk factor, recurrence, efficacy of antiepileptic drug. J Neurol Sci. 2015;359(1–2):318–22.
39. Claassen J, Riviello Jr JJ, Silbergleit R. Emergency neurological life support: status epilepticus. Neurocrit Care. 2015;23(Suppl 2):136–42.
40. Claassen J, Jetté N, Chum F, et al. Electrographic seizures and periodic discharges after intracerebral hemorrhage. Neurology. 2007;69:1356–65.
41. Vespa PM, O'Phelan K, Shah M, et al. Acute seizures after intracerebral hemorrhage: a factor in progressive midline shift and outcome. Neurology. 2003;60:1441–6.
42. Brüning T, Awwad S, Al-Khaled M. Do early seizures indicate survival of patients with nontraumatic intracerebral hemorrhage? Cerebrovasc Dis. 2015;41(1–2):68–73.
43. De Herdt V, Dumont F, Hénon H, et al. Early seizures in intracerebral hemorrhage: incidence, associated factors, and outcome. Neurology. 2011;77(20):1794–800.
44. Broderick J, Connolly S, Feldmann E, et al. Guidelines for the management of spontaneous intracerebral hemorrhage in adults: 2007 update: a guideline from the American Heart Association/American

Stroke Association Stroke Council, High Blood Pressure Research Council, and the Quality of Care and Outcomes in Research Interdisciplinary Working Group. Stroke. 2007;38:2001–23.

45. Steiner T, Kaste M, Forsting M, et al. Recommendations for the management of intracranial haemorrhage—Part I: spontaneous intracerebral haemorrhage. The European stroke initiative writing committee and the writing committee for the EUSI executive committee. Cerebrovasc Dis. 2006;22:294–316.

46. Hemphill 3rd JC, Greenberg SM, Anderson CS, et al. Guidelines for the management of spontaneous intracerebral hemorrhage: a guideline for healthcare professionals from the American heart association/American stroke association. Stroke. 2015;46(7):2032–60.

47. Naidech AM, Garg RK, Liebling S, et al. Anticonvulsant use and outcomes after intracerebral hemorrhage. Stroke. 2009;40:3810–5.

48. Gilad R, Boaz M, Dabby R, Sadeh M, Lampl Y. Are post intracerebral hemorrhage seizures prevented by anti-epileptic treatment? Epilepsy Res. 2011;95(3):227–31.

49. Sheth KN, Martini SR, Moomaw CJ, et al. Prophylactic antiepileptic drug use and outcome in the ethnic/racial variations of intracerebral hemorrhage study. Stroke. 2015;46(12):3532–5.

50. Niedermeyer E. Cerebrovascular disorders and EEG. In: Niedermeyer E, Lopes da Silva F, (eds). Electroencephalography. 5th. Baltimore: Urban & Schwarzenberg, 2005. p. 339–362.

51. Hirose G, Saeki M, Kosoegawa H, et al. Delta waves in the EEGs of patients with intracerebral hemorrhage. Arch Neurol. 1981;38:170–5.

52. Jasper HH, Van Buren J. Interrelationship between cortex and subcortical structures: clinical electroencephalographic studies. Electroencephalogr Clin Neurophys. 1953;4:168–88.

53. Loeb C, Rosadini G, Poggio GF. Electroencephalograms during coma; normal and borderline records in 5 patients. Neurology. 1959;9:610–8.

54. Brown Jr RD, Wiebers DO, Torner JC, O'Fallon WM. Frequency of intracranial hemorrhage as a presenting symptom and subtype analysis: a population-based study of intracranial vascular malformations in Olmsted Country, Minnesota. J Neurosurg. 1996;85:29–32.

55. Ogilvy CS, Stieg PE, Awad I, Brown Jr RD, Kondziolka D, Rosenwasser R, et al. AHA Scientific Statement: Recommendations for the management of intracranial arteriovenous malformations: a statement for healthcare professionals from a special writing group of the Stroke Council, American Stroke Association. Stroke. 2001;32.1458–71.

56. Crawford PM, West CR, Shaw MD, Chadwick DW. Cerebral arteriovenous malformations and epilepsy: factors in the development of epilepsy. Epilepsia. 1986;27:270–5.

57. Mast H, Mohr JP, Osipov A, Pile-Spellman J, Marshall RS, Lazar RM, et al. 'Steal' is an unestablished mechanism for the clinical presentation of cerebral arteriovenous malformations. Stroke. 1995;26:1215–20.

58. Murphy MJ. Long-term follow-up of seizures associated with cerebral arteriovenous malformations. Results Ther Arch Neurol. 1985;42:477–9.

59. Osipov A, Koennecke HC, Hartmann A. Seizures in cerebral arteriovenous malformations: type, clinical course, and medical management. Interv Neuroradiol. 1997;3:37–41.

60. Turjman F, Massoud TF, Sayre JW, Vinuela F, Guglielmi G, Duckwiler G. Epilepsy associated with cerebral arteriovenous malformations: a multivariate analysis of angioarchitectural characteristics. AJNR Am J Neuroradiol. 1995;16:345–50.

61. Josephson CB, Leach JP, Duncan R, Roberts RC, Counsell CE, Salman RAS. Seizure risk from cavernous or arteriovenous malfor-

mations: prospective population based study. Neurology. 2011;76:1548–54.

62. Hoh BL, Chapman PH, Loeffler JS, Carter BS, Ogilvy CS. Results of multimodality treatment for 141 patients with brain arteriovenous malformations and seizures: factors associated with seizure incidence and seizure outcomes. Neurosurgery. 2002;51:303–9. discussion 309–311.

63. Yeh HS, Privitera MD. Secondary epileptogenesis in cerebral arteriovenous malformations. Arch Neurol. 1991;48:1122–4.

64. Kraemer DL, Awad IA. Vascular malformations and epilepsy: clinical considerations and basic mechanisms. Epilepsia. 1994;35(Suppl 6):S30–43.

65. Piepgras DG, Sundt Jr TM, Ragoowansi AT, Stevens L. Seizure outcome in patients with surgically treated cerebral arteriovenous malformations. J Neurosurg. 1993;78:5–11.

66. Yeh HS, Tew Jr JM, Gartner M. Seizure control after surgery on cerebral arteriovenous malformations. J Neurosurg. 1993;78:12–8.

67. Josephson CB, Sauro K, Wiebe S, Clement F, Jette N. Medical vs invasive therapy in AVM-related epilepsy: systematic review and meta-analysis. Neurology. 2016 Jan 5;86(1):64–71.

68. Chang EF, Gabriel RA, Potts MB, Garcia PA, Barbaro NM, Lawton MT. Seizure characteristics and control after microsurgical resection of supratentorial cerebral cavernous malformations. Neurosurgery. 2009;65(1):31–7. discussion 7–8

69. Moran NF, Fish DR, Kitchen N, Shorvon S, Kendall BE, Stevens JM. Supratentorial cavernous haemangiomas and epilepsy: a review of the literature and case series. J Neurol Neurosurg Psychiatry. 1999;66(5):561–8.

70. Kondziolka D, Lunsford LD, Kestle JRW. The natural history of cerebral cavernous malformations. J Neurosurg. 1995;83(5):822–4.

71. Bruno A, Qualls C. Risk factors for intracerebral and subarachnoid hemorrhage among Hispanics and non-Hispanic whites in a New Mexico community. Neuroepidemiology. 2000;19:227–32.

72. Englot DJ, Han SJ, Lawton MT, Chang EF. Predictors of seizure freedom in the surgical treatment of supratentorial cavernous malformations. J Neurosurg. 2011;115(6):1169–74.

73. Williamson A, Patrylo PR, Lee S, Spencer DD. Physiology of human cortical neurons adjacent to cavernous malformations and tumors. Epilepsia. 2003;44(11):1413–9.

74. Awad IA, Robinson Jr JR, Mohanty S, Estes ML. Mixed vascular malformations of the brain: clinical and pathogenetic considerations. Neurosurgery. 1993;33(2):179–88. discussion 188

75. Ruan D, Yu XB, Shrestha S, Wang L, Chen G. The role of hemosiderin excision in seizure outcome in cerebral cavernous malformation surgery: a systematic review and meta-analysis. PLoS One. 2015;10(8):e0136619.

76. Sussman ES, Connolly Jr ES. Hemorrhagic transformation: a review of the rate of hemorrhage in the major clinical trials of acute ischemic stroke. Front Neurol. 2013;4:69.

77. Beghi E, D'Alessandro R, Beretta S, et al. Incidence and predictors of acute symptomatic seizures after stroke. Neurology. 2011;77(20):1785–93.

78. Procaccianti G, Zaniboni A, Rondelli F, Crisci M, Sacquegna T. Seizures in acute stroke: incidence, risk factors and prognosis. Neuroepidemiology. 2012;39(1):45–50.

79. Zhang C, Wang X, Wang Y, et al. Risk factors for post-stroke seizures: a systematic review and meta-analysis. Epilepsy Res. 2014;108(10):1806–16.

80. Jung S, Schindler K, Findling O, et al. Adverse effect of early epileptic seizures in patients receiving endovascular therapy for acute stroke. Stroke. 2012;43(6):1584–90.

Traumatic Brain Injury and Critical Care Seizures

Georgia Korbakis, Paul M. Vespa, and Andrew Beaumont

Introduction

Traumatic brain injury (TBI) is a serious public health concern in the United States. An estimated 1.7 to 2 million people suffer TBI annually leading to 1,365,000 emergency department visits per year. Of these visits, 275,000 result in hospitalization and 52,000 in death [1–3]. This incidence equates to one hospitalization per 1000 people each year [2]. Many of these patients are admitted to the intensive care unit (ICU) for initial stabilization and monitoring. The lifetime medical care costs of head injuries occurring in the United States in 1985 were estimated to total $4.5 billion, including $3.5 billion of hospital costs [4]. Seizures are a well-known complication of TBI with reported incidences for convulsive seizures ranging from 2 to 12% [5–13] and up to 33 % for nonconvulsive seizures [14, 15]. The incidence of seizures is higher in severe TBI and also with penetrating injury [6, 16]. Post-traumatic seizures are classified into immediate (<24 h), early, and late based on the relationship between the time of injury and time of seizure onset. The mechanisms that generate post-traumatic seizures are not known and there may be differences in the pathophysiology of early and late seizures. Post-traumatic epilepsy is defined as two or more unprovoked seizures following injury and must be viewed in a different perspective as a single post-TBI seizure [17].

One of the main goals of ICU care in TBI should be the prevention of physiological stresses that can worsen the initial injury. These secondary insults include hypoxia, hypo-tension, hyper-/hypoglycemia, hypo-/hyperperfusion, and neurotoxicity. Seizures are known to cause intense metabolic stress and also release significant quantities of neurotransmitters. Vespa et al. examined continuous EEG (cEEG) and microdialysis from ten patients with severe TBI and seizures with a matched cohort of ten patients without seizures [18]. Seizures were associated with a higher mean intracranial pressure and a higher mean lactate/pyruvate ratio.

Seizures therefore represent a potential for secondary insult, and some data demonstrates that seizures are associated with a worse outcome in TBI [19]. Thus, it is important to recognize seizures in patients with TBI and to treat them aggressively; care must also be given to diagnose nonconvulsive seizures promptly. Their significance in affecting outcome post-TBI is unknown, but they may be a potential risk factor for poor prognosis [20]. In addition, patients with recognized risk factors for post-traumatic seizures should receive anticonvulsant prophylaxis.

This chapter will review data regarding the incidence of post-traumatic seizures, particularly in the ICU population. Methods for diagnosing post-traumatic seizures will be reviewed, along with experimental data and current hypotheses regarding their pathophysiology. Methods of treating seizures in TBI and current recommendations for seizure prophylaxis will be discussed.

Incidence of Seizures in Traumatic Brain Injury

Estimates of the incidence of post-traumatic seizures have varied widely, ranging from 2 to 16% [6, 7, 13] of patients with clinically apparent seizures. These studies used clinical evidence of seizure activity for establishing the diagnosis, but electrographic seizures with minimal to no clinical correlation may be even more common. A recent prospective, non-randomized, non-blinded study using cEEG monitoring in the ICU found that 22% of moderately to severely injured TBI patients experienced seizures [14]. This study by Vespa et al.

G. Korbakis (✉) • P.M. Vespa
Department of Neurosurgery, UCLA David Geffen School of Medicine, 757 Westwood Blvd, RR UCLA # 6236, Los Angeles, CA 90095, USA
e-mail: georgiakorbakis@gmail.com; Pvespa@mednet.ucla.edu

A. Beaumont
Department of Neurosurgery, Aspirus Spine and Neuroscience Institute, Aspirus Wausau Hospital, 425 Pine Ridge Blvd #300, Wausau, WI 54401, CA, USA
e-mail: andrew.beaumont@aspirus.org

© Springer International Publishing AG 2017
P.N. Varelas, J. Claassen (eds.), *Seizures in Critical Care*, Current Clinical Neurology, DOI 10.1007/978-3-319-49557-6_11

examined 94 patients with moderate to severe TBI for up to 14 days post-injury. Of the 22% of patients with seizures, 52% had nonconvulsive or clinically silent seizures, and one third of the group had status epilepticus. Interestingly, except for one patient without any clinical seizure activity, the patients with status epilepticus had minimal clinical signs including rhythmic facial twitching, eyelid fluttering, and irregular myoclonus that could easily be missed. All patients with status epilepticus died, compared with a 24% mortality rate in the non-seizure group. Another study by Ronne-Engstrom and Winkler using cEEG in 70 patients with TBI found a 33% incidence of seizures with onset 1–5 days after injury [21]. 35% of the patients with seizures had persistent seizure activity requiring propofol or barbiturate sedation. Older age and low-energy trauma were risk factors for developing seizures.

The incidence of post-traumatic epilepsy is reported to vary according to injury severity. Annegers et al. followed 4541 cases of traumatic brain injury in Olmsted County, MN, from 1935 to 1984 and calculated seizure risk [5]. The relative risk of seizures was 1.5 (95% confidence interval 1.0–2.2) after mild injuries, but with no increase after 5 years, 2.9 (95% confidence interval 1.9–4.1) after moderate injuries, and 17.2 (95% confidence interval 12.3–23.6) after severe injuries. Significant risk factors for the development of post-traumatic seizures were brain contusion with subdural hematoma, skull fracture, loss of consciousness or amnesia of greater than 24 h, and age over 65 years. Englander et al. found a 12% incidence of post-traumatic seizures in 647 TBI patients followed over 24 months [16]. The highest cumulative probability for late seizures included biparietal contusions (66%), dural penetration (62.5%), multiple intracranial procedures (36.5%), multiple subcortical contusions (33.4%), evacuated subdural (27.8%), midline shift >5 mm (25.8%), and multiple cortical contusions (25%). In addition, Glasgow Coma Scale (GCS) was correlated with seizure incidence: GCS 3–8 had a cumulative seizure probability of 16.8%, whereas GCS 9–12 had 24.3% and GCS 13–15 had 8.0%. In a large prospective, randomized, double-blind seizure prophylaxis study from Seattle, Temkin et al. reported independent risk factors from Cox regression multivariate models. Five factors emerged as increasing seizure risk in this population: early seizures (within 7 days), coma for over 1 week, dural penetration, depressed skull fracture not surgically treated, and one or more nonreactive pupil [22]. These findings are in agreement with Annegers et al. who described that brain contusion, skull fractures, and prolonged amnesia or unconsciousness (>24 h) are injury patterns associated with a higher incidence of seizures [6]. Additionally, age ≥65 was also a risk factor for seizure development. In a more recent study, an overall incidence of post-traumatic seizures of 6.33% (95% CI 3.96–8.69) was found in 411 patients followed for 5 years with rates for early seizures of 1.95% and late seizures at 4.38% [23]. The patients with severe injury, defined as intracerebral hemorrhage/contusion, loss of con-

sciousness, or amnesia >24 h, were more likely to develop post-traumatic seizures. Interestingly, there were no statistically significant differences between age and GCS score. The rates of post-traumatic seizures in the civilian population are lower than those based on military populations. In the Vietnam Head Injury Study, 53 % of veterans who had penetrating head injuries developed post-traumatic epilepsy, and half of those patients still had seizures 15 years after injury. However, the relative risk of developing epilepsy in these patients dropped from 580 times higher than the general age-matched population in the first year after TBI to 25 times higher after 10 years [8]. A study looking at the more recent Afghanistan and Iraq war veterans again identified penetrating head injuries as having the strongest association of epilepsy development with an odds ratio of 18.77 (95 % CI 9.21–38.23) [24]. Figure 11.1 shows examples of injuries associated with post-traumatic seizures.

Other factors that can predispose to the development of post-traumatic seizures include age (incidence is higher in the pediatric population [25] and the elderly [6]), history of alcohol abuse, previous seizures, and a family history of seizures [5]. Genetic predisposition to post-TBI seizures is an interesting issue that has not been well addressed to date. Similar injuries lead to a wide variety of seizure incidence and frequency. Not all studies agree on the genetic predisposition. Jennett found that family history of epilepsy was more common in patients aged less than 16 years with late post-TBI seizures [26]. In the Vietnam Head Injury Study, this factor was not predictive of either early or late seizures [8]. In another study examining genetic susceptibility to epilepsy, seizure incidence among relatives of patients with post-TBI seizures was not higher than among the general population [27]. In a prospective study of late post-traumatic seizures after moderate and severe TBI, 106 patients were examined for the ApoE locus by restriction fragment length polymorphism analysis [28]. Twenty-one patients had at least one late post-TBI seizure. The relative risk of late post-TBI seizures for patients with the ε4 allele was 2.41 (95 % CI 1.15–5.07, p = 0.03). Of note, the presence of this allele was not associated with an unfavorable outcome. Genetic variations of inhibitory neurotransmitters and pathways are also being evaluated as risk factors for post-traumatic seizure development. A 2010 study by Wagner et al. found certain adenosine A1 receptor gene variations to be associated with increased susceptibility of early and late seizures [29]. Darrah et al. found increased risk of post-traumatic seizures between 1 week and 6 months post-injury in patients with a particular polymorphism of the glutamic acid decarboxylase (GAD) 1 gene [30]. Identifying these genetic variations has important implications in both targeting the appropriate patient population to treat with anticonvulsants and helping to determine the pathophysiology of post-traumatic epilepsy.

In studies examining post-traumatic seizures, an arbitrary definition of early and late is commonly used. Early seizures

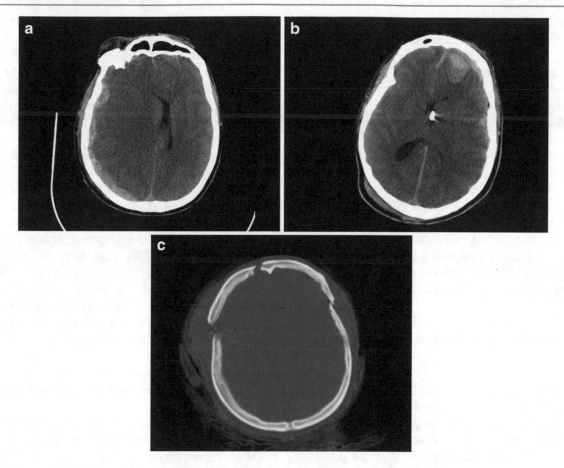

Fig. 11.1 CT examples of findings associated with post-traumatic seizures. (**a**) Right subdural hematoma. (**b**) Left frontal contusion. (**c**) Multiple skull fractures

are defined as occurring in the first 7 days after injury and late seizures occur after this point. Early seizure incidence ranges from 2.1 % to 16.9 % [6, 26, 31]. The incidence of late seizures ranges from 1.9 to 30 % [17]. However, this classification is potentially too restrictive. Many TBI patients remain critical in the ICU for longer than 7 days; it would be unreasonable to consider a seizure on the tenth hospital day a "late" seizure. Some studies have extended the acute period to include the first month post-injury. This approach, however, is not ideal, since the underlying cause of seizures in the first week after injury is most likely different from the cause of seizures occurring in the first month or indeed in the first year after injury. Seizures in the first week are more likely related to neurochemical and metabolic derangements, whereas later seizures may be related to the formation of glial scar leading to cortical irritation. Also, there is a significant occurrence of seizures at the scene of both mild and severe TBIs [32, 33]. These immediate seizures are more likely related to the direct disruption of cortical and subcortical connections as a result of percussive forces on the brain and less likely the result of neurochemical or metabolic derangements. However, classifying the timing of onset of post-traumatic seizures is important for both trying to under-

stand their pathophysiology and also in trying to define factors that can predict their occurrence.

A second important goal of dividing seizures by time of occurrence is to evaluate whether early seizures can predict the occurrence of late seizures or the development of a long-term seizure disorder. Early seizures are linked with late seizure development. The increased risk for late seizures after early seizures is independent of the actual number of seizures occurring during the first week after TBI [17]. Not all studies, however, report an increased incidence of late seizures after early post-TBI seizures. A large retrospective study by Annegers et al. utilized multivariate analysis and found that early seizures are not an independent risk factor for late post-traumatic epilepsy, and most likely early seizures are a marker of injury severity sufficient to cause late epilepsy [5]. Another interesting observation is that the incidence of late seizures after early post-TBI seizures is dependent on the age of the patient. Children less than 16 years old may not be at increased risk for late seizures regardless of the early seizure type [5, 17]. Additionally, there is some evidence that immediate seizures occurring at the scene of the trauma are not linked with any increased risk of developing late seizures [32].

The incidence of post-traumatic seizures differs in the pediatric population. The overall incidence is higher than in adults [6, 25, 31]. Early post-traumatic seizures occur slightly more commonly with reported incidence rates of 9–15% [12, 34–36]. As with adults, there is a close correlation between injury severity and the incidence of any type of seizures. Hahn et al. demonstrated that the incidence of post-traumatic seizures was seven times greater in children with severe TBI and GCS <8, compared with milder injury and higher GCS score [34]. Young age is also an important risk factor for seizures, with younger age having higher risk [35–37]. The occurrence of early seizures in severe TBI is also higher than the adult population, with reported incidences as high as 38.7% in one study, which classified severe TBI as GCS 3–8 [35]. Furthermore, early seizures tend to occur even earlier in children; up to 50–80% of early seizures in the pediatric population occur in the first 24 h after injury [25, 38].

Experimental Approaches to Post-traumatic Seizures

Immediate post-traumatic seizures have been described in several experimental models of traumatic brain injury including the impact acceleration model of diffuse TBI, the lateral fluid percussion model [39], and models of cortical contusion [40, 41]. One study monitored EEG for 2 h post-injury in rodents exposed to cortical contusion, and generalized seizure activity was recorded in 14 out of 17 cases, at a mean time of 67 s after trauma [41]. Concurrent microdialysis measured a consistent increase in aspartate, taurine, glutamate, and glycine; however, it is not clear if this represented a cause or a consequence of the seizures. Longer-term behavioral studies in experimental TBI have not demonstrated any significant evidence of clinical seizure activity [42, 43]. This finding is at odds with the clinical behavior of TBI, and it may relate to differences in seizure thresholds between rodents and humans, though the difference may also be explained by the heterogeneity of models of TBI. For example, a study utilizing the lateral fluid percussion model found that nearly half of rats developed clinical epilepsy with a latency of 7 weeks to 1 year post-injury [39]. Another study using the controlled cortical injury and lateral fluid percussion injury models demonstrated that while the rate of delayed seizures is low (3–9%), over 70% of mice had spontaneous epileptiform discharges up to 9 months post-injury with the majority showing increased seizure susceptibility when compared to controls [44]. This ongoing hyperexcitability plays a role in post-traumatic epileptogenesis.

The origin of post-traumatic seizures is not known and improved understanding requires a good experimental model. Studies have evaluated in vivo seizure activity, in vitro seizure activity in brain tissue from injured animals, and in vitro seizure activity in brain tissue injured in vitro. In vivo models have focused on either direct observation of seizures or stimulation of seizures by cortical injection of ferrous chloride [45]; the latter technique is thought to mimic cortical accumulation of blood breakdown products and causes recurrent focal epileptiform discharges. One of the in vitro approaches used isolated hippocampal slices from the brains of injured animals, followed by in vitro electrophysiological recording [46]. In vitro models of traumatic brain injury have difficulty in reproducing a meaningful level of trauma. Models have included scraping hippocampal slices or stretching neurons grown in culture [47, 48]. Combining all these techniques, Golarai et al. examined changes in the rodent brain after weight drop injury to the somatosensory cortex [49]. They found an early selective cell loss in the dentate gyrus and area CA3 of the hippocampus, a persistently enhanced susceptibility to pentylenetetrazole-induced seizures for up to 15 weeks after injury and an abnormal hyperexcitability in the granule cell and molecular layers of the dentate gyrus.

Pathophysiology of Post-traumatic Seizures

The pathophysiological mechanisms causing post-traumatic seizures are not well understood, and there is likely some variation depending on the time of onset after injury. Post-traumatic seizures should be thought of as primary and secondary. Primary post-traumatic seizures are most likely to occur immediately after injury and are caused by direct effects of the brain injury itself. Secondary seizures are caused by other epileptogenic factors not directly related to the injury, such as fever, inflammation, metabolic and electrolyte abnormalities, or drug reactions. Late seizures are explained by structural changes such as neurogenesis and synaptic plasticity [50]. Primary and secondary seizures are related in that the injury itself may contribute to a reduction in seizure threshold, therefore increasing the epileptogenicity of the factors that can cause secondary and late seizures.

A cascade of metabolic and neurochemical events characterize traumatic brain injury, starting at the time of injury and continuing throughout the acute and subacute phases. Many of these changes are potentially epileptogenic, including hyperglycolysis [51]; extracellular elevation of glutamate (and other amino acids, particularly aspartate) [52, 53]; transient flux of ions including sodium, calcium, and potassium [54]; and altered cerebral blood flow [55]. Traumatic brain injury also triggers a series of cellular repair mechanisms such as axonal sprouting, necessary for functional recovery; however, some of these processes may subsequently lead to hyperexcitability and epileptogenesis [56].

In the acute phase, elevations in extracellular excitatory amino acids can cause widespread depolarization that may reach seizure threshold. Loss of inhibitory neurons may promote generation of a seizure focus. Ionic transients may shift the cell membrane equilibrium potential either causing action potential generation or a reduction in the stimulus threshold required to generate an action potential. Changes in extracellular pH can also shift the membrane potential as alkalosis tends to cause depolarization. The most widely studied theory involves the massive rise in levels of the excitatory neurotransmitter, glutamate, which then triggers a series of changes in calcium homeostasis, cell signaling pathways including NMDA receptor activation, and eventually cell death [57].

Seizures arising in the more chronic phases of injury are less likely caused by acute changes in cellular physiology. These late seizures are more likely related to the influence of glial scars, breakdown products of hemoglobin, death of inhibitory interneurons, or disruption of neuronal connections with formation of abnormal neosynapses with greater excitatory potential [58].

A change in the balance of inhibitory and excitatory neurons may also play a role in seizure development. Loss of hippocampal hilar neurons and subsequent hyperexcitability has been identified in injured animals [59]. A phenomenon known as "mossy fiber sprouting" in which granule cells in the dentate nucleus sprout axons to nearby granule cells forming new connections has been recurrently demonstrated in animal models of post-traumatic epilepsy [39, 60]. These changes occur in the hippocampus ipsilateral to the injury and are correlated with the severity of injury. A pathology study in humans undergoing temporal lobectomy for post-traumatic epilepsy also identified hippocampal cell loss in 94 % of patients and, to some extent, mossy fiber sprouting in all specimens [61]. Using another mouse model of TBI, the neocortical "undercut," Jin et al. demonstrated that these new connections lead to increased excitatory connectivity upon layer V pyramidal neurons [62]. This cortical reorganization contributes to development of post-traumatic epilepsy.

Epileptogenesis may not be entirely a neuronal phenomenon. It is known that glial membrane channels participate in ionic homeostasis [63] especially at times of neuronal activity. In particular, glial cells buffer levels of extracellular potassium, and failure of this mechanism can result in increased neuronal excitability and seizures [64]. Electrophysiological recordings in hippocampal slices from experimentally injured brains have demonstrated reductions in inward and outward potassium currents and abnormal accumulation of extracellular potassium. Abnormal glial buffering of potassium may represent another mechanism of post-traumatic seizure development [46].

Breakdown of the blood-brain barrier and inflammation are key features of TBI and may also play a role in seizure development. Direct damage to the blood-brain barrier causes increased permeability of foreign substances such as blood proteins, complement, and reactive oxygen species [50]. One study by Seiffert et al. exposed rat cortex to bile salts causing breakdown of the blood-brain barrier and extravasation of serum albumin. Brain slices were then recorded, and abnormal epileptiform activity was seen in 69% of the treated slices compared to only 10% of the sham-operated controls [65]. Focal EEG abnormalities correlated to areas of blood-brain barrier breakdown have also been demonstrated in human brains following injury [66]. Furthermore, a release of cytokines and chemokines occurs within minutes of injury and leads to accumulation of immune cells in the damaged brain and long-term microglial activation [67]. While these inflammatory mediators also play a protective role and are important for neural repair, the complex pathways require further study to determine potential targets for post-traumatic epileptogenesis.

The impact of seizures on macroscopic physiological parameters in traumatic brain injury has not been well studied. In a study using cEEG monitoring in ICU patients with severe TBI [14], the incidence of raised ICP was similar in both seizure and non-seizure patients. The mean ICP was higher in the seizure group (15.6 vs 11.8 mmHg, $p < 0.001$); however, this finding may simply reflect seizures occurring in the most severely injured patients. A separate analysis comparing ICP values in individual patients on seizure days and non-seizure days demonstrated no significant difference. Furthermore, serial trends of ICP in the hours before and after seizure events did not demonstrate a clear seizure-related effect. Seizures can cause profound hypotension and hypoxia (in the non-ventilated patient), and prolonged myoclonic and tonic-clonic activity can lead to excess tissue and serum lactate levels and acidosis. Moreover, seizures have been found to contribute to altered cerebral metabolism in TBI patients. A study of 34 severe TBI patients found that seizures and periodic epileptiform discharges were associated with lower cerebral microdialysis glucose and elevated lactate/pyruvate ratio indicating metabolic crisis, which then normalized during the non-ictal period [68]. Of particular interest in this study was the finding that periodic discharges, thought by some to be benign, were also associated with metabolic crisis. These factors may constitute secondary insults, known to worsen outcome after TBI [69], and may represent new therapeutic targets.

Diagnosis of Seizures

The occurrence of seizures can be suspected by clinical activity but EEG confirmation is required. The clinical appearance of early seizures in the ICU includes generalized tonic-clonic and focal seizures. Complex partial seizures may also occur, but documentation of these in an intubated, sedated patient is difficult. Focal seizures can appear as rhythmic myoclonic activity or as a more subtle finding, such as a facial twitch [14]. Seizures may also manifest as a decrease in mental status, and any workup for this problem after TBI should include an evaluation for seizures with EEG. Seizures may be masked in the ICU population by the use of neuromuscular blocking agents, and therefore, caution should be taken when using these agents in patients who are at higher risk of post-traumatic seizures and cEEG should be considered.

The EEG can be utilized in different ways for diagnosing post-traumatic seizures. The simplest method is to obtain an EEG in a patient clinically suspected of having seizures. However, this EEG is a snapshot of the injured brain's electrical activity. If it does not capture a single seizure event or nonconvulsive status, then seizure diagnosis relies on being able to identify abnormal interictal activity. If there is a significant delay in obtaining the EEG, then seizure activity may not be seen and the diagnostic yield of the study is compromised. Few studies have examined the benefit of frequent screening EEGs or cEEG monitoring. Dawson et al. obtained serial short-duration EEGs in 45 brain-injured patients every few days during the first 14 days and found a 25% incidence of seizures by EEG criteria [70]. Vespa et al. examined the role of cEEG monitoring in moderate to severe TBI and found a 22% incidence of seizures among 94 patients admitted to the ICU [14]. More importantly, 52% of the patients with seizures had no clinical evidence of seizure activity. Additionally, in the subgroup with no clinical or electrographic seizures, 10% of patients had epileptiform and nonepileptiform activity. Epileptiform activity included isolated spikes or sharp waves and/or repetitive sharp waves. Pseudoperiodic lateralized epileptiform discharges (PLEDs) were also seen in patients without other evidence of seizures. Nonepileptiform EEG abnormalities observed in these patients included symmetric disorganized slowing, asymmetrical disorganized delta waves with a focus, intermittent rhythmic delta activity, absence of sleep potentials, and progressive loss of EEG amplitude with burst suppression. The latter was associated with impending brain death. Other EEG abnormalities were observed, including increased beta activity, amplitude suppression, and burst suppression. These patterns were seen in both the seizure and non-seizure groups and are related to sedative hypnotics such as midazolam or propofol. Other studies have described a loss of EEG reactivity to external stimuli and loss of spontaneous variability [71–74]. A reactive EEG has been shown to be a good prognostic factor for recovery of consciousness after TBI [75].

Power spectral analysis has also been used to examine prognosis in TBI. Poor prognosis is frequently associated with unvarying activity and a predominance of delta band activity (1–3 Hz) [71]. Additionally, the percent alpha variability (a quantitative EEG trend analyzing the variability in alpha power compared to total power over time) has been evaluated

in moderate to severe TBI. Vespa et al. found that patients with reduced percent alpha variability (values less than 0.1) in the first 3 days after injury had a high likelihood of poor outcome, defined as Glasgow Outcome Scale score of 1 and 2, at the time of discharge [76]. Variable spectral patterns are associated with better prognosis [71, 77] as are persistence or return of a peak in the alpha or theta frequency [78, 79]. Figure 11.2 shows examples of various seizures on EEG.

The increased use of cEEG monitoring in intensive care units has led to new recommendations. The Neurocritical Care Society recommends cEEG for all comatose patients, not just limited to intracranial pathology given the high rate of nonconvulsive status epilepticus in critically ill patients. Additionally, cEEG monitoring should be initiated within 1 h of suspected status epilepticus onset, and monitoring should continue for at least 48 h in comatose patients [80]. Similarly, the European Society of Intensive Care Medicine recommends EEG to rule out nonconvulsive status epilepticus in brain-injured patients and for those with unexplained alterations in consciousness who lack primary brain injury [81].

The urgency of ordering EEG when seizures are suspected after TBI has to be considered, as well. In one study, 23 emergent EEGs (EmEEG), defined as a study performed in less than 1 h from request, were ordered mainly in post-TBI ICU patients [82]. The reason for ordering the test was to rule out convulsive status epilepticus in 12 patients, nonconvulsive status epilepticus in six patients, and seizures in another six patients. Clinical seizures before the test were observed in three patients, and suspicious clinical activity (unclear to the observers if it represented seizures) was observed in 12 additional patients. The EmEEG showed convulsive status epilepticus in three patients, nonconvulsive status in two patients, and epileptiform activity or electrographic seizures in four patients. Half of the patients were already on antiepileptic therapy when the test was performed. As previously mentioned, the emergent need for EEG has been incorporated into the Neurocritical Care Society guidelines for management of status epilepticus [80].

In addition to raw data, the EEG can be analyzed in a variety of ways and is important in identifying and making determinations regarding seizures. Many studies have focused on compressed spectral array and other quantitative methods, whereas the highest yield of information comes from both trend analysis and examination of the raw EEG data. Vespa et al. used frequency analysis by fast Fourier transform in the ICU, followed by examination of twominute epochs that were evaluated for any increases in total power [14]. Any epoch in which increased spectral power was observed had the raw EEG data analyzed for evidence of seizures. The trend analysis was therefore used to flag periods where seizures might have occurred, and this approach allowed a more focused examination of the raw EEG. While quantitative EEG can be useful and provide

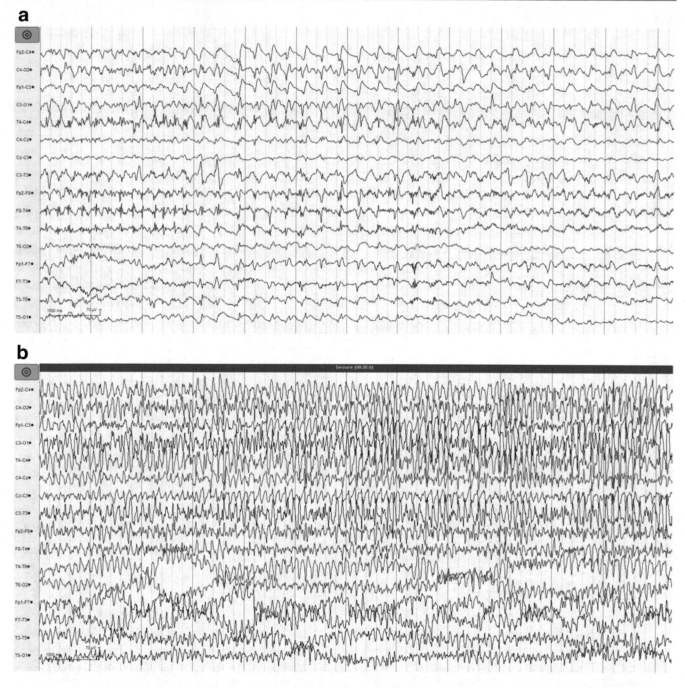

Fig. 11.2 EEG examples of seizures in TBI. (**a**) Generalized spike and wave activity. (**b**) Generalized The caption for Fig 11.2 b should be "generalizedseizure" and not "generalized epileptiform discharges. (**c**) Focal right frontocentral seizure, (*i*) beginning of seizure with faster frequencies on the right (*red*), (*ii*) progression of seizure with increasing amplitude of right-sided discharges, (*iii*) slowing of right-sided seizure activity, (*iv*) conclusion of seizure followed by attenuation of EEG

ci

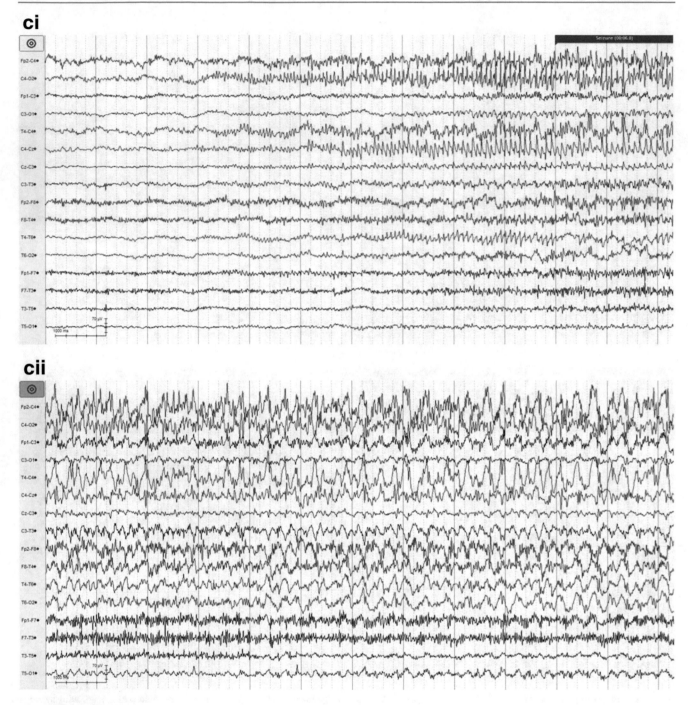

cii

Fig. 11.2 (continued)

ciii

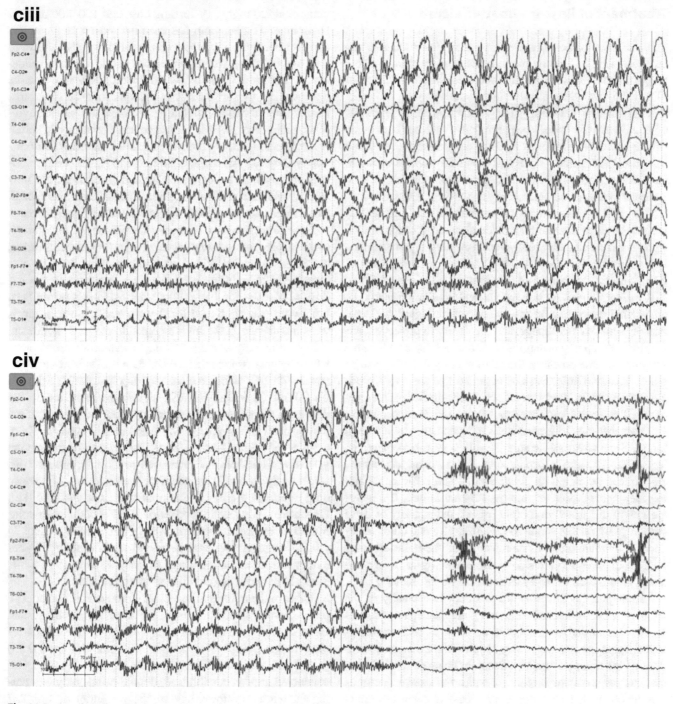

civ

Fig. 11.2 (continued)

additional information, it must be analyzed with caution and only by those skilled in clinical EEG interpretation [83].

Intracranial EEG monitoring is another diagnostic tool to identify seizures that are not visible on scalp EEG. These devices come in the form of subdural strip electrodes or intracortical depth electrodes and have a similar safety profile compared to other brain monitors [84]. Waziri et al. performed intracortical EEG and compared findings to scalp EEG in 14 patients. Ten patients with depth electrode place-

ment had electrographic seizures, and six of these had no corresponding ictal activity on the scalp EEG [85]. A more recent study of 34 severe TBI patients using both surface and depth electrode EEG found a high rate of electrographic epileptiform activity (seizures or periodic discharges) in 21 patients (62%). In nine of these 21 patients, the activity was only visible on the depth electrode [68]. The use of intracranial EEG monitoring may provide a higher sensitivity for detecting post-traumatic seizures.

Treatment of Post-traumatic Seizures

There are two principal goals of treating post-traumatic seizures in the ICU. Firstly, in the acute post-traumatic period, the goal should be rapid cessation of seizure activity in order to prevent secondary physiological and biochemical insults that may lead to worsening injury. Secondly, further episodes of seizure activity should be prevented. There has been some debate about whether prevention of early seizures can result in a lower incidence of late post-traumatic seizures. Studies have also addressed whether long-term prophylaxis with antiepileptic agents is indicated, and this will be discussed below.

The initial management of seizures in the critically ill brain-injured patient should include close observation of vital signs to ensure adequate oxygenation and end-organ perfusion and adherence to ACLS/ATLS guidelines for assessment of ABC (airway, breathing, and circulation). In the non-intubated TBI patient, intubation and mechanical ventilation should be considered depending on the severity of the injury, the duration of mental status change, and the ability to protect the airway [86]. Vasopressors may also be indicated for hemodynamic support. An assessment of the seizure's origin should also be made. It should not always be assumed that seizures are primarily related to the brain injury. Critically ill patients are exposed to a wide variety of metabolic and pharmacological stressors that may trigger seizures independently of any brain injury. Such stressors include hypoglycemia, hyponatremia, hypocalcemia, hypophosphatemia, hypoxemia, hypocarbia, alcohol/recreational drug withdrawal, fever, infection including meningoencephalitis, and hepatorenal failure. If seizures are newly diagnosed in a brain-injured patient, any of these complicating factors should be evaluated for and corrected as needed. Furthermore, a combination of these factors may interact in an additive fashion with the injury to trigger seizures, where each factor by itself would be insufficient.

Initial pharmacotherapy for seizures is typically in the form of a benzodiazepine. Lorazepam, diazepam, or midazolam are available and should be given as an intravenous bolus. Prolonged seizures may require higher doses or continuous infusions of either midazolam or propofol. Seizures that are recurrent or ongoing despite the above measures should be treated as status epilepticus. If seizures remain refractory, then escalation to barbiturates may be necessary. If an infusion is started, cEEG monitoring should be ordered with a goal of achieving EEG burst suppression (see chapter on Treatment of Status Epilepticus in Critical Care).

A patient not currently on anticonvulsants should be started on one, typically phenytoin or fosphenytoin (15–20 mg/kg IV loading dose and 300–400 mg/day IV or enteral, with frequent assessment of serum levels and a goal of 10–20 mg/dl). Additional agents include levetiracetam (1000–3000 mg IV loading dose and 1000–4000 mg/day IV or enteral), valproic acid (15–20 mg/kg IV loading dose and 600–3000 mg/day IV or enteral), lacosamide (200–400 mg IV loading dose and 200–600 mg/day IV or enteral), or phe-

nobarbital (20 mg/kg IV loading dose and 100–800 mg/day IV or enteral). Phenytoin has been the most widely studied and has benefits over other agents including the ability to load rapidly, the ability to titrate dose to effect, and the widespread ability to follow serum levels. Negative factors against phenytoin are the risk of Stevens-Johnson syndrome, cardiac complications including hypotension and arrhythmias, reliance on hepatic clearance and variability in serum levels due to complex pharmacokinetics, and therefore difficulty targeting the therapeutic range [87]. The newer anticonvulsants such as levetiracetam and lacosamide are now widely available and have minimal drug interactions though these agents are not as well studied in the TBI population.

Several studies have examined the efficacy of anticonvulsants in preventing early seizures. The largest prospective, randomized, double-blind, placebo-controlled trial to date examined 404 brain-injured patients given phenytoin prophylaxis or placebo for 1 year after traumatic brain injury [11]. Follow-up was continued for 2 years and phenytoin levels were maintained in the high therapeutic range. A significant reduction in early seizures (<7 days) was observed. Patients receiving phenytoin had a 3.6% incidence of seizures as compared with 14.2 % in the placebo group ($p < 0.001$, risk ratio 0.27, 95% CI 0.12–0.62). No significant reduction in the development of late seizures was reported. By the end of the first year, 21.5% of phenytoin-treated patients and 15.7% of the placebo patients had seizures. By the end of the second year, these numbers had increased to 27.5 % and 21.1 %, respectively ($p > 0.2$). In addition, the incidence of adverse drug effects in the first 2 weeks of treatment was low [88]. Hypersensitivity reactions occurred in 2.5% of the phenytoin-treated patients as compared to 0% of the placebo patients ($p = 0.12$). Other studies have also confirmed the ability of phenytoin to reduce the incidence of early seizures [89], while others have shown no significant difference [90].

Other anticonvulsants have been evaluated; Glötzner et al. prospectively studied a group of 139 severe TBI patients and found a lower probability of early seizures in the carbamazepine-treated group when compared to placebo ($p < 0.05$) [91]. There was no difference in late seizures. Temkin et al. conducted another randomized, double-blind study comparing phenytoin to valproic acid for the prevention of post-TBI seizures [92]. In this study, 132 patients were randomized to receive either phenytoin or valproic acid. The early seizure rate was higher on valproic acid; however, the number was small and not statistically significant.

There is little information available regarding the use of levetiracetam in traumatic brain injury. Jones et al. reported on data collected from 32 cases of severe TBI treated with levetiracetam and compared with a historical cohort of 41 cases treated with phenytoin monotherapy [93]. Their data suggests that levetiracetam has an equivalent protective benefit as compared with phenytoin within the numbers of patients analyzed, but that it might be associated with a higher number of abnormalities on EEG and therefore may be associated with a higher tendency for seizures. A larger prospective study of 813 TBI patients showed no significant difference in clinical seizure rate, mortality, or adverse drug reactions when either phenytoin or levetiracetam was used for early post-traumatic seizure prophylaxis [94]. Another study also compared levetiracetam versus phenytoin when used for seizure prophylaxis in adults with TBI and found similar rates of early EEG-confirmed seizure activity (28% in the levetiracetam group vs. 29% in the phenytoin group) [95]. Additionally, daily costs when levetiracetam was used were also lower when compared to phenytoin therapy and drug level monitoring. Some studies have shown less short-term complications such as fevers [96] and improved long-term outcomes [97] when levetiracetam is used over phenytoin.

Several studies have examined the role of seizure prophylaxis in preventing late-onset post-traumatic seizures, and only one study has found a beneficial effect of long-term seizure prophylaxis [89]. This study was not blinded or placebo controlled, however. Thirty-four patients with severe TBI were randomized to receive phenytoin for 3 months and were compared with 52 untreated severe TBI patients. After 2 years, 6% of patients treated with phenytoin developed post-traumatic epilepsy as compared with 42% of the untreated group. McQueen et al. evaluated 164 patients in a prospective, randomized, double-blind study comparing phenytoin and placebo and found no beneficial effect in the reduction of late seizures [98]. Temkin et al. in their large well-controlled study of 404 patients did not find any reduction in late post-traumatic seizures with phenytoin [11]. Studies of other agents including carbamazepine [91] and phenobarbital [99] have also been unable to demonstrate any clear benefit on the incidence of late seizures.

Magnesium has also been considered for post-traumatic seizure prophylaxis and neuroprotection. In a double-blind, randomized, controlled trial, Temkin et al. evaluated 499 moderate to severe TBI patients with either low-dose versus high-dose magnesium or placebo for 5 days and assessed for a composite primary outcome including seizures. Most patients also received phenytoin as prophylaxis. Magnesium showed no overall positive effect, and in fact there was a trend toward worse outcomes in the magnesium group with no effect on early or late seizures [100].

Clearly the occurrence of seizures needs to be rapidly recognized and treated in brain-injured patients. The clinical evidence at present supports the use of seizure prophylaxis for the prevention of early seizures (<7 days from injury), but does not support long-term administration of anticonvulsants for the prevention of late-onset seizures [101–103]. Specific risk factors for developing post-traumatic seizures have been identified including GCS <10, depressed skull fracture, cortical contusion, subdural/epidural hematomas, intracerebral hematoma, penetrating injury, focal deficit, or prolonged amnesia (>24 h) [5, 22]. It is recommended that particular attention be given to seizure prophylaxis in the subgroup of brain-injured patients with these pathologies.

Outcome of Seizures Complicating TBI

It is pertinent to ask whether the benefits of seizure prophylaxis on early seizures reported in the literature translate into improved mortality or morbidity. Few studies have specifically addressed outcomes in relation to seizure prophylaxis [11, 89, 91, 98]. No study to date has demonstrated any improvement in mortality as a result of administering anticonvulsants. A meta-analysis of several studies described a pooled relative risk of 1.08 (95 % CI 0.79–1.46) for all-cause mortality in anticonvulsant-treated vs. placebo or standard care, implying treatment has no effect on mortality [103]. Two studies have examined outcome in surviving patients in relation to seizure prophylaxis. Glötzner et al. found a worse outcome in the treated group (RR 1.49, 95% CI 1.06–2.08, $p = 0.183$) [91], and Temkin et al. found no overall effect of seizure prophylaxis on patient outcome (RR 0.96, 95% CI 0.72–1.39, $p = 0.75$) [11]. Another study using continuous EEG monitoring in critically ill ICU patients did not find any differences in either mortality or outcome at the time of discharge between the groups of patients with or without seizures [14]. However, six patients were identified who had status epilepticus, of which three were found to be in nonconvulsive status. All six of the patients ultimately died, two due to sepsis after control of status epilepticus, three from progressive neurological deterioration and brain death, and one from late respiratory arrest. Clearly, the occurrence of status epilepticus is a grave prognostic sign in the traumatically brain-injured patient, and the high risk of nonconvulsive status suggests that EEG recording should be more frequently utilized in this patient population.

Finally, the potential benefit for using antiseizure prophylaxis after TBI has to be weighed against the potential risk for impeding recovery of brain function. Secondary analysis of the trial by Temkin et al. [11] using phenytoin as prophylaxis found impaired neuropsychological testing at 1 month in severe TBI patients who remained on phenytoin pharmacotherapy [104]. More recently, Bhullar et al. assessed functional outcomes for severe blunt TBI patients who either received or did not receive seizure prophylaxis with phenytoin [105]. Ninety-three patients were reviewed, and patients who received phenytoin had a significantly longer hospital stay and worse functional outcome at discharge based on the Glasgow Outcome Scale and modified Rankin Scale. This concept has been applied to animal models of TBI. Pitkänen et al. studied the effect of lacosamide on a rat model of TBI using the lateral fluid-percussion method [106]. The group treated with lacosamide lagged behind the control group in motor function, but there was no significant impairment in the structural or cognitive parameters. Finally, Lu et al. studied a dextromethorphan derivative in a rat model of TBI and found both antiseizure and anti-inflammatory effects [107]. Rats had epidural EEG electrodes implanted and then underwent a penetrating ballistic-like brain injury operation.

When nonconvulsive status epilepticus was detected, the animals were injected with either study drug or placebo, and a significant reduction in duration and frequency of seizure activity was seen. In summary, future studies are needed to determine which anticonvulsant may provide the greatest benefit by preventing seizures with the lowest risk of impaired functional outcomes or ideally for identifying agents that may promote neuroprotection.

Conclusions

Seizures may occur in up to 22% of ICU patients with severe traumatic brain injury. There is a relatively high risk of nonconvulsive seizures in this population. Seizures may exacerbate the injury process and disrupt both patient care and family coping. Therefore, seizures should be recognized quickly and treated promptly. The clinician should have a high index of suspicion for seizures, especially in patients with clearly defined risk factors for seizure development. Continuous EEG monitoring should be considered in those patients who are considered to be at high risk of clinical or subclinical seizures. Seizure prophylaxis with anticonvulsants is supported by the literature for the prevention of early seizures (defined as <7 days post-injury) but not for late seizures. Phenytoin primarily has been used in this setting and both found to be efficacious in preventing early seizures. More experience is being gained with newer agents, such as levetiracetam and lacosamide. Anticonvulsants have not been found to reduce the incidence of developing late post-traumatic seizures, and therefore prolonged prophylaxis with anticonvulsants is not currently supported (Tables 11.1 and 11.2).

Table 11.1 Risk factors for developing early and late post-traumatic seizures

Risk factor	Increased risk for seizures	
	Early	Late
Acute intracerebral hematoma	+	+
Acute subdural hematoma	+	+
LOC or post-TBI amnesia >30 min	+	
LOC or post-TBI amnesia >24 h		+
Younger age (children)	+	
Older age (> 65 years)		+
Diffuse cerebral edema (children)	+	
Depressed/linear skull fracture	+	+
Metal fragment retention	+	+
Focal neurological deficits	+	+
Persistent EEG changes (>1 month)		+
Early post-TBI seizures		+
Chronic alcoholism		+

LOC loss of consciousness, + risk factor has been shown to increase the risk of seizures at the specified time point. Adapted from Frey [17]

Table 11.2 Summary of studies in the literature that examine prophylaxis against the risk of early and late seizures following traumatic brain injury and the anticonvulsant drug used (DPH, dilantin/phenytoin; CBZ, carbamazepine; PB, phenobarbital; VPA, valproic acid; LEV, levetiracetam)

Study	Drug used	Early seizures	Late seizures
Young et al. (1983) [90]	DPH	0.99 (0.27–3.61)	
Young et al. (1983) [108]	DPH		1.29 (0.56–3.0)
McQueen et al. (1983) [98]	DPH		1.09 (0.41–2.86)
Glötzner et al. (1983) [91]	CBZ	0.37 (0.18–0.78)*	0.71 (0.39–1.3)
Temkin et al. (1990) [11]	DPH	0.25 (0.11–0.57)*	1.3 (0.82–2.08)
Pechadre et al. (1991) [89]	DPH		0.14 (0.03–0.55)
Manaka et al. (1992) [99]	PB		1.38 (0.54–3.5)
Temkin et al. (1999) [92]	VPA	2.9 (0.7–13.3)	1.4 (0.8–2.4)
Szaflarski et al. (2010) [97]	LEVᵗ	0.88 (0.24–3.28)	
Inaba et al. (2013) [94]	LEVᵗ	1 (0.33-3.08)	

Values represent relative risk with the 95 % confidence interval in parentheses
*significant with $p < 0.05$
$t$when compared to DPH

References

1. Sosin DM, Sniezek JE, Thurman DJ. Incidence of mild and moderate brain injury in the United States, 1991. Brain Inj. 1996;10(1):47–54.
2. Thurman D, Guerrero J. Trends in hospitalization associated with traumatic brain injury. JAMA. 1999;282(10):954–7.
3. Sosin DM, Sniezek JE, Waxweiler RJ. Trends in death associated with traumatic brain injury, 1979 through 1992. JAMA. 1995;273(22):1778–80.
4. Thurman DJ, Alverson C, Dunn KA, Guerrero J, Sniezek JE. Traumatic brain injury in the United States: a public health perspective. J Head Trauma Rehabil. 1999;14(6):602–15.
5. Annegers JF, Grabow JD, Kurland LT, Laws Jr ER. The incidence, causes, and secular trends of head trauma in Olmsted County, Minnesota, 1935-1974. Neurology. 1980;30(9):912–9.
6. Annegers JF, Hauser WA, Coan SP, Rocca WA. A population-based study of seizures after traumatic brain injuries. N Engl J Med. 1998;338(1):20–4.
7. Lee ST, Lui TN, Wong CW, Yeh YS, Tzaan WC. Early seizures after moderate closed head injury. Acta Neurochir. 1995;137(3–4):151–4.
8. Salazar AM, Jabbari B, Vance SC, Grafman J, Amin D, Dillon JD. Epilepsy after penetrating head injury. I. Clinical correlates: a report of the Vietnam Head Injury Study. Neurology. 1985;35(10):1406–14.
9. Hauser WA. Prevention of post-traumatic epilepsy. N Engl J Med. 1990;323(8):540–2.
10. Hauser WA, Tabaddor K, Factor PR, Finer C. Seizures and head injury in an urban community. Neurology. 1984;34(6):746–51.
11. Temkin NR, Dikmen SS, Wilensky AJ, Keihm J, Chabal S, Winn HR. A randomized, double-blind study of phenytoin for the prevention of post-traumatic seizures. N Engl J Med. 1990;323(8):497–502.
12. Black P, Shepard RH, Walker AE. Outcome of head trauma: age and post-traumatic seizures. Ciba Found Symp. 1975;34:215–26.

13. Scholtes FB, Renier WO, Meinardi H. Generalized convulsive status epilepticus: causes, therapy, and outcome in 346 patients. Epilepsia. 1994;35(5):1104–12.

14. Vespa PM, Nuwer MR, Nenov V, Ronne-Engstrom E, Hovda DA, Bergsneider M, et al. Increased incidence and impact of nonconvulsive and convulsive seizures after traumatic brain injury as detected by continuous electroencephalographic monitoring. J Neurosurg. 1999;91(5):750–60.

15. Claassen J, Mayer SA, Kowalski RG, Emerson RG, Hirsch LJ. Detection of electrographic seizures with continuous EEG monitoring in critically ill patients. Neurology. 2004;62(10):1743–8.

16. Englander J, Bushnik T, Duong TT, Cifu DX, Zafonte R, Wright J, Hughes R, Bergman W. Analyzing risk factors for late posttraumatic seizures: a prospective, multicenter investigation. Arch Phys Med Rehabil. 2003;84(3):365–73.

17. Frey LC. Epidemiology of posttraumatic epilepsy: a critical review. Epilepsia. 2003;44(Suppl 10):11–7.

18. Vespa PM, Miller C, McArthur D, Eliseo M, Etchepare M, Hirt D, Glenn TC, Martin N, Hovda D. Nonconvulsive electrographic seizures after traumatic brain injury result in intracranial pressure and metabolic crisis. Crit Care Med. 2007;35(12):2830–6.

19. Wiedemayer H, Triesch K, Schäfer H, Stolke D. Early seizures following non-penetrating traumatic brain injury in adults: risk factors and clinical significance. Brain Inj. 2002;16(4):323–30.

20. Vespa P. Continuous EEG monitoring for the detection of seizures in traumatic brain injury, infarction, and intracerebral hemorrhage: to detect and protect. J Clin Neurophysiol. 2005;22(2):99–106.

21. Ronne-Engrstrom E, Winkler T. Continuous EEG monitoring in patients with traumatic brain injury reveals a high incidence of epileptiform activity. Acta Neurol Scand. 2006;114(1):47–53.

22. Temkin NR. Risk factors for posttraumatic seizures in adults. Epilepsia. 2003;44(Suppl 10):18–20.

23. Najafi MR, Tabesh H, Hosseini H, Akbari M, Najafi MA. Early and late posttraumatic seizures following traumatic brain injury: a five-year follow up survival study. Adv Biomed Res. 2015;4:82. doi:10.4103/2277-9175.156640.

24. Pugh MJ, Orman JA, Jaramillo CA, Salinsky MC, Eapen BC, Towne AR, Amuan ME, Roman G, McNamee SD, Kent TA, McMillan KK, Hamid H, Grafman JH. The prevalence of epilepsy and association with traumatic brain injury in veterans of the Afghanistan and Iraq wars. J Head Trauma Rehabil. 2015;30(1):29–37.

25. Mansfield RT. Head injuries in children and adults. Crit Care Clin. 1997;13(3):611–28.

26. Jennett WB, Lewin W. Traumatic epilepsy after closed head injuries. J Neurol Neurosurg Psychiatry. 1960;23:295–301.

27. Ottman R, Lee JH, Risch N, Hauser WA, Susser M. Clinical indicators of genetic susceptibility to epilepsy. Epilepsia. 1996;37(4):353–61.

28. Diaz-Arrastia R, Gong Y, Fair S, Scott KD, Garcia MC, Carlile MC, Agostini MA, Van Ness PC. Increased risk of late posttraumatic seizures associated with inheritance of APOE epsilon4 allele. Arch Neurol. 2003;60(6):818–22.

29. Wagner AK, Miller MA, Scanlon J, Ren D, Kochanek PM, Conley YP. Adenosine A1 receptor gene variants associated with posttraumatic seizures after severe TBI. Epilepsy Res. 2010;90(3):259–72.

30. Darrah SD, Miller MA, Ren D, Hoh NZ, Scanlon J, Conley YP, Wagner AK. Genetic variability in glutamic acid decarboxylase genes: associations with post-traumatic seizures after severe TBI. Epilepsy Res. 2013;103:180–94.

31. Desai BT, Whitman S, Coonley-Hoganson R, Coleman TE, Gabriel G, Dell J. Seizures and civilian head injuries. Epilepsia. 1983;24(3):289–96.

32. McCrory PR, Bladin PF, Berkovic SF. Retrospective study of concussive convulsions in elite Australian rules and rugby league footballers: phenomenology, aetiology, and outcome. BMJ. 1997;314(7075):171–4.

33. McCrory PR, Berkovic SF. Video analysis of acute motor and convulsive manifestations in sport-related concussion. Neurology. 2000;54(7):1488–91.

34. Hahn YS, Fuchs S, Flannery AM, Barthel MJ, McLone DG. Factors influencing posttraumatic seizures in children. Neurosurgery. 1988;22(5):864–7.

35. Lewis RJ, Yee L, Inkelis SH, Gilmore D. Clinical predictors of post-traumatic seizures in children with head trauma. Ann Emerg Med. 1993;22(7):1114–8.

36. Ong LC, Dhillon MK, Selladurai BM, Maimunah A, Lye MS. Early post-traumatic seizures in children: clinical and radiological aspects of injury. J Paediatr Child Health. 1996;32(2):173–6.

37. Hahn YS, Chyung C, Barthel MJ, Bailes J, Flannery AM, McLone DG. Head injuries in children under 36 months of age. Demography and outcome. Childs Nerv Syst. 1988;4(1):34–40.

38. Hendrick EB, Harris L. Post-traumatic epilepsy in children. J Trauma. 1968;8(4):547–56.

39. Kharatishvili I, Nissinen JP, McIntosh TK, Pitkänen A. A model of posttraumatic epilepsy induced by lateral fluid-percussion brain injury in rats. Neuroscience. 2006;140(2):685–97.

40. Marmarou A, Foda MA, van den Brink W, Campbell J, Kita H, Demetriadou K. A new model of diffuse brain injury in rats. Part I: pathophysiology and biomechanics. J Neurosurg. 1994;80(2):291–300.

41. Nilsson P, Ronne-Engstrom E, Flink R, Ungerstedt U, Carlson H, Hillered L. Epileptic seizure activity in the acute phase following cortical impact trauma in rat. Brain Res. 1994;637(1–2):227–32.

42. Beaumont A, Marmarou A, Czigner A, Yamamoto M, Demetriadou K, Shirotani T, Marmarou C, Dunbar J. The impact-acceleration model of head injury: injury severity predicts motor and cognitive performance after trauma. Neurol Res. 1999;21(8):742–54.

43. Hamm RJ, Pike BR, Temple MD, O'Dell DM, Lyeth BG. The effect of postinjury kindled seizures on cognitive performance of traumatically brain-injured rats. Exp Neurol. 1995;136(2):143–8.

44. Bolkvadze T. Pitkänen. Development of post-traumatic epilepsy after controlled cortical impact and lateral fluid-percussion-induced brain injury in the mouse. J Neurotrauma. 2012;29(5):789–812.

45. Willmore LJ. Post-traumatic epilepsy: cellular mechanisms and implications for treatment. Neurology. 1990;31(Suppl 3):S67–73.

46. D'Ambrosio R, Maris DO, Grady MS, Winn HR, Janigro D. Impaired K(+) homeostasis and altered electrophysiological properties of post-traumatic hippocampal glia. J Neurosci. 1999;19(18):8152–62.

47. Rzigalinski BA, Weber JT, Williughby KA, Ellis EF. Intracellular free calcium dynamics in stretch-injured astrocytes. J Neurochem. 1998;70(6):2377–85.

48. Yang L, Benardo LS. Valproate prevents epileptiform activity after trauma in an in vitro model in neocortical slices. Epilepsia. 2000;41(12):1507–13.

49. Golarai G, Greenwood AC, Feeney DM, Connor JA. Physiological and structural evidence for hippocampal involvement in persistent seizure susceptibility after traumatic brain injury. J Neurosci. 2001;21(21):8523–37.

50. Hunt RF, Boychuk JA, Smith BN. Neural circuit mechanisms of post-traumatic epilepsy. Front Cell Neurosci. 2013;7:89. doi:10.3389/fncel.2013.00089.

51. Bergsneider M, Hovda DA, Shalmon E, Kelly DF, Vespa PM, Martin NA, et al. Cerebral hyperglycolysis following severe traumatic brain injury in humans: a positron emission tomography study. J Neurosurg. 1997;86(2):241–51.

52. Bullock R, Zauner A, Myseros JS, Marmarou A, Woodward JJ, Young HF. Evidence for prolonged release of excitatory amino acids in severe human head trauma. Relationship to clinical events. Ann N Y Acad Sci. 1995;765:290–7.

53. Goodman JC, Valadka AB, Gopinath SP, Cormio M, Robertson CS. Lactate and excitatory amino acids measured by microdialysis are decreased by pentobarbital coma in head-injured patients. J Neurotrauma. 1996;13(10):549–56.

54. Nilsson P, Hillered L, Olsson Y, Sheardown MJ, Hansen AJ. Regional changes in interstitial K+ and Ca2+ levels following cortical compression contusion trauma in rats. J Cereb Blood Flow Metab. 1993;13(2):183–92.

55. DeWitt DS, Prough DS, Taylor CL, Whitley JM. Reduced cerebral blood flow, oxygen delivery, and electroencephalographic activity after traumatic brain injury and mild hemorrhage in cats. J Neurosurg. 1992;76(5):812–21.

56. Prince DA, Parada I, Scalise K, Graber K, Shen F. Epilepsy following cortical injury: cellular and molecular mechanisms as targets for potential prophylaxis. Epilepsia. 2009;50(Suppl 2):30–40.

57. Weber JT. Altered calcium signaling following traumatic brain injury. Front Pharmacol. 2012;3:60. doi:10.3389/fphar.2012.00060.

58. McKinney RA, Debanne D, Gahwiler BH, Thompson SM. Lesion-induced axonal sprouting and hyperexcitability in the hippocampus in vitro: implications for the genesis of posttraumatic epilepsy. Nat Med. 1997;3(9):990–6.

59. Lowenstein DH, Thomas MJ, Smith DH, McIntosh TK. Selective vulnerability of dentate hilar neurons following traumatic brain injury: a potential mechanistic link between head trauma and disorders of the hippocampus. J Neurosci. 1992;12(12):4846–53.

60. Hunt RF, Scheff SW, Bn S. Regionally localized recurrent excitation in the dentate gyrus of a cortical contusion model of posttraumatic epilepsy. J Neurophysiol. 2010;103(3):1490–500.

61. Swartz BE, Houser CR, Tomiyasu U, Walsh GO, DeSalles A, Rich JR, Delgado-Escueta A. Hippocampal cell loss in posttraumatic human epilepsy. Epilepsia. 2006;47(8):1373–82.

62. Jin X, Prince DA, Huguenard JR. Layer V pyramidal neurons of chronically injured epileptogenic neocortex in rats. J Neurosci. 2006;26(18):4891–900.

63. Ballanyi K, Grafe P, ten Bruggencate G. Ion activities and potassium uptake mechanisms of glial cells in guinea–pig olfactory cortex slices. J Physiol. 1987;382:159–74.

64. Janigro D, Gasparini S, D'Ambrosio R, McKhann G, DiFrancesco D. Reduction of K+ uptake in glia prevents long-term depression maintenance and causes epileptiform activity. J Neurosci. 1997;17(8):2813–24.

65. Seiffert E, Dreier JP, Ivens S, Bechmann I, Tomkins O, Heinemann U, Friedman A. Lasting blood-brain barrier disruption induces epileptic focus in the rat somatosensory cortex. J Neurosci. 2004;24(36):7829–36.

66. Korn A, Golan H, Melamed I, Pascual-Marqui R, Friedman A. Focal cortical dysfunction and blood-brain barrier disruption in patients with postconcussion syndrome. J Clin Neurophysiol. 2005;22(1):1–9.

67. Morganti-Kossmann MC, Rancan M, Otto VI, Stahel PF, Kossmann T. Role of cerebral inflammation after traumatic brain injury: a revisited concept. Shock. 2001;16(3):165–77.

68. Vespa P, Tubi M, Claassen J, Blanco M, McArthur D, Velazquez AG, et al. Metabolic crisis occurs with seizures and periodic discharges after brain trauma. Ann Neurol. 2016. doi: 10.1002/ana.24606

69. Chesnut RM, Marshall LF, Klauber MR, Blunt BA, Baldwin N, Eisenberg HM, et al. The role of secondary brain injury in determining outcome from severe head injury. J Trauma. 1993;34(2):216–22.

70. Dawson RE, Webster JE, Gurdjian ES. Serial electroencephalography in acute head injuries. J Neurosurg. 1951;8(6):613–30.

71. Bricolo A, Turazzi S, Faccioli F, Odorizzi F, Sciaretta G, Erculiani P. Clinical application of compressed spectral array in long-term EEG monitoring of comatose patients. Electroencephalogr Clin Neurophysiol. 1978;45(2):211–25.

72. Hutchinson DO, Frith RW, Shaw NA, Judson JA, Cant BR. A comparison between electroencephalography and somatosensory evoked potentials for outcome prediction following severe head injury. Electroencephalogr Clin Neurophysiol. 1991;78(3):228–33.

73. Rumpl E, Lorenzi E, Hackl JM, Gerstenbrand F, Hengl W. The EEG at different stages of acute secondary traumatic midbrain and bulbar brain syndromes. Electroencephalogr Clin Neurophysiol. 1979;46(5):487–97.

74. Synek VM. Revised EEG coma scale in diffuse acute head injuries in adults. Clin Exp Neurol. 1990;27:99–111.

75. Logi F, Pasqualetti P, Tomaiuolo F. Predict recovery of consciousness in post-acute severe brain injury: the role of EEG reactivity. Brain Inj. 2011;25(10):972–9.

76. Vespa PM, Boscardin WJ, Hovda DA, McArthur DL, Nuwer MR, Martin NA, et al. Early and persistent impaired percent alpha variability of continuous electroencephalography monitoring as predictive of poor outcome after traumatic brain injury. J Neurosurg. 2002;97(1):84–92.

77. Sironi VA, Ravagnati L, Signoroni G. Diagnostic and prognostic value of EEG compressed spectral analysis in post-traumatic coma. In: Villani R, Papo I, Giovanelli M, editors. Advances in Neurotraumatology. Amsterdam: Excerpta Medica; 1982. p. 328–30.

78. Cant BR, Shaw NA. Monitoring by compressed spectral array in prolonged coma. Neurology. 1984;34(1):35–9.

79. Steudel WI, Kruger J. Using the spectral analysis of the EEG for prognosis of severe brain injuries in the first post-traumatic week. Acta Neurochir Suppl (Wien). 1979;28(1):40–2.

80. Brophy GM, Bell R, Claassen J, Alldredge B, Bleck TP, Glauser T, et al. Guidelines for the evaluation and management of status epilepticus. Neurocrit Care. 2012;17(1):3–23.

81. Claassen J, Taccone FS, Horn P, Holtkamp M, Stocchetti N, Oddo M. Recommendations on the use of EEG monitoring in critically ill patients: consensus statement from the neurointensive care section of the ESICM. Intensive Care Med. 2013;39(8):1337–51.

82. Varelas PN, Spanaki MV, Hacein-Bey L, Hether T, Terranova B, EEG E. Indications and diagnostic yield. Neurology. 2003;61(5):702–4.

83. Nuwer M. Assessment of digital EEG, quantitative EEG, and EEG brain mapping: report of the American Academy of Neurology and the American Clinical Neurophysiology Society. Neurology. 1997;49(1):277–92.

84. Claassen J, Vespa P. Electrophysiologic monitoring in acute brain injury. Neurocrit Care. 2014;21:S129–47.

85. Waziri A, Claassen J, Stuart RM, Arif H, Schmidt JM, Mayer SA, et al. Intracortical electroencephalography in acute brain injury. Ann Neurol. 2009;66(3):366–77.

86. Roppolo LP, Walters K. Airway management in neurological emergencies. Neurocrit Care. 2004;1(4):405–14.

87. McCluggage LK, Voils SA, Bullock MR. Phenytoin toxicity due to genetic polymorphism. Neurocrit Care. 2009;10(2):222–4.

88. Haltiner AM, Newell DW, Temkin NR, Dikmen SS, Winn HR. Side effects and mortality associated with use of phenytoin for early posttraumatic seizure prophylaxis. J Neurosurg. 1999;91(4):588–92.

89. Pechadre JC, Lauxerois M, Colnet G, Commun C, Dimicoli C, Bonnard M, et al. Prevention of late post-traumatic epilepsy by phenytoin in severe brain injuries. 2 years' follow-up. Presse Med. 1991;20(18):841–5.

90. Young B, Rapp RP, Norton JA, Haack D, Tibbs PA, Bean JR. Failure of prophylactically administered phenytoin to prevent early posttraumatic seizures. J Neurosurg. 1983;58(2):231–5.

91. Glötzner FL, Haubitz I, Miltner F, Kapp G, Pflughaupt KW. Seizure prevention using carbamazepine following severe brain injuries. Neurochirurgia. 1983;26(3):66–79.

92. Temkin NR, Dikmen SS, Anderson GD, Wilensky AJ, Holmes MD, Cohen W, et al. Valproate therapy for prevention of posttraumatic seizures: a randomized trial. J Neurosurg. 1999;91(4):593–600.

93. Jones KE, Puccio AM, Harshman KJ, Falcione B, Benedict N, Jankowitz BT, et al. Levetiracetam versus phenytoin for seizure prophylaxis in severe traumatic brain injury. Neurosurg Focus. 2008;25(4):E3.

94. Inaba K, Menaker J, Branco BC, Gooch J, Okoye OT, Herrold J, et al. A prospective multicenter comparison of levetiracetam versus phenytoin for early posttraumatic seizure prophylaxis. J Trauma Acute Care Surg. 2013;74(3):766–71.

95. Caballero GC, Hughes DW, Maxwell PR, Green K, Gamboa CD, Barthol CA. Retrospective analysis of levetiracetam compared to phenytoin for seizure prophylaxis in adults with traumatic brain injury. Hosp Pharm. 2013;48(9):757–61.

96. Gabriel WM, Rowe AS. Long-term comparison of GOS-E scores in patients treated with phenytoin or levetiracetam for posttraumatic seizure prophylaxis after traumatic brain injury. Ann Pharmacother. 2014;48(11):1440–4.

97. Szaflarski JP, Sangha KS, Lindsell CJ, Shutter LA. Prospective, randomized, single-blinded comparative trial of intravenous levetiracetam versus phenytoin for seizure prophylaxis. Neurocrit Care. 2010;12(2):165–72.

98. McQueen JK, Blackwood DH, Harris P, Kalbag RM, Johnson AL. Low risk of late post-traumatic seizures following severe head injury: implications for clinical trials of prophylaxis. J Neurol Neurosurg Psychiatry. 1983;46(10):899–904.

99. Manaka S. Cooperative prospective study on posttraumatic epilepsy: risk factors and the effect of prophylactic anticonvulsant. Jpn J Psychiatry Neurol. 1992;46(2):311–5.

100. Temkin NR, Anderson GD, Winn HR, Ellenbogen RG, Britz GW, Schuster J, et al. Magnesium sulfate for neuroprotection after traumatic brain injury: a randomised controlled trial. Lancet Neurol. 2007;6(1):29–38.

101. Foundation BT, American Association of Neurological Surgeons, Congress of Neurological Surgeons, The Joint Section on Neurotrauma and Critical Care. Guidelines for the management of severe traumatic brain injury. XIII. Antiseizure prophylaxis. J Neurotrauma. 2007;24(Suppl 1):S83–6.

102. Chang BS, Lowenstein DH. Practice parameter: antiepileptic drug prophylaxis in severe traumatic brain injury. Report of the Quality Standards Subcommittee of the American Academy of Neurology. Neurology. 2003;60(1):10–6.

103. Thompson K, Pohlmann-Eden B, Campbell LA, Abel H. Pharmacological treatments for preventing epilepsy following traumatic head injury. Cochrane Database Syst Rev. 2015;8:CD009900 10.1002/14651858.CD009900.pub2

104. Dikmen SS, Temkin NR, Miller B, Machamer J, Winn HR. Neurobehavioral effects of phenytoin prophylaxis of posttraumatic seizures. JAMA. 1999;265(10):1271–7.

105. Bhullar IS, Johnson D, Paul JP, Kerwin AJ, Tepas JJ, Frykberg ER. More harm than good: antiseizure prophylaxis after traumatic brain injury does not decrease seizure rates but may inhibit functional recovery. J Trauma Acute Care Surg. 2014;76(1):54–60.

106. Pitkänen A, Immonen R, Ndode-Ekane X, Gröhn O, Stöhr T, Nissinen J. Effect of lacosamide on structural damage and functional recovery after traumatic brain injury in rats. Epilepsy Res. 2014;108(4):653–65.

107. Lu XC, Shear DA, Graham PB, Bridson GW, Uttamsingh V, Chen Z, Leung LY, Tortella FC. Dual therapeutic effects of C-10068, a dextromethorphan derivative, against post-traumatic nonconvulsive seizures and neuroinflammation in a rat model of penetrating ballistic-like brain injury. J Neurotrauma. 2015;32(20):1621–32.

108. Young B, Rapp RP, Norton JA, Haack D, Tibbs PA, Bean JR. Failure of prophylactically administered phenytoin to prevent late posttraumatic seizures. J Neurosurg. 1983;58(2):236–41.

Brain Tumors and Critical Care Seizures

Panayiotis N. Varelas, Jose Ignacio Suarez,
and Marianna V. Spanaki

Introduction

Primary and metastatic brain tumors are frequently associated with seizures and epilepsy.

In the intensive care unit (ICU), three categories of patients with brain tumors may be brought to the intensivist's attention related to seizures. (1) Some of these patients, especially if the seizures recur or are associated with significant cerebral edema, hemorrhage, signs of increased intracranial pressure, or pending herniation, will end up being admitted to the ICU and spend anywhere from one day to few days of monitoring. In all these cases, the members of the ICU team will be the first ones to address at least the acute, short-term management of seizures. (2) The second large category includes postoperative patients after brain tumor resection, who spend at least one day in the ICU for observation. These patients may have no history of seizures or may have exhibited one or more seizures in the ICU, and appropriate treatment should be prescribed. Therefore, an important issue to be addressed in the postoperative period, if patients are seizure-free, is whether they need prophylactic antiepileptic drug (AED) treatment during their ICU or hospital stay. (3) The third category includes patients with known and already treated brain tumors, who are admitted because of refractory seizures or status epilepticus (SE) or who have an unexplained change in mental status and are found to be in nonconvulsive status epilepticus.

There are not many data regarding the ICU stay and management of these patients. A study by Ziai et al. addressed only postoperative issues. In this retrospective study, only 23/158 (15%) postoperative tumor patients had a >24 h stay in the NICU at the Johns Hopkins Hospital [1]. Independent predictors of >1-day stay in the NICU were a high tumor severity index (comprising preoperative radiologic characteristics of tumor location, mass effect, and midline shift), an intraoperative fluid score (comprising estimated blood loss, total volume of crystalloid, and other colloid/hypertonic solutions administered), and postoperative intubation. Seizures were preoperatively present in 15/158 (9.5%) patients. Five patients (3.2%) had postoperative seizures. More patients who stayed longer had seizures postoperatively (2/135 patients in group 1 [$\leq$24 h NICU stay] vs 3/23 patients in group 2 [>24 h NICU stay], odds, 95% CI, 10, 1.6–62.5, $P = 0.02$). NICU resource use was reviewed in detail for 134 of 135 patients who stayed in the unit for $\leq$1 day. A total of 226 NICU interventions were performed in 69 (51%) patients. Fifteen (6.6%) were related to IV AED administration, but this was never done after the first 16 postoperative hours. This study provides valuable information regarding incidence of ICU seizures in brain tumor patients and use of ICU resources to treat them, but the results cannot be necessarily generalized to other ICUs.

A more recent study of 105 pediatric patients admitted to a pediatric ICU after brain tumor resection showed that the majority (69.5%) stayed there for <1 day. The presence of preoperative seizures was more common in the <1 day group, with 25 (34%) patients reporting seizures compared to 3 (9%) in the >1-day group. Eleven patients had new-onset seizures. Development of new seizures was more common in the >1-day group. Seizures were not independent predictors of longer PICU stay [2].

P.N. Varelas (✉)
Departments of Neurology and Neurosurgery, Henry Ford Hospital, 2799 West Grand Blvd, Detroit, MI 48202, USA

Department of Neurology, Wayne State University, Detroit, MI, USA
e-mail: varelas@neuro.hfh.edu

J.I. Suarez
Baylor College of Medicine, Houston, TX 77030, USA
e-mail: jisuarez@bcm.edu

M.V. Spanaki
Henry Ford Hospital, Detroit, MI 48202, USA

Wayne State University, Detroit, MI 48202, USA
e-mail: mspanak1@hfhs.org

© Springer International Publishing AG 2017
P.N. Varelas, J. Claassen (eds.), *Seizures in Critical Care*, Current Clinical Neurology, DOI 10.1007/978-3-319-49557-6_12

Incidence

Overall, the incidence of brain tumors is 4% in patients with epilepsy [3]. Conversely, seizure occurrence remains a major morbidity problem in patients with intracranial tumors. Between 30 and 50% of patients with brain tumors present with seizures, and an additional 30% will later develop seizures [3]. Between one third and more than half of patients with brain tumors present with seizures as the initial symptom [4]. In 2424 glioblastoma cases in the Swedish National Cancer Registry, seizures had an odds ratio of 31.6 (95% confidence interval 24.7–40.3) to be present at diagnosis [5]. Approximately 30–70% of patients with primary brain tumors will have seizures at some point throughout their disease [6–9]. Similarly, about 40% of all patients with metastatic brain tumors will have a seizure during their disease [10, 11]. Half of these seizures will be simple or partial complex seizures and the other half secondary generalized seizures [12–14]. Brain tumors are rarely associated with primary generalized seizures.

SE, either convulsive or nonconvulsive, can also occur in patients with brain tumors. Overall, SE is observed in about 12% of patients with glioblastomas [15]. In a study from the University of Virginia, 555 patients were admitted with a diagnosis of SE over a 7-year period. Fifty patients had a concurrent diagnosis of cancer, 28 (5%) of whom had SE related to the tumor or treatment [16]. In another study, 10.5% of patients with newly diagnosed glioblastoma multiforme and initial postsurgery seizures presented in SE. Two cases of nonconvulsive SE were noted in patients who had been weaned off AEDs from the time of surgery, and two cases of convulsive SE were observed in patients that had never been treated with AEDs [17].

Among the primary brain tumors, the highest incidence of seizures is found in patients with low-grade gliomas (65–85%, first clinical symptom in 70–90% at an average age of 38–40 years) [15], gangliogliomas (80–90%, at an average age of 17–21 years) [18], and dysembryoplastic neuroectodermal tumors (DNET, 100%, at an average age of 15 years) [3, 19]. High-grade IV tumors (glioblastomas) have an incidence of about 30–62% (average age at presentation 60 years), in about two thirds at presentation and in one third developing during the course of the disease [3, 6, 20]. In a recent systematic review of meningiomas, preoperative seizures were observed in 29.2% of 4709 patients with supratentorial meningiomas and were significantly predicted by male sex, absence of headache, peritumoral edema, and non-skull base location. After surgery, seizure freedom was achieved in 69.3% of 703 patients with preoperative epilepsy and was more than twice as likely in those without peritumoral edema. Of 1085 individuals without preoperative epilepsy who underwent resection, new postoperative seizures were seen in 12.3% of patients [21].

Other studies have estimated the incidence of seizures with metastatic tumors at 35% [22–24]. Melanoma, chorio-carcinoma, lung cancer, and breast cancer are tumors frequently metastasizing to the brain and associated with hemorrhage and seizures. Among metastatic tumors, melanoma seems to have the highest incidence of seizures.

Conversely, based on a study from the Cleveland Clinic, among patients with intractable chronic epilepsy, the most common types of tumors discovered were ganglioglioma in 49/127 (39%) of cases and low-grade astrocytoma in 48/127 (38%) of cases [25]. Pleomorphic xanthoastrocytoma, DNET tumors, and oligodendroglioma were also tumors frequently associated with epilepsy. As already mentioned, it seems likely that low-grade, well-differentiated gliomas have higher incidence of seizures than more aggressive glioblastomas or anaplastic astrocytomas [3, 26]. A similar distinction may be true for age: children have low-grade tumors and epilepsy as the primary, if only, sign, compared to middle-aged or elderly adults who have higher-grade tumors and more neurological focality [3].

Different brain areas are also characterized by varying susceptibility to seizures. For example, among patients with gliomas, seizures occur in 59% of frontal tumors, 42% of parietal tumors, 35% of temporal tumors, and 33% of occipital tumors [27]. Using a summed-statistic image showing the aggregate location of 124 tumors, Lee et al. demonstrated that smaller tumors, those growing less quickly and those located in the superficial cortical areas, especially temporal or frontal lobes or the insula, have a higher incidence of seizures [28]. Similar observations suggest that the limbic and temporal lobe, primary and supplementary motor (M-I, M-II) areas, and primary and secondary somatosensory (S-I, S-II opercula and insula) areas have the lowest thresholds for seizures [26]. In contrast, the occipital lobe has a much higher threshold [29]. Tumors in the subcortical areas, such as thalamus and posterior fossa, are much less epileptogenic as well.

Clinical Presentation

Besides focal neurological deficits, altered mental status, headache and signs of increased intracranial pressure (nausea, vomiting, papilledema), and seizures are one of the most common presentations in patients with brain tumors [30]. A first, unprovoked seizure in an adult is always concerning for an intracranial tumor, until proven otherwise [31].

The timing of their presentation is important to know. Seizure onset is usually within the first 24 h postoperatively [32, 33] and, therefore, may be witnessed during the ICU patient stay. Patients who had seizures preoperatively are at a higher risk of developing postoperative seizures [34]. The type of the seizures does not seem to be different pre- and postoperatively [33, 34].

High-frequency seizures (>4 seizures per month) or SE are observed in 18% and 12% patients with brain tumors, respectively [35]. SE occurred either at the time of tumor diagnosis (29%) or during tumor progression (23%). However, an almost equal percentage of SE occurred, while the tumor was stable (23%) [16].

Not all seizures have the same presentation: several seizure types have been reported and mainly reflect the location of the lesion. Most characteristic are the hypothalamic hamartomas, which are associated with gelastic seizures (sudden outburst of laughter or crying with no apparent cause) and precocious puberty, but these are rare phenomena, representing 0.8% of all admissions for video EEG in a recent study [36]. Parasagittal meningiomas may present with generalized seizures when located in the anterior one third of the sagittal sinus, whereas meningiomas of the middle third usually present with focal seizures, at times following a Jacksonian marching pattern. Simple or partial seizures characterized by olfactory, gustatory and epigastric auras, depersonalization, feelings of fear, and pleasure are usually an indication of temporal lobe pathology. Complex partial seizures with repetitive psychomotor movements (e.g., masticatory), impairment of consciousness, or déjà vu phenomena are also associated with the temporal lobe. Delusions and psychotic behavior have been reported with frontal lobe tumors [37]. Lesions involving the frontal eye fields are associated with turning of the eyes and head to one side (contraversive or ipsiversive, depending on the side of turning compared to the lesion). Parietal lobe tumors are associated with sensory seizures, and occipital lobe tumors can cause seizures with visual phenomena such as seeing lights, colors, and geometric patterns [31].

Because some tumors present with nonconvulsive seizures or SE, a clinical presentation of decreased or altered mental status, including coma, should not be attributed to the tumor per se, but an evaluation with EEG should be undertaken to exclude this treatable cause. Five patients out of 84 (6%) with cancer and altered mental status (coma or delirium) were found to be on NCSE by EEG in an Italian study. None of these patients had brain metastases: one was aphasic, two patients treated with ifosfamide had absence, and two patients treated with cisplatin had complex partial status epilepticus. All had rapid recovery after antiepileptic treatment [38]. In another study, four patients never diagnosed before with metastatic CNS disease presented with altered mental status. All patients had abnormal neuroimaging of the brain were in NCSE by EEG and were treated with fosphenytoin IV. In two patients, the NCSE resolved, but in the other two, despite an initial mental status improvement, status recurred and both eventually died after 5 and 20 days, respectively [39]. Not all patients with tumors and NCSE are comatose. In a retrospective study, 26 episodes of NCSE were identified in 25 patients (4%). Eleven patients had primary brain tumor, twelve systemic cancer, and two had both. At diagnostic EEG, 18 were awake, 3 were lethargic, and only 5 patients were comatose [40]. Moreover, many patients have subclinical or a combination of clinical and subclinical seizures. In a recent study of 1101 brain tumor patients, 259 (24%) had an EEG and 24

(2%) had NCSE. The vast majority of seizures captured were subclinical with 13 patients (54%) having only subclinical seizures. Treatment resolved NCSE in 22 patients (92%) with accompanying clinical improvement in 18 (75%) of those patients [41].

Pathophysiology

The pathogenic mechanisms of epileptogenesis in patients with brain tumors are not fully understood [26] and beyond the scope of this chapter. Several excellent reviews are available for the interested reader [3, 42, 43].

The location, as well as the histopathology which correlates with the infiltrative potential, is an important factor determining the clinical presentation of the tumors [44]. Tumors that tend to cause hemorrhage, necrosis, inflammation, and ischemia have a higher incidence of seizures. Focal hypoxia, mass effect and edema, decreased blood-brain barrier, and altered levels of excitatory amino acids all have been postulated to play a role in epileptogenesis. Hemosiderin deposition in cortical areas preoperatively, as assessed by susceptibility-weighted MRI sequence, also correlates with the development of seizures [45]. Different types of tumors may cause seizures through different mechanisms. Some tumors, like DNETs and gangliogliomas, with significantly higher seizure frequencies, have been associated with intrinsic epileptogenic properties. Brain tumors are also thought to alter the dendritic, axonal, and synaptic plasticity of the neurons and in this way contribute to epileptogenesis [46, 47].

At a molecular level, sodium channels in tumor cells may play a role in epileptogenesis, since these channels are responsible for generating action potentials more frequently than others, thus making cells such as those in glioblastoma intrinsically hyperexcitable [48, 49]. Inhibitory (GABA, taurine), as well as excitatory amino acid (glutamate, aspartate) deregulation, may also contribute to the process [50–52]. Raised glutamate concentrations in tumor and peritumor tissue and increased expression of peritumor system X_c^- (a major glutamate transport protein on astrocyte membranes, i.e., a cysteine/glutamate exchange complex) have been shown to be independent predictors of preoperative seizures [53]. Phosphorylation of the extrasynaptic NMDA receptor 2B subunit has also been reported in human peritumoral tissue. This receptor change increases its permeability for Ca^{++} influx and subsequently mediates neuronal overexcitation and seizure activity [54]. Downregulation of glutamine synthetase, an enzyme found deficient in sclerotic hippocampi of patients with temporal lobe epilepsy, has also been found in astrocytes of patients with high-grade gliomas, resulting in glutamate accumulation and seizure generation [55]. Increased levels of Fe^{++} in peritumoral brain tissue convey a potential for paroxysmal epileptogenic activity, which may be the reason why hemosiderin deposition increases the risk for seizures [45]. Alterations in the glial gap junctions have been observed in the cortex surrounding glial tumors [26]. Astrocytes also play a role in the induction and maturation of epileptogenesis. Aquaporin-4 (AQP-4), expressed by astrocyte end feet abutting microvessels, has been found with altered expression levels and redistribution in glioblastoma multiforme, a possible cause for the edema that often surrounds the tumor mass. AQP-4 expression, but not AQP-4 mRNA levels, were more frequently detected on the glioblastoma cell membranes from specimens of patients with seizures than from individuals without, implying a posttranslational mechanism [56].

All these mechanisms may be present and may work in parallel in the process of epileptogenesis. However, the individual's susceptibility to different homeostatic changes (systemic or regional) and their contribution in reducing the seizure threshold probably make up for the extensive variability noted in patients with similar findings, but different clinical presentations. Recently, the influence of genes on seizure presentation was mapped by location of the tumor, with the hypothesis being that the influence of gene expression on tumor-associated seizures is regional (gene expression may play a significant role in determining epileptogenicity in certain regions of the brain, whereas it may play little role in other regions, where the location of tumor may predominate the determination of epileptogenicity). Using gene expression imaging tools, a 9-set gene expression profile predicting long-term survivors was assigned to the location of the tumors and evaluated for seizures. Through this gene expression imaging analysis, brain regions with significantly lower expression of OLIG2 and RTN1 in patients with tumor-associated seizures were found [57].

Iatrogenic contribution is another entity that ICU specialists should be aware of. The route of drug administration in the ICU is important, besides their epileptogenic potential (see chapter Drugs Used for the Critically Ill and Critical Care Seizures). For example, patients with primary brain lymphoma receiving intrathecal chemotherapy have a 47% incidence of seizures [58]. Even IV contrast has been implicated in the generation of seizures in a patient with primary brain tumor [59].

Systemic cancer can metastasize to the brain and produce seizures as their first manifestation. Intracranial metastases usually originate from embolization of neoplastic cells to the brain, commonly in terminal arterial supply territories, such as the gray-white matter junction. However, systemic cancer may induce seizures through additional noninvasive mechanisms: coagulopathy and stroke (sinus thrombosis); nonbacterial thrombotic endocarditis with cerebral emboli; systemic metabolic derangements, such as hypomagnesemia [60] or hyponatremia [61]; opportunistic infections after chemotherapy; or direct toxicity of chemotherapeutic agents to the brain [62, 63] are few of the potential pathogenetic mechanisms for which treatment is available. Paraneoplastic syndromes, such as limbic encephalopathy with anti-Hu antibodies, can also be associated with seizures preceding the diagnosis of cancer [64]. More recently, autoantibodies against NMDA receptors which can also present with seizures or intractable epilepsy have been associated with ovarian teratomas in young women [65].

Some patients with cancer and altered mental status may be in NCSE (Fig. 12.1). EEG or continuous video EEG may be necessary to evaluate these patients and reach the correct diagnosis. If seizures become refractory to antiepileptic treatment, development of multidrug resistance proteins in tumor beds may be the cause. The multidrug resistance gene MDR1 (ABCB1, P-glycoprotein [Pgp]) and multidrug resistance-related proteins (MRP, ABCC1) are expressed in the cells forming many blood-brain and blood-CSF barriers and contribute to decreased transport into the brain parenchyma of drugs such as phenytoin, carbamazepine, phenobarbital, lamotrigine, and felbamate (levetiracetam is not a substrate for MDR1, and gabapentin may be moved out of the brain via a nonspecific transporter) [3]. These proteins are overexpressed in the cells of patients with glioma [66], focal cortical dysplasia, and ganglioglioma [67]. In a clinicopathologic study of 35 patients with gliomas and epilepsy, the authors observed MRP1 expression in tumor and endothelial cells, MRP3 and Pgp expression mainly in endothelial cells, and glutathione transferase – π (GST-pi) predominantly in tumor cells. MRP1 and MRP3 were more expressed in high-grade than in low-grade gliomas. There was a trend of a better outcome in seizure control associated with a lower expression of MRP1 and MRP3. MRP3 was statistically more expressed in tumor cells of high-grade than low-grade gliomas, more expressed in tumor bed than in periphery, and less expressed in patients with complete response to AEDs [68].

Evaluation of Patients with ICU Seizures

Most of the seizures associated with primary or metastatic CNS tumors are of focal onset (Figs. 12.2 and 12.3) with or without secondary generalization. These patients may progress to convulsive status and permanent neurologic damage. Brain tumors are not intrinsic and can lead to seizures associated with increased blood volume, intracranial pressure, and tissue displacement, resulting in cerebral herniation. Posturing in this case has to be differentiated from a seizure. Seizures due to brain tumors must also be differentiated from intermittent episodes of increased intracranial pressure with plateau waves, which cause headache, diplopia and other visual disturbances, fluctuation of mental status, motor deficits, or dystonic or opisthotonic postures.

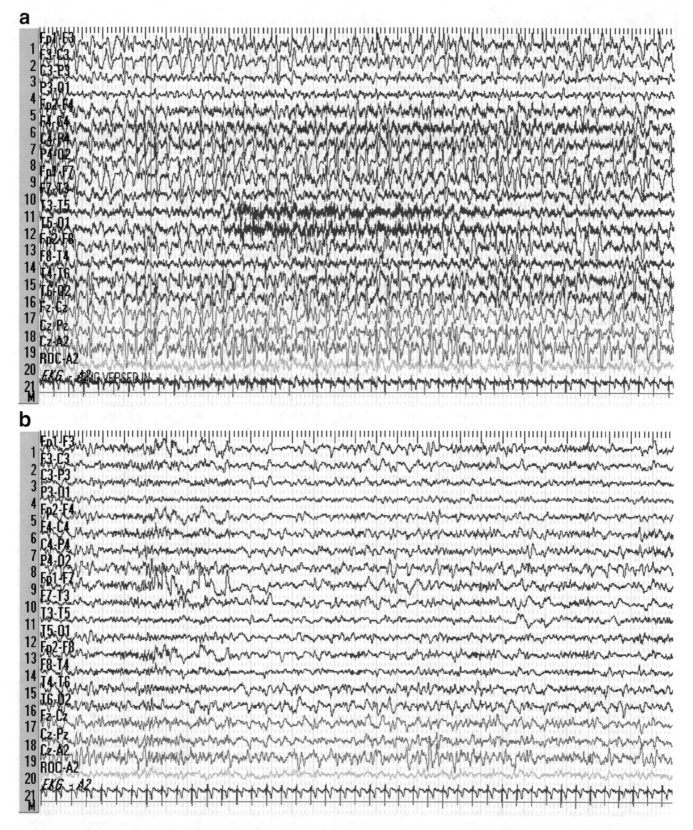

Fig. 12.1 A 63-year-old man with metastatic squamous cell carcinoma of the tonsils to the brain. Patient had two large metastases, one in the right parieto-occipital area (resected, with recurrence) and one in the left frontal area, status post whole brain radiation and chemotherapy. He was admitted to the NICU for change in mental status: drowsy, able to say only "Eeeh" with minimal stimulation, moving all four extremities, but not following commands. No toxic or metabolic reason was present in the work-up. Patient was on phenytoin with therapeutic levels. (**a**) EEG: nearly continuous triphasic waves over both frontal regions on a theta/delta background. (**b**) EEG after 2 mg of midazolam IV were administered: marked attenuation of the background, including the triphasic waves. The patient was placed on lorazepam 1 mg po tid. Two days later, his mental status had improved, and he was able to carry some conversation. Despite that, he was transferred to palliative care where he expired 9 days later

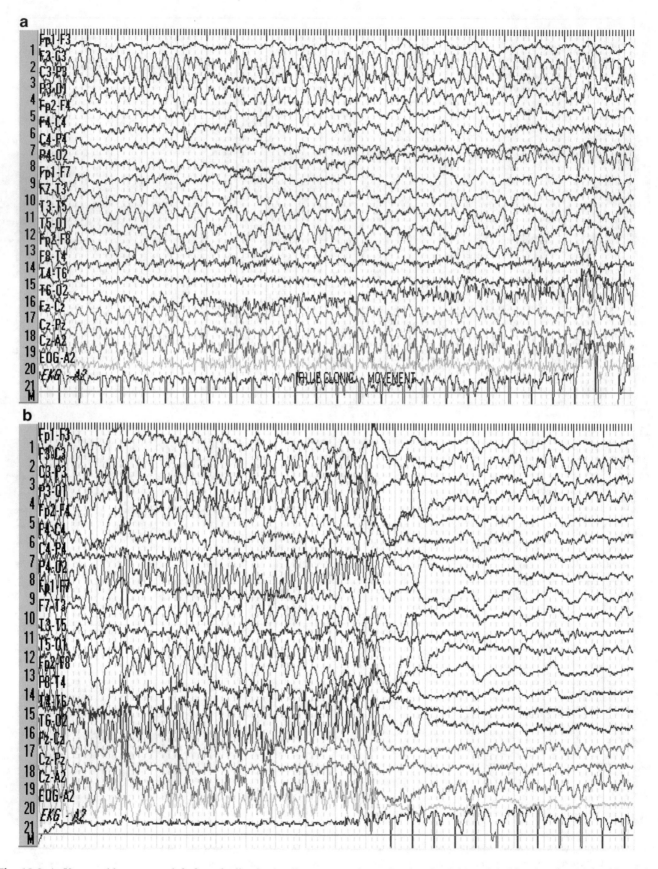

Fig. 12.2 A 59-year-old man post left frontal oligodendroglioma resection 7 days earlier, and readmitted to the NICU because of significant edema, presents with intermittent episodes of right upper extremity clonic activity lasting for 15–60 s. (**a**) EEG revealing left frontocentral epileptiform discharges at a frequency of 2–3 Hz pro-

gressing to involve the right occipital head region (right side of the epoque). (**b**) EEG 30 s later: abrupt cessation of spike and slow-wave activity with subsequent attenuation of the record. The patient responded to IV lorazepam 1 mg and extra phenytoin to correct the low levels

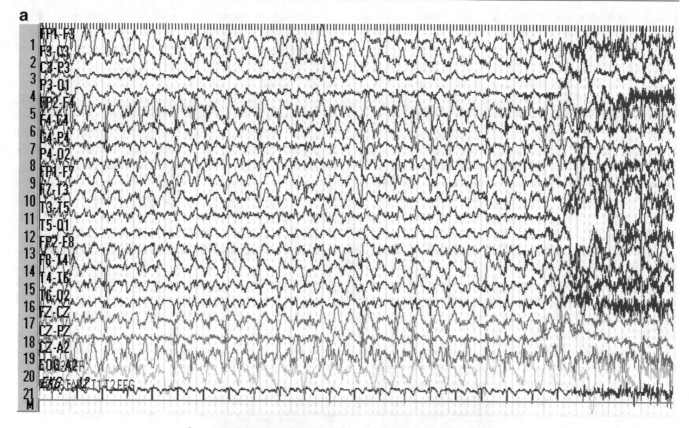

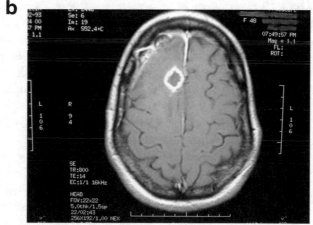

Fig. 12.3 A 48-year-old woman admitted for frequent paroxysmal episodes of staring and found to host a lesion on the CT of the head. (**a**) EEG showing rhythmic sharp waves maximally over the right fronto-central region. The patient was unresponsive with head and eyes turned to the left during this event (**b**) Gadolinium-enhanced T1-weighted MRI of the head showing a ring-enhancing lesion on the right frontal lobe. The lesion was resected and found to be a metastasis

A patient who has a sudden change of mental status postoperatively after brain tumor resection will need to be evaluated for hemorrhage, edema, infarction, as well as seizures, clinical or subclinical. In parallel with a head CT, MRI, and the appropriate workup for other common critical care causes of encephalopathy (see above), an EEG will confirm whether the patient is having nonconvulsive seizure activity and may also help in assessing the appropriate response to treatment. In a study of 102 patients with meningioma resection, Rothoerl et al. reported normal preoperative 30-minute EEGs in 49% and normal postoperative EEGs in 33.3%. Thirty-two percent of patients had preoperative and 15% postoperative seizures. Of those with preoperative seizures, 53% had complete seizure resolution postoperatively. Dominant hemispheric localization and pre-or postoperative headache were associated with postoperative seizures. Interestingly, the pre- or postoperative EEG findings were not associated with postoperative seizures in this series [69]. This may be due to the short period of EEG recording, which may have missed significant abnormalities more easily picked up on a longer or continuous EEG. The role of continuous EEG (cEEG) monitoring in this ICU population has not been well established, but there is growing evidence of its utility in diagnosing NCSE in tumor patients. Jordan monitored 124 NICU patients with cEEG and reported that 34% of them had nonconvulsive seizures and 27% were in NCSE. Among the 11 patients with brain tumors, six (54%) had nonconvulsive seizures. Overall, cEEG played a decisive or contributing role in the ICU management in 81% of brain tumor patients in a later report with additional patients by the same author [70, 71]. NCSE was reported in two patients with non-Hodgkin's lymphoma presenting with mutism and confusional state after ifosfamide (an alkylating agent, structurally an isomer of cyclophosphamide) infusion [72]. Another patient with glioblastoma multiforme was treated with IV tirapazamine and brain irradiation. After CT scan was performed with intravenous contrast medium, the patient became aphasic, and the EEG showed NCSE. IV lorazepam and a loading dose of phenytoin resolved the symptoms [59]. In the aforementioned study by Marcuse, out of 259 patients with brain tumors and an EEG, 24 (9.2%) had NCSE. Because 13 patients had only subclinical seizures and the vast majority of seizures captured in the rest were also subclinical, these patients would have never been diagnosed and treated without an EEG or CEEG [41].

If an EEG is not considered and an MRI is performed in a patient with cancer and mental status change, abnormalities that may be attributed to seizures can be found. These may alarm the intensivist and after an EEG is performed contribute to the correct diagnosis. This is the case of four patients with primary or metastatic brain tumors from Memorial Sloan Kettering Cancer Center, who had been intermittently confused or unresponsive 1–7 days before the MRI: the MRI showed cortical hyperintensity on FLAIR, T2-weighted, or diffusion-weighted images, with or without leptomeningeal enhancement on T1 with gadolinium. In two of these patients who had 18 F positron emission tomography, hypermetabolism was shown in the abnormal cortical MRI locations. All patients and another eight were in NCSE on the EEG, and all except for one improved clinically after receiving antiepileptic drugs. Repeat MRI 1–4 weeks later showed complete resolution of abnormalities in three patients and improvement in the fourth patient [73]. These results emphasize the need for electroencephalographic emergent evaluation of tumor patients with unexplained change in the neurological examination in the ICU.

Treatment

Prophylactic Administration of AEDs

The issue of prophylactic treatment of patients with brain tumors is very complex. If a seizure has already occurred, there is little doubt for the value of AEDs [74] to avoid esca-

lation to more refractory seizures or SE, but when the patient has never exhibited epileptic phenomena, such a treatment becomes more controversial. Efficacy of the treatment has to be balanced with adverse events associated with the chosen drugs. Despite the best efforts, a significant percentage of patients still have breakthrough seizures, and the response to the treatment is very unpredictable. Several reasons have to be considered: lack of AEDs to have an effect on a vast array of physiologic derangements induced by brain tumors, difficulty maintaining appropriate AEDs levels, and tumor progression or recurrence [26, 75]. In fact, in a recent retrospective study of postoperative patients with brain tumors, the odds of seizure for patients on prophylactic AED was 1.62 times higher than those not on AED, although the difference was not significant [76]. Likewise, AED use is not without adverse effects, some of them potentially serious, like severe Stevens-Johnson syndrome [77]. Moreover, there is evidence supporting increased frequency and severity of side effects from these drugs in this specific patient population: in a meta-analysis of studies examining prophylactic AED use in patients with newly diagnosed brain tumors, 23.8% (range 5–38%) of treated patients experienced side effects that were severe enough to lead to change or discontinuation of the medications. This incidence is higher than that in the general population and should make physicians sceptic about the real need for using them [74]. Unfortunately, personal preference and previous training or experience of physicians may be more important in making the decision than clinical evidence for pros and cons. According to a study conducted in Rhode Island, 55% of participating physicians gave AED prophylaxis, but the percentage differed according to the subspecialty: 33% of radiation oncologists, 50% of oncologists, 53% of neurologists, and 81% of neurosurgeons [74, 78].

The effect of surgery on seizures has been studied in numerous trials. The effect of craniotomy per se, with the meningeal or parenchymal injury that ensues, on seizure occurrence cannot be easily separated from the very effect the tumor induces. Most of the available studies were performed in mixed tumor and non-tumor patients; therefore, the conclusions may not be applicable to the former. In the next sections, we will review some of the most important studies regarding craniotomy, all including tumor patients, because these data are pertinent to the decisions that an intensivist has to make. Subsequently, we will present the data regarding prophylactic AED use specifically in patients with brain tumors.

Kvam et al. showed that out of 538 post-craniotomy patients, 23 had postoperative seizures. Out of these 23 patients, only 5 had seizures preoperatively. The authors suggested a preoperative loading dose of 10 mg/kg of phenytoin, followed by a postoperative dose of 5 mg/kg/day [32]. A study more pertinent to the ICU was conducted in Taiwan [79]. Three hundred seventy-four patients post-craniotomy were randomized to receive phenytoin (15 mg/kg IV during surgery, followed by 3–6 mg/kg/day for 3 days) or placebo. The group receiving phenytoin had two early postoperative seizures, and the placebo group had nine, but the difference was not statistically significant. Eighty percent of the seizures occurred within 20 min after surgery. Thus, the authors recommended that prophylactic anticonvulsant medication be given at least 20 min before completion of wound closure. This view was not shared by the authors of a subsequent large prospective study, who did not recommend prophylactic AEDs after supratentorial craniotomy. In this study, 276 post-craniotomy patients were randomized to receive carbamazepine or phenytoin for 6 or 24 months or no treatment [80]. The three treatment groups did not overall differ in the risk of seizures, but there was a nonsignificant 10% reduction of seizures in the two groups which received AEDs. Meningiomas had the highest risk for seizures (75% by 4 years) and pituitary tumors the lowest (21% by 4 years). Longer operations, those associated with dissection of the lesion away from the surface of the brain, and left-sided or bilateral lesions also carried a higher risk. Early seizures (within 1 week) after craniotomy did not increase the likelihood of late epilepsy. In a systematic review of seizures and meningiomas, however, no difference in the rate of new postoperative seizures was observed with or without perioperative prophylactic anticonvulsants [21]. Adding to the debate are the results of a prospective, stratified, randomized, double-blind Dutch study that compared 300 mg phenytoin/day to 1500 mg valproate/day given for 1 year in 100 post-craniotomy patients. Fourteen patients had postoperative seizures, but there was no difference in seizure incidence between the two groups [81]. Finally, a meta-analysis of six controlled studies addressing the issue showed a tendency of prophylactic AEDs to prevent postoperative convulsions in patients without preexisting seizures, but this effect did not reach statistical significance [82].

Several studies have examined the need for AED use, either prophylactically or after surgery, usually in mixed primary or metastatic brain tumor populations. In a double-blind, randomized study of phenytoin (100 mg tid) vs placebo in 281 post-craniotomy patients, the phenytoin group had significantly fewer seizures (12.9% vs 18.4%), and highest protection was present between days 7 and 72. However, the subgroup analysis of 81 patients with brain tumors and craniotomy showed that 21% of patients treated with phenytoin had seizures versus only 13% of nontreated (odds ratio 1.8, 95% CI 0.6–6.1). Only the meningioma subgroup in this study had slightly lower risk for seizures in the treated versus placebo patients. Therefore, based on these results, the recommendations for phenytoin prophylaxis should not apply to brain tumors [83].

In a subsequent Italian study, 65/128 (51%) patients with supratentorial brain tumors had preoperative seizures and were treated with AEDs. Those without preoperative seizures were randomized to receive phenobarbital or phenytoin as prophylactic treatment or no treatment. No significant difference in seizure incidence was found between patients treated (7%) and those not treated (18%). The authors suggested short-term preventive antiepileptic treatment after surgery in patients without preoperative seizures and continuation of postoperative treatment in patients with preoperative epilepsy [84].

Other AEDs have also been used. Glantz et al. conducted a well-designed randomized, double-blind, placebo-controlled study comparing the incidence of first seizures in 74 valproate versus placebo-treated patients with newly diagnosed supratentorial brain tumors. The drug and placebo groups did not differ significantly in the incidence of seizures (35% in the valproate and, surprisingly, 24% in the placebo-treated group). Based on these results, no prophylactic treatment with valproate could be recommended [78].

Finally, a prospective, randomized, unblinded study from Canada examined the effect of prophylactic phenytoin administration in newly diagnosed patients with primary and metastatic brain tumors without prior seizures. Seizures occurred in 26% of all patients, 24% in the treated, and 28% in the nontreated group (odds ratio 0.82, 95% CI 0.3–2) [85].

Based on the aforementioned evidence, there is no clear benefit of prophylactic use of AEDs perioperatively [86]. However, a short-term perioperative course even of enzyme inducers (e.g., one dose at the end of the surgery; it takes 1–2 weeks of therapy to develop enzyme induction) or a short-term course of the AEDs (which have a safer profile) may be a reasonable research endeavor for the future.

Similarly, reports on patients exclusively with metastatic brain tumors do not support the use of prophylactic anticonvulsants [10, 87]. In a large retrospective analysis of 195 patients with metastatic brain tumors, Cohen et al. reported that 18% of patients presented with seizures. Of the remaining seizure-free patients, 40% were treated prophylactically with AEDs (phenytoin in >90%). During a follow-up period of up to 59 weeks, 10% of patients developed late seizures. The incidence of seizures did not differ between treated (13.1%) and untreated (11.1%) groups. However, this study is flawed due to the fact that two thirds of patients with seizures had subtherapeutic AED levels. The authors did not advocate AED use, unless the patient has the first seizure [10]. This is in accord to a more recent meta-analysis of adult patients with metastatic tumors without a seizure ever, where prophylactic AED treatment was not recommended [88].

Likewise, a meta-analysis evaluated five trials with specific inclusion criteria (patients with a neoplasm, either primary glial tumors, cerebral metastases, or meningiomas, but no history of epilepsy) who were randomized to either an AED or placebo. The three AEDs studied were phenobarbital, phenytoin, and valproic acid. This meta-analysis confirmed the lack of antiepileptic benefit at 1 week and at 6 months of follow-up. In addition, the AEDs had no effect on seizure prevention for specific tumor pathology [89].

Summarizing the above information, the Quality Standards Subcommittee of the American Academy of Neurology published a meta-analysis of 12 studies, which had addressed the issue of prophylactic antiepileptic treatment for newly diagnosed brain tumor patients. Four were randomized and eight were cohorts. Only one study showed significant difference between treated and untreated groups and, actually, favored the untreated. The overall odds ratio from the randomized trials was 1.09, 95% CI 0.63–1.89 ($P = 0.8$) for seizure incidence and 1.03, 0.74–1.44 ($P = 0.9$) for seizure-free survival. Therefore, the subcommittee recommended no prophylactic use of AED on patients with newly diagnosed brain tumors. Tapering and discontinuing the AEDs was appropriate after the first postoperative week in those patients without a seizure (who were, nevertheless, treated before). Although not excluding the possibility that some subgroups of brain tumor patients may be at a higher risk for seizures (melanoma, hemorrhagic or multiple metastatic lesions, tumors located near the Rolandic fissure, slow-growing primary brain tumors), the subcommittee did not find any reason for prophylaxis in those patients either [74]. This guideline has been retired by the AAN Board of Directors on June 4, 2012, but until a new guideline is published, one should consider this evidence still as the best available, especially since newer studies have not disputed its recommendations [86, 90]. Likewise, these recommendations extend to secondary brain tumors.

In a systematic review of adult patients with solid metastases, never having experienced a seizure due to their metastatic brain disease, routine prophylactic use of anticonvulsants was not recommended [88]. As with primary brain tumors, however, some subgroups of metastatic tumors may have higher incidence of seizures and may benefit from AEDs. For example, in a retrospective study of 105 patients with brain tumors using susceptibility-weighted MRI to detect hemosiderin deposition preoperatively, Roelcke et al. found a significant correlation between cortical hemosiderin deposition and the presence of seizures in the subgroup of patients with brain metastasis [45]. This finding has not been replicated in longitudinal studies; though, neither the effect of any AED in this subgroup is known.

How often these guidelines are followed is questionable, with some data showing that there is a discordance between the recommendations and the current practice. In a recent study from Brazil, for example, 70.2% of seizure-naïve patients with primary brain tumors had received primary prophylaxis with AEDs [91].

Treatment of Seizures in the ICU

Treatment of seizures or SE in patients with brain tumors follows the general guidelines that are presented in the chapter Management of Status Epilepticus and Critical Care Seizures. There are, however, several important details regarding these complex patients that the intensivist should master.

Firstly, one should not forget that seizure control may be influenced by the evolution of the brain tumor and its treatment [92]. Secondly, surgery may be a potent treatment modality in patients with refractory epilepsy and brain tumors, because studies have shown that resection of the epileptogenic zone due to brain tumors may lead to seizure freedom or significant control of seizures in 56–90% of patients [35, 93–96].

Thirdly, interactions between the various medications are a major problem and can lead to unforeseen complications. AEDs, especially those affecting the cytochrome P450 system, may affect the metabolism of chemotherapeutic agents used for the treatment of metastatic or primary brain tumors (Table 12.1). These agents have a narrow therapeutic window and real potential for toxicity or lethal side effects, if their level is increased by an additional agent or to lose their anticancer efficacy and reduce the chance for remission, if their level is decreased. Usually, the addition of phenytoin, carbamazepine, phenobarbital, and other inducer AEDs reduces the levels or efficacy of cyclophosphamide, methotrexate, adriamycin, nitrosoureas, paclitaxel, etoposide, topotecan, irinotecan, thiotepa, and corticosteroids [74, 92, 97]. Therefore, when these inducing agents are used, the chemotherapeutic agents' dosage should be increased. Conversely, when these AEDs are stopped, and since induction is a reversible phenomenon, the anticancer agent dose should be decreased [92]. Oxcarbazepine has lower interaction potential, but can reduce the levels of anticancer drugs, such as imatinib [98]. For the ICU, lamotrigine, topiramate, and zonisamide, lacking parenteral formulations and requiring slow-dose titration remain in a disadvantage [92]. Valproic acid, being an inhibitor, can have the opposite effect and increase the chemotherapeutic agents' levels and lead to higher toxicity from these agents or myelosuppression [99]. There are also some data showing increased postoperative bleeding with valproic acid and that makes some neurosurgeons reluctant to operate with this drug on board [92, 100]. This negative effect of valproic acid on platelets, however, has not been confirmed in subsequent analyses. In a study of 35 patients with glioblastoma, platelet count <100.000/mm^3 was only associated with accumulated temozolomide and not independently with valproic acid [101]. More recently, no hematologic toxicity could be proven in patients with glioblastoma multiforme treated with radiochemotherapy and use of levetiracetam or valproic acid [102]. Interaction between valproic acid and warfarin with resulting elevation of the international normalized ratio and bleeding at the tumor bed has been reported in glioblastoma multiforme and requires caution when both drugs are coadministered [103]. On the other hand, valproic acid may also have beneficial effects in patients with seizures due to brain tumors via direct or indirect antitumor properties (see below) and decreased refractoriness to seizure control via suppression of the multidrug resistance gene MDR1 [104].

Table 12.1 Hepatic metabolism of common chemotherapeutic agents and antiepileptics (modified from [92, 105])

Chemotherapeutic drug	Hepatic cytochrome P system used
Corticosteroids	CYP3A4
Vinca alkaloids	CYP3A4
Etoposide/teniposide	CYP3A4
Tamoxifen	CYP1A2, CYP2D6
Cyclophosphamide	CYP2B
Nitrosoureas	CYP3A4, CYOC19, CYP2D6
Taxanes	CYP3A4, CYP2C8
Irinotecan	CYP3A4
Busulfan	CYP3A4
Doxorubicin	CYP3A4
Cisplatin	CYP3A4, CYP2E1
Methotrexate	80–90% renally excreted unchanged
Antiepileptic drug	
Phenytoin	CYP3A4, inducer
Phenobarbital	CYP3A4, inducer
Carbamazepine	CYP3A4, inducer
Oxcarbazepine	CYP3A4 weak inducer
Valproic acid	CYP3A4, inhibitor
Lamotrigine	Non-inducer
Levetiracetam	Non-inducer

Fourthly, competition for binding to plasma proteins may be important with several of those medications, especially in states of hypoalbuminemia, not uncommon in the ICU or during chemotherapy. Measuring the free levels of drugs and adjusting the dose can be useful in order to avoid toxicity or subtherapeutic levels.

Lastly, regarding the steroids, either their dose should be increased or the patient should be switched to one of the newer, non-inducing AEDs (lamotrigine, levetiracetam, zonisamide, vigabatrin, and gabapentin). These newer drugs are either renally excreted (levetiracetam, zonisamide, gabapentin, vigabatrin) or, if hepatically metabolized, either non-inducers of the cytochrome P system (lamotrigine) or mild inducers (oxcarbazepine) [30, 105].

Overall, the intensivist should be cautious because, contrary to the aforementioned data, there have also been studies showing improved outcomes in patients with brain tumors exposed to enzyme-inducing AEDs [106–108]. One possible explanation is that patients with brain tumors and seizures are diagnosed earlier and therefore may have a better prognosis because of that reason [43, 92].

On the other hand, enzyme inhibitors, such as valproic acid, may lead to better outcomes in these patients. Weller et al. analyzed the survival data of patients with glioblastoma enrolled in a randomized study and treated with radiotherapy alone versus radiotherapy plus temozolomide. Patients receiving valproic acid alone (97 [16.9%]) appeared to derive more survival benefit from temozolomide/radiotherapy (hazard ratio [HR], 95% confidence intervals 0.39, 0.24–

0.63) than patients receiving an enzyme-inducing AED only (HR 0.69, 0.53–0.90) or patients not receiving any AED (HR 0.67, 0.49–0.93). Valproic acid did not confer any survival advantage in the radiotherapy-alone arm and was more likely to induce thrombocytopenia and leukopenia [99]. Potential explanations of this effect are either decreased clearance of temozolomide by valproic acid-induced enzymatic inhibition or direct potentiation by valproic of the temozolomide effect [92]. These positive effects of the combination of temozolomide and valproic acid on survival were also found in a more recent Dutch study of patients with glioblastoma [20] and in a Brazilian study of children with a variety of brain tumors [109]. In a recent systematic review of valproic acid in patients with glioblastoma, a prolonged survival was confirmed [110].

Chemotherapy per se may have additional effects on seizure control. Newer chemotherapeutic agents, such as temozolomide, may decrease seizure frequency in 50–60% or lead to seizure freedom in 20–40% of treated patients, but the mechanism is unclear [111, 112]. In a retrospective study, seizure frequency in patients with low-grade gliomas and intractable epilepsy was analyzed before and after treatment with temozolomide in 69 patients. There was a significant difference in >50% seizure reduction frequency between patients receiving temozolomide (59%) and those who did not receive temozolomide (13%). Seven patients (18%) in the temozolomide group displayed this improvement independent of AED adjustment compared with no patient in the control group, a significant difference [113].

Newer AEDs are believed to have a more favorable safety profile; fewer interactions with other drugs and some are also available in an IV formulation, all useful characteristics for their use in the ICU. Levetiracetam belongs to this group of newer AEDs and has a favorable profile for use in patients with brain tumors [114]. There are data that the addition of levetiracetam (1–4 g/day) to older AEDs in patients with refractory seizures can lead to reduction of seizures by 65–90%. In fact, 44–46% of patients in these small case series (a total 86 patients included) were switched to levetiracetam monotherapy later on [115–117]. In a prospective small study of 17 patients with brain tumors (mostly glioblastoma multiforme), levetiracetam monotherapy achieved ≥50% seizure reduction in 91.7% of them. A total of 92 drug interactions were avoided by using levetiracetam (instead of using phenytoin as a comparison), with dexamethasone, acetaminophen, and fentanyl being the most common interacting drugs [118]. In another older small study of 14 patients with brain tumors, addition of gabapentin (0.3–2.4 g/day) to phenytoin, carbamazepine, or clobazam led to 100% seizure reduction and 57% seizure freedom [119]. More recently, lacosamide, a newer AED with minimal drug interactions and renal excretion, had been used in a retrospective study of patients with primary brain tumors. This drug was an add-on for recurrent seizures in 74% of patients and used due to previous drug toxicity in another 23%. Lacosamide, in daily doses ranging from 100 to 600 mg, led to decreased seizure frequency in 66% and stable seizure frequency in 30% of patients. Seizure frequency also decreased in 4 out of 12 (33.3%) patients where lacosamide was not used concomitantly with any other AED. No toxicity was seen in 77% of patients [120]. In another study of 14 patients with brain tumor-associated seizures, who had already been treated with other AEDs and who had not experienced adequate seizure control, the mean seizure number in the last month prior to the introduction of lacosamide was 15.4. After the introduction of this drug, the mean seizure number was reduced to 1.9/month. Lacosamide mean dosage was of 332.1 mg/day (min 100 max 400 mg/day) and the overall responder rate was 78.6%. Only one patient discontinued the drug because of side effects (dizziness and blurred vision) [121].

Chemotherapeutic agents or corticosteroids can also affect the metabolism of several AEDs, increasing or decreasing their levels [122–124]. This may explain the subtherapeutic levels of these drugs in the studies that evaluated their prophylactic use [10, 78, 84, 85]. Phenytoin concentrations may become toxic after withdrawal of dexamethasone [125], probably due to slower hepatic metabolism of the former. Poor seizure control may result from the combinations of phenytoin with cisplatin or corticosteroids and valproic acid with methotrexate. Increased toxicity of AEDs can occur when phenytoin is combined with 5-fluorouracil [126]. In addition, several chemotherapeutic agents may have proconvulsant activity on their own [38, 72] (see chapter Drugs Used for the Critically Ill and Critical Care Seizures), and the intensivist should be aware that the aforementioned studies of prophylactic AED use did not control for the presence of specific chemotherapeutic agents.

An interesting aspect of the antiepileptic drug use in patients with cancer is their potential for antineoplastic or immunosuppressive effect [92, 99, 127–130]. Valproate is exhibiting inherent antitumor activity through inhibition of histone deacetylase (which leads to cell differentiation, growth arrest, and apoptosis of cancer cells, including gliomas) [42, 96, 110, 126, 131] and tumor angiogenesis [132].

Similarly to valproic acid, carbamazepine and its metabolite carbamazepine-10,11-epoxide have also been shown to act as histone deacetylase inhibitors, although less consistently in the literature [42]. Levetiracetam enhances p53-mediated inhibition of O-methylguanine-DNA methyltransferase (MGMT; a DNA repair protein that confers resistance to alkylating agents) and sensitizes glioblastoma cells to temozolamide [133]. Phenytoin on the other hand may lead to immunosuppression, but clinical studies examining this effect are not available. Neutropenia secondary to myelosuppressive chemotherapy may worsen with carbamazepine, an adverse effect that should be monitored very carefully [134].

Gabapentin may also ameliorate chemotherapeutic-induced nausea, and this may be of additional benefit in patients with seizures and breast cancer [135].

Interaction between AEDs and irradiation treatment offered to the brain or spine may lead to dermatologic complications. Skin rash in patients treated with phenytoin and brain irradiation may herald Stevens-Johnson syndrome [76, 136], and valproic acid has been implicated in Rowell's syndrome (lupus erythematosus associated with erythema multiforme-like lesions) [137]. One retrospective study, however, of 289 patients with brain tumors treated with AEDs and radiation found only one (0.3%) patient who developed erythema multiforme. Phenytoin was associated with milder rashes in 22% of patients, a higher incidence than the usual 5–10%. These rashes did not appear to be related to radiation, because they usually occurred before its initiation [138]. More recently, in a retrospective analysis of 544 adults with glioblastoma, valproic acid (but not levetiracetam) use during radiation therapy was associated with improved overall survival, independently of Radiation Therapy Oncology Group recursive partitioning analysis (RTOG RPA) class, seizure history, and concurrent temozolomide use [139]. This contrasts to the aforementioned study, where valproic acid did not confer any survival advantage in the radiotherapy-alone arm [99].

Based on the above safety profile, interactions with chemotherapeutic agents, and the fact that for partial seizures in adults with or without secondary generalization, the International League Against Epilepsy considers levetiracetam (as well as phenytoin, carbamazepine, and zonisamide) level A anticonvulsant and valproic acid level B [140], levetiracetam is considered the preferred monotherapy choice for patients with brain tumors [43]. Similarly, levetiracetam may be effective in patients with brain metastases [141] or meningiomas and seizures [43]. For patients with glioblastoma multiforme, valproic acid confers survival benefit and may be used. If seizures are not optimally controlled with either valproic acid or levetiracetam monotherapy, a polytherapy of both valproic acid and levetiracetam is preferable over sequential trials of antiepileptic monotherapy. If this combination is still suboptimal, experts suggest as an add-on either zonisamide, lacosamide, or lamotrigine [43].

Summarizing these data, individualized treatment in the ICU and afterwards is probably best. Factors that should be considered before one decides if and when to treat the patient and which medications to use including the histopathology of the tumor, the location of the mass, the presence of preexisting epilepsy, the extent of additional injury incurred by craniotomy, the involvement of other important organs metabolizing the drugs, the nutritional state of the patient, the pharmacological interactions between the agents, and the ability of the patient to tolerate side effects of the treatment.

Outcome

Overall, surgical excision of the tumor results in improved control of seizures, and the more extensive the resection of gliomas, the lower the postoperative seizure frequency, in most studies [26]. A recurrence or worsening of seizures following first-line antitumor treatment predicts progression of GBM in two thirds of patients, an association less evident with low-grade gliomas [14, 43, 142]. In low-grade gliomas, however, favorable postoperative seizure control factors are the presence of generalized seizures, surgery within <1 year from presentation, gross tumor resection, and successful preoperative control of seizures [43, 143].

There are data supporting a better outcome in patients with brain tumors and seizures [26, 43, 92, 144]. In a retrospective study from Johns Hopkins, 56% of 544 patients, who underwent first-time resection for glioblastoma multiforme, lost their functional independence at a median of 10 months (IQR 6–16 months). Preoperative seizures were one of the factors independently associated with prolonged functional independence (odds ratio 0.606, 95% CI 0.431–0.832) [145]. This information can be of some help in the discussions the intensivist may have with the patients or relatives in the ICU.

References

1. Ziai WC, Varelas PN, Zeger SL, Mirski MA, Ulatowski JA. Neurologic intensive care resource use after brain tumor surgery: an analysis of indications and alternative strategies. Crit Care Med. 2003;31:2782–7.
2. Spentzas T, Escue JE, Patters AB, Varelas PN. Brain tumor resection in children: neurointensive care unit course and resource utilization. Pediatr Crit Care Med. 2010;11:718–22.
3. van Breemen MS, Wilms EB, Vecht CJ. Epilepsy in patients with brain tumours: epidemiology, mechanisms, and management. Lancet Neurol. 2007;6:421–30.
4. Posti JP, Bori M, Kauko T, et al. Presenting symptoms of glioma in adults. Acta Neurol Scand. 2015;131:88–93.
5. Fisher JL, Palmisano S, Schwartzbaum JA, Svensson T, Lonn S. Comorbid conditions associated with glioblastoma. J Neuro-Oncol. 2014;116:585–91.
6. LeBlanc F, Rasmussen T. Cerebral seizures and brain tumors. In: Vinken PJBG, editor. Handbook of clinical neurology. Amsterdam: North-Holland; 1974. p. 295–301.
7. Cascino G. Epilepsy and brain tumors: implications to treatment. Epilepsia. 1990;31(Suppl 3):S37–44.
8. Bartolomei J, Christopher S, Vives K, Spencer DD, Piepmeier JM. Low grade gliomas of chronic epilepsy: a distinct clinical and pathological entity. J Neuro-Oncol. 1997;34:79–84.
9. McKeran R, Thomas DGT. The clinical study of gliomas. In: Thomas D, Graham DL, editors. Brain tumors: scientific basis, clinical investigation and current therapy. Baltimore: Lippincott; 1980. p. 194–230.
10. Cohen N, Strauss G, Lew R, Silver R, Recht L. Should prophylactic anticonvulsants be administered to patients with newly diagnosed cerebral metastases? A retrospective analysis. J Clin Oncol. 1988;6:1621–4.
11. Simonescu M. Metastatic tumors of the brain. A follow-up study of 195 patients with neurosurgical considerations. J Neurosurg. 1960;17:361–73.
12. Ketz E. Brain tumors and epilepsy. In: Vinken P, Bruyn GW, (ed). Handbook of clinical neurology. Amsterdam: North-Holland 1974. p. 254–269.
13. Moots P, Maciunas RJ, Eisert DR, Parker RA, Laporte K, Abou-Khalil B. The course of seizure disorders in patients with malignant gliomas. Arch Neurol. 1995;52:717–24.
14. Chaichana KL, Parker SL, Olivi A, Quinones-Hinojosa A. Long-term seizure outcomes in adult patients undergoing primary resection of malignant brain astrocytomas. J Neurosurg. 2009;111:282–92. Clinical article
15. Kerkhof M, Vecht CJ. Seizure characteristics and prognostic factors of gliomas. Epilepsia. 2013;54(Suppl 9):12–7.
16. Cavaliere R, Farace E, Schiff D. Clinical implications of status epilepticus in patients with neoplasms. Arch Neurol. 2006;63:1746–9.
17. Wychowski T, Wang H, Buniak L, Henry JC, Mohile N. Considerations in prophylaxis for tumor-associated epilepsy: prevention of status epilepticus and tolerability of newer generation AEDs. Clin Neurol Neurosurg. 2013;115:2365–9.
18. Compton JJ, Laack NN, Eckel LJ, Schomas DA, Giannini C, Meyer FB. Long-term outcomes for low-grade intracranial ganglioglioma: 30-year experience from the Mayo Clinic. J Neurosurg. 2012;117:825–30.
19. Thom M, Toma A, An S, et al. One hundred and one dysembryoplastic neuroepithelial tumors: an adult epilepsy series with immunohistochemical, molecular genetic, and clinical correlations and a review of the literature. J Neuropathol Exp Neurol. 2011;70:859–78.
20. Kerkhof M, Dielemans JC, van Breemen MS, et al. Effect of valproic acid on seizure control and on survival in patients with glioblastoma multiforme. Neuro-Oncology. 2013;15:961–7.
21. Englot DJ, Magill ST, Han SJ, Chang EF, Berger MS, McDermott MW. Seizures in supratentorial meningioma: a systematic review and meta-analysis. J Neurosurg 20151;24(6):1552–61.
22. Whittle I, Beaumont A. Seizures in patients with supratentorial oligodendroglial tumours; clinicopathological features and management considerations. Acta Neurochir. 1995;135:19–24.
23. Rasmussen T, Blundell J. Epilepsy and Brain tumours. Clin Neurosurg. 1959;7:138–58.
24. Hoefer P, Schlesinger EB, Peress HH. Seizures in patients with brain tumours. Res Nerv Ment Dis Proceed. 1947;26:50–8.
25. Morris H, Estes ML, Prayson RA, et al. Frequency of different tumor types encountered in the Cleveland Clinic epilepsy surgery program. Epilepsia. 1996;37:96.
26. Beaumont A, Whittle IR. The pathogenesis of tumour associated epilepsy. Acta Neurochir. 2000;142:1–15.
27. Scott G, Gibberd FB. Epilepsy and other factors in the prognosis of gliomas. Acta Neurol Scand. 1980;61:227–39.
28. Lee JW, Wen PY, Hurwitz S, et al. Morphological characteristics of brain tumors causing seizures. Arch Neurol. 2010;67:336–42.
29. Mahaley MJ, Dudka L. The role of anticonvulsant medications in the management of patients with anaplastic gliomas. Surg Neurol. 1981;16:399–401.
30. Englot DJ, Berger MS, Chang EF, Garcia PA. Characteristics and treatment of seizures in patients with high-grade glioma: a review. Neurosurg Clin N Am. 2012;23:227–35. vii-viii
31. Victor M, Ropper AH. Principles of neurology. 7th ed. New York: McGraw-Hill; 2001.
32. Kvam D, Loftus CM, Copeland B, Quest DO. Seizures during the immediate postoperative period. Neurosurgery. 1983;12:14–7.
33. Lee S, Lui TN, Chang CN, Cheng WC. Early postoperative seizures after posterior fossa surgery. J Neurosurg. 1990;73:541–4.
34. Fukamachi A, Koizumi H, Nukui H. Immediate postoperative seizures—incidence and computed tomographic findings. Surg Neurol. 1985;24:671–6.

35. Michelucci R, Pasini E, Meletti S, et al. Epilepsy in primary cerebral tumors: the characteristics of epilepsy at the onset (results from the PERNO study—Project of Emilia Romagna Region on Neuro-Oncology). Epilepsia. 2013;54(Suppl 7):86–91.

36. Kovac S, Diehl B, Wehner T, et al. Gelastic seizures: incidence, clinical and EEG features in adult patients undergoing video-EEG telemetry. Epilepsia. 2015;56:e1–5.

37. Sato T, Takeichi M, Abe M, Tabuchi K, Hara T. Frontal lobe tumor associated with late-onset seizure and psychosis: a case report. Jpn J Psychiatry Neurol. 1993;47:541–4.

38. Cocito L, Audenino D, Primavera A. Altered mental state and nonconvulsive status epilepticus in patients with cancer. Arch Neurol. 2001;58:1310.

39. Blitshteyn S, Jaeckle KA. Nonconvulsive status epilepticus in metastatic CNS disease. Neurology. 2006;66:1261–3.

40. Spindler M, Jacks LM, Chen X, Panageas K, DeAngelis LM, Avila EK. Spectrum of nonconvulsive status epilepticus in patients with cancer. J Clin Neurophysiol. 2013;30:339–43.

41. Marcuse LV, Lancman G, Demopoulos A, Fields M. Nonconvulsive status epilepticus in patients with brain tumors. Seizure. 2014;23:542–7.

42. Gefroh-Grimes HA, Gidal BE. Antiepileptic drugs in patients with malignant brain tumor: beyond seizures and pharmacokinetics. Acta Neurol Scand. 2016;133:4–16.

43. Vecht CJ, Kerkhof M, Duran-Pena A. Seizure prognosis in brain tumors: new insights and evidence-based management. Oncologist. 2014;19:751–9.

44. Ettinger A. Structural causes of epilepsy. Tumors, cysts, stroke, and vascular malformations. Neurol Clin. 1994;12:41–56.

45. Roelcke U, Boxheimer L, Fathi AR, et al. Cortical hemosiderin is associated with seizures in patients with newly diagnosed malignant brain tumors. J Neuro-Oncol. 2013;115:463–8.

46. McKinney R, Debanne D, Gahwiler BH, et al. Lesion induced axonal sprouting and hyperexcitability in the hippocampus in vitro. Implications for the genesis of posttraumatic epilepsy. Nat Med. 1997;3:990–6.

47. Gray W, Sundstrom LE. Kainic acid increases the proliferation of granule cell progenitors in the dentate gyrus of the rat. Brain Res. 1998;790:52–9.

48. Patt S, Labrakakis C, Bernstein M, et al. Neuron-like physiological properties of cells from human oligodendroglial tumors. Neuroscience. 1996;71:601–11.

49. Labrakakis C, Patt S, Weydt P, et al. Action potential generating cells in human glioblastoma. J Neuropathol Exp Neurol. 1997;56:243–54.

50. Goldstein D, Nadi NS, Stull R, Wyler AR, Porter RJ. Levels of catechols in epileptogenic and nonepileptogenic regions of the human brain. J Neurochem. 1988;50:225–9.

51. Kish S, Dixon LM, Sherwin AL. Aspartic acid aminotransferase activity is increased in actively spiking compared with nonspiking cortex. J Neurol Neurosurg Psychiatry. 1988;51:552–6.

52. Sherwin A, Vernet O, Dubeau F, Olivier A. Biochemical markers of excitability in human neocortex. Can J Neurol Sci. 1991;18:640–4.

53. Yuen TI, Morokoff AP, Bjorksten A, et al. Glutamate is associated with a higher risk of seizures in patients with gliomas. Neurology. 2012;79:883–9.

54. Gao X, Wang H, Cai S, et al. Phosphorylation of NMDA 2B at S1303 in human glioma peritumoral tissue: implications for glioma epileptogenesis. Neurosurg Focus. 2014;37:E17.

55. Rosati A, Marconi S, Pollo B, et al. Epilepsy in glioblastoma multiforme: correlation with glutamine synthetase levels. J Neuro-Oncol. 2009;93:319–24.

56. Isoardo G, Morra I, Chiarle G, et al. Different aquaporin-4 expression in glioblastoma multiforme patients with and without seizures. Mol Med. 2012;18:1147–51.

57. Lee JW, Norden AD, Ligon KL, et al. Tumor associated seizures in glioblastomas are influenced by survival gene expression in a region-specific manner: a gene expression imaging study. Epilepsy Res. 2014;108:843–52.

58. Neuwelt E, Goldman DL, Dahlborg SA, et al. Primary CNS lymphoma treated with osmotic blood-brain barrier disruption: prolonged survival and preservation of cognitive function. J Clin Oncol. 1991;9:1580–90.

59. Lukovits TG, Fadul CE, Pipas JM, Williamson PD. Nonconvulsive status epilepticus after intravenous contrast medium administration. Epilepsia. 1996;37:1117–20.

60. van de Loosdrecht AA, Gietema JA, van der Graaf WT. Seizures in a patient with disseminated testicular cancer due to cisplatin-induced hypomagnesaemia. Acta Oncol. 2000;39:239–40.

61. McDonald GA, Dubose Jr TD. Hyponatremia in the cancer patient. Oncology. 1993;7:55–64. discussion 7–8; 70–1

62. Meropol NJ, Creaven PJ, Petrelli NJ, White RM, Arbuck SG. Seizures associated with leucovorin administration in cancer patients. J Natl Cancer Inst. 1995;87:56–8.

63. Delanty N, Vaughan CJ, French JA. Medical causes of seizures. Lancet. 1998;352:383–90.

64. Dalmau J, Graus F, Rosenblum MK, Posner JB. Anti-Hu—associated paraneoplastic encephalomyelitis/sensory neuronopathy. A clinical study of 71 patients. Medicine. 1992;71:59–72.

65. Lancaster E. The diagnosis and treatment of autoimmune encephalitis. J Clin Neurol. 2016;12:1–13.

66. Calatozzolo C, Gelati M, Ciusani E, et al. Expression of drug resistance proteins Pgp, MRP1, MRP3, MRP5 and GST-pi in human glioma. J Neuro-Oncol. 2005;74:113–21.

67. Aronica E, Gorter JA, Jansen GH, et al. Expression and cellular distribution of multidrug transporter proteins in two major causes of medically intractable epilepsy: focal cortical dysplasia and glioneuronal tumors. Neuroscience. 2003;118:417–29.

68. Calatozzolo C, Pollo B, Botturi A, et al. Multidrug resistance proteins expression in glioma patients with epilepsy. J Neuro-Oncol. 2012;110:129–35.

69. Rothoerl RD, Bernreuther D, Woertgen C, Brawanski A. The value of routine electroencephalographic recordings in predicting postoperative seizures associated with meningioma surgery. Neurosurg Rev. 2003;26:108–12.

70. Jordan KG. Nonconvulsive status epilepticus in acute brain injury. J Clin Neurophysiol. 1999;16:332–40. discussion 53

71. Jordan KG. Continuous EEG monitoring in the neuroscience intensive care unit and emergency department. J Clin Neurophysiol. 1999;16:14–39.

72. Primavera A, Audenino D, Cocito L. Ifosfamide encephalopathy and nonconvulsive status epilepticus. Can J Neurol Sci. 2002;29:180–3.

73. Hormigo A, Liberato B, Lis E, DeAngelis LM. Nonconvulsive status epilepticus in patients with cancer: imaging abnormalities. Arch Neurol. 2004;61:362–5.

74. Glantz MJ, Cole BF, Forsyth PA, et al. Practice parameter: anticonvulsant prophylaxis in patients with newly diagnosed brain tumors. Report of the Quality Standards Subcommittee of the American Academy of Neurology. Neurology. 2000;54:1886–93.

75. Schaller B, Ruegg SJ. Brain tumor and seizures: pathophysiology and its implications for treatment revisited. Epilepsia. 2003;44:1223–32.

76. Ansari SF, Bohnstedt BN, Perkins SM, Althouse SK, Miller JC. Efficacy of postoperative seizure prophylaxis in intra-axial brain tumor resections. J Neuro-Oncol. 2014;118:117–22.

77. Cockey GH, Amann ST, Reents SB, Lynch Jr JW. Stevens-Johnson syndrome resulting from whole-brain radiation and phenytoin. Am J Clin Oncol. 1996;19:32–4.

78. Glantz MJ, Cole BF, Friedberg MH, et al. A randomized, blinded, placebo-controlled trial of divalproex sodium prophylaxis in adults with newly diagnosed brain tumors. Neurology. 1996;46:985–91.

79. Lee S, Lui TN, Chang CN, Cheng WC, Wang DJ, Heimbarger RF, Lin CG. Prophylactic anticonvulsants for prevention of immediate and early postcraniotomy seizures. Surg Neurol. 1989;31:361–4.
80. Foy PM, Chadwick DW, Rajgopalan N, Johnson AL, Shaw MD. Do prophylactic anticonvulsant drugs alter the pattern of seizures after craniotomy? J Neurol Neurosurg Psychiatry. 1992;55:753–7.
81. Beenen LF, Lindeboom J, Kasteleijn-Nolst Trenite DG, et al. Comparative double blind clinical trial of phenytoin and sodium valproate as anticonvulsant prophylaxis after craniotomy: efficacy, tolerability, and cognitive effects. J Neurol Neurosurg Psychiatry. 1999;67:474–80.
82. Kuijlen JM, Teernstra OP, Kessels AG, Herpers MJ, Beuls EA. Effectiveness of antiepileptic prophylaxis used with supratentorial craniotomies: a meta-analysis. Seizure. 1996;5:291–8.
83. North JB, Penhall RK, Hanieh A, Frewin DB, Taylor WB. Phenytoin and postoperative epilepsy- a double blind study. J Neurosurg. 1983;58:672–7.
84. Franceschetti S, Binelli S, Casazza M, et al. Influence of surgery and antiepileptic drugs on seizures symptomatic of cerebral tumours. Acta Neurochir. 1990;103:47–51.
85. Forsyth PA, Weaver S, Fulton D, et al. Prophylactic anticonvulsants in patients with brain tumour. Can J Neurol Sci. 2003;30:106–12.
86. Rowe AS, Goodwin H, Brophy GM, et al. Seizure prophylaxis in neurocritical care: a review of evidence-based support. Pharmacotherapy. 2014;34:396–409.
87. Hung S, Hilsenbeck S, Feun L. Seizure prophylaxis with phenytoin in patients with brain metastasis. Proc Am Soc Clin Oncol. 1991;10:327.
88. Mikkelsen T, Paleologos NA, Robinson PD, et al. The role of prophylactic anticonvulsants in the management of brain metastases: a systematic review and evidence-based clinical practice guideline. J Neuro-Oncol. 2010;96:97–102.
89. Sirven JI, Wingerchuk DM, Drazkowski JF, Lyons MK, Zimmerman RS. Seizure prophylaxis in patients with brain tumors: a meta-analysis. Mayo Clin Proc. 2004;79:1489–94.
90. Sayegh ET, Fakurnejad S, Oh T, Bloch O, Parsa AT. Anticonvulsant prophylaxis for brain tumor surgery: determining the current best available evidence. J Neurosurg. 2014;121:1139–47.
91. de Oliveira JA, Santana IA, Caires IQ, et al. Antiepileptic drug prophylaxis in primary brain tumor patients: is current practice in agreement to the consensus? J Neuro-Oncol. 2014;120:399–403.
92. Perucca E. Optimizing antiepileptic drug treatment in tumoral epilepsy. Epilepsia. 2013;54(Suppl 9):97–104.
93. Zentner J, Hufnagel A, Wolf HK, et al. Surgical treatment of neoplasms associated with medically intractable epilepsy. Neurosurgery. 1997;41:378–86. discussion 86-7
94. Britton JW, Cascino GD, Sharbrough FW, Kelly PJ. Low-grade glial neoplasms and intractable partial epilepsy: efficacy of surgical treatment. Epilepsia. 1994;35:1130–5.
95. Maschio M. Brain tumor-related epilepsy. Curr Neuropharmacol. 2012;10:124–33.
96. Weller M, Stupp R, Wick W. Epilepsy meets cancer: when, why, and what to do about it? Lancet Oncol. 2012;13:e375–82.
97. Patsalos PN, Froscher W, Pisani F, van Rijn CM. The importance of drug interactions in epilepsy therapy. Epilepsia. 2002;43:365–85.
98. Pursche S, Schleyer E, von Bonin M, et al. Influence of enzyme-inducing antiepileptic drugs on trough level of imatinib in glioblastoma patients. Curr Clin Pharmacol. 2008;3:198–203.
99. Weller M, Gorlia T, Cairncross JG, et al. Prolonged survival with valproic acid use in the EORTC/NCIC temozolomide trial for glioblastoma. Neurology. 2011;77:1156–64.
100. Cannizzaro E, Albisetti M, Wohlrab G, Schmugge M. Severe bleeding complications during antiepileptic treatment with valproic acid in children. Neuropediatrics. 2007;38:42–5.
101. Simo M, Velasco R, Graus F, et al. Impact of antiepileptic drugs on thrombocytopenia in glioblastoma patients treated with standard chemoradiotherapy. J Neuro-Oncol. 2012;108:451–8.
102. Tinchon A, Oberndorfer S, Marosi C, et al. Haematological toxicity of Valproic acid compared to Levetiracetam in patients with glioblastoma multiforme undergoing concomitant radio-chemotherapy: a retrospective cohort study. J Neurol. 2015;262:179–86.
103. Yoon HW, Giraldo EA, Wijdicks EF. Valproic acid and warfarin: an underrecognized drug interaction. Neurocrit Care. 2011;15:182–5.
104. Vecht CJ, Wagner GL, Wilms EB. Interactions between antiepileptic and chemotherapeutic drugs. Lancet Neurol. 2003;2:404–9.
105. Rios O, French JA. Interactions between antiepileptic drugs and chemotherapeutic agents. Profiles Seizure Manage. 2004;3:5–8.
106. Groves MD, Puduvalli VK, Conrad CA, et al. Phase II trial of temozolomide plus marimastat for recurrent anaplastic gliomas: a relationship among efficacy, joint toxicity and anticonvulsant status. J Neuro-Oncol. 2006;80:83–90.
107. Jaeckle KA, Ballman K, Furth A, Buckner JC. Correlation of enzyme-inducing anticonvulsant use with outcome of patients with glioblastoma. Neurology. 2009;73:1207–13.
108. Reardon DA, Egorin MJ, Quinn JA, et al. Phase II study of imatinib mesylate plus hydroxyurea in adults with recurrent glioblastoma multiforme. J Clin Oncol. 2005;23:9359–68.
109. Felix FH, de Araujo OL, da Trindade KM, Trompieri NM, Fontenele JB. Survival of children with malignant brain tumors receiving valproate: a retrospective study. Childs Nerv Syst. 2013;29:195–7.
110. Yuan Y, Xiang W, Qing M, Yanhui L, Jiewen L, Yunhe M. Survival analysis for valproic acid use in adult glioblastoma multiforme: a meta-analysis of individual patient data and a systematic review. Seizure. 2014;23:830–5.
111. Brada M, Viviers L, Abson C, et al. Phase II study of primary temozolomide chemotherapy in patients with WHO grade II gliomas. Ann Oncol. 2003;14:1715–21.
112. Pace A, Vidiri A, Galie E, et al. Temozolomide chemotherapy for progressive low-grade glioma: clinical benefits and radiological response. Ann Oncol. 2003;14:1722–6.
113. Sherman JH, Moldovan K, Yeoh HK, et al. Impact of temozolomide chemotherapy on seizure frequency in patients with low-grade gliomas. J Neurosurg. 2011;114:1617–21.
114. Fonkem E, Bricker P, Mungall D, et al. The role of levetiracetam in treatment of seizures in brain tumor patients. Front Neurol. 2013;4:153.
115. Newton HB, Dalton J, Goldlust S, Pearl D. Retrospective analysis of the efficacy and tolerability of levetiracetam in patients with metastatic brain tumors. J Neuro-Oncol. 2007;84:293–6.
116. Wagner GL, Wilms EB, Van Donselaar CA, Vecht CJ. Levetiracetam: preliminary experience in patients with primary brain tumours. Seizure. 2003;12:585–6.
117. Maschio M, Albani F, Baruzzi A, et al. Levetiracetam therapy in patients with brain tumour and epilepsy. J Neuro-Oncol. 2006;80:97–100.
118. Usery JB, Michael 2nd LM, Sills AK, Finch CK. A prospective evaluation and literature review of levetiracetam use in patients with brain tumors and seizures. J Neuro-Oncol. 2010;99:251–60.
119. Perry JR, Sawka C. Add-on gabapentin for refractory seizures in patients with brain tumours. Can J Neurol Sci. 1996;23:128–31.
120. Saria MG, Corle C, Hu J, et al. Retrospective analysis of the tolerability and activity of lacosamide in patients with brain tumors: clinical article. J Neurosurg. 2013;118:1183–7.

121. Maschio M, Dinapoli L, Mingoia M, et al. Lacosamide as add-on in brain tumor-related epilepsy: preliminary report on efficacy and tolerability. J Neurol. 2011;258:2100–4.

122. Sylvester RK, Lewis FB, Caldwell KC, Lobell M, Perri R, Sawchuk RA. Impaired phenytoin bioavailability secondary to cisplatinum, vinblastine, and bleomycin. Ther Drug Monit. 1984;6:302–5.

123. Neef C, de Voogd-van der Straaten I. An interaction between cytostatic and anticonvulsant drugs. Clin Pharmacol Ther. 1988;43:372–5.

124. Gattis WA, May DB. Possible interaction involving phenytoin, dexamethasone, and antineoplastic agents: a case report and review. Ann Pharmacother. 1996;30:520–6.

125. Ruegg S. Dexamethasone/phenytoin interactions: neurooncological concerns. Swiss Med Wkly. 2002;132:425–6.

126. Vecht CJ, Wagner GL, Wilms EB. Treating seizures in patients with brain tumors: Drug interactions between antiepileptic and chemotherapeutic agents. Semin Oncol. 2003;30:49–52.

127. Bittigau P, Sifringer M, Genz K, et al. Antiepileptic drugs and apoptotic neurodegeneration in the developing brain. Proc Natl Acad Sci U S A. 2002;99:15089–94.

128. Blaheta RA, Cinatl Jr J. Anti-tumor mechanisms of valproate: a novel role for an old drug. Med Res Rev. 2002;22:492–511.

129. Bardana Jr EJ, Gabourel JD, Davies GH, Craig S. Effects of phenytoin on man's immunity. Evaluation of changes in serum immunoglobulins, complement, and antinuclear antibody. Am J Med. 1983;74:289–96.

130. Kikuchi K, McCormick CI, Neuwelt EA. Immunosuppression by phenytoin: implication for altered immune competence in brain-tumor patients. J Neurosurg. 1984;61:1085–90.

131. Li XN, Shu Q, Su JM, Perlaky L, Blaney SM, Lau CC. Valproic acid induces growth arrest, apoptosis, and senescence in medulloblastomas by increasing histone hyperacetylation and regulating expression of p21Cip1, CDK4, and CMYC. Mol Cancer Ther. 2005;4:1912–22.

132. Osuka S, Takano S, Watanabe S, Ishikawa E, Yamamoto T, Matsumura A. Valproic acid inhibits angiogenesis in vitro and glioma angiogenesis in vivo in the brain. Neurol Med Chir. 2012;52:186–93.

133. Bobustuc GC, Baker CH, Limaye A, et al. Levetiracetam enhances p 53-mediated MGMT inhibition and sensitizes glioblastoma cells to temozolomide. Neuro-Oncology. 2010;12:917–27.

134. Weissman DE. Glucocorticoid treatment for brain metastases and epidural spinal cord compression: a review. J Clin Oncol. 1988;6:543–51.

135. Guttuso Jr T, Roscoe J, Griggs J. Effect of gabapentin on nausea induced by chemotherapy in patients with breast cancer. Lancet. 2003;361:1703–5.

136. Eralp Y, Aydiner A, Tas F, Saip P, Topuz E. Stevens-Johnson syndrome in a patient receiving anticonvulsant therapy during cranial irradiation. Am J Clin Oncol. 2001;24:347–50.

137. Esteve E, Favre A, Martin L. Post-radiotherapy eruption in a patient treated with valproic acid. Rowell's syndrome? Ann Dermatol Venereol. 2002;129:901–3.

138. Mamon HJ, Wen PY, Burns AC, Loeffler JS. Allergic skin reactions to anticonvulsant medications in patients receiving cranial radiation therapy. Epilepsia. 1999;40:341–4.

139. Barker CA, Bishop AJ, Chang M, Beal K, Chan TA. Valproic acid use during radiation therapy for glioblastoma associated with improved survival. Int J Radiat Oncol Biol Phys. 2013;86:504–9.

140. Glauser T, Ben-Menachem E, Bourgeois B, et al. Updated ILAE evidence review of antiepileptic drug efficacy and effectiveness as initial monotherapy for epileptic seizures and syndromes. Epilepsia. 2013;54:551–63.

141. Maschio M, Dinapoli L, Gomellini S, et al. Antiepileptics in brain metastases: safety, efficacy and impact on life expectancy. J Neuro-Oncol. 2010;98:109–16.

142. You G, Sha ZY, Yan W, et al. Seizure characteristics and outcomes in 508 Chinese adult patients undergoing primary resection of low-grade gliomas: a clinicopathological study. Neuro-Oncology. 2012;14:230–41.

143. Chang EF, Potts MB, Keles GE, et al. Seizure characteristics and control following resection in 332 patients with low-grade gliomas. J Neurosurg. 2008;108:227–35.

144. Smith DF, Hutton JL, Sandemann D, et al. The prognosis of primary intracerebral tumours presenting with epilepsy: the outcome of medical and surgical management. J Neurol Neurosurg Psychiatry. 1991;54:915–20.

145. Chaichana KL, Halthore AN, Parker SL, et al. Factors involved in maintaining prolonged functional independence following supratentorial glioblastoma resection. J Neurosurg. 2011;114:604–12. Clinical article

Lauren Koffman, Matthew A. Koenig, and Romergryko Geocadin

Introduction

The increasing success of cardiopulmonary resuscitation (CPR) in reviving individuals from cardiac and respiratory arrest has generated an upsurge in hospital admissions for patients in post-resuscitative coma. The immediate post-resuscitation period is marked by the highest risk of hemodynamic instability, recurrent arrest, and prognostic uncertainty. Cardiac intensive care units in the United States have become accustomed to facing the challenge of managing seizures and myoclonus in the setting of hypoxic-ischemic coma. Despite the common occurrence of this problem, clinical and basic science research in this area has been sparse, and several important questions remain unanswered. Do seizures exacerbate brain damage in hypoxic-ischemic coma? How aggressively should they be treated and with which agents? Can some seizure types offer prognostic information that impacts the decision to withdraw care? How does TTM and TH affect post-cardiac arrest care and prognostication related to seizures? How should encephalography be used to guide therapy and care? This review will provide a comprehensive presentation of existing literature related to this problem.

L. Koffman (✉) • R. Geocadin
Department of Neurology, Johns Hopkins
University School of Medicine, Baltimore, MD, USA

Department of Anesthesiology and Critical Care Medicine,
Johns Hopkins University School of Medicine,
Baltimore, MD, USA
e-mail: lkoffma1@jhmi.edu; rgeocad95@jhmi.edu

M.A. Koenig
Neuroscience Institute, The Queens Medical Center,
Honolulu, HI, USA
e-mail: mkoenig95@gmail.com

Epidemiology

A large proportion of patients who are comatose after cardiac arrest have seizures; Nielsen et al. reported seizures in 24% of patients in their large (765 patients) prospective observational multinational registry of patients resuscitated from out-of-hospital cardiac arrest [1]. In a referral population of 114 patients who survived CPR for over 24 h, Krumholz et al. [2] described seizures in 44%. Thirty-five percent of patients had myoclonus alone or in association with other seizure types. Status epilepticus was found in 32%, the majority of which was either status myoclonus (SM) alone or a combination of SM and generalized tonic-clonic (GTC) status epilepticus, which the authors termed myoclonic status epilepticus. In prospective [3] and retrospective [4] studies of all comatose patients admitted after CPR, Snyder et al. found that one-third of patients experienced seizures, the majority of which had more than one seizure type. Myoclonic seizures were described in 19%, partial seizures in 19%, and GTC seizures in 6% of the total population. The incidence of myoclonic seizures was bimodal, with the majority beginning within 12 h after CPR and the remainder delayed by several days [3]. In the classic outcome study by Levy et al. [5], 15% of patients in hypoxic-ischemic coma experienced generalized convulsions, while 10% had isolated myoclonus. The post-hypoxic syndrome of action myoclonus described by Lance and Adams [6] can occur within a few days of cardiac arrest, but the incidence rate among survivors has never been studied.

Mani et al. [7] conducted one of the first investigations of the frequency and onset of seizures in comatose post-cardiac arrest patients treated with TH. Although it was a small (38 patients) single center study, there were many noteworthy findings. A total of 23% of patients had electrographic seizures with a median onset of 19 h from arrest. Of this group 56% had seizure onset prior to rewarming and 78% had status epilepticus [7]. The early onset of seizures in the comatose post-cardiac arrest population is supported by Rittenberger et al. who found nonconvulsive status epilepticus (NCSE) in

© Springer International Publishing AG 2017
P.N. Varelas, J. Claassen (eds.), *Seizures in Critical Care*, Current Clinical Neurology, DOI 10.1007/978-3-319-49557-6_13

12% of patients with out-of-hospital cardiac arrest that underwent TH [8]. Twenty-five percent of these patients were in NCSE upon initiation of EEG monitoring, reiterating the early onset of epileptiform activity from the time of arrest.

Pathophysiology

Pathological and Chemical Changes in Hypoxic-Ischemic Injury and Seizures

Experimental animal studies have provided insights into the mechanism of epileptogenesis in hypoxic-ischemic coma. Adenosine triphosphate (ATP)-sensitive potassium channels (K_{ATP}) are activated by hypoxic stress, resulting in protective cellular hyperpolarization by inward rectifying potassium currents [9]. K_{ATP} knockout mice subjected to brief episodes of hypoxia are more susceptible to generalized seizures [9]. The highest concentration of K_{ATP} channels is located within the substantia nigra pars reticulata (SN_{PR}), which acts as a central gating system for the propagation of generalized seizures [9]. In prolonged hypoxia-ischemia, SN_{PR} may be damaged and the gating function of the K_{ATP} receptors may be lost. Alternatively, hypoxic depletion of ATP could result in loss of the inward rectifying potassium current and failure to block seizure propagation at the SN_{PR} [9].

Prolonged generalized seizures induce permanent neuronal injury that shares some characteristics with global hypoxia. Excess glutamate release activates N-methyl-D-aspartate (NMDA) receptors resulting in intracellular accumulation of calcium and early apoptosis [10]. When mitochondrial energy stores are depleted during hypoxic and ischemic states, the cytotoxicity of NMDA receptor activation is markedly potentiated [11]. Experimental blockade of the NMDA receptor inhibits neuronal toxicity even though it does not shorten the duration of the seizure [12].

Pathological studies of uncomplicated seizures in humans report either no neuronal injury or ischemic cell changes limited to the hippocampus, particularly the Sommer sector (H1) [13]. After prolonged status epilepticus, the cortex may show laminar ischemic changes similar to hypoxic-ischemic encephalopathy with or without involvement of the cerebellar Purkinje cells [13]. Experimental data from well-oxygenated baboons with chemically induced status epilepticus showed cortical damage but limited cerebellar pathology [14]. In mechanically ventilated rats, prolonged seizures produced cellular changes limited to the substantia nigra pars reticulata (SN_{PR}), hypothalamus, and globus pallidus [15, 16]. Damage to the white matter and deep gray matter structures other than the hippocampus is not typically demonstrated in adult humans in the absence of concomitant hypoxia or ischemia [13]. Pathological changes demonstrated in global hypoxia-ischemia, on the other hand, involve all neuronal layers of the cortex, subcortical gray matter structures, cerebellum, and spinal cord in human autopsy series [17].

Animal data have been important in studying whether seizures exacerbate hypoxic-ischemic neuronal injury. Young et al. studied extracellular inhibitory and excitatory amino acid concentrations in juvenile rabbits with hypoxia alone, seizures alone, and seizures after hypoxia [18]. They found no increase in glutamate or GABA with hypoxia or seizures. When seizures were preceded by a period of hypoxia, however, there was a dramatic increase in both glutamate and GABA [18]. Concomitant hypoxia and seizures potentiate neuronal excitotoxicity, and excess glutamate release may lower the seizure threshold. In neonatal rats subjected to 3 h of unilateral stagnant hypoxia, CSF concentrations of glutamate and GABA were elevated [19]. When these rats were subjected to prolonged status epilepticus, the concentration of GABA increased further but glutamate did not [19]. These findings suggest that glutamate neurotoxicity in the setting of hypoxia-ischemia was not enhanced by seizures. Several pathological studies of global hypoxic-ischemic insults in neonatal rats found no further increase in lesion size after status epilepticus [19–21]. In newborn rats with limited hypoxic-ischemic lesions from unilateral carotid ligation, however, status epilepticus resulted in heightened neuronal injury [22]. It is believed that prolonged global hypoxia-ischemia results in such devastating neurological injury that the additional damage caused by seizures, if present, may be pathologically undetectable [22].

Myoclonus in Hypoxic-Ischemic Coma

Many clinicians ascribe SM in the setting hypoxic-ischemic coma to agonal neuronal firing that is a fragment of GTC status epilepticus [23–25]. Celesia et al. [25] speculated that hypoxic-ischemic destruction of the neocortex, cerebellum, and subcortical gray matter disrupts the normal propagation and regulation of tonic-clonic seizure activity, resulting in SM. They note that hypoxic damage to the neocortical laminar and intralaminar nuclei disrupts Jacksonian seizure progression, while destruction of the thalamic relay system prevents generalization to GTC convulsions [25].

Pathological data were provided in several case series of patients with SM in post-anoxic coma [23–25]. In the Young et al. series [23], damage was seen in all layers of the cerebral cortex, hippocampus, basal ganglia, cerebellar Purkinje cells, and spinal cord gray matter. These findings are more reflective of severe hypoxic-ischemic injury than neuronal damage from status epilepticus [23]. In the Celesia et al. series [25], the only two patients with Ammon's horn sclerosis—reflective of neuronal damage from status epilepticus—had GTC status epilepticus prior to the development of SM. In the study by Wijdicks et al. [24], post-anoxic patients with SM showed significantly greater involvement of all cortical laminae than those who died without SM. The damage in the hippocampus and cerebellum was not significantly different between the two groups. These data were interpreted to reflect that patients with SM had suffered greater anoxic brain injury [24], but the study was not designed to discern whether or not myoclonic seizures contributed to this injury.

Lance-Adams Syndrome

Although, in their classic paper describing the post-hypoxic syndrome of action myoclonus, Lance and Adams [6] implicated damage to the ventrolateral thalamic nuclei as the causative lesion, subsequent reports have focused on impaired serotonin neurotransmission and lesions in the caudal medulla and cortex. Many patients with Lance-Adams syndrome have low cerebrospinal fluid (CSF) concentrations of serotonin metabolites [26, 27]. Rat models of post-hypoxic myoclonus demonstrate impaired neurotransmission at 5-HT$_{1B}$ and 5-HT$_{2A/2B}$ receptors [28, 29]. Myoclonus is often attenuated by treatment with 5-hydroxytryptophan (5-HTP), valproic acid, and clonazepam—substances which are known to enhance serotonergic neurotransmission—in both the rat [30] and human [31]. Excess CSF serotonin metabolites, exacerbation of myoclonus with serotonin agonists, and amelioration with the serotonin antagonist methysergide was reported in a single patient with severe hypercarbic respiratory arrest [32]. The exact role of serotonin in Lance-Adams syndrome remains unclear.

Clinical Presentation

Generalized Tonic-Clonic (GTC) Seizures

GTC seizures following CPR were reported in 16 of 114 cardiac arrest survivors in the Krumholz prospective series [2]. GTC status epilepticus occurred in conjunction with myoclonus in 17% of patients, a constellation Krumholz et al. termed myoclonic status epilepticus. The majority of these seizure episodes began within 5 h (range 1–12) of cardiac arrest and lasted an average of 17.5 h (range 2–48). All patients were profoundly comatose at seizure onset. In the same series, respiratory arrests were more frequently implicated in myoclonic status epilepticus than cardiac arrests [2]. Snyder et al. [4] reported GTC seizures in 4 of their 63 patients in coma after CPR in another prospective series. The majority of these seizure episodes occurred in close proximity to the administration of lidocaine. One of these patients had GTC convulsions simultaneous with myoclonus.

Focal and Complex Partial Seizures

Focal and complex partial seizures following CPR have not been extensively reported in the literature. Krumholz et al. [2] mention that 3 of the 114 cardiac arrest survivors studied developed focal motor seizures. Snyder et al. [4] reported

complex and simple partial seizures in 12 of their 63 patients in hypoxic-ischemic coma. Most patients were profoundly comatose at the onset of seizures. Partial seizures typically began within the first 12 h after arrest but could be delayed 2–4 days [4]. The majority of seizure episodes lasted less than 48 h, but a few patients had recurrence of partial seizures after 4–6 days. The majority of patients with partial seizures had other types of seizures as well, including GTC seizures and myoclonus.

Myoclonus

Cortical, reticular, segmental, generalized, reflex, and action myoclonus have all been described as sequelae to hypoxic-ischemic encephalopathy [2, 4, 6, 23–25, 33–40]. Cortical myoclonus is felt to be a fragment of focal seizures, with myoclonic jerks involving only a small number of adjacent muscle groups [41]. It preferentially involves distal appendicular structures, typically affecting agonist and antagonist muscle groups simultaneously, and may be multifocal [41]. Cortical myoclonus occurs spontaneously but may be accentuated by volitional movement (action myoclonus) or somatosensory stimulation (reflex myoclonus) [41]. The movements are typically preceded by time-locked EEG discharges at the sensorimotor cortex. Reticular myoclonus is felt to be a fragment of generalized epilepsy, with myoclonic jerks involving the entire body [41]. Axial structures and proximal muscle groups are preferentially involved, and the jerks may also be triggered by movement or somatosensory stimuli [41]. Reticular myoclonus is believed to result from lesions of the nucleus reticularis gigantocellularis in the caudal medulla [41]. EEG spikes are generalized and follow the movement, suggestive of a subcortical discharge referred to the cortex [41]. Primary generalized myoclonus involves synchronous jerks of the distal appendicular muscles time-locked to generalized cortical discharges on EEG [41]. SM is any form of epileptic myoclonus that persists for greater than 30 min. Segmental myoclonus is felt to be a non-epileptic brainstem or spinal cord reflex resulting in isolated, non-rhythmic jerks of axial structures with no EEG correlate.

Snyder et al. [4] reported myoclonic seizures in 12 of their 63 CPR survivors. Most patients had synchronous, symmetric jerks involving the face, adductors of the thighs, and flexors of the arms. Others had asynchronous, asymmetric jerks involving the extremities alone. Myoclonus occurred in 30% of CPR survivors in the Krumholz et al. series [2], the majority of whom (78%) had generalized or multifocal cortical myoclonus with co-occurrence of other seizure types. Segmental myoclonus involving the eyes, palate, and pharynx was noted in several patients. In the Young et al. series [23], myoclonic jerks were always bilaterally synchronous and involved the face, particularly the eyelids. The extraocular muscles could be involved as well [23, 24]. Limb jerks occurred variably and simultaneous to facial movements.

Myoclonic jerks occasionally involve the diaphragm and interfere with mechanical ventilation [23]. Myoclonus typically begins within 12 h of cardiopulmonary arrest with a mean duration around 24 h [2, 4, 24, 25]. A sub-group of patients develop myoclonus only 3–5 days after arrest and it persists for days to weeks [4]. Spontaneous myoclonus typically occurs at a frequency of a jerk every 1–5 s [25]. Stimulus sensitivity has been reported in many patients [4, 23–25, 34, 35, 37], with increased jerks on tracheal suctioning, touch, painful stimuli, or loud noise. Stereotyped myoclonic jerks have also been reported with episodic hypotension [24]. One group reported reticular myoclonus in synchrony to the carotid pulse that was ablated by carotid sinus massage [40].

Lance-Adams Syndrome

Some mention must be made of Lance-Adams syndrome because it may evolve while the patient remains in the intensive care unit [6, 42, 43]. In the original Lance and Adams case series [6], 3 of the 4 patients began experiencing myoclonus during the first few days after resuscitation while they remained in post-anoxic coma. "Generalized myoclonus was a feature of the early stages of the illness soon after the episode of hypoxia but after a few days, when consciousness was regained and the patients' condition stabilized, the movements became restricted in site and all tendency to rhythmicity was lost" [6]. In one series, 9 of 14 patients first experienced myoclonus within days of the hypoxic event, and—in all but one—myoclonic jerks were first noted during coma [43]. After arousal from coma, Lance and Adams' [6] patients had normal or near-normal intellect, subtle cerebellar signs, and labile mood. The myoclonic jerks were brief, variable in amplitude, and typically comprised a series of contractions of agonist and antagonist groups. Myoclonus was usually limited to the activated limb, but occasionally spread contralaterally or ipsilaterally. It could be enhanced by emotional states or sensory stimuli such as pinprick, touch, tendon tap, or loud noise. Post-anoxic myoclonus can show characteristics of either cortical or reticular myoclonus and sometimes both [43–48]. The majority of patients in one series [43] had cortical discharges on EEG preceding and time-locked to myoclonic jerks. These jerks were predominantly distal and limited to the part of the body involved in the volitional movement. Myoclonic jerks involved the facial muscles in several patients, interfering with swallowing and speaking. Other patients had stimulus-sensitive myoclonic jerks that were bilateral, synchronous, and predominantly involving axial structures, suggestive of reticular reflex myoclonus [43]. One case report [45] described a patient who developed both cortical action myoclonus and reticular reflex myoclonus after CPR.

Laboratory Investigation

Electroencephalography

EEG has been the mainstay of clinical investigation in postanoxic seizures. In a study [49] from a single university center by Varelas et al., cardiorespiratory arrest was the indication for ordering an emergent EEG in 11% (29 out of 261) of cases. EEG was ordered to rule out status epilepticus in 23 patients and seizures in 3 patients. Preceding suspicious clinical activity was reported in 65% and previously witnessed seizures in 10%. Twenty-one patients were already receiving antiepileptic medications when the study was ordered. Generalized slowing was the most common emergent EEG finding (11 cases), followed by convulsive status epilepticus (8 cases), epileptiform discharges (4 cases), and nonconvulsive status epilepticus (3 cases). In the multivariate analysis of all emergent EEGs in this study, history of cardiopulmonary arrest was the only independent predictor of convulsive or NCSE [49].

The presence of multiple various rhythmic and fluctuating patterns in EEG activity in the critically ill has created a challenge for those caring for patients, as well as researchers who wish to evaluate the presence and significance of these patterns. There has been a movement to clarify these patterns recently, with the development of a more standardized nomenclature [50]. After implementation of these guidelines, high interrater agreement was shown for the interpretation of critical care EEG monitoring [51]. Despite these interpretation challenges in the intensive care unit, EEG remains a valuable tool for comatose individuals [52].

It is recommended that EEG monitoring be performed, with frequent interpretation for patients that remain comatose after return of spontaneous circulation (ROSC; Class I, LOE C-Limited Data) [53]. If continuous EEG monitoring is not available, intermittent routine EEG studies are recommended. These guidelines are based on a high prevalence of epileptiform activity (12–22%), including both seizures and NCSE, in comatose patients after cardiac arrest [8, 54, 55].

Krumholz et al. [2] found epileptiform discharges in 58% of survivors with clinical seizures or myoclonus and 88% of those with myoclonic status epilepticus. Epileptiform discharges were rare in CPR survivors without clinical seizures or myoclonus (9%). Burst suppression was also seen more frequently (76%) in patients with myoclonic status epilepticus [2]. EEG characteristics of the various types of seizures after hypoxic-ischemic injury have also been described. Snyder et al. [4] commented that the most common finding in patients with partial seizures was diffuse slowing, with spike activity and rhythmic slowing occurring in the minority of patients. The EEG findings in comatose patients with myoclonus are highly variable. The most frequently reported patterns include burst suppression, diffuse slowing, isoelectric tracing, periodic spikes and polyspike/slow-wave complexes, and alpha coma [2, 4, 23–25, 33–35]. The most common tracing in most series is diffuse slowing with or without periodic spikes or polyspike complexes [33]. The interval between complexes is stable for a given patient but ranges from 0.5 to 5 s [33]. The complexes may or may not be time-locked to the myoclonic jerks [23, 25]. In stimulus-sensitive myoclonus, tactile and auditory stimulation elicit bursts of generalized spike-polyspike complexes that precede and are time-locked to clinical myoclonus [25, 35]. Burst suppression is the second most frequently reported pattern [33]. The bursts typically last 1–10 s and are separated by prolonged periods of suppression ranging 5–25 s [33]. One series reported periods of inter-burst suppression lasting as long as 2–4 min [35]. Burst-suppression patterns in hypoxic-ischemic coma without myoclonus have typical intervals around 15 s [56], and prolonged suppression in this scenario may reflect more profound brain injury [33]. As described above, patients with Lance-Adams syndrome follow 3 EEG patterns: focal time-locked spikes that precede the myoclonus (cortical myoclonus), generalized non-time-locked spike-and-slow-wave complexes that follow the myoclonus (reticular myoclonus), and no abnormal EEG activity (segmental myoclonus) [43–48]. EEG has also been used for prognostic purposes after cardiopulmonary arrest [57–59]. In a systematic review of EEG data [60], five out of six studies demonstrated 100% specificity for poor outcome in CPR survivors with burst-suppression or isoelectric patterns within the first week. The likelihood ratio for poor outcome with these EEG patterns was 9.0 (95% CI 2.5–33.3) [60].

Electromyography

Electromyography (EMG) may be useful in delineating reticular myoclonus from cortical myoclonus in patients with Lance-Adams syndrome, especially in conjunction with EEG. Patients with cortical myoclonus demonstrate EMG discharges that occur in a rostrocaudal distribution, are time-locked to cortical spikes on EEG, follow them, and have conduction delays similar to direct cortical stimulation of the motor tract [6, 41]. Patients with reticular myoclonus involving the cranial nerves demonstrate a caudorostral distribution of EMG discharges originating in the caudal medulla that are not time-locked to and normally precede cortical EEG spikes [41, 44, 47].

Somatosensory Evoked Potentials

Somatosensory evoked potentials (SSEP) have prognostic utility in post-anoxic coma and have contributed to clinical research in Lance-Adams syndrome. They have not been studied in acute post-anoxic myoclonus per se. Bilateral absence of early cortical N20 SSEP responses portends poor outcome in hypoxic-ischemic coma when conducted at 24–72 h after arrest or rewarming [56, 61–67] with a low false-positive rate (FPR 1%; 95% CI, 0–3%, Class IIa, LOE B-nonrandomized) [53]. Benefits of using SSEP include minimal influence of medications and metabolic derangements [56], but this testing does require a high level of technical skill, and care must be taken to minimize muscle artifact. SSEP has also been useful in studying Lance-Adams syndrome. Patients with cortical action myoclonus often demonstrate abnormally large evoked potentials in the sensorimotor cortex, whereas patients with reticular myoclonus do not [41, 43, 45, 46]. These data have been used to support the hypothesis that cortical reflex myoclonus results from hyperexcitability of the sensory input to a cortical reflex arc [41].

Brain Imaging

Brain imaging has been extensively studied in patients after cardiopulmonary arrest, but not in the subpopulation with hypoxic-ischemic seizures and myoclonus. Torbey et al. [59] demonstrated the loss of distinction between the gray and white matter on CT scan immediately after cardiac arrest. A gray matter to white matter Hounsfield unit ratio <1.18 at the level of the basal ganglia predicted death in this small retrospective study [68]. In one series, brain CT scans done at various times after cardiopulmonary arrest were grossly normal in 77% of all comatose patients with or without subsequent seizures [24]. Cerebral edema and hypodensities in the deep cortical white matter, cerebellum, thalamus, and cortical watershed areas occurred more frequently in those patients with myoclonus than in those without myoclonus. More recently it has been discovered that bilateral hippocampal hyperintensities on MRI diffusion-weighted imaging (DWI) and fluid-attenuated inversion recovery (FLAIR) indicate a poor prognosis for comatose cardiac arrest survivors, although this was demonstrated on a small sample size [69]. Brain MRI has been studied in survivors of cardiac arrest and in status epilepticus, but not in the subpopulation with both seizures and cardiorespiratory arrest. One small study of CPR survivors [70] showed restricted diffusion in the basal ganglia, cerebellum, and cortex on the day of arrest. Diffusion was restricted mostly in the cortical and subcortical gray matter between 24 h and 13 days and in the white matter between 14 and 20 days. After 21 days, diffusion-weighted imaging was normal [70]. In the absence of hypoxic or ischemic insults, status epilepticus is known to induce T2- and diffusion-weighted hyperintensities and T1-weighted hypointensities as well as contrast enhancement in the involved cortex, adjacent subcortical white matter, and hippocampus [71]. These changes represent cortical cytotoxic edema and subcortical vasogenic edema that typically reverses when seizures are controlled [71]. For more information on differentiating MRI changes between ischemic stroke and status epilepticus, please refer to the Chap. 9.

Brain imaging is poorly studied in CPR survivors with seizures. In one series, brain MRI and CT in patients with Lance-Adams syndrome were normal in one-third of patients, showed cortical or cerebellar infarcts in one-third, and showed mild cortical and cerebellar atrophy in the remaining third [43].

Cerebrospinal Fluid Analysis

There is no evidence to support the evaluation of cerebrospinal fluid in the setting of acute hypoxic-ischemic seizures in humans [53]. In Lance-Adams syndrome, conflicting data have been reported with regard to concentrations of serotonin metabolites, as described above. The majority of patients have depressed serotonin metabolites and often respond clinically and biochemically to serotonin precursors and agonists like 5-HTP, clonazepam, and valproic acid [27, 31]. Those patients with elevated CSF serotonin metabolites tend to respond to serotonin antagonists like methysergide [32].

Differential Diagnosis

Many conditions that cause cardiopulmonary arrest may also lower the seizure threshold. This understanding is especially important if prolonged seizures are taken as an indication of severe irreversible brain injury that may influence the decision to limit medical care. Patients with a previous diagnosis of epilepsy may present in status epilepticus after a relatively brief episode of hypoxia. Preexisting epilepsy may not be known at the initial point of care, and baseline antiepileptic drug levels may be helpful in this regard. Drugs given to patients during the resuscitation may trigger or lower seizure threshold. Lidocaine, used as part of the standard Advanced Cardiac Life Support protocol, is well known to induce seizures at serum levels >9 µg/ml [72–74]. Propafenone, although rarely used in cardiac arrest, has also been reported to lower the seizure threshold [75]. Streptokinase, prourokinase, and tissue-type plasminogen activator given during acute myocardial infarction may also induce seizures [76]. Although rarely used in the modern management of asthma, theophylline administered for respiratory arrest secondary to status asthmaticus is epileptogenic [77]. Stimulants, tricyclic antidepressants, and cocaine can potentially cause arrhythmic cardiac arrest and seizures [68, 73, 78, 79]. Alcohol-, barbiturate-, and benzodiazepine-withdrawal seizures must be considered in the first few days of admission in alcoholics and sedative users who present with respiratory or cardiac arrest.

Penicillins, fluoroquinolones, and other antibiotics used in the ICU setting may trigger seizures. Rapid withdrawal of anesthetic agents, such as propofol and barbiturates, may also precipitate prolonged seizures and post-propofol myoclonus is a well-described phenomenon [80]. For more details on drug-induced seizures, review the Chap. 20

Metabolic derangements, such as hyponatremia and hypomagnesemia, are common in patients with congestive heart failure, intrinsic renal disease, the syndrome of inappropriate antidiuretic hormone release (SIADH), and diuretic users. If severe, hyponatremia may produce obtundation—with or without focal neurological deficits—and seizures. Profound hypoglycemia in insulin users may also precipitate coma and seizures in the setting of cardiopulmonary arrest. Seizures in encephalopathic patients may be difficult to clinically distinguish from shivering, rigors, hyperekplexia, and reflex startle responses [41, 45]. EEG, with or without paralytic medications, may be helpful in this regard. Specific discussion on the role of metabolic and systemic derangement in seizure disorder is provided elsewhere in this book.

Treatment

General Considerations

Seizures are most likely to occur during the first day after cardiopulmonary arrest. This is a period of hemodynamic instability, prognostic uncertainty, and high risk of recurrent arrest. Cardiac arrest and profound hypotension often cause hepatic and renal damage, which may alter the metabolism and excretion of resuscitative and anticonvulsant medications. Drugs used to control these—often highly refractory—seizures may have untoward effects on cardiac rhythm, blood pressure, and level of consciousness. Intravenous phenytoin is well known to induce hypotension and may trigger arrhythmias such as ventricular fibrillation, complete heart block, bradycardia, and asystole. Divalproex sodium, phenytoin, and barbiturates can precipitate hepatic injury that may be especially problematic in the setting of shock liver. Divalproex sodium and phenytoin also have significant interactions with many antiarrhythmic agents, including lidocaine and amiodarone. Intravenous benzodiazepines and barbiturates may also induce hypotension and may interfere with neurological examination such that a falsely poor prognosis is given in patients with shock liver and untested blood levels.

Simple and Complex Partial Seizures

Simple and complex partial seizures have not been demonstrated to cause neuronal injury in most case series and may not require aggressive management in post-anoxic coma. In the Snyder et al. case series [4], few patients had partial seizures in isolation, and most patients had good seizure control with phenytoin alone, phenobarbital alone, or both. The decision to treat partial seizures in comatose patients must be individualized, weighing the ease of treatment versus the low risk of exacerbated neuronal injury in this setting.

Generalized Tonic-Clonic Seizures

GTC seizures are well known to cause progressive neuronal injury after 30 min [9, 12, 13]. They typically begin during the first day after cardiopulmonary arrest, a period in which the ultimate prognosis remains unclear. The pathological data in post-anoxic patients with GTC status epilepticus is limited, but one series [25] did demonstrate Ammon's horn sclerosis – typical of epileptic neuronal injury—in two such patients. GTC status epilepticus should be managed aggressively in these patients—particularly when it occurs early in the hospital course—as detailed elsewhere in this book (chapter on "Management of Status Epilepticus and Critical Care Seizures"). To what extent this management may change the outcome after hypoxic-ischemic injury is unknown.

Myoclonus

Isolated epileptic myoclonus and segmental myoclonus are not harmful and do not require treatment unless they interfere with mechanical ventilation or clinical care. Whether or not SM exacerbates the brain damage caused by hypoxic-ischemic encephalopathy remains unclear. Most clinicians argue that SM represents agonal neuronal activity that reflects neurological devastation. A review of the literature for this publication found five patients [6, 25, 39, 81] who developed SM during post-anoxic coma and had good neurological outcomes. Importantly, all of these patients appear to have suffered respiratory arrest as opposed to cardiac arrest. Several case series focused purely on cardiac arrest [2, 4, 24, 33, 38] report uniform mortality or vegetative state in post-anoxic SM. It is unclear, however, whether these results reflect a "self-fulfilling prophesy" as SM itself may be used as an argument to withdraw supportive care [24, 38]. Although pathological studies from patients with SM after cardiopulmonary arrest show greater cortical involvement than similar patients without SM [24], it is unclear whether SM is reflective or causative of this injury. SM is often refractory to treatment short of pharmacological coma. Medications employed with varying degrees of success include phenytoin, phenobarbital, levetiracetam, valproic acid, and benzodiazepines [2, 4, 23–25, 33, 35, 36, 38].

The AHA 2015 guidelines note the importance in distinguishing myoclonus from status myoclonus [53]. The term status myoclonus was defined as continuous repetitive myoclonic jerks with a duration of greater than 30 min. The presence of status myoclonus in subjects that underwent TTM within 72–120 h after ROSC is predictive of a poor outcome with a 0% FPR (CI 0–4%) [8, 82, 83]. Cardiac arrest survivors who do not undergo TTM still have a poor outcome when status myoclonus is present within 72 of arrest (FPR 0%, CI 0–14%) [2, 84]. Differentiation must be made between myoclonus and status myoclonus, as a subset of myoclonus patients have been reported to have good outcomes when there is an early onset and prolonged myoclonus that evolves later into the action myoclonus of the Lance-Adams syndrome [53].

Nonconvulsive Status Epilepticus

NCSE should be treated immediately once recognized. The Neurocritical Care Society has proposed a set of guidelines for the treatment of SE and NCSE based on current evidence and consensus of expert opinion [85]. Treatment is divided into categories such as emergency, urgent, and refractory medications. These guidelines also provide detailed information regarding the nomenclature of SE, refractory SE, and their associated prognoses.

Prophylactic Antiepileptic Drug Use

To date, there is no evidence to support the use of prophylactic antiepileptic drugs in the setting of post-anoxic coma. In the Brain Resuscitation Clinical Trial [86], comatose survivors of cardiac arrest were randomized to standard care with or without a loading dose of thiopental. There was no statistically significant difference in outcome between the two groups. Another randomized clinical trial [54] compared the use of diazepam to placebo, both given shortly after ROSC, with no significant difference in outcome. Routine use of prophylactic antiepileptic medications is not recommended, since the risk of adverse effects outweighs potential benefits [53, 87].

Supportive Management

A relatively benign intervention in any seizure type is the optimization of factors that affect systemic function such as electrolytes, medications, and infections. Correction of hypoglycemia, hyponatremia, hypocalcemia, and hypomagnesemia may reduce the risk of recurrent cardiac events and seizures. As with any severe neurological injury, serum glucose levels should be normalized using insulin as needed. Acid-base disturbances should be optimized with appropriate adjustments to the mechanical ventilator. Discontinuation of proconvulsant medications should be undertaken if possible.

Prognosis and Outcomes

The prognostic significance of seizures in hypoxic-ischemic coma has been a source of controversy in the literature. Levy's classic study of a general population of patients in hypoxic-ischemic coma failed to demonstrate poorer outcomes in the subpopulation with seizures of any type [5]. Although Snyder et al. [3] showed 17% survival in hypoxic-ischemic coma patients with myoclonus and 32% survival with seizures versus 43% survival without any seizure activity, the difference failed to reach statistical significance. Likewise, there was only a trend toward higher incidence of excellent outcome in survivors without seizure than in patients who had any form of seizure activity [3]. Another large study by Krumholz et al. [2] showed that seizures or myoclonus per se is not significantly related to outcome, but convulsive status epilepticus and myoclonic status epilepticus confer poor outcome as judged by survival and recovery of consciousness [1].

In 2006, the American Academy of Neurology (AAN) published a practice parameter for the prediction of outcome in comatose survivors of cardiac arrest [88]. Subtle changes have been made in the most recent guidelines, presented by the AHA in 2015 [53]. Prognostication after cardiac arrest should be rendered using evidence-based practices as provided by those AAN and AHA post-cardiac arrest care guidelines.

Other testing may also be used in conjunction with clinical exam to assist in prognostication. Neuron-specific enolase (NSE) and S100B are serum biomarkers that should not be used alone to prognosticate but may be used in conjunction with other prognostic testing. When NSE and S100B are elevated more than 72 h from cardiac arrest, they support a poor neurologic outcome (Class IIb, LOE B-NR) [53]. Prognostication should always be multimodal when possible, due to the low sensitivity of individual tests, with as much reduction of confounders as possibly [89]. Testing should not be conducted until at least 72 h from ROSC, or in the TTM era, 72 h from rewarming. Caution should be used when interpreting these biomarkers from patients that have undergone cooling, as the kinetics are unknown and may be affected by hypothermia [53].

Hypothermia and Seizures After Resuscitation from Cardiac Arrest

Two well-designed randomized-controlled clinical trials have demonstrated that therapeutic hypothermia improves neurological recovery [90, 91]. Current treatment protocols for hypothermia after cardiac arrest have been based on the study designs of those landmark clinical trials and typically aim at initiation of hypothermia within 4 h of CPR, a target temperature of 32–34° C, maintenance of therapy for 12–24 h, and a period of gradual rewarming [91, 92]. The majority of patients experience shivering during the hypothermia maintenance period that requires either sedation, paralysis, or both [91]. The use of long-acting paralytic agents has the obvious potential to mask convulsive seizures, leading some to recommend continuous EEG monitoring during the hypothermia period to aid seizure recognition [93, 94].

Since therapeutic hypothermia has become protocolized for post-cardiac arrest, care data have emerged on the presence of epileptic activity in this patient population. Amorim et al. [95] conducted a study investigating patients that underwent TTM and, per protocol, received continuous EEG monitoring for at least 48 h. A total of 120 subjects were enrolled, and only EEG patterns of patients that survived to hospital discharge were analyzed. Abnormal EEG patterns were dichotomized into either "malignant EEG patterns (MEPs)" or burst suppression (SB). The MEPs included seizures, status epilepticus, myoclonic status epilepticus, and generalized periodic discharges. Results showed that MEPs and SB were found in 15.8 and 18.3% of survivors, respectively. Of these subjects, two with MEPs and eight with SB had a good neurologic outcome, defined as CPC (cerebral performance category) of 1 or 2. The presence of MEPs was not, however, an independent predictor of poor neurologic outcome. Given these findings, burst-suppression patterns, once previously thought to be a predictor of poor outcome, should perhaps not be used alone as an independent factor for predicting poor outcome.

Aside from ictal activity, it is important to investigate for EEG reactivity, which is useful in predicting outcome. The absence of EEG reactivity to external stimulation at 72 h from arrest, and persistent burst suppression after rewarming, predicts poor outcome [53]. Oddo and Rossetti [96] conducted a prospective cohort study in 134 patients that underwent TH after cardiac arrest to investigate predictors of outcome. Using a multivariable ordinal logistic regression, they found that the absence of EEG reactivity, incomplete recovery of brainstem reflexes at normothermia, and NSE greater than 33 µg/L were independent predictors of poor outcome (defined as CPC 3–5). Furthermore, the combination of these three findings has 100% specificity for poor outcome.

The Future of EEG and Post-cardiac Arrest Seizures

As technology continues to develop and more clinicians have access to EEG capabilities, there still remains a need for frequent interpretation of data. For those who are comatose and often sedated and paralyzed, it is ideal to have continuous EEG monitoring to assist in detecting and treating underlying electrographic seizure activity. Reduced EEG montages with trend analysis [97] have been proposed but need to be validated with large-scale studies in the future.

Additionally, there should be a consensus among neurologists regarding a consistent nomenclature for EEG patterns described in post-cardiac arrest patients. Once there is a widely accepted system for defining and classifying patterns, it could be used to devise a cohesive consensus statement as to each pattern and their respective prognostic neurologic outcome.

Lastly, the concept of the "self-fulfilling prophecy" should also not be underestimated. The presence of epileptiform activity and seizures post cardiac arrest has been traditionally associated with poor neurologic outcome. There is a paucity of randomized clinical trials for the treatment of SE in general, with even less evidence for SE in the post-cardiac

arrest population. As post-cardiac arrest care continues to progress, we should support more efforts to develop novel therapies targeting the specific pathophysiology of this condition, and their efficacy should be evaluated with generation of higher level of evidence data [98].

Case 1. Nonconvulsive status in a patient with post-anoxic myoclonus. Forty-three-year-old white man was admitted after drowning. He was found in the bottom of a lake, where he stayed for approximately 15 min. He was initially pulseless and without breathing. MRI was performed and shown below (Figs. 13.1 and 13.2). In the ICU he developed continuous

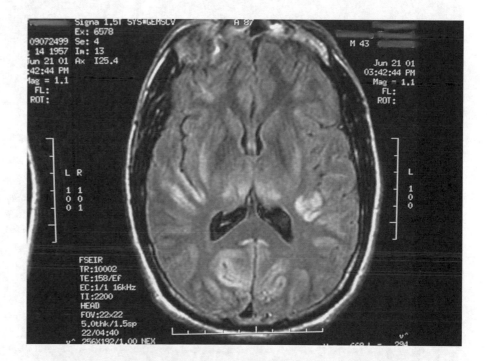

Fig. 13.1 DWI MRI of the brain 29 h later demonstrating diffuse abnormalities, especially in the basal ganglia, thalamus, insular and occipital cortices

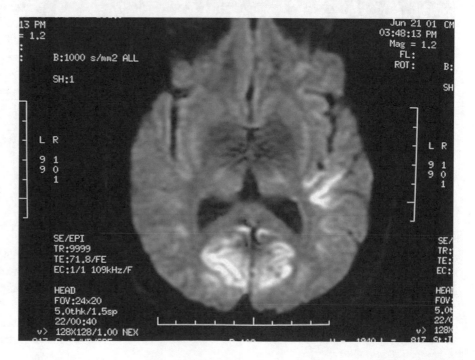

Fig. 13.2 DWI MRI of the brain 29 h later demonstrating diffuse abnormalities, especially in the basal ganglia, thalamus, insular and occipital cortices

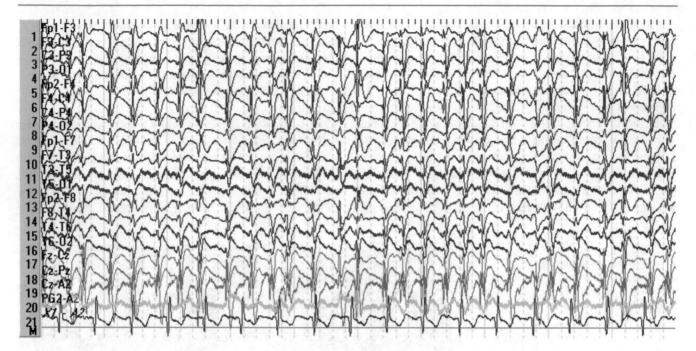

Fig. 13.3 Continuous EEG monitoring demonstrating bi-hemispheric continuous runs of sharp and slow waves, which did not correlate with myoclonic jerking or clinical convulsions

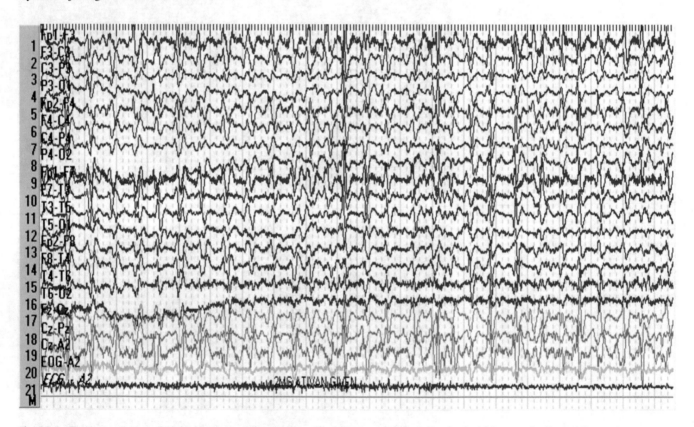

Fig. 13.4 Continuous bursts of triphasic wave activity at a rate of 1–2 Hz, occasionally intermixed with bursts of spike activity

bilateral and synchronous myoclonic jerks in the upper and lower extremities. EEG monitoring was performed. (Fig. 13.3). In addition, the patient who had several generalized tonic-clonic convulsions were suppressed by phenytoin and valproic acid. The patient regained only brainstem reflex function and eventually expired in palliative care 12 days after extubation.

Case 2. Nonconvulsive status epilepticus. Seventy-five-year-old woman was involved in a car accident, with admission GCS of 15, and developed multi-organ failure after a protracted ICU stay. She had a cardiac arrest in the ICU, after which she never regained consciousness. An EEG was performed to rule out nonconvulsive status epilepticus (Figs. 13.4 and 13.5).

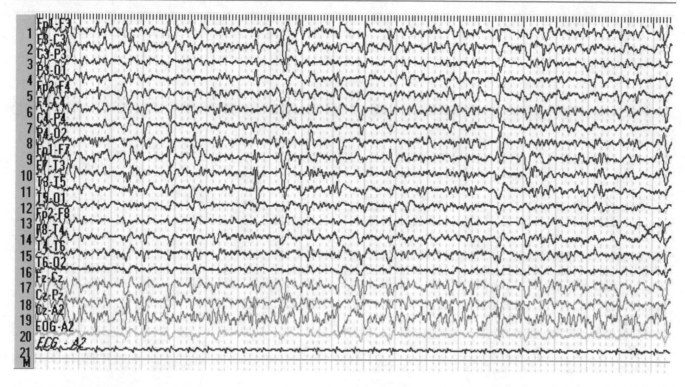

Fig. 13.5 Significant decrease of the epileptiform activity after intravenous administration of 2 mg lorazepam. The patient did not have any clinical improvement and remained in coma

Fig. 13.6 CT of the head showing a small centrum semiovale subacute lacune (white arrow), but paucity of other significant radiologic injuries. No MRI was ever performed due to the prolonged and severe critical condition of the patient

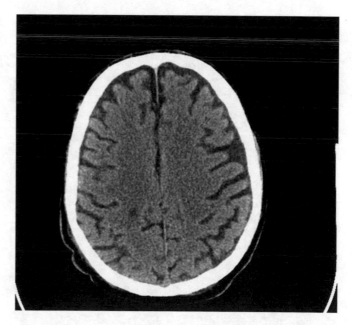

Case 3. Seventy-year-old man s/p coronary artery bypass (×3 vessels), with complicated course in the cardiac-ICU (hemodynamic instability with prolonged hypotension). CT head was done (Fig. 13.6) and showed a small lacunar infarct. Four days after his surgery, he developed generalized tonic-clonic status epilepticus and was placed on pentobarbital coma under continuous EEG monitoring. EEG monitoring showed evolving electrographic seizures from the right (Figs. 13.7, 13.8, 13.9, and 13.10). He never regained consciousness, but the status epilepticus resolved after more than a month in barbiturate coma. Because of skin ulceration under the electrode placement areas, the continuous EEG had to be stopped.

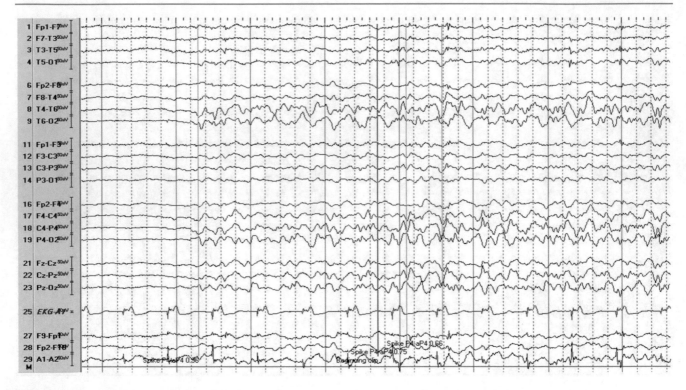

Fig. 13.7 Electrographic seizure, beginning from the parieto-temporo-occipital areas of the right hemisphere

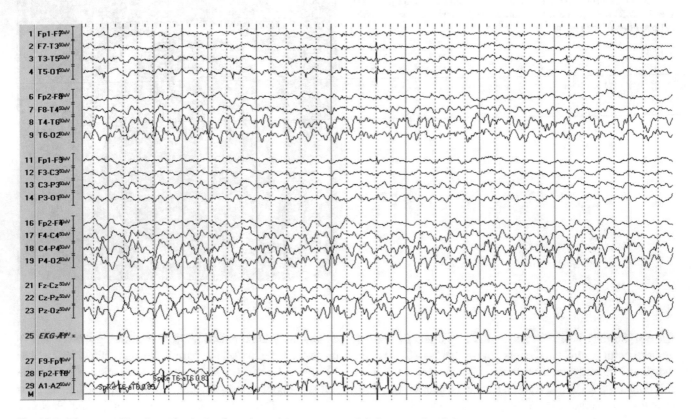

Fig. 13.8 Electrographic seizure, beginning from the parieto-temporo-occipital areas and evolving

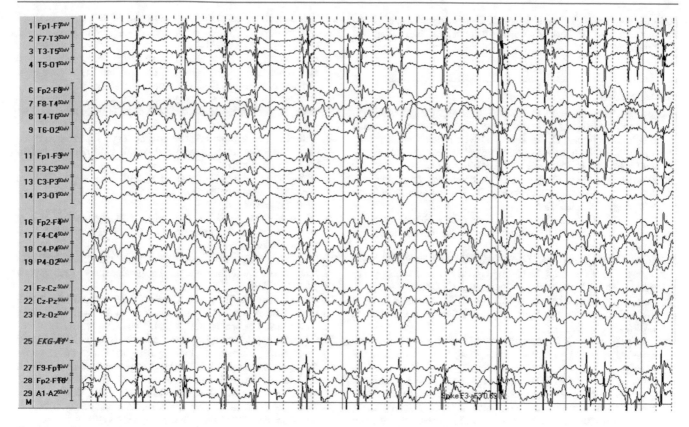

Fig. 13.9 Electrographic seizure, see in two previous figures now speading to the left hemisphere

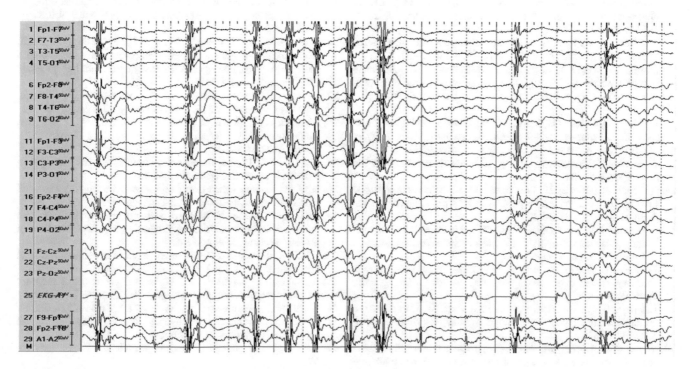

Fig. 13.10 Electrographic seizure, seen in three previous figures now ending

Acknowledgments The authors would like to acknowledge Dr. Ernst Niedermeyer and Dr. Peter Kaplan for their helpful suggestions and EEG tracings.

References

1. Nielsen N, Sunde K, Hovdenes J, Riker RR, Rubertsson S, Stammet P, Nilsson F, Friberg H, Network H. Adverse events and their relation to mortality in out-of –hospital cardiac arrest patients treated with hypothermia. Crit Care Med. 2011;39:57–64.
2. Krumholz A, Stern BJ, Weiss HD. Outcome from coma after cardiopulmonary resuscitation: relation to seizures and myoclonus. Neurology. 1988;38:401–5.
3. Snyder BD, Ramirez-Lassepas M, Lippert DM. Neurologic status and prognosis after cardiopulmonary arrest: I. a retrospective study. Neurology. 1977;27:807–11.
4. Snyder BD, Hauser WA, Loewenson RB, Leppik IE, Ramirez-Lassepas M, Gumnit RJ. Neurologic prognosis after cardiopulmonary arrest: III. seizure activity. Neurology. 1980;30:1292–7.
5. Levy DE, Caronna JJ, Singer BH, Lapinski RH, Frydman H, Plum F. Predicting outcome from hypoxic-ischemic coma. JAMA. 1985;253:1420–6.
6. Lance JW, Adams RD. The syndrome of intention or action myoclonus as a sequel to hypoxic encephalopathy. Brain. 1963;86:111–36.
7. Mani R, Schmitt SE, Mazer M, Putt ME, Gaieski DF. The frequency and timing of epileptiform activity on continuous electroencephalogram in comatose post-cardiac arrest syndrome patients treated with therapeutic hypothermia. Resuscitation. 2012;83:840–7.
8. Rittenberger JC, Popescu A, Brenner RP, Guyette FX, Callaway CW. Frequency and timing of nonconvulsive status epilepticus in comatose post-cardiac arrest subjects treated with hypothermia. Neurocrit Care. 2012;16(1):114–22.
9. Yamada K, Ji JJ, Yuan H, Miki T, Sato S, Horimoto N, Shimizu T, Seino S, Inagaki N. Protective role of ATP-sensitive potassium channels in hypoxia-induced generalized seizure. Science. 2001;292:1543–6.
10. Meldrum BS. Epileptic brain damage: a consequence and cause of seizures. Neuropathol Appl Neurobiol. 1997;23:185–202.
11. Novelli A, Reilly JA, Lysko PG, Henneberry RC. Glutamate becomes neurotoxic via the N-methyl-D-aspartate receptor when intracellular energy levels are reduced. Brain Res. 1988;451:205–12.
12. Fariello RG, Golden GT, Smith GG, Reyes PF. Potentiation of kainic acid epileptogenicity and sparing from neuronal damage by an NMDA receptor antagonist. Epilepsy Res. 1989;3:206–13.
13. Norman RM. The neuropathology of status epilepticus. Med Sci Law. 1964;4:46–51.
14. Meldrum BS, Brierley JB. Prolonged epileptic seizures in primates: ischemic cell change and its relation to ictal physiological events. Arch Neurol. 1973;28:10–7.
15. O'Connell BK, Towfighi J, Kofke WA, Hawkins RA. Neuronal lesions in mercaptopropionic acid-induced status epilepticus. Acta Neuropathol. 1988;77:47–54.
16. Nevander G, Ingvar M, Auer R, Siesjö BK. Status epilepticus in well-oxygenated rats causes neuronal necrosis. Ann Neurol. 1985;18:281–90.
17. Brierley JB. Cerebral hypoxia. In: Blackwood W, Corsellis JAN, editors. Greenfield's neuropathology. Edinburgh: Edward Arnold; 1976. p. 43–85.
18. Young RSK, During MJ, Aquila WJ, Tendler D, Ley E. Hypoxia increases extracellular concentrations of excitatory and inhibitory neurotransmitters in subsequently induced seizure: in vivo microdialysis study in the rabbit. Exp Neurol. 1992;117:204–9.
19. Cataltepe O, Vannucci RC, Heitjan DF, Towfighi J. Effect of status epilepticus on hypoxic-ischemic brain damage in the immature rat. Pediatr Res. 1995;38:251–7.
20. Hayakawa T, Higuchi Y, Nigami H, Hattori H. Zonisamide reduces hypoxic-ischemic brain damage in neonatal rats irrespective of its anticonvulsant effect. Eur J Pharmacol. 1994;257:131–6.
21. Towfighi J, Housman C, Mauger D, Vannucci RC. Effect of seizures on cerebral hypoxic-ischemic lesions in immature rats. Dev Brain Res. 1999;113:83–95.
22. Wirrell EC, Armstrong EA, Osman LD, Yager JY. Prolonged seizures exacerbate perinatal hypoxic-ischemic brain damage. Pediatr Res. 2001;50:445–54.
23. Young GB, Gilbert JJ, Zochodne DW. The significance of myoclonic status epilepticus in postanoxic coma. Neurology. 1990;40:1843–8.
24. Wijdicks EFM, Parisi JE, Sharbrough FW. Prognostic value of myoclonus status in comatose survivors of cardiac arrest. Ann Neurol. 1994;35:239–43.
25. Celesia GG, Grigg MM, Ross E. Generalized status myoclonicus in acute anoxic and toxic-metabolic encephalopathies. Arch Neurol. 1988;45:781–4.
26. Guilleminault C, Tharp BR, Cousin D. HVA and 5-HIAA CSF measurements and 5-HTP trials in some patients with involuntary movements. J Neurol Sci. 1973;18:435–41.
27. Chadwick D, Hallet M, Harris R, Jenner P, Reynolds EH, Marsden CD. Clinical, biochemical, and physiological features distinguishing myoclonus responsive to 5-HTP, tryptophan with monoamine oxidase inhibitor, and clonazepam. Brain. 1977;100:455–87.
28. Jaw SP, Hussong MJ, Matsumoto RR, Truong DD. Involvement of 5-HT$_2$ receptors in posthypoxic stimulus-sensitive myoclonus in rats. Pharmacol Biochem Behav. 1994;49:129–31.
29. Pappert EJ, Goetz CG, Vu TQ, Ling ZD, Leurgans S, Raman R, Carvey PM. Animal model of posthypoxic myoclonus: effects of serotonergic antagonists. Neurology. 1999;52:16–21.
30. Truong DD, Matsumoto RR, Schwartz PH, Hussong MJ, Wasterlain CG. Novel rat cardiac arrest model of posthypoxic myoclonus. Mov Disord. 1994;9:201–6.
31. De Lean J, Richardson JC, Hornykiewicz O. Beneficial effect of serotonin precursors in postanoxic action myoclonus. Neurology. 1976;26:863–8.
32. Gimenez-Roldan S, Mateo D, Muradas V, De Yeben JG. Clinical, biochemical, and pharmacologic observation in a patient with postasphyxic myoclonus: association with serotonin hyperactivity. Clin Neuropharmacol. 1988;11(2):151–60.
33. Jumao-as A, Brenner RP. Myoclonic status epilepticus: a clinical and electroencephalographic study. Neurology. 1990;40:1199–202.
34. Niedermeyer E, Bauer G, Burnite R, Reichenbach D. Selective stimulus-sensitive myoclonus in acute cerebral anoxia. Arch Neurol. 1977;34:365–8.
35. Van Cott AC, Blatt I, Brenner RP. Stimulus-sensitive seizures in postanoxic coma. Epilepsia. 1996;37:868–74.
36. Wolf P. Periodic synchronous and stereotyped myoclonus with postanoxic coma. J Neurol. 1977;215(1):39–47.
37. Kanemoto K, Ozawa K. A case of post-anoxic encephalopathy with initial massive myoclonic status followed by alternating Jacksonian seizures. Seizure. 2000;9:352–5.
38. Wijdicks EFM, Young GB. Myoclonus status in comatose patients after cardiac arrest. The Lancet. 1994;343:1642–3.
39. Arnoldus EPJ, Lammers GJ. Postanoxic coma: good recovery despite myoclonus status. Ann Neurol. 1995;38:697–8.
40. Hanakawa T, Hashimoto S, Iga K, Segawa Y, Shibasaki H. Carotid brainstem myoclonus after hypoxic brain damage. J Neurol Neurosurg Psychiatry. 2000;69:672–4.
41. Hallett M. The pathophysiology of myoclonus. TINS. 1987;10:69–73.
42. Harper SJ, Wilkes RG. Posthypoxic myoclonus (the Lance-Adams syndrome) in the intensive care unit. Anaesthesia. 1991;46:199–201.

43. Werhahn KJ, Brown P, Thompson PD, Marsden CD. The clinical features and prognosis of chronic posthypoxic myoclonus. Mov Disord. 1997;12:216–20.
44. Hallett M, Chadwick D, Adam J, Marsden CD. Reticular reflex myoclonus: a physiological type of human post-hypoxic myoclonus. J Neurol Neurosurg Psychiatry. 1977;40:253–64.
45. Brown P, Thompson PD, Rothwell JC, Day BL, Marsden CD. A case of postanoxic encephalopathy with cortical action and brainstem reticular reflex myoclonus. Mov Disord. 1991;6:139–44.
46. Witte OW, Niedermeyer E, Arendt G, Freund HJ. Post-hypoxic action (intention) myoclonus: a clinico-electroencephalographic study. J Neurol. 1988;235:214–8.
47. Lance JW, Adams RD. Negative myoclonus in posthypoxic patients: historical note. Mov Disord. 2001;16:162–3.
48. Fahn S. Posthypoxic action myoclonus: literature review update. Adv Neurol. 1986;43:157–69.
49. Varelas PN, Spanaki MV, Hacein-Bey L, Hether T, Terranova B. Emergent EEG: indications and diagnostic yield. Neurology. 2003;61:702–4.
50. Hirsch LJ, LaRoche SM, Gaspard N, Gerard E, Svoronos A, Herman ST, Mani R, Arif H, Jette N, Minazad Y, Kerrigan JF, Vespa P, Hantus S, Claassen J, Young GB, So E, Kaplan PW, Nuwer MR, Fountain NB, Drislane FW. American Clinical Neurophysiology Society's Standardized Critical Care EEG Terminology: 2012 version. J Clin Neurophysiol. 2013;30:1–27.
51. Gaspard N, Hirsch LJ, LaRoche SM, Hahn CD, Westover MB, Critical Care EEG Monitoring Research Consortium. Interrater agreement for critical care EEG terminology. Epilepsia. 2014;9:1366–73.
52. Herman ST, Abend NS, Bleck TP, Chapman KE, Drislane FW, Emerson RG, Gerard EE, Hahn CD, Husain AM, Kaplan PW, LaRoche SM, Nuwer MR, Quigg M, Riviello JJ, Schmitt SE, Simmons LA, Tsuchida TN, Hirsch LJ, Critical Care Continuous EEG Task Force of the American Clinical Neurophysiology Society. Consensus statement on continuous EEG in critically ill adults and children, part I: indications. J Clin Neurophysiol. 2015;32:87–95.
53. Callaway CW, Donnino MW, Fink EL, Geocadin RG, Golan E, Kern KB, Leary M, Meurer WJ, Peberdy MA, Thompson TM, Zimmerman JL. Part 8: post-cardiac arrest care: 2015 American Heart Association Guidelines update for cardiopulmonary resuscitation and emergency cardiovascular care. Circulation. 2015;132:S465–82.
54. Longstreth WT, Fahrenbruch CE, Olsufka M, Walsh TR, Copass MK, Cobb LA. Randomized clinical trial of magnesium, diazepam, or both after out-of-hospital cardiac arrest. Neurology. 2002;59: 506–14.
55. Tomte O, Draegni T, Mangschau A, Jacobsen D, Auestad B, Sunde K. A comparison of intravascular and surface cooling techniques in comatose cardiac arrest survivors. Crit Care Med. 2011;39:443–9.
56. Beydoun A, Yen CE, Drury I. Variance of interburst intervals in burst suppression. Electroencephalogr Clin Neurophysiol. 1991;79: 435–9.
57. Chen R, Bolton CF, Young GB. Prediction of outcome in patients with anoxic coma: a clinical and electro-physiologic study. Crit Care Med. 1996;24:672–8.
58. Binnie CD, Prior PF, Lloyd DSL, Scott DF, Margison JH. Electroencephalographic prediction of fatal anoxic brain damage after resuscitation for cardiac arrest. Br Med J. 1970;4:265–8.
59. Møller M, Holm B, Sindrup E, Lyager NB. Electroencephalographic prediction of anoxic brain damage after resuscitation from cardiac arrest in patients with acute myocardial infarction. Acta Med Scand. 1978;203:31–7.
60. Zandbergen EGJ, de Haan RJ, Stoutenbeek CP, Koelman JHTM, Hijdra A. Systematic review of early prediction of poor outcome in anoxic-ischaemic coma. The Lancet. 1998;352:1808–12.
61. Ahmed I. Use of somatosensory evoked responses in the prediction of outcome from coma. Clin Electroencephalogr. 1988;19:78–86.

62. Bassetti C, Bomio F, Mathis J, Hess CW. Early prognosis in coma after cardiac arrest: a prospective clinical, electrophysiological, and biochemical study of 60 patients. J Neurol Neurosurg Psychiatry. 1996;61:610–5.
63. Brunko E, Zegers de Beyl D. Prognostic value of early cortical somatosensory evoked potentials after resuscitation from cardiac arrest. Electroencephalogr Clin Neurophysiol. 1987;66:14–24.
64. Kano T, Shimoda O, Morioka T, Yagishita Y, Hashiguchi A. Evaluation of the central nervous function in resuscitated comatose patients by multilevel evoked potentials. Resuscitation. 1992;23: 235–48.
65. Rothstein TL, Thomas EM, Sumi SM. Predicting outcome in hypoxic-ischemic coma. A prospective clinical and electrophysiologic study. Electoencephalogr Clin Neurophysiol. 1991;79:101–7.
66. Walser H, Mattle H, Keller HM, Janzer R. Early cortical median nerve somatosensory evoked potentials. Prognostic value in anoxic coma. Arch Neurol. 1985;42:32–8.
67. Madl C, Kramer L, Yeganehfar W. Detection of nontraumatic comatose patients with no benefit of intensive care treatment by recording of sensory evoked potentials. Arch Neurol. 1996;53:512–6.
68. Torbey MT, Selim M, Knorr J, Bigelow C, Recht L. Quantitative analysis of the loss of distinction between gray and white matter in comatose patients after cardiac arrest. Stroke. 2000;31:2163–7.
69. Greer DM, Scripko PD, Wu O, Edlow BL, Bartscher J, Sims JR, Camargo EE, Singhal AB, Furie KL. Hippocampal magnetic resonance imaging abnormalities in cardiac arrest are associated with poor outcome. J Stroke Cerebrovasc Dis. 2013;22:899–905.
70. Arbelaez A, Castillo M, Mukherji SK. Diffusion-weighted MR imaging of global cerebral anoxia. Am J Neuroradiol. 1999;20:999–1007.
71. Kim JA, Chung JI, Yoon PH, Kim DI, Chung TS, Kim EJ, Jeong EK. Transient MR signal changes in patients with generalized tonic-clonic seizure or status epilepticus: periictal diffusion-weighted imaging. Am J Neuroradiol. 2001;22:1149–60.
72. Ye JH, Ren J, Krnjevic K, Liu PL, McArdle JJ. Cocaine and lidocaine have additive inhibitory effects on GABA A current of acutely dissociated hippocampal pyramidal cells. Brain Res. 1999;821:26–32.
73. Barat SA, Abdel-Rahman MS. Decreased cocaine- and lidocaine-induced seizure response by dextromethorphan and DNQX in rat. Brain Res. 1997;756:179–83.
74. DeToledo JC. Lidocaine and seizures. Ther Drug Monit. 2000;22:320–2.
75. Kerns W, English B, Ford M. Propafenone overdose. Ann Emerg Med. 1994;81:35–9.
76. Caramelli P, Mutarelli EG, Caramelli B, Tranchesi B, Pileggi F, Schaff M. Neurological complications after thrombolytic treatment for acute myocardial infarction: emphasis on unprecedented manifestations. Acta Neurol Scand. 1992;85:331–3.
77. Cooling DS. Theophylline toxicity. J Emerg Med. 1993;11: 415–25.
78. Hollander JE. The management of cocaine-associated myocardial ischemia. N Eng J Med. 1995;333:1267–72.
79. Koppel BS, Samkoff L, Daras M. Relation of cocaine use to seizures and epilepsy. Epilepsia. 1996;37:875–8.
80. Tam MK, Irwin MG, Tse ML, Lui YW, Law KI, Ng PW. Prolonged myoclonus after a single bolus dose of propofol. Anesthesia. 2009;64:1254–7.
81. Goh WC, Heath PD, Ellis SJ, Oakley PA. Neurological outcome prediction in a cardiorespiratory arrest survivor. Br J Anaesth. 2002;88:719–22.
82. Fugate JE, Wijdicks EFM, Mandrekar J, Claassen DO, Manno EM, White RD, Bell MR, Rabinstein AA. Predictors of neurologic outcome in hypothermia after cardiac arrest. Ann Neurol. 2010;68:907–14.
83. Samaniego EA, Mlynash M, Caulfield AF, Eyngorn I, Wijman CA. Sedation confounds outcome prediction in cardiac arrest survivors treated with hypothermia. Neurocrit Care. 2011;15:113–99.

84. Zandbergen EG, Hijdra A, Koelman JH, Hart AA, Vos PE, Verbeek MM, de Haan RJ, PROPAC Study Group. Prediction of poor outcome within the first 3 days of post anoxic coma. Neurology. 2006;66:62–8.

85. Brophy GM, Bell R, Claassen J, Alldredge B, Bleck TP, Glauser T, LaRoche SM, Riviello JJ, Shutter L, Sperling MR, Treiman DM, Vespa PM, Neurocritical Care Society Status Epilepticus Guideline Writing Committee. Guidelines for the evaluation and management of status epilepticus. Neurocrit Care. 2012;17:2–23.

86. Brain Resuscitation Clinical Trial I Study Group. Randomized clinical study of thiopental loading in comatose survivors of cardiac arrest. N Eng J Med. 1986;314:397–403.

87. Nolan JP, Soar J, Cariou A, Cronberg T, Moulaert VR, Deakin CD, Bottiger BW, Friberg H, Sunde K, Sandroni C. European Resuscitation Council and European Society of Intensive Care Medicine 2015 guidelines for post-resuscitation care. Intensive Care Med. 2015;41:2039–56.

88. Wijdicks EFM, Hijdra A, Young GB, Bassetti CL, Wiebe S. Practice parameter: prediction of outcome in comatose survivors after cardiopulmonary resuscitation (an evidence-based review). Neurology. 2006;67:203–10.

89. Sandroni C, Geocadin RG. Neurological prognostication after cardiac arrest. Curr Opin Crit Care. 2015;21:209–14.

90. The Hypothermia After Cardiac Arrest Study Group. Mild therapeutic hypothermia to improve the neurologic outcome after cardiac arrest. N Eng J Med. 2002;346:549–56.

91. Bernard SA, Gray TW, Buist MD, et al. Treatment of comatose survivors of out-of-hospital cardiac arrest with induced hypothermia. N Eng J Med. 2002;346:557–63.

92. Nolan JP, Morley PT, Vanden Hoek TL, Hickey RW. Therapeutic hypothermia after cardiac arrest: ILCOR advisory statement. Resuscitation. 2003;57:231–7.

93. Rundgren M, Rosén I, Friberg H. Amplitude-integrated EEG (aEEG) predicts outcome after cardiac arrest and induced hypothermia. Intensive Care Med. 2006;32:836–42.

94. Hovland A, Nielsen EW, Kluver J, Salvesen R. EEG should be performed during induced hypothermia. Resuscitation. 2006;68:143–6.

95. Amorim E, Rittenberger JC, Baldwin ME, Callaway CW, Popescu A, Post Cardiac Arrest Service. Malignant EEG patterns in cardiac arrest patients treated with targeted temperature management who survive to hospital discharge. Resuscitation. 2015;90:127–32.

96. Oddo M, Rossetti AO. Early multimodal outcome prediction after cardiac arrest in patients treated with hypothermia. Crit Care Med. 2014;42:1340–7.

97. Friberg H, Westhall E, Rosen I, Rundgren M, Nielsen N, Cronberg T. Clinical review: continuous and simplified electroencephalography to monitor brain recovery after cardiac arrest. Critical Care. 2013;17:233.

98. Geocadin RG, Ritzl EK. Seizures and status epilepticus in post cardiac arrest syndrome: therapeutic opportunities to improve outcome or basis to withhold life sustaining therapies? Resuscitation. 2012;83:791–2.

Fulminant Hepatic Failure, Multiorgan Failure and Endocrine Crisis and Critical Care Seizures

14

Julian Macedo and Brandon Foreman

Abbreviations

ADH	Antidiuretic hormone or vasopressin
AED	Antiepileptic drug
BBB	Blood-brain barrier
BUN	Blood urea nitrogen
cEEG	Continuous electroencephalography
CSF	Cerebrospinal fluid
DDS	Dialysis disequilibrium syndrome
DI	Diabetes insipidus
DKA	Diabetic ketoacidosis
FLF	Fulminant hepatic failure
GABA	γ-aminobutyric acid
GC	Guanidino compounds
ICU	Intensive care unit
INR	International normalized ratio
MRI	Magnetic resonance imaging
NHS	Nonketotic hyperosmolar state
NMDA	N-Methyl-D-aspartic acid
OR	Operating room
PCR	Polymerase chain reaction
PRES	Posterior reversible encephalopathy syndrome
PTH	Parathyroid hormone
RCVS	Reversible cerebral vasoconstriction syndrome
SIADH	Syndrome of inappropriate antidiuretic hormone
WD	Wilson's disease

J. Macedo
University of Cincinnati Medical Center,
Cincinnati, OH 45267-0517, USA
e-mail: macedojn@ucmail.uc.edu

B. Foreman (✉)
University of Cincinnati Medical Center,
Cincinnati, OH 45267-0517, USA

Department of Neurology and Rehabilitation Medicine,
University of Cincinnati, 231 Albert Sabin Way, Cincinnati,
OH 45267-0517, USA
e-mail: brandon.foreman@uc.edu

Introduction

Seizures and encephalopathy may be associated with organ failure and endocrine dysfunction in the critically ill as a result of biochemical abnormalities (e.g., hypoglycemia), vascular alterations, cellular dysfunction, or abnormal protein processing. Commonly, multiple mechanisms act together to create brain dysfunction. In this chapter, we will discuss specific organ failure syndromes' pathophysiologic effects on the brain, their electroclinical correlates, and the available literature regarding seizures and their treatment.

Hepatic Failure

Background

Fulminant liver failure (FLF) occurs in 1:100,000 in the developed world [1]. In the Unites States, drug-induced toxicity remains the leading cause of acute and fulminant liver failure, primarily due to the overuse of acetaminophen [1]. Other common causes of FLF include hepatitis viruses, ischemic hepatitis, and other idiosyncratic drug reactions; approximately 20% of those with FLF have no known cause. The mortality associated with FLF is 57% without transplantation and 33 % overall; infection and cerebral edema are the leading causes of death [2].

While FLF affects virtually every organ system, the definition of FLF requires the development of *brain dysfunction* as a presenting symptom along with severe acute liver injury without preexisting cirrhosis or other liver diseases. Hepatic encephalopathy is graded clinically (Table 14.1), and seizures have been reported in all stages of liver failure. Seizures may be seen in up to one-third of patients with acute liver failure and are more common in those who present with a greater degree of hepatic encephalopathy (Grades III/IV) [4, 5].

© Springer International Publishing AG 2017
P.N. Varelas, J. Claassen (eds.), *Seizures in Critical Care*, Current Clinical Neurology, DOI 10.1007/978-3-319-49557-6_14

Table 14.1 West Haven Criteria for grading hepatic encephalopathy

Grade	Symptoms
0	No abnormality present
I	Short-term memory loss, reversal of sleep/wake cycle
II	Asterixis, apathy, inappropriate behavior, confusion, lethargy
III	Stupor, marked confusion, incoherent speech
IV	Comatose

Adapted from [3]

Pathophysiology

Several pathophysiologic mechanisms appear to underlie the effects of FLF on the brain and may contribute to the development of seizures. The hallmark pathological feature of hepatic encephalopathy is astrocytic swelling. Astrocytes are rich in the enzyme *glutamine synthetase*, which catalyzes the conversion of ammonia to glutamine. When hepatic failure occurs, excessive ammonia is available for metabolism by *glutamine synthetase*. Intracellular glutamine accumulates, causing astrocytic swelling, breakdown of the blood-brain barrier (BBB), and cytotoxic edema [6].

Excessive glutamate, a major excitatory neurotransmitter, has been implicated in the development of seizures [7]. FLF models have demonstrated decreased GLT-1, a glutamate transport protein present on astrocytes [8] leading to reduced glutamate reuptake. Glycine, which activates excitatory *n-methyl-* d *-aspartate (NMDA)* receptors, has also been implicated. A similar animal model of FLF demonstrated decreased expression of Glyt-1, a glycine transport channel. Cerebral microdialysis in these animals revealed approximately three times the extracellular glycine concentration compared to controls [9].

Increased GABA-ergic tone may also play a role in both encephalopathy and, by inhibiting interneuron populations, the development of seizures. Flumazenil, a GABA antagonist, transiently improves neurological function in patients with hepatic encephalopathy, but randomized controlled trials have not demonstrated durable improvements in recovery or survival [10]. In astrocytic tissue samples, reuptake of GABA is inhibited by ammonia at concentrations associated with the development of hepatic encephalopathy [11]. Rabbit models of FLF have shown that the activity of the GABA-metabolizing enzyme *GABA-transaminase* is decreased, further supporting a role for excessive GABA activity [12].

Diagnosis

Seizures in the critically ill, particularly those in the medical or surgical intensive care unit, are typically nonconvulsive [13–15] and require continuous EEG (cEEG) monitoring in order to achieve sufficient sensitivity [15, 16]. In the early stages of hepatic encephalopathy, movement disorders such as asterixis/myoclonus may be difficult to distinguish from ictal movements such as clonus. cEEG, which includes video recording, is crucial to elucidate shaking or jerking spells observed in the ICU environment. Further complicating the clinical observation of seizures in patients with hepatic failure, patients with more severe hepatic encephalopathy (Grades III/IV) often require mechanical ventilation, analgosedation, and/or paralysis. These mask clinical seizure activity, and therefore the threshold for considering cEEG monitoring in patients with organ failure, including those with FLF, must remain low [17].

The background EEG of patients with liver failure is traditionally characterized by three stages correlating to the depth of coma [18]. Grade I/II encephalopathy is associated with θ frequency background slowing. As encephalopathy progresses, δ frequency slowing becomes more pronounced. Generalized, symmetric, and periodic waves described as "triphasic" in morphology appear—classically with a positive-polarity dominant second or third phase, a frontal predominance, and an anterior-posterior lag (Fig. 14.1). These were originally described in close association with liver failure [5], but subsequently these generalized periodic discharges with triphasic morphology have been reported across a variety of conditions including other organ failure syndromes and as the ictal pattern in some patients with seizures [19, 20]. The presence of generalized periodic discharges of any kind, including those with triphasic morphology, is highly associated with nonconvulsive seizures [21, 22], and others have observed that indeed seizures are more common in liver failure with brain dysfunction during this second stage. A third stage, consisting of a diffuse, asynchronous polymorphic δ pattern, is observed in the most severe stage of hepatic coma.

The largest series to date retrospectively studied 118 of 526 patients admitted with a diagnosis of hepatic encephalopathy undergoing EEG. EEGs were typically "routine" and not continuous 24 h EEG. 18 patients (15%) were noted to have epileptiform abnormalities on EEG, and electrographic status epilepticus (SE) was observed in five patients (4%). Epileptiform activity was related to clinical deterioration or death, suggesting an association with poor prognosis [23]. More recently, medical and surgical ICU cohorts undergoing cEEG have not shown a relationship between acute hepatic failure and the presence of periodic discharges or seizures [13, 14].

After transplant, epileptiform abnormalities may increase in incidence during the first 7 days, with an incidence of seizures up to 42 % [24]. Mechanisms by which seizures occur posttransplant may be related to immunosuppressant medications or withdrawal from GABA-ergic metabolites, both pharmacologic and endogenous, that occur with a newly functioning liver [25].

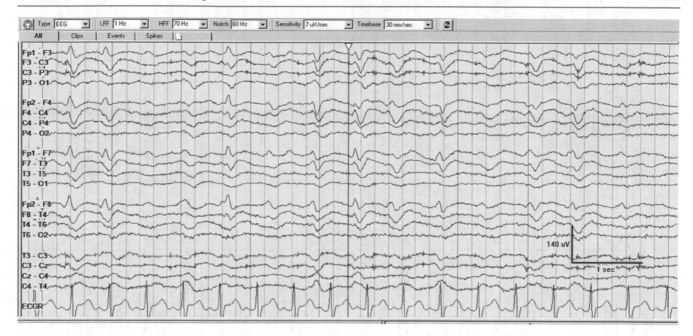

Fig. 14.1 Grade III encephalopathy including generalized periodic discharges with triphasic morphology. 41-year-old man with nonalcoholic steatohepatitis with cirrhosis and variceal bleeding. cEEG performed 4 days after transjugular intrahepatic portosystemic shunt procedure with increasing ammonia to 330 μg/dL and Grade III hepatic encephalopathy. The EEG background demonstrated predominantly delta frequency slowing with frequent, very brief runs of triphasic-appearing waveforms occurring at approximately regular intervals. These gradually resolved as mental status improved

Management

As with any seizures in the critically ill, initial steps in management include an assessment for readily reversible causes. Particularly in organ failure and endocrine crises, biochemical derangements such as hypoglycemia or hyponatremia are seen frequently and may act as a precipitant for seizures to develop. If these have been addressed, the choice of antiepileptic drug (AED) itself may be complicated: with the exception of levetiracetam, vigabatrin, pregabalin, topiramate, and gabapentin, almost all AEDs undergo some degree of hepatic conversion (Table 14.2). Further, patients with liver dysfunction exhibit several relevant physiologic changes that may also impact the decision about which AED to choose (Table 14.3).

Acute seizures and particularly SE should be treated as medical emergencies [26]. Benzodiazepines form the first line of therapy based on two randomized controlled trials for SE in the prehospital setting [27, 28]. Although benzodiazepines are extensively metabolized by the liver (Table 14.2), they are not considered hepatotoxic as a class and therefore are considered safe to use as first line in those with acute liver failure. Benzodiazepines with shorter $t_{1/2}$ such as lorazepam might avoid prolonged sedation and therefore may be preferred as an initial benzodiazepine. Further, lorazepam is metabolized by glucuronidation (along with older benzodiazepines oxazepam and temazepam), and therefore although liver failure may affect its overall clearance, there are no active metabolites formed that may prolong effects of the medication, as is the case with diazepam.

Several AEDs are known to have to direct hepatotoxic effects on the liver, particularly phenytoin and phenobarbital, which may rarely cause toxic or hypersensitivity hepatitides. Valproic acid is a short-chain branched carboxylic acid with multiple active metabolites, including 4-ene-valproic acid, which may exhibit hepatotoxicity. Through metabolites formed via the carnitine shuttle, hypocarnitinemia and hyperammonemia may develop even in those with normal liver function [29]. Valproic acid should be avoided in patients with hepatic failure where possible, and supplementation with L-carnitine should be considered if hyperammonemia or other signs of hepatic failure occur in the setting of valproic acid use [30].

Despite the association between liver failure with brain dysfunction and the development of seizures or epileptiform abnormalities on EEG, routine prophylaxis with AEDs is not currently recommended. Two studies have investigated the role of phenytoin for prophylactic use in hepatic failure [4, 31]. One study of 42 patients with Grade III/IV encephalopathy used the cerebral function monitor, a limited montage EEG-based signal processing method used in the OR or ICU setting. Electrographic seizures were documented in 15% of those randomized to phenytoin prophylaxis compared to 32% without phenytoin. Of the 25 that died, 19 were autopsied; significantly fewer in the prophylaxis group had cerebral edema [4]. However, in another study of 42 patients, no difference in clinical seizures, clinical manifestations of cerebral edema, or survival was observed when phenytoin was used prophylactically [31]. When cerebral edema and

Table 14.2 Pharmacology of Antiepileptic Drugs

Name	Routes of administration	Hepatic metabolism[a]	Renal elimination[b]	Protein binding (%)	Dialyzable	Adverse effects	Serum concentration available	Special considerations
Phenytoin	IV, oral	++++	+	80–95	N	Arrhythmia, agranulocytosis, ataxia, hepatitis	Y	Nonlinear kinetics, weight-based dosing
Carbamazepine	Oral	++++	+	75–90	Y	Dizziness, drowsiness, nausea, hyponatremia, anemia, agranulocytosis, skin reactions	Y	Autoinduction metabolism, major CYP3A4 substrate
Oxcarbazepine	Oral	++++	++	40	No data	Hyponatremia, dizziness, drowsiness, nausea	Y	At steady-state concentrations the extended release product is not bioequivalent to the same daily dose of immediate release product
Eslicarbazepine	Oral	++	+++	<40	Y (metabolites)	Hyponatremia, diplopia, blurred vision, hypertension, skin reactions	Y	
Zonisamide	Oral	+++	++	40	Y	Metabolic acidosis, increased BUN, nephrolithiasis, agranulocytosis, aplastic anemia	Y	Use not recommended with GFR < 50 mL/minute; monitor patients for suicidality
Lamotrigine	Oral	++++	+	55	Y	Skin reactions, visual disturbance	Y	
Lacosamide	IV, oral	+++	++	<15	Y	EKG changes, diplopia, blurred vision	Y	
Ethosuximide	Oral	++++	+	0–5	Y	Blood dyscrasias, skin reactions, systemic lupus erythematosus	Y	
Benzodiazepines								
Diazepam	IV, oral	++++	+	98	N	Hypotension, amnesia, drowsiness, urinary incontinence, apnea	N	Active metabolite
Midazolam	IV, oral	++++	+	97	N	Hypotension, drowsiness	N	
Lorazepam	IV, oral	++++	+	85–93	N	Hypotension, sedation, dizziness	N	IV: Risk of propylene glycol toxicity
Clonazepam	Oral	++++	+	85	N	Ataxia, drowsiness, edema	N	
Clobazam	Oral	++++	+	80–90	N	Drowsiness, lethargy, sialorrhea, URTI, fever	N	
Pentobarbital	IV	++++	+	45–70	N	Bradycardia, hypotension, hepatotoxicity	Y	
Phenobarbital	IV, oral	++++	++	20–40	Y	Drowsiness, sedation, ataxia, cognitive and behavioral changes	Y	
Primidone	Oral	++++	+++	30	Y	Drowsiness, sedation, ataxia	Y	
Tiagabine	Oral	++++	+	96	N	Dizziness, asthenia, lack of energy, somnolence	Y	
Vigabatrin	Oral	+	++++	0	Y	Vision loss, anemia, somnolence, neuropathy, edema	N	
Gabapentin	Oral	+	++++	<3	Y	Dizziness, drowsiness, ataxia	Y	
Pregabalin	Oral	+	++++	0	Y	Peripheral edema, dizziness, somnolence, weight gain	Y	
Valproate	IV, oral	++++	+	80–90	N	Headache, drowsiness, dizziness, N/V, thrombocytopenia, alopecia, tremor	Y	Nonlinear kinetics, weight-based dosing
Felbamate	Oral	+++	++	22–25	No data	Somnolence, dizziness, anorexia, N/V	Y	
Topiramate	Oral	+	+++	15–41	Y	Paresthesias, drowsiness, dizziness, weight loss	Y	
Levetiracetam	IV, oral	+	+++	<10	Y	Headache, behavioral problems, drowsiness, irritability	Y	
Ketamine	IV	+++	+	60	N	Hypertension, tachycardia, emergence reaction (hallucinations, excitement, etc.)	N	Weight-based dosing
Propofol	IV	++	+	97–99	N	Hypotension, hyperlipidemia, propofol-related infusion syndrome	N	
Perampanel	Oral	++++	+	95–96	No data	Dizziness, drowsiness, headache, hostility, falls	Y	
Rufinamide	Oral	++++	+	34	N	Shortened QT interval, headache, drowsiness, dizziness	Y	Weight-based dosing; absorption increases with food
Ezogabine	Oral	++++	++	80	No data	Urinary retention, retinal abnormalities, QT prolongation	Y	May falsely elevate serum/urine bilirubin

Table Courtesy Shaun P. Keegan, PharmD, BCPS

[a]+ 0–25%; ++ 26–50%; +++ 51–75%; ++++ 76%–100%

[b]Based on clearance of parent drug or active metabolites

Table 14.3 Metabolic changes associated with fulminant liver failure

Physiologic Alteration	Effect
Increased blood flow to liver (early)	Increased drug metabolism
Hepatocyte death and P450 dysfunction	Increased circulating levels of hepatically metabolized antiepileptic drugs
Decreased synthetic function	Hypoalbuminemia and increased free levels of protein-bound antiepileptic drugs
Enhanced sensitivity to hepatotoxic side effects	Decreased tolerance of certain hepatically metabolized antiepileptic drugs

intracranial hypertension are present, prophylactic AEDs in general may serve to optimize patients who might otherwise not be operative candidates for liver transplantation. Given the potential for toxicity, larger studies are warranted before phenytoin is used as a primary agent; the authors prefer levetiracetam in those with hepatic failure. The authors recommend AEDs only for those patients with confirmed clinical or electrographic seizure activity, for those with EEG patterns highly associated with seizures (e.g., periodic discharges), or as prophylaxis in those in coma with global cerebral edema or other signs of elevated intracranial pressure.

Hepatic Conditions Associated with Seizures

Wilson's Disease

Wilson's disease (WD) is an autosomal recessive disorder of copper metabolism that results from abnormalities in the *ATP7B* gene. WD results in the deposition of copper in the brain, liver, and cornea (referred to as Kayser-Fleischer rings). Patients may manifest myriad symptoms ranging from primarily neuropsychiatric to purely hepatic [32]. Patients with WD develop chronic seizures at a rate of 6–8%, substantially more than the incidence of epilepsy in the general population. Nearly three-quarters will develop seizures upon initiation of chelation treatment or shortly thereafter [33, 34].

The pathophysiology of seizures in WD may be related to (a) a relative pyridoxine deficiency specifically during chelation with penicillamine, (b) direct toxicity from liberated copper, or (c) deafferentation of subcortical white matter tracts from the overlaying cortex caused by large copper deposits. Early literature suggested that rats treated with penicillamine chelation became pyridoxine deficient and were more likely to develop seizures [35]. Others have countered that neurotoxicity associated with the mobilization of copper during chelation contributes to the seizures seen during and just after treatment [33]. Cavitary lesions in subcortical white matter, caudate, or putamen may be seen on MRI or autopsy and may predict the development of refractory seizures [36–38]. Once therapy is complete, the majority, 84.5% of patients in one series, experience substantial improvement in seizure frequency [33]. The authors suggest pyridoxine supplementation in conjunction with AEDs in the treatment of seizures that occur in patients undergoing chelation therapy.

Reye's Syndrome

Reye's syndrome is a rare, rapidly progressive encephalopathy marked by liver dysfunction. Viruses, including influenza, coxsackie, measles, and varicella, are epidemiologically linked with Reye's syndrome [39], which develops with co-exposure to salicylates. Though mostly a pediatric illness, adult cases have been reported [39, 40]. Clinically, Reye's syndrome begins with confusion and somnolence and progresses to seizures and coma. Fatty infiltration of the abdominal viscera, hepatomegaly, and cerebral edema are observed, but icteric changes are mild or absent. Cases are extraordinarily rare, and while the pathogenesis is not well understood, electron microscopy studies of rat liver hepatocytes have demonstrated uncoupling of oxidative phosphorylation, swelling, and cell permeability when exposed to salicylates [41]. Outcomes of patients with Reye's syndrome have been associated with the degree of background slowing on electroencephalography (EEG), with those demonstrating diffuse slowing ultimately succumbing to their illness [42, 43]. Seizures have been considered a poor prognostic marker and are observed in approximately half of patients [43], although a good outcome has been reported in a patient with Reye's syndrome and SE [44].

Hepatic Porphyrias

The hepatic porphyrias (including acute intermittent porphyria, *ALA dehydratase* deficiency porphyria, variegate porphyria, and hereditary coproporphyria) are caused by various enzymatic deficiencies in the heme synthesis pathway, with resulting accumulation of porphyrin precursors. Reported incidence of seizures may be as high as 5 % in those who present with symptoms of an acute porphyric attack [45]. Proposed mechanisms leading to encephalopathy and seizures involve δ-aminolevulinic acid crossing the BBB and (1) affecting GABA, and possibly glutamate, receptors, (2) inducing oxidative stress/oxygen radical damage, and (3) inhibiting the neuronal Na$^+$/K$^+$ ATPase [46]. Treatment of seizures related to porphyria starts with hematin infusions which terminate further porphyrogenesis by inhibiting *ALA synthetase*, thus correcting the underlying pathology.

Several commonly used AEDs may induce, or worsen, porphyric attacks in patients with hepatic porphyrias, primarily by inducing cytochrome p450 isoenzyme metabolism and accelerating the generation of heme pathway byproducts.

AEDs that exacerbate porphyrias:

- Phenobarbital
- Phenytoin
- Valproic acid
- Carbamazepine
- Lamotrigine
- Topiramate
- Tiagabine
- Ethosuximide
- Diazepam

These AEDs should be avoided or stopped immediately. Non-hepatically cleared AEDs such as, gabapentin [47] and levetiracetam [45] are preferred. Clonazepam has been used successfully [48] after failure of phenytoin and valproic acid, but refractory SE has been reported [49], in which case propofol may be used as a preferred continuous intravenous anesthetic agent instead of pentobarbital and perhaps even midazolam, which has been shown to induce prophyrogenesis even at relatively low concentrations [50, 51]. Interestingly, the GABA-ergic and antioxidant effects of melatonin may benefit patients with porphyrias: a small series found that patients with seizures had decreased urinary excretion of melatonin compared to those without seizures [52].

Renal Failure

Background

Renal failure, specifically acute kidney injury, is a common clinical problem encountered in the ICU. Renal failure is associated with increased length of hospital stay, resource utilization, and mortality [53]. Acute kidney injury occurs in up to 25% of those hospitalized in an ICU [54], though this estimation may be higher depending on the definition used; approximately 6% will require renal replacement therapy [55].

Current definitions of acute kidney injury exist from several groups (Table 14.4). All use serum creatinine and urine output as principle markers of renal compromise. As renal clearance decreases, azotemia develops, and while the absolute level of azotemia does not appear to correspond with changes in neurological functioning, the rapidity and degree of renal dysfunction correspond both to encephalopathy and increasing seizure risk. Encephalopathy may initially manifest as fatigue, forgetfulness, or decreased attention, but progresses to include bifrontal dysfunction and finally frank delirium with tremulousness or asterixis/myoclonus, hallucinations, and obtundation. Between 2 and 10% of those with

Table 14.4 Definitions of acute kidney injury (AKI)

Group	Definition	Reference
Kidney Disease: Improving Global Outcome (KDIGO)	1. Increase in serum Cr of 0.3 mg/dL developing over <48 h or >50% over 7 days OR 2. Urine output of <0.5 mL/kg/h for >6 h	[56]
Acute Kidney Injury Network (AKIN)	1. Increase in serum Cr of 0.3 mg/dL or >50% developing over <48 h OR 2. Urine output of <0.5 mL/kg/h for >6 h	[57]
Risk, Injury, and Failure (RIFLE)	1. Increase in serum Cr of >50% developing over <7 days OR 2. Urine output of <0.5 mL/kg/h for >6 h	[58]

renal failure requiring dialysis and up to one-third of patients with acute uremic encephalopathy are reported to have seizures or SE, most in later stages of encephalopathy [59, 60].

Pathophysiology

Blood urea nitrogen (BUN) is commonly used to evaluate renal function, and its removal from serum is directly associated with improved patient mortality [61]. By itself, urea does not appear to be toxic despite its nominal association with uremic encephalopathy. However, its presence acts as a surrogate marker of failed renal clearance, with unmeasured metabolites more likely contributing to the neurologic findings seen in uremic encephalopathy.

Both excitatory and inhibitory neurotransmitters become disrupted when organic substances are not adequately filtered. In particular, guanidino compounds (GC) such as *guanidinosuccinic acid* have been reported to be increased in the brain and cerebrospinal fluid (CSF) [61–63]. By complex interactions with GABA, glycine, and NMDA receptors, GCs may contribute both to encephalopathy and the development of seizures. *Methylguanidine* has been shown to inhibit neuronal Na^+/K^+ ATPase as well and therefore may have a direct effect on neurotransmission or seizure propagation. Azotemia has been linked with dysfunction of the neuronal Na^+/K^+ ATPase, as well as the Na^+/Ca^{++} exchange mechanism and the ATP-dependent calcium transport system [64, 65]. Experimental introduction of GCs directly into CSF has been shown to induce tonic-clonic activity in animal models in a dose-related fashion [66].

Evidence suggests total brain calcium is increased in renal failure [63]. This is likely the result of parathyroid hormone (PTH)-sensitive neuronal calcium transporters. Increased serum phosphate levels act to lower serum calcium in renal failure, stimulating PTH secretion (secondary hyperparathyroidism). Calcium excess is linked to neuronal hyperexcitability, and the relationship between calcium/hyperparathyroidism and neuronal dysfunction has been supported using canine models [67]. After induction of uremia, increases in EEG power and bursting (paroxysms of high-amplitude delta activity/total duration of the record) have been reported. In those with EEG changes, total brain calcium was noted to be significantly elevated. Interestingly, animals in whom parathyroidectomy was performed prior to induction of uremia lacked electroencephalographic abnormalities, suggesting a distinct role of parathyroid hormone in the pathogenesis of encephalopathy associated with renal failure.

In addition to the clearance of organic compounds and the regulation of calcium, the kidney is central to the homeostasis of vascular tension and volume management through maintenance of fluid and solute balance, in part through its endocrine function via the renin-angiotensin axis.

Alternations in kidney function, and particularly in filtration rates, may manifest as malignant hypertension. Often severe, renal failure-related hypertension may be associated with cerebral vascular dysfunction, loss of cerebral autoregulation, and the reversible posterior leukoencephalopathy syndrome (PRES). In a series of 15 patients with PRES, nine had had a documented creatinine values >1.2 (range: 1.2–16.1), of whom seven developed clinical seizures [68].

Several medications may contribute to seizure development in patients with renal failure, many with common use in ICU care.

Selected common ICU drugs associated with seizures in renal failure:

- Acyclovir and valacyclovir
- Antihistamines (diphenhydramine, cimetidine)
- Baclofen
- Bupropion
- Carbapenems (imepenem, ertapenem, and meropenem)
- Cephalosporins (cefazolin, cefepime, ceftazidime, and ceftriaxone)
- Clozapine
- Cyclosporine
- Isoniazid
- Lithium
- Meperidine
- Metronidazole
- Penicillins
- Polymyxin B
- Quinolones
- Tramadol
- Tranexamic acid
- Tricyclics

Figure 14.2 demonstrates a case of a patient in renal failure, clozapine toxicity, and NCSE.

The cephalosporins (particularly cefepime), carbapenems, and penicillins have all been implicated in seizure development, possibly by competitively antagonizing GABA receptor sites [69–71]. Adequately adjusting doses of renally cleared antibiotics based on glomerular filtration rate should mitigate the risk for such complications; however, the expertise of a clinical pharmacist is required to ensure adequate antibiotic concentrations. Acyclovir and its prodrug valacyclovir may also induce seizures [72] during treatment for encephalitis. Neurotoxicity may be distinguished from symptoms of encephalitis by the absence of fever, headache, focal neurological signs, and a lack of EEG patterns suggestive of temporal encephalitis, namely, lateralized periodic discharges [73]. Patients taking baclofen who develop renal failure may develop encephalopathy and coma—even in low doses [74]. While seizures are uncommon, the encephalopathy is severe, and EEG may demonstrate generalized periodic discharges that are challenging to distinguish from ictal activity. If neurotoxicity is suspected, discontinuation of the medication and potentially hemodialysis may help reduce ongoing neurotoxicity, although responses may not be immediate due to central nervous system accumulation.

Diagnosis

The background EEG in uremic encephalopathy begins with generalized slowing, often θ or δ slowing, sometimes with bilateral, frontally predominant sharp-wave complexes. As the encephalopathy progresses, slowing becomes more prominent, and generalized periodic discharges with triphasic morphology may be observed with an incidence similar to that of hepatic encephalopathy [75]. In chronic renal failure, absolute and relative EEG changes occur with fluctuations in serum values of BUN, potassium, and calcium—with the greatest degree of electroencephalographic correlation occurring with BUN values [76]. Most (70 %) exhibit at least one abnormal EEG. EEG in those with acute renal failure is almost uniformly abnormal suggesting that compensatory mechanisms may exist for those with chronic renal failure [77]. We know of no series that has documented the prevalence of seizures in adults specifically with acute renal failure, although a study of 107 children admitted with renal failure reported 15 % having clinical seizures [78]. In retrospective series of adult patients in the medical or surgical ICU, the presence of acute or chronic renal failure alone does not confer an independent risk for periodic discharges or seizures, although the degree of encephalopathy was not stratified [13, 14].

Because patients with acute or chronic renal failure may be at risk to develop intracranial hemorrhages (subdural hematomas, intracerebral hemorrhage), new onset seizures and focality in the neurological examination should always mandate neuroimaging of the brain and/or spine.

Management

As with liver failure, renal failure induces a variety of metabolic derangements that may cause seizures either directly (e.g., hyponatremia) or indirectly (e.g., hypercalcemia leading to PRES). Once these have been addressed, the choice or dosing of AEDs may be limited by physiologic changes that occur during renal failure (Table 14.2 and Table 14.5). The primary treatment of renal failure with brain dysfunction is either correction of the underlying cause for the renal failure or hemodialysis.

In those requiring dialysis, dosage adjustments are important to maintain therapeutic AED levels and avoid toxicity. For most AEDs that are partially renally cleared, dosage

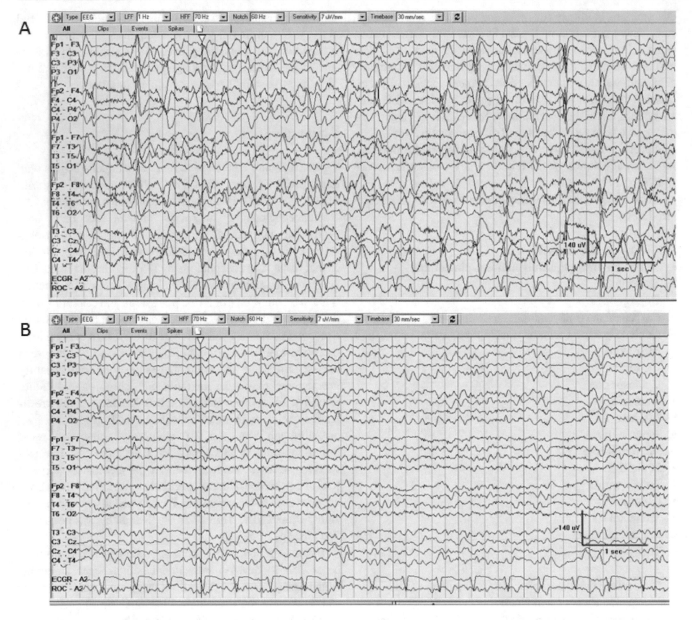

Fig. 14.2 Status epilepticus due to clozapine toxicity in renal failure. 58-year-old woman with schizoaffective disorder on home clozapine presented unresponsive with acute on chronic renal failure (Cr 1.9, BUN 32) in the setting of sepsis with hypoglycemia. Despite correction of hypoglycemia and appropriate antibiotics, she remained comatose. Clozapine levels were supratherapeutic at 1987 ng/mL. (**a**) Initial cEEG demonstrated nonconvulsive status epilepticus comprised of continuous high-amplitude 2–3 Hz generalized sharp-wave complexes. (**b**) Lorazepam was administered with improvement in both the background EEG and clinical exam. Levetiracetam was started, and clozapine was stopped with gradual improvement of mental status over several days

Table 14.5 Metabolic changes associated with renal failure

Physiologic alteration	Effect
Decreased glomerular filtration rate	Variable clearance of renally cleared antiepileptic drugs
Larger volume of distribution (V_d) due to edema	Difficulty achieving appropriate dose
Decreased serum protein due to protein loss nephropathy	Increased free levels of protein-bound antiepileptic drugs
Requirement for dialysis	Rapid clearance of renally cleared antiepileptic drugs

adjustments are relatively straightforward and require a fixed reduction in dose alone. AEDs that are protein bound may experience fluctuations in serum concentration after dialysis. For instance, although phenytoin is up to 95 % protein bound, intensive dialysis may remove nearly half of the total body stores [79]. For AEDs that are completely renally cleared (gabapentin, pregabalin, topiramate, and levetiracetam), a dose is required immediately after intermittent hemodialysis to restore adequate drug concentrations. Levetiracetam is amenable to loading in this fashion, and an intravenous formulation makes this feasible. Vigabatrin is not recommended in those with renal failure due to the potential for irreversible vision loss. By contrast, continuous renal replacement therapy typically requires a similar dosage adjustment as recommended for a glomerular filtration rate of <30; no loading doses are required due to the continuous nature of this form of dialysis.

Dialysis Disequilibrium Syndrome (DDS)

Dialysis disequilibrium syndrome (DDS) is a condition thought to occur as the result of osmotic shifts and changes in pH that occur with dialysis [80, 81]. Reports of symptoms range from mild (headaches, cramps, and nausea) to more severe symptoms (delirium, myoclonus, seizures, and cardiac arrhythmias). With the "reverse urea effect," it is hypothesized that urea is removed more slowly from intracellular compartment than from blood during dialysis. With the delay in brain urea clearance, an osmotic gradient between plasma and the brain leads to cerebral edema. CT evidence supports the observation of cerebral free water movement into cortex during dialysis [82]. Further, a paradoxical drop in the pH of CSF and cortex has been reported during hemodialysis [83].

Historically, DDS was attributed to exceedingly rapid, frequent dialysis sessions outstripping the cerebral tissue's normal osmoregulatory and pH balance mechanisms. Modern intensive care units focus on slower rate utilization and more frequent sessions when intermittent hemodialysis is employed. Occasionally, osmotically acting solutes may be considered as additives to the dialysate (urea, glycerol) when slower rates and more frequent sessions fail to obviate symptoms. Yet, cerebral edema, herniation, and death may still occur with modern techniques [81]. After acute brain injury, guidelines recommend continuous methods of renal replacement therapy [84] to allow slower osmolar changes and to mitigate swings in intracranial volume or pH. A recent series of four patients who developed progressive herniation after undergoing hemodialysis highlights the risk of DDS even today, even with continuous renal replacement therapy [81].

Sepsis

Background and Pathophysiology

Severe sepsis and septic shock occur in three-quarters of a million individuals in the United States each year. Approximately 10 % of primary ICU admissions are thought to be related to the treatment of severe sepsis [85]. More than 70 % of those with sepsis develop delirium, encephalopathy, or other symptoms of cerebral dysfunction [86–88]. Sepsis with brain failure sufficient to cause coma increases the risk

of mortality by a factor of three [86]. Once brain dysfunction occurs, there are long-standing cognitive and functional consequences beyond the acute illness [89].

The term severe sepsis and systemic inflammatory response syndrome (SIRS) have been abandoned in the new consensus definitions, which include definitions of sepsis and septic shock only. According to those [90]:

- Sepsis is defined as life-threatening organ dysfunction caused by a dysregulated host response to infection. Organ dysfunction can be identified as an acute change in total Sequential Organ Failure Assessment (SOFA) score ≥2 points consequent to the infection.
- Septic shock is a subset of sepsis in which underlying circulatory and cellular/metabolic abnormalities are profound enough to substantially increase mortality. Patients with septic shock can be identified with a clinical construct of sepsis with persisting hypotension requiring vasopressors to maintain MAP ≥ 65 mm Hg and having a serum lactate level >2 mmol/L (18 mg/dL) despite adequate volume resuscitation.

A variety of mechanisms have been proposed to explain the neurological effects of sepsis, including neurotoxic or inflammatory mediators, cerebral autoregulatory dysfunction, cytokine release, and increased excitatory neurotransmitters [91]. Leukoencephalopathy and ischemic infarcts are the most commonly observed radiographic abnormalities in sepsis, suggesting breakdown of the BBB and local tissue ischemia resulting from inflammatory mediators [92]. By creating end-organ damage, including renal or hepatic injury, sepsis also employs the secondary mechanisms of brain failure as discussed above.

Diagnosis and Management

The background EEG in sepsis is similar to that seen during renal failure or hepatic failure. First, mild diffuse slowing develops, followed by increasing δ frequency slowing with or without generalized periodic discharges with triphasic morphology. In a study of 125 patients in a medical ICU, 39 % developed burst suppression, a pattern of background suppression punctuated by bursts of higher-frequency activity that reflects cortical hyperexcitability and is associated with deep sedation, severe brain injury, or both. The presence of burst suppression patterns on EEG has been shown to be an independent predictor of death at 6 months [93].

In a retrospective series including 58 patients with sepsis in a surgical ICU, 16 % experienced nonconvulsive seizures; coma and prior clinical seizures were predictors of seizures on EEG [14]. In the medical ICU, a series including 60 % of patients admitted with sepsis, 22 % had periodic discharges or seizures. Only sepsis predicted the presence or absence of these epileptiform abnormalities on multivariate analysis [13]. In the only prospective study of cEEG in sepsis, 98 patients with 100 episodes of sepsis were studied. Twenty-five episodes were associated with periodic discharges, of which 11 (44 %) had nonconvulsive seizures. No patient had nonconvulsive seizures without periodic discharges. Lack of EEG reactivity was associated with significantly higher 1-year mortality (mean survival 3.3, 95 % CI 1.8–4.9 versus 7.5, 6.4–8.7 months in those with EEG reactivity). Interestingly, the presence of periodic discharges or nonconvulsive seizures was not a predictor of mortality (mean survival 6.2, 5.2–7.6 versus 6.4, 4.1–8.2 months for those without them) [88]. Although periodic discharges and seizures have been independently associated with poor outcome in some other series [13, 14], mortality associated with sepsis is largely related to its underlying severity. Larger studies are required to determine the impact of periodic discharges or seizures on cognitive functioning or functional outcome.

Because coma is a primary predictor of nonconvulsive seizures [16, 88], encephalopathy and particularly coma in patients with sepsis should prompt consideration for cEEG. In a series of patients admitted to the medical ICU with coma of unclear cause, 8 % were found to be in nonconvulsive SE [94]. In addition to EEG, a lumbar puncture in selected cases may be required to exclude meningitis as the etiology of coma or seizures in septic and especially bacteremic patients. Neuroimaging before the LP should be always considered in ICU patients with encephalopathy and poor cooperation during the neurological evaluation.

There are no guidelines regarding the treatment of seizures, but consideration of other end-organ dysfunction as discussed above is warranted. In general, we recommend against the use of pentobarbital and phenobarbital in patients with sepsis, as barbiturates inhibit neutrophil chemotaxis, impairing the immune system's ability to fight serious infection [95, 96]. We also recommend against routine seizure prophylaxis in sepsis.

Thyrotoxicosis and Thyroid Disorders

Background

Thyrotoxicosis is a disorder that results from excess circulating free thyroxine (FT4) and free triiodothyronine (FT3). Graves' disease is the single most common etiology of thyrotoxicosis, but other etiologies exist including pituitary adenoma, thyroid replacement overdose, postoperative thyroiditis, and amiodarone thyroiditis [97]. Between 0.2% and 9% in patients with thyrotoxicosis will develop seizures [98]. Seizures may be focal or generalized and SE has been reported [99]. A related antibody-mediated disorder,

Hashimoto's encephalopathy or steroid-responsive encephalopathy associated with autoimmune thyroiditis (SREAT), is associated with encephalopathy and seizures in the presence of elevated titers of anti-thyroglobulin or anti-thyroperoxidase antibodies [100].

Hypothyroidism, and particularly myxedema coma, is not typically associated with seizures, although seizures have been reported as a presenting symptom [101]. The encephalopathy associated with hypothyroidism, including coma, may rarely be in part due to nonconvulsive seizures. Thyroid replacement is the treatment of choice for hypothyroidism-related seizures when they occur.

In the setting of thyrotoxicosis, hypermetabolic changes occur throughout the body, yet oxygen metabolism in the brain remains unchanged [102], making cortical hypermetabolism less likely as a cause for seizures. Instead, activation of nuclear thyroid hormone receptors may modulate gene expression, and extra- and intracellular electrolyte concentrations are altered when exposed to thyroid hormones, suggesting that excess thyroid hormone may modulate neuronal excitability [103]. Thyroid hormones may also directly modulate GABA-ergic tone, leading to relative hyperexcitability [104, 105]. Finally, reductions in thyrotropin-releasing hormone remove a potential endogenous antiepileptic mechanism: direct injection of thyrotropin-releasing hormone into the hippocampus of a rat kindling model reduced seizure duration and afterdischarges [106].

Diagnosis and Management

The background EEG during thyrotoxicosis is frequently abnormal. In a series of 44 patients admitted with a diagnosis of thyrotoxicosis, only 32 % had normal EEG background [107]. The most common findings were generalized slow activity, but focal slowing and excess fast activity were also noted. Treatment led to restoration of normal background in two-thirds. Others have found similar nonspecific slowing, but a distinctive electroencephalographic pattern unique to thyrotoxicosis complicated by seizures is described as excess slow activity in the temporal regions, in addition to fast, high-amplitude sharp-wave activity in the frontal regions [98, 99, 108].

Treatment of seizures related to thyrotoxicosis requires concomitant treatment of the underlying and potentially fatal endocrine disorder. Prevention of thyroid hormone conversion to its active form using methimazole along with corticosteroids is required, usually along with ablation of any culprit thyroid lesions. Beta blockers are indicated for symptomatic control of anxiety and tachyarrhythmias. In one case, high doses of propranolol were thought to contribute to clinical seizure development [109]. If Hashimoto's encephalopathy is suspected, a course of pulse-dose steroids is the treatment of choice.

Seizures are treated using standard AEDs. Hepatically metabolized, enzyme-inducing AEDs (particularly carbamazepine and phenytoin) have been associated with decreased total and free T4 levels in those on chronic monotherapy for epilepsy [110] and should be avoided in those with hypothyroidism or in those undergoing ablation who may require supplemental thyroxine.

Diabetes Mellitus

Background

It is estimated that nearly 30 million Americans have diabetes, with approximately 8 million unaware of their diagnosis [111]. Critically ill patients may develop stress hyperglycemia in response to the presence of acute illness [112]. Strict glycemic control in the surgical but not medical ICU may be associated with better outcomes: a significant decrease in mortality was reported when strict blood glucose goals of <110 mg/dl were implemented in a population of critically ill patients in one study [113]. However, critically ill stroke and traumatic brain injury patients failed to demonstrate a difference in functional outcome at 3 months with intensive insulin therapy [114]. After severe brain injuries, "normal" glucose targets may lead to brain energy crisis characterized by lowered cerebral glucose and elevated lactate/pyruvate levels [115].

Glucose levels that are too low or too high may cause seizures and brain dysfunction. Hypoglycemia is associated with focal or generalized seizures, usually as glucose falls below 40 mg/dL. Hypoglycemic seizures respond to concentrated glucose infusion but rarely to conventional AEDs. Many patients present instead with hyperglycemia, either in the nonketotic hyperosmolar state (NHS) or diabetic ketoacidosis (DKA). Patients with epilepsy who experience hyperglycemia tend to have more severe seizures and have a higher frequency of SE at the time of presentation [116].

Nonketotic Hyperosmolar State (NHS)

Several cases of NHS with seizures have been reported in the literature; up to 25 % develop seizures in the setting of hyperosmolar hyperglycemia [117]. The most commonly reported seizure types include partial motor seizures and epilepsia partialis continua (EPC), but tonic-clonic seizures have been observed. *Kinesiogenic or reflex seizures* are seizures associated with NHS. They are induced by movement and usually followed by a refractory period, during which movement will not activate seizures. In seven patients with NHS and seizures, three developed kinesiogenic seizures caused by walking or by having the patient move a limb [118].

The exact pathogenesis of seizure in NHS is not well understood. Dehydration induced by the hyperosmolar state may cause areas of focal ischemia prone to developing ictal discharges [119]. MRI demonstrates changes consistent with focal ischemia in some patients with NHS. These changes are transient, and resolution may occur with correction of the underlying metabolic derangements [120]. On the other hand, some patients have normal MRI at the time of seizure occurrence [117, 118]. Hyperglycemia may increase the metabolism of GABA, leading to relative hyperexcitability [118] as an alternative mechanism.

Diabetic Ketoacidosis (DKA)

Only a few cases of seizures acutely caused by DKA have been reported in the literature [121, 122]. This discrepancy is thought to occur as the result of the antiepileptic effect of ketosis. GABA is thought to increase as a result of intracellular acidosis created by ketosis, resulting in an increased seizure threshold. The ketogenic diet is an established treatment in patients with epilepsy [123].

Treatment of patients either with NHS or with DKA is aimed at correcting hyperglycemia, restoring volume while slowly correcting any coexistent hyponatremia. Benzodiazepines are used as first-line therapy while glucose levels and other metabolic abnormalities are addressed. Older literature has implicated phenytoin in creating insulin resistance leading to hyperglycemia, but long-term AEDs are not required for seizures provoked solely by poor glycemic control.

Pituitary Hormones

Antidiuretic Hormone

Antidiuretic hormone (ADH) is critical to maintaining euvolemia, serum osmolality, and serum sodium concentrations. Also called vasopressin, ADH also promotes peripheral vasoconstriction and maintenance of blood pressure. Excess ADH results in the syndrome of inappropriate ADH (SIADH) caused by a variety of critical illnesses.

Causes of syndrome of inappropriate antidiuretic hormone (SIADH):

- Drug induced (carbamazepine, oxcarbazepine)
- Encephalomeningitis
- Hereditary
- Hypopituitarism
- Malignancy (small cell lung carcinoma)
- Stroke (ischemic, subarachnoid, or intraventricular hemorrhage)

- Transsphenoidal surgery
- Trauma
- Severe pain

By promoting permeability of free water in the kidney's distal collecting tubule and collecting duct, significant hyponatremia may develop, which can precipitate seizures. Typically, treatment options restrict free water. In some cases, fluid restriction may be relatively contraindicated (e.g., patients with subarachnoid hemorrhage experiencing delayed cerebral ischemia). In such cases, vasopressin receptor antagonists such as conivaptan or tolvaptan [124], may be useful to induce free water diuresis (aquaresis), increasing sodium without restricting access to volume. Rapid correction of sodium (>8–12 mEq/L/day) may lead to the syndrome of central pontine or extrapontine myelinolysis which itself may rarely cause seizures.

Central diabetes insipidus (DI) occurs when ADH secretion is reduced. Clinically, this manifests as polyuria with decreased urine specific gravity, hypernatremia, and increased serum osmolality. Although diabetes insipidus does not cause seizures per se, the rate of sodium correction can create a relative hyperosmolar state within the brain parenchyma which may result in cerebral edema and potentially seizures, especially in young children. Treatment of DI consists of exogenous desmopressin and hypotonic fluids under close monitoring, with a goal correction rate of 10 mEq/L/day.

Sex Hormones

Estrogen and progesterone have important effects on the development of seizures. Estrogens are both neuroexcitatory and neuroinhibitory [125, 126], although relative increases in estrogen are thought to underlie the increase in seizure frequency that occurs in women with catamenial epilepsy. Estrogen replacement therapy has conversely been reported to improve seizure control during menopause in some women [127]. There is no evidence that oral contraceptives increase the risk of seizures in women with epilepsy, although protein-bound and hepatically metabolized AEDs and contraceptive-dose hormone therapies exhibit significant interactions and initiation of contraception may reduce the effective dose of lamotrigine particularly, thus precipitating seizures.

Progesterone by contrast appears to have anticonvulsant properties. Seizures are less common during phases of the normal menstrual cycle with higher levels of progesterone. Seizure frequency may be exacerbated by the administration of finasteride, which blocks progesterone synthesis [128]. More recently, allopregnanolone, a progesterone metabolite, was found to positively modulate δ-subunit $GABA_A$ receptors

by promoting tonic currents in the hippocampus [129]. Although extracellular GABA receptors become insensitive to benzodiazepines in chronic epilepsy and in SE, they remain sensitive to progesterone-derivative neurosteroids [130–133], providing a promising therapeutic target for the treatment of refractory SE (the ongoing Phase III STATUS trial; Clinicaltrials.gov Identifier: NCT02477618).

Parathyroid Hormones

The parathyroid glands maintain calcium homeostasis. Seizures may occur at the extremes of calcemic states as discussed above. Patients with hypoparathyroidism presenting with isolated hypocalcemia develop seizures in 25–30%; up to 70% of those with concurrent symptoms related to hypocalcemia will have a seizure [134]. Treating with intravenous calcium in conjunction with benzodiazepines is effective; in patients with hypocalcemia, even small corrections in ionized calcium may terminate seizures.

Symptoms of hyperparathyroidism are related to hypercalcemia and may include bone and abdominal pain, nephrolithiasis, and altered mental status, including coma. While hypercalcemia rarely causes seizures, hypercalcemia-induced hypertensive encephalopathies associated with either PRES or RCVS have been reported [135, 136] (see Chapter for electrolytes and ICU seizures).

Adrenal Hormones

The adrenal glands are responsible for physiologic secretion of cortisol and catecholamines in response to trophic hormones. During periods of physiologic stress, elevations of both cortisol and catecholamines occur. However, in the critically ill, compensatory catecholamine release and their normal phasic peaks and troughs may be blunted and insufficient to maintain normal homeostasis [137]. Relative cortisol insufficiency is therefore considered when symptoms of hypotension, hypoglycemia, and hyponatremia occur. However, these derangements are gradual and rarely sufficient to provoke seizures.

In contrast, the *forme pleine* of catecholamine release occurs in patients with pheochromocytoma, a catecholamine-secreting adrenal malignancy. The majority, nearly three-quarters, of those with pheochromocytoma experience neurological symptoms. Seizures were reported in 5 of the 93 patients described in one series [138]. Seizures may occur in the setting of hypertensive emergency or as a result of intracranial hemorrhage, PRES [139], or RCVS spectrum vasculopathy [138]. Blood pressure control and pheochromocytoma resection are enough to control seizures, if no causative underlying hemorrhagic lesion is present.

References

1. Bernal W, Wendon J. Acute Liver Failure. N Engl J Med. 2013;369:2525–34.
2. Ostapowicz G, Fontana RJ, Schiødt FV, Larson A, Davern TJ, Han SHB, et al. Results of a prospective study of acute liver failure at 17 tertiary care centers in the United States. Ann Intern Med. 2002;137:947–54.
3. Cash WJ, McConville P, McDermott E, McCormick PA, Callender ME, McDougall NI. Current concepts in the assessment and treatment of hepatic encephalopathy. QJM. 2010;103:9–16.
4. Ellis AJ, Wendon JA, Williams R. Subclinical Seizure Activity and Prophylactic Phenytoin Infusion in Acute Liver Failure: A Controlled Clinical Trial. Hepatology. 2000;32:536–41.
5. Foley JM, Watson CW, Adams RD. Significance of the electroencephalographic changes in hepatic coma. Trans Am Neurol Assoc. 1950;51:161–5.
6. Aldridge DR, Tranah EJ, Shawcross DL. Pathogenesis of Hepatic Encephalopathy: Role of Ammonia and Systemic Inflammation. J Clin Exp Hepatol. 2015;5:S7–20.
7. Butterworth RF. Pathogenesis of Hepatic Encephalopathy and Brain Edema in Acute Liver Failure. J. Clin. Exp. Hepatol. 2015;5:S96–103.
8. Knecht K, Michalak A, Rose C, Rothstein JD, Butterworth RF. Decreased glutamate transporter (GLT-1) expression in frontal cortex of rats with acute liver failure. Neurosci Lett. 1997;229:201–3.
9. Zwingmann C, Desjardins P, Hazell A, Chatauret N, Michalak A, Butterworth RF. Reduced expression of astrocytic glycine transporter (Glyt-1) in acute liver failure. Metab Brain Dis. 2002;17:263–73.
10. Ahboucha S, Butterworth RF. Role of Endogenous Benzodiazepine Ligands and Their GABA-A-Associated Receptors in Hepatic Encephalopathy. Metab Brain Dis. 2005;20:425–37.
11. Bender AS, Norenberg MD. Effect of ammonia on GABA uptake and release in cultured astrocytes. Neurochem Int. 2000;36:389–95.
12. Ferenci P, Jacobs R, Pappas SC, Schafer DF, Jones EA. Enzymes of cerebral GABA metabolism and synaptosomal GABA uptake in acute liver failure in the rabbit: evidence for decreased cerebral GABA-transaminase activity. J Neurochem. 1984;42:1487–90.
13. Oddo M, Carrera E, Claassen J, Mayer SA, Hirsch LJ. Continuous electroencephalography in the medical intensive care unit*. Crit Care Med. 2009;37:2051–6.
14. Kurtz P, Gaspard N, Wahl AS, Bauer RM, Hirsch LJ, Wunsch H, et al. Continuous electroencephalography in a surgical intensive care unit. Intensive Care Med. 2014;40:228–34.
15. Westover MB, Shafi MM, Bianchi MT, Moura LMVR, O'Rourke D, Rosenthal ES, et al. The probability of seizures during EEG monitoring in critically ill adults. Clin Neurophysiol Off J Int Fed Clin Neurophysiol. 2015;126:463–71.
16. Claassen J, Mayer SA, Kowalski RG, Emerson RG, Hirsch LJ. Detection of electrographic seizures with continuous EEG monitoring in critically ill patients. Neurology. 2004;62:1743–8.
17. Brophy GM, Bell R, Claassen J, Alldredge B, Bleck TP, Glauser T, et al. Guidelines for the evaluation and management of status epilepticus. Neurocrit Care. 2012;17:3–23.
18. Bickford RG, Butt HR. Hepatic coma: the electroencephalographic pattern. J Clin Invest. 1955;34:790–9.
19. Sutter R, Kaplan PW. Uncovering clinical and radiological associations of triphasic waves in acute encephalopathy: a case-control study. Eur J Neurol. 2014;21:660–6.
20. Karnaze DS, Bickford RG. Triphasic waves: a reassessment of their significance. Electroencephalogr Clin Neurophysiol. 1984;57:193–8.

21. Foreman B, Claassen J, Khaled KA, Jirsch J, Alschuler DM, JohnWittman J, et al. Generalized periodic discharges in the critically ill: a case-control study of 200 patients. Neurology. 2012;79:1951–60.
22. Foreman B, Mahulikar A, Tadi P, Claassen J, Szaflarski J, Halford JJ, et al. Generalized periodic discharges and "triphasic waves": a blinded evaluation of inter-rater agreement and clinical significance. Clin Neurophysiol. 2016;127:1073–80.
23. Ficker DM, Westmoreland BF, Sharbrough FW. Epileptiform abnormalities in hepatic encephalopathy. J Clin Neurophysiol Off Publ Am Electroencephalogr Soc. 1997;14:230–4.
24. Wszolek ZK, Steg RE. Seizures after orthotopic liver transplantation. Seizure. 1997;6:31–9.
25. Baraldi M, Avallone R, Corsi L, Venturini I, Baraldi C, Zeneroli ML. Natural endogenous ligands for benzodiazepine receptors in hepatic encephalopathy. Metab Brain Dis. 2009;24:81–93.
26. Claassen J, Silbergleit R, Weingart SD, Smith WS. Emergency Neurological Life Support: Status Epilepticus. Neurocrit Care. 2012;17:73–8.
27. Alldredge BK, Gelb AM, Isaacs SM, Corry MD, Allen F, Ulrich S, et al. A comparison of lorazepam, diazepam, and placebo for the treatment of out-of-hospital status epilepticus. N Engl J Med. 2001;345:631–7.
28. Silbergleit R, Durkalski V, Lowenstein D, Conwit R, Pancioli A, Palesch Y, et al. Intramuscular versus intravenous therapy for prehospital status epilepticus. N Engl J Med. 2012;366:591–600.
29. McCall M, Bourgeois JA. Valproic Acid-Induced Hyperammonemia: A Case Report. J Clin Psychopharmacol. 2004;24:521–6.
30. Lheureux PE, Penaloza A, Zahir S, Gris M. Science review: Carnitine in the treatment of valproic acid-induced toxicity–what is the evidence? Crit Care. 2005;9:431.
31. Bhatia V, Batra Y, Acharya SK. Prophylactic phenytoin does not improve cerebral edema or survival in acute liver failure—a controlled clinical trial. J Hepatol. 2004;41:89–96.
32. Lorincz MT. Neurologic Wilson's disease. Ann N Y Acad Sci. 2010;1184:173–87.
33. Dening TR, Berrios GE, Walshe JM. Wilson's disease and epilepsy. Brain. 1988;111:1139–55.
34. Prashanth LK, Sinha S, Taly AB, Mahadevan A, Vasudev MK, Shankar SK. Spectrum of epilepsy in Wilson's disease with electroencephalographic, MR imaging and pathological correlates. J Neurol Sci. 2010;291:44–51.
35. Smith CK, Mattson RH. Seizures in Wilson's disease. Neurology. 1967;17:1121–3.
36. Meenakshi-Sundaram S, Mahadevan A, Taly AB, Arunodaya GR, Swamy HS, Shankar SK. Wilson's disease: A clinico-neuropathological autopsy study. J Clin Neurosci. 2008;15:409–17.
37. Shukla R, Desai P, Vinod P. Wilson's disease presenting as status epilepticus. J Assoc Physicians India. 2006;54:887–9.
38. Türk-Börü U, Kocer A, Alp R, Gümüş M, Gümüş M. Status epilepticus in a case with Wilson's disease during D-pencillamine treatment. Swiss Med Wkly. 2003;133:446–7.
39. Morse RS, Holmes AW, Levin S. Reye's syndrome in an adult. Am J Dig Dis. 1975;20:1184–90.
40. Atkins JN, Haponik EF. Reye's syndrome in the adult patients. Am J Med. 1979;67:672–8.
41. You K. Salicylate and mitochondrial injury in Reye's syndrome. Science. 1983;221:163–5.
42. Aoki Y, Lombroso C. Prognostic value of electroencephalography in Reye's syndrome. Neurology. 1973;23:333–43.
43. Barr RE, Ackmann JJ, Harrington GJ, Varma RR, Lewis JD, Casper JT. Computerized evaluation of electroencephalographic changes accompanying exchange transfusion in Reye's syndrome. Electroencephalogr Clin Neurophysiol. 1977;42:466–79.
44. Arai M. [A case of adult Reye's syndrome with favorable outcome despite status epilepticus]. Rinshō Shinkeigaku Clin. Neurology. 1996;36:1256–8.

45. Solinas C, Vajda FJ. Epilepsy and porphyria: new perspectives. J Clin Neurosci. 2004;11:356–61.

46. Simon NG, Herkes GK. The neurologic manifestations of the acute porphyrias. J Clin Neurosci. 2011;18:1147–53.

47. Hahn M, Gildemeister OS, Krauss GL, Pepe JA, Lambrecht RW, Donohue S, et al. Effects of new anticonvulsant medications on porphyrin synthesis in cultured liver cells: potential implications for patients with acute porphyria. Neurology. 1997;49:97–106.

48. Suzuki A, Aso K, Ariyoshi C, Ishimaru M. Acute intermittent porphyria and epilepsy: safety of clonazepam. Epilepsia. 1992;33:108–11.

49. Bonkowsky HL, Sinclair PR, Emery S, Sinclair JF. Seizure management in acute hepatic porphyria: risks of valproate and clonazepam. Neurology. 1980;30:588–92.

50. Bhatia R, Vibha D, Srivastava MV, Prasad K, Tripathi M, Bhushan SM. Use of propofol anesthesia and adjunctive treatment with levetiracetam and gabapentin in managing status epilepticus in a patient of acute intermittent porphyria. Epilepsia. 2008;49:934–6.

51. Lambrecht RW, Gildemeister OS, Pepe JA, Tortorelli KD, Williams A, Bonkovsky HL. Effects of antidepressants and benzodiazepine-type anxiolytic agents on hepatic porphyrin accumulation in primary cultures of chick embryo liver cells. J Pharmacol Exp Ther. 1999;291:1150–5.

52. Bylesjö I, Forsgren L, Wetterberg L. Melatonin and epileptic seizures in patients with acute intermittent porphyria. Epileptic Disord Int Epilepsy J Videotape. 2000;2:203–8.

53. Hoste EA, Clermont G, Kersten A, Venkataraman R, Angus DC, De Bacquer D, et al. RIFLE criteria for acute kidney injury are associated with hospital mortality in critically ill patients: a cohort analysis. Crit Care. 2006;10:R73.

54. Tolwani A. Continuous Renal-Replacement Therapy for Acute Kidney Injury. N Engl J Med. 2012;367:2505–14.

55. Bagshaw SM, George C, Dinu I, Bellomo R. A multi-centre evaluation of the RIFLE criteria for early acute kidney injury in critically ill patients. Nephrol Dial Transplant. 2007;23:1203–10.

56. Kellum JA, Lameire N, KDIGO AKI, Guideline Work Group. Diagnosis, evaluation, and management of acute kidney injury: a KDIGO summary (Part 1). Crit Care Lond Engl. 2013;17:204.

57. Mehta RL, Kellum JA, Shah SV, Molitoris BA, Ronco C, Warnock DG, et al. Acute kidney injury network: report of an initiative to improve outcomes in acute kidney injury. Crit Care. 2007;11:R31.

58. Bellomo R, Ronco C, Kellum JA, Mehta RL, Palevsky P, Acute Dialysis Quality Initiative workgroup. Acute renal failure – definition, outcome measures, animal models, fluid therapy and information technology needs: the Second International Consensus Conference of the Acute Dialysis Quality Initiative (ADQI) Group. Crit. Care Lond. Engl. 2004;8:R204–12.

59. Lacerda G, Krummel T, Hirsch E. Neurologic Presentations of Renal Diseases. Neurol Clin. 2010;28:45–59.

60. Foreman B, Hirsch LJ. Epilepsy Emergencies: Diagnosis and Management. Neurol Clin. 2012;30:11–41.

61. Vanholder R, Glorieux G, De Smet R, Lameire N. New insights in uremic toxins. Kidney Int. 2003;63:S6–10.

62. De Deyn PP, Vanholder R, Eloot S, Glorieux G. Guanidino compounds as uremic (neuro)toxins. Semin Dial. 2009;22:340–5.

63. Smogorzewski MJ. Central nervous dysfunction in uremia. Am J Kidney Dis. 2001;38:S122–8.

64. Fraser CL, Sarnacki P, Arieff AI. Calcium transport abnormality in uremic rat brain synaptosomes. J Clin Invest. 1985;76:1789.

65. Fraser CL, Sarnacki P, Arieff AI. Abnormal sodium transport in synaptosomes from brain of uremic rats. J Clin Invest. 1985;75:2014.

66. D'Hooge R, Pei YQ, Marescau B, De Deyn PP. Convulsive action and toxicity of uremic guanidino compounds: behavioral assessment and relation to brain concentration in adult mice. J Neurol Sci. 1992;112:96–105.

67. Guisado R, Arieff AI, Massry SG, Lazarowitz V, Kerian A. Changes in the electroencephalogram in acute uremia. Effects of parathyroid hormone and brain electrolytes. J Clin Invest. 1975;55:738–45.

68. Hinchey J, Chaves C, Appignani B, Breen J, Pao L, Wang A, et al. A reversible posterior leukoencephalopathy syndrome. N Engl J Med. 1996;334:494–500.

69. Chatellier D, Jourdain M, Mangalaboyi J, Ader F, Chopin C, Derambure P, et al. Cefepime-induced neurotoxicity: an underestimated complication of antibiotherapy in patients with acute renal failure. Intensive Care Med. 2002;28:214–7.

70. Martínez-Rodríguez JE, Barriga FJ, Santamaria J, Iranzo A, Pareja JA, Revilla M, et al. Nonconvulsive status epilepticus associated with cephalosporins in patients with renal failure. Am J Med. 2001;111:115–9.

71. Ohtsuki S, Asaba H, Takanaga H, Deguchi T, Hosoya K, Otagiri M, et al. Role of blood–brain barrier organic anion transporter 3 (OAT3) in the efflux of indoxyl sulfate, a uremic toxin: its involvement in neurotransmitter metabolite clearance from the brain. J Neurochem. 2002;83:57–66.

72. Bates D. Valacyclovir neurotoxicity: two case reports and a review of the literature. Aust J Hosp Pharm. 2002;55:123–7.

73. Rashiq S, Briewa L, Mooney M, Giancarlo T, Khatib R, Wilson FM. Distinguishing acyclovir neurotoxicity from encephalomyelitis. J Intern Med. 1993;234:507–11.

74. Chen KS, Bullard MJ, Chien YY, Lee SY. Baclofen toxicity in patients with severely impaired renal function. Ann Pharmacother. 1997;31:1315–20.

75. Brenner RP. The interpretation of the EEG in stupor and coma. Neurologist. 2005;11:271–84.

76. Hughes JR. Correlations between EEG and chemical changes in uremia. Electroencephalogr Clin Neurophysiol. 1980;48:583–94.

77. Fraser CL, Arieff AI. Nervous system complications in uremia. Ann Intern Med. 1988;109:143–53.

78. Rufo Campos M, Vázquez Florido AM, Madruga Garrido M, Fijo J, Sánchez Moreno A, Martín GJ. Renal failure as a factor leading to epileptic seizures. Pediatriia. 2002;56:212–8.

79. Frenchie D, Bastani B. Significant removal of phenytoin during high flux dialysis with cellulose triacetate dialyzer. Nephrol Dial Transplant. 1998;13:817–8.

80. Arieff AI. Dialysis disequilibrium syndrome: current concepts on pathogenesis and prevention. Kidney Int. 1994;45:629–35.

81. Osgood M, Compton R, Carandang R, Hall W, Kershaw G, Muehlschlegel S. Rapid unexpected brain herniation in association with renal replacement therapy in acute brain injury: caution in the neurocritical care unit. Neurocrit Care. 2015;22:176–83.

82. La Greca G, Biasioli S, Chiaramonte S, Dettori P, Fabris A, Feriani M, et al. Studies on brain density in hemodialysis and peritoneal dialysis. Nephron. 1982;31:146–50.

83. Arieff AI, Guisado R, Massry SG, Lazarowitz VC. Central nervous system pH in uremia and the effects of hemodialysis. J Clin Invest. 1976;58:306.

84. Davenport A. Practical guidance for dialyzing a hemodialysis patient following acute brain injury. Hemodial Int Int Symp Home Hemodial. 2008;12:307–12.

85. Angus DC, Linde-Zwirble WT, Lidicker J, Clermont G, Carcillo J, Pinsky MR, et al. Epidemiology of severe sepsis in the United States: analysis of incidence, outcome, and associated costs of care. Crit Care Med Baltim. 2001;29:1303–10.

86. Eidelman LA, Putterman D, Putterman C, Sprung CL. The spectrum of septic encephalopathy: definitions, etiologies, and mortalities. JAMA. 1996;275:470–3.

87. Siami S, Annane D, Sharshar T. The Encephalopathy in Sepsis. Crit Care Clin. 2008;24:67–82.

88. Gilmore EJ, Gaspard N, Choi HA, Cohen E, Burkart KM, Chong DH, et al. Acute brain failure in severe sepsis: a prospective study

in the medical intensive care unit utilizing continuous EEG monitoring. Intensive Care Med. 2015;41:686–94.

89. Pandharipande PP, Girard TD, Jackson JC, Morandi A, Thompson JL, Pun BT, et al. Long-Term Cognitive Impairment after Critical Illness. N Engl J Med. 2013;369:1306–16.

90. Singer M, Deutschman CS, Seymour CW, Shankar-Hari M, Annane D, Bauer M, et al. The third international consensus definitions for sepsis and septic shock (Sepsis-3). JAMA. 2016; 315:801.

91. Ebersoldt M, Sharshar T, Annane D. Sepsis-associated delirium. Intensive Care Med. 2007;33:941–50.

92. Polito A, Eischwald F, Maho A-L, Azabou E, Annane D, Chretien F, et al. Pattern of brain injury in the acute setting of human septic shock. Crit Care. 2013;17:R204.

93. Watson PL, Shintani AK, Tyson R, Pandharipande PP, Pun BT, Ely EW. Presence of electroencephalogram burst suppression in sedated, critically ill patients is associated with increased mortality. Crit Care Med. 2008;36:3171–7.

94. Towne AR, Waterhouse EJ, Boggs JG, Garnett LK, Brown AJ, Jr S, et al. Prevalence of nonconvulsive status epilepticus in comatose patients. Neurology. 2000;54:340.

95. Nishina K, Akamatsu H, Mikawa K, Shiga M, Maekawa N, Obara H, et al. The inhibitory effects of thiopental, midazolam, and ketamine on human neutrophil functions. Anesth Analg. 1998;86:159–65.

96. Mikawa K, Akamatsu H, Nishina K, Shiga M, Obara H, Niwa Y. Inhibitory effects of pentobarbital and phenobarbital on human neutrophil functions. J Intensive Care Med. 2001;16:79–87.

97. Weetman AP. Thyrotoxicosis. Medicine (Baltimore). 2009;37: 430–5.

98. Song T-J, Kim S-J, Kim GS, Choi Y-C, Kim W-J. The prevalence of thyrotoxicosis-related seizures. Thyroid. 2010;20:955–8.

99. Radetti G, Dordi B, Mengarda G, Biscaldi I, Larizza D, Severi F. Thyrotoxicosis presenting with seizures and coma in two children. Am J Dis Child. 1993;147:925–7.

100. Henchey R, Cibula J, Helveston W, Malone J, Gilmore RL. Electroencephalographic findings in Hashimoto's encephalopathy. Neurology. 1995;45:977–81.

101. Bryce GM, Poyner F. Myxoedema presenting with seizures. Postgrad Med J. 1992;68:35–6.

102. Sokoloff L, Wechsler RL, Mangold R, Balls K, Kety SS. Cerebral blood flow and oxygen consumption in hyperthyroidism before and after treatment. J Clin Invest. 1953;32:202.

103. Hoffmann G, Dietzel I. Thyroid hormone regulates excitability in central neurons from postnatal rats. Neuroscience. 2004;125:369–79.

104. Martin JV, Padron JM, Newman MA, Chapell R, Leidenheimer NJ, Burke LA. Inhibition of the activity of the native γ-aminobutyric acidA receptor by metabolites of thyroid hormones: correlations with molecular modeling studies. Brain Res. 2004;1004:98–107.

105. Puia G, Losi G. Thyroid hormones modulate GABAA receptor-mediated currents in hippocampal neurons. Neuropharmacology. 2011;60:1254–61.

106. Wan RQ, Noguera EC, Weiss SR. Anticonvulsant effects of intrahippocampal injection of TRH in amygdala kindled rats. Neuroreport. 1998;9:677–82.

107. Skanse B, Nyman GE. Thyrotoxicosis as a cause of cerebral dysrhythmia and convulsive seizures. Acta Endocrinol. 1956;22: 246–63.

108. Li Voon Chong JS, Lecky BR, Macfarlane IA. Recurrent encephalopathy and generalised seizures associated with relapses of thyrotoxicosis. Int J Clin Pract. 2000;54:621–2.

109. Smith DL, Looney TJ. Seizures secondary to thyrotoxicosis and high-dosage propranolol therapy. Arch Neurol. 1983;40:457–8.

110. Svalheim S, Sveberg L, Mochol M, Taubøll E. Interactions between antiepileptic drugs and hormones. Seizure. 2015;28:12–7.

111. Centers for Disease Control and Prevention. National diabetes statistics report: estimates of diabetes and its burden in the United States. Atlanta, GA: U.S. Department of Health and Human Services; 2014.

112. Dungan KM, Braithwaite SS, Preiser J-C. Stress hyperglycaemia. Lancet. 2009;373:1798–807.

113. Van G, Berghe MD, Wouters P, Weekers F, Verwaest C, Bruyninckx F, et al. Intensive insulin therapy in critically ill patients. N Engl J Med. 2001;345:1359–67.

114. Green DM, O'Phelan KH, Bassin SL, Chang CWJ, Stern TS, Asai SM. Intensive versus conventional insulin therapy in critically ill neurologic patients. Neurocrit Care. 2010;13:299–306.

115. Oddo M, Schmidt JM, Carrera E, Badjatia N, Connolly ES, Presciutti M, et al. Impact of tight glycemic control on cerebral glucose metabolism after severe brain injury: a microdialysis study. Crit Care Med. 2008;36:3233–8.

116. Huang C-W, Tsai J-J, Ou H-Y, Wang S-T, Cheng J-T, Wu S-N, et al. Diabetic hyperglycemia is associated with the severity of epileptic seizures in adults. Epilepsy Res. 2008;79:71–7.

117. Çokar Ö, Aydin B, Özer F. Non-ketotic hyperglycaemia presenting as epilepsia partialis continua. Seizure. 2004;13:264–9.

118. Hennis A, Corbin D, Fraser H. Focal seizures and non-ketotic hyperglycaemia. J Neurol Neurosurg Psychiatry. 1992;55:195–7.

119. Singh BM, Strobos RJ. Epilepsia partialis continua associated with nonketotic hyperglycemia: clinical and biochemical profile of 21 patients. Ann Neurol. 1980;8:155–60.

120. Raghavendra S, Ashalatha R, Thomas SV, Kesavadas C. Focal neuronal loss, reversible subcortical focal T2 hypointensity in seizures with a nonketotic hyperglycemic hyperosmolar state. Neuroradiology. 2007;49:299–305.

121. Martínez-Fernández R, Gelabert A, Pablo MJ, Carmona O, Molins A. Status epilepticus with visual seizures in ketotic hyperglycemia. Epilepsy Behav. 2009;16:660–2.

122. Placidi F, Floris R, Bozzao A, Romigi A, Baviera ME, Tombini M, et al. Ketotic hyperglycemia and epilepsia partialis continua. Neurology. 2001;57:534–7.

123. Martin K, Jackson CF, Levy RG, Cooper PN. Ketogenic diet and other dietary treatments for epilepsy. Cochrane Database Syst Rev. 2016;2:CD001903.

124. Wright WL, Asbury WH, Gilmore JL, Samuels OB. Conivaptan for hyponatremia in the neurocritical care unit. Neurocrit Care. 2009;11:6–13.

125. Velíšková J. The role of estrogens in seizures and epilepsy: The bad guys or the good guys? Neuroscience. 2006;138:837–44.

126. Velíšková J, De Jesus G, Kaur R, Velíšek L. Females, their estrogens, and seizures: females, their estrogens, and seizures. Epilepsia. 2010;51:141–4.

127. Peebles CT, McAuley JW, Moore JL, Malone HJ, Reeves AL. Hormone replacement therapy in a postmenopausal woman with epilepsy. Ann Pharmacother. 2000;34:1028–31.

128. Frye CA, Bayon LE. Seizure activity is increased in endocrine states characterized by decline in endogenous levels of the neurosteroid 3α, 5α-THP. Neuroendocrinology. 1998;68:272–80.

129. Carver C, Reddy DS. Neurosteroid structure-activity relationships for functional activation of extrasynaptic delta-GABA-A receptors. J Pharmacol Exp Ther. 2016;357:188–204. doi: 10.1124/jpet.115.229302.

130. Frye CA. The neurosteroid 3 alpha, 5 apha-THP has antiseizure and possible neuroprotective effects in an animal model of epilepsy. Brain Res. 1995;696:113–20.

131. Toner I, Taylor KM, Newman S, Smith PLC. Cerebral functional changes following cardiac surgery: neuropsychological and EEG assessment. Eur J Cardiothorac Surg. 1998;13:13–20.

132. Maguire JL, Stell BM, Rafizadeh M, Mody I. Ovarian cycle–linked changes in GABAA receptors mediating tonic inhibition alter seizure susceptibility and anxiety. Nat Neurosci. 2005;8:797–804.

133. Reddy K, Reife R, Cole AJ. SGE-102: A novel therapy for refractory status epilepticus. Epilepsia. 2013;54:81–3.

134. Castilla-Guerra L, del Carmen F-MM, López-Chozas JM, Fernández-Bolaños R. Electrolytes disturbances and seizures. Epilepsia. 2006;47:1990–8.

135. Chen T-H, Huang C-C, Chang Y-Y, Chen Y-F, Chen W-H, Lai S-L. Vasoconstriction as the etiology of hypercalcemia-induced seizures. Epilepsia. 2004;45:551–4.

136. Camara-Lemarroy CR, Gonzalez-Moreno EI, Ortiz-Corona JJ, Yeverino-Castro SG, Sanchez-Cardenas M, Nuñez-Aguirre S, et al. Posterior reversible encephalopathy syndrome due to malignant hypercalcemia: physiopathological considerations. J Clin Endocrinol Metab. 2014;99:1112–6.

137. Marik PE, Zaloga GP. Adrenal insufficiency in the critically ill. Chest. 2002;122:1784–96.

138. Anderson NE, Chung K, Willoughby E, Croxson MS. Neurological manifestations of phaeochromocytomas and secretory paragangliomas: a reappraisal. J Neurol Neurosurg Psychiatry. 2013;84:452–7.

139. Majic T, Aiyagari V. Cerebrovascular manifestations of pheochromocytoma and the implications of a missed diagnosis. Neurocrit Care. 2008;9:378–81.

Organ Transplant Recipients and Critical Care Seizures

Deena M. Nasr, Sara Hocker, and Eelco F.M. Wijdicks

Introduction

Seizures are the second most common central nervous system complication in solid organ transplant recipients. They are second to encephalopathy in liver, intestinal, and lung transplantation and stroke in cardiac and renal transplant recipients [1]. The incidence of seizures among solid organ transplant (SOT) recipients is wide with reports ranging from 1 to 13%, and 2 to 20% in hematopoietic stem cell transplant (HSCT) recipients [2, 3] (Table 15.1). Such a wide disparity in prevalence is not easily explained and may be related to a premorbid condition, use of certain immunosuppressive drugs, and control of hypertension causing posterior reversible encephalopathy syndrome. In most series it is unclear how the diagnosis of seizures was made or confirmed.

Seizures may be focal or generalized in onset. They are essentially a non-specific symptom of cerebral dysfunction. In the setting of organ transplantation, they may result from drug-induced neurotoxicity, metabolic/electrolyte disturbances, central nervous system (CNS) infections, malignant hypertension, ischemic or hemorrhage stroke, or CNS malignancy.

The general approach to the evaluation of seizures in this population differs little from the general population. The priorities are: (1) to abort the seizure in order to minimize neurologic and systemic morbidity, (2) to minimize seizure recurrence by identifying and treating the etiology when possible, and (3) to determine if there is need for long-term antiepileptic drugs (AEDs). A few additional considerations specific to this patient population also apply and are outlined in this chapter.

Initial Patient Evaluation and Treatment

In the acute setting, the primary goal is to abort the seizure. Because most seizures are self-limited, there is a tendency to think that most patients will not require emergent treatment and can be observed, however, seizures in these fragile postoperative patients may lead to major systemic complications (aspiration, myocardial demand ischemia, rhabdomyolysis). We opt for a short two week course with an antiepileptic with a good safety profile such as levetiracetam. Obviously in the case of recurrent seizures or status epilepticus, emergent pharmacologic treatment with intravenous AEDs is recommended.

Most post-transplant seizures respond to first line treatment with benzodiazepines with preferred agents being lorazepam or midazolam [4]. When seizures continue despite benzodiazepine administration efforts should be made to rapidly identify and correct any readily reversible precipitating factors (i.e., severe hyponatremia) and a second line intravenous AED should be administered. Options include phenytoin, fosphenytoin, valproic acid, phenobarbital, or levetiracetam [5].

The next step is to find a possible cause of the seizure (Table 15.2). This is especially pertinent in transplant patients who are immunosuppressed with antirejection medications and therefore at higher risk for infections and neurotoxicity related to the antirejection drugs. Investigation of serum electrolyte levels including magnesium, sodium, calcium,

D.M. Nasr
Department of Neurology, Mayo Clinic, Rochester, MN, USA
e-mail: Nasr.Deena@mayo.edu

S. Hocker (✉)
Division of Critical Care Neurology, Mayo Clinic,
200 First Street S.W., Rochester, MN 55905, USA
e-mail: Hocker.Sara@mayo.edu

E.F.M. Wijdicks
Division of Critical Care Neurology, Mayo Clinic,
Rochester, MN, USA
e-mail: Wijde@mayo.edu

© Springer International Publishing AG 2017
P.N. Varelas, J. Claassen (eds.), *Seizures in Critical Care*, Current Clinical Neurology, DOI 10.1007/978-3-319-49557-6_15

Table 15.1 Incidence of seizures in organ transplant patients

Transplant organ	Incidence of seizures (%)
Liver	4–8 [79–82]
Bone marrow transplant	2–20 [2–3, 83–85]
Heart	2–9 [76, 86–88]
Kidney	2–6 [1, 89]
Lung	6–10 [90–91]
Pancreas	13 [92]
Intestinal	17 [93]

Table 15.2 Possible causes of seizures in transplant recipients

Cerebrovascular events	**Malignancy**
• Arterial ischemic infarcts	• B-cell lymphoma
• Intracranial hemorrhage	• Post-transplant
• Cerebral venous thrombosis	lymphoproliferative disorder
CNS infection	**Medication induced**
Bacterial	**neurotoxicity**
• Nocardia	*Antirejection agents*
• Listeria	• CNIs: Tacrolimus, cyclosporin A
• Tuberculosis	• OKT3 (muronmonab-CD3)
Viral	• Chemotherapy: busulfan and
• JC virus	carmustine
• Herpes Viruses (HSV,	*Antibiotics*
CMV, VZV, EBV, HHV-6)	• Quinolone Class
Fungal	• Carbapenem class
• Aspergillus	*Analgesics*
• Candida	• Meperidine
• Cryptococcus	**Metabolic derangements**
Parasite	• Hyponatremia
• Toxoplasmosis	• Hypocalcemia
	• Hypomagnesemia
	• Hypoglycemia
	• Hyperammonemia

and glucose as well as a complete blood count with differential, ammonia, blood cultures, and antirejection medication levels should be performed.

Because seizures are comparatively more common in CNS infections associated with transplantations an infectious evaluation should be initiated if seizures occur one month after transplantation (CNS infections are exceedingly rare in the postoperative period). A history of preceding headache, confusion, signs of increased intracranial pressure including transient visual obscurations, morning headaches, or signs of meningismus on examination justifies a lumbar puncture but immunosuppressed post-transplant patients should undergo neuroimaging prior to lumbar puncture. Empiric antimicrobial therapy should be started while neuroimaging and lumbar puncture are performed.

Because of their immunosuppressed status, imaging is strongly considered in these patients, even when a clear trigger (i.e., severe hypocalcemia) is present. A non-contrast CT is the first investigational step to rule out the presence of a lesion that may require emergent intervention. Non-contrast CT can also be useful in detecting the typical vasogenic edema of posterior reversible encephalopathy syndrome

(PRES) (Fig. 15.1), a mass-like lesion such as brain abscess, intracerebral hemorrhage, or diffuse cerebral edema.

If initial investigations are unrevealing, MRI with contrast can be considered. Smaller brain abscesses, empyema, septic emboli, pachymeningeal or leptomeningeal enhancement, brainstem infarctions, radiologic signs of PRES, and central pontine myelinolysis are more readily identified on MRI compared with CT [5].

An electroencephalogram (EEG) is not performed in most settings due to the fact that the majority of seizures last less than 1 min and patients recover quickly from these seizures. However, patients who remain persistently encephalopathic following a seizure will need an urgent EEG in order to determine if the patient is in nonconvulsive status epilepticus. Because undefined rhythmic movements are so common in the postoperative period an EEG can also be useful to characterize the nature of uncertain "spells" of unresponsiveness or abnormal movements. For example, to differentiate multifocal myoclonus (seen in metabolic encephalopathy) or tremors from seizures in unresponsive patients or in patients awakening from anesthesia [5].

Seizures in Transplant Patients: Specific Causes

Drug-Induced Seizures

Immunosuppressant agents such as cyclosporine, tacrolimus, mycophenolate mofetil, and corticosteroids are universally administered following organ transplantation to reduce the risk of rejection and improve graft survival. In the acute post-transplant period, induction agents can be used including thymoglobulin, OKT3, and basiliximab. These are followed with maintenance steroids, mycophenolate mofetil, or calcineurin inhibitors such as cyclosporine or tacrolimus. Most transplant patients are then continued on a long-term regimen consisting of a calcineurin inhibitor or mycophenolate mofetil [6].

Because of the narrow therapeutic windows of antirejection drugs and the higher propensity for metabolic derangements in the post-transplant period, drug toxicity from calcineurin inhibitors or mycophenolate mofetil can be considered as a potential cause for seizures. Post-transplant drug-induced encephalopathy affects up to 40% of patients with the incidence peaking within the early postoperative period due to high loading doses [7, 8]. Drug toxicity from antirejection agents is the most common cause of seizures and is the cause in about 25% of cases [9]. The calcineurin inhibitors have been mostly responsible for most drug-induced seizures due to their mechanism of action. They inhibit calcium signaling pathways that are essential to T-cell activations. However, calcineurin also plays an essential role

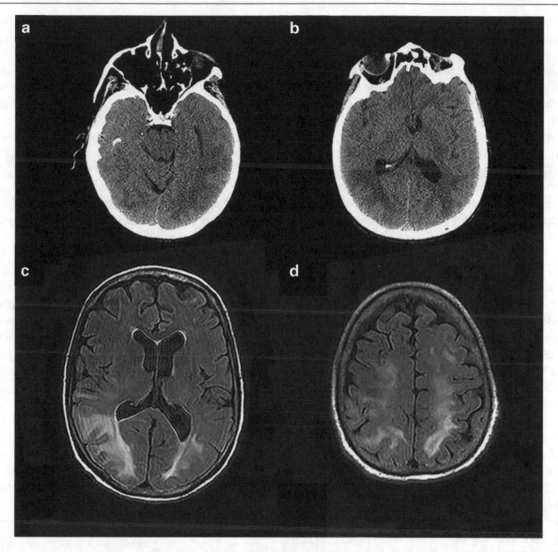

Fig 15.1 (**a, b**) Computed tomography and (**c, d**) magnetic resonance imaging fluid attenuated inversion recovery (FLAIR/T2 weighted sequences demonstrating a typical pattern of vasogenic edema associ-ated with PRES). The edema is bilateral, asymmetric, predominantly subcortical, and preferentially affecting the posterior regions and frontal lobes

in regulating neuron excitability, blood–brain barrier permeability, and sympathetic activation [9]. The neurotoxic effects of calcineurin inhibitors may be potentiated by pre-existing disruption of the blood–brain barrier in the perioperative period due to hepatic encephalopathy or perioperative hypotension [10]. Ultimately, these disruptions can lead to vasogenic edema, posterior reversible encephalopathy syndrome (PRES), and seizures.

The diagnostic criteria for CNI induced toxicity include development of seizures or encephalopathy in patients receiving CNIs who have high serum trough levels of the drug at the time of symptoms onset and rapid increase in drug levels prior to symptomatic presentation. Neurotoxicity from CNIs is more commonly seen in the first month of post-transplant care due to the higher intravenous dosing [11]. Postural tremors and headaches are the most common

symptoms encountered and can be seen with tacrolimus neurotoxicity. However, both tacrolimus and cyclosporine neurotoxicity can manifest with focal or generalized tonic-clonic seizures that can be seen with or without the presence of posterior reversible encephalopathy syndrome (PRES). Risk factors for CNI toxicity include hepatic dysfunction, hypertension, low magnesium levels, and administration of medications such as corticosteroids, amphotericin, and gan-ciclovir which inhibit drug metabolism [12]. While it is important to monitor drug levels during the early phase of maintenance immunosuppression while on these therapies, it has been demonstrated that no correlation exists between seizures and drug levels themselves [13]. Rather, it is the rapid increase in drug levels that is thought to be a provoking cause. In addition, levels of metabolites, rather than the drug itself, can be associated with seizures.

Over the past several years, there has been a switch from cyclosporine to tacrolimus as the antirejection agent of choice in organ transplant patients. Tacrolimus is associated with lower rates of hypertension, acute rejection, and possibly a better neurotoxicity profile as compared to cyclosporine. The incidence of seizures is similar when comparing the two drugs [14].

Newer agents such as sirolimus and everolimus have been introduced to be used as either first line agents or calcineurin inhibitor (CNI) sparing agents in cases of neurotoxicity. Despite their similar appearing names, these medications are mammalian target of rapamycin (mTOR) inhibitors, not CNIs. There has not been any compelling evidence to suggest that sirolimus itself potentiates seizures. However, there have been few case reports of PRES associated with sirolimus, predominantly in association with hypertensive crises [15, 16].

In cases of neurotoxicity, the primary treatment strategy is reducing the dose or changing the offending agent [17, 13, 18]. This decision should not be taken lightly as it puts the transplanted organ at potential risk for rejection. Various strategies exist for restarting the antirejection transplant regimen including transitioning one CNI to another or an alternative agent such as an mTOR inhibitor or muromonab-CD3 (OKT3) [19]. OKT3 is a murine immunoglobulin monoclonal antibody that is rarely used today for very limited indications such as acute steroid-resistant rejection of allogenic renal, cardiac and liver transplant patients. Neurotoxicity is uncommon with the most commonly reported manifestation being the development of an aseptic meningitis within 72 h of administration [20]. It is in this context that seizures have, rarely, been reported.

Busulfan is commonly used to condition patients in preparation of hematopoietic stem cell transplantation. This agent has been frequently reported to cause seizures in HSCT patients. This complication typically occurs in the 3rd or 4th day of administration and appears to be dose dependent [21, 22]. Although hard evidence is lacking regarding seizure prophylaxis, it has become a generally accepted practice when initiating high-dose busulfan. This is complicated by the fact that the seizure prophylaxis must not have any interaction or toxicity with the conditioning regimen, interfere with the donor cells, or interact with other medications that the patient is receiving. Phenytoin is not an ideal agent for prevention of seizures in this setting due to the risk of toxicity and its ability to induce busulfan metabolism. Current data support the use of benzodiazepines such as clonazepam or lorazepam as seizure prophylaxis. Levetiracetam is another promising agent due to its limited drug–drug interactions and adverse effects.

A number of other agents, both chemotherapeutic and immunosuppressive, have been associated with seizures in transplant patients. Carmustine is a chemotherapeutic agent used in preparation of HSCT. This agent has been associated with seizures in a number of studies [23, 24]. Azathioprine and mycophenolate mofetil have also been associated with seizures in the post-transplant setting [25].

Many antibiotics used to treat infections in immunosuppressed patients are associated with reductions in seizure threshold. Quinolone antibiotics have a variable effect on the seizure threshold. Trovafloxacin has the greatest potential for seizure induction and levofloxacin has the lowest rate of seizure induction. Imipenem and meropenem have also been associated with seizures in prior studies [26, 27]. While the overall risk of seizures in these patients is low, close monitoring of transplant patients on these drugs is recommended [27] and they should probably be avoided entirely in patients with pre-existing epilepsy [28].

Post-transplant pain is often managed with opioid medications such as meperidine [29]. Meperidine has a high central nervous system depressant effect, however, its metabolite is normeperidine, which has twice the CNS neurotoxic effect of meperidine and is a CNS excitatory agent. Accumulation of normeperidine in the CNS can result in generalized seizures, myoclonus, tremors, and hyperreflexia. These effects cannot be reversed by opioid antagonists. Risk factors for meperidine related seizures include hepatic or renal dysfunction [30].

Management in the setting of drug-induced seizures is primarily cessation of the drug after which recurrent seizures are not expected. If seizures recur after the suspected causal drug has been discontinued and sufficient time to allow five half-lives of the drug has passed, an alternative cause for the seizures should be sought.

Acute Metabolic Change

An acute metabolic change should be considered in all patients with post-transplant seizures as in many cases, these disturbances are easily reversible. Metabolic disturbances can result from acute electrolyte imbalances in the early postoperative period. Delayed onset idiopathic hyperammonemia has also been reported and can result in refractory seizures, however, this rare complication is not easily reversible [31].

Hyponatremia and hypo-osmolality can contribute to seizures in the early postoperative period [32]. In one study of seizures in children who seized within 24 h following a kidney transplant, the patients with seizures had more pronounced shifts in sodium levels and serum osmolality that those without seizures [32]. Renal transplant patients are particularly prone to hyponatremia and shifts in serum osmolality due to their high rates of postoperative polyuria. This is due to renal tubular dysfunction and can be exacerbated by aggressive fluid resuscitation. Severe hyponatremia as a result of post-transplant polyuria can result in generalized tonic-clonic seizures [33]. Low sodium levels have also been associated with seizure events in cystic fibrosis patients following lung transplant [34] and rapid changes in sodium levels have been associated with seizures in liver transplant patients [35]. Treatment is often correction with hypertonic saline, however, care must be taken to not reverse the hyponatremia too quickly otherwise the patient will be at risk for the development of central pontine myelinolysis (CPM) [36, 37].

Hypomagnesemia is another well-established risk factor for seizures in the post-transplant population [35]. This is especially true in the liver transplant population where hypomagnesemia is an independent risk factor of seizures as well as in patients receiving small bowel transplants and HSCT [35, 38, 39]. Hypomagnesemia can potentiate the effects of drug-induced neurotoxicity [40] and can also result from cyclosporine induced renal wasting [41, 42]. Hypomagnesemia frequently presents with muscle weakness prior to its more serious manifestations such as behavioral changes and seizures. Reversal of the electrolyte deficiency is the only way to prevent further seizures in these patients.

Hypocalcemia is another side effect of CNIs such as cyclosporine. Like hypomagnesemia, it is due to increased excretion of the electrolyte in the urine. Hypocalcemia occurs with a nadir level at about one week post-transplant [43]. Hypocalcemia has been shown to be a predictor of PRES in patients with chronic kidney disease, including transplant patients [44].

Hypoglycemia induced seizures are also not uncommon and may be most likely to occur in patients receiving combined pancreas-renal transplants.

Idiopathic hyperammonemia is a rare complication in organ transplant recipients but is often devastating [31, 45]. This most commonly occurs while patients are severely neutropenic. Patients present with acute lethargy, confusion, seizures, and then progress to coma. Serologic evaluation demonstrates ammonia levels over 200 μmol/L with mild elevation of liver enzymes [45]. Patients with liver failure or who are receiving valproic acid can also experience high serum ammonia levels. Imaging evaluation of these patients demonstrates diffuse cerebral edema. There are no pharmacologic treatments for idiopathic hyperammonemia although some have reported success with lactulose, nonabsorbable antibiotics, dialysis or sodium benzoate for trapping, and removal of ammonia [31, 46].

CNS Infections

Infections most commonly occur one to six months following solid organ transplantation [47]. In the first month following the transplant, patients are at high risk for pneumonia or wound infection. Patients with hematopoietic stem cell transplant are at higher risk of opportunist infections in the first month as they are under maximal immunosuppression during this period. This is in contrast to solid organ transplant patients who are not on maximal therapy until about 1 month following the transplant. Beyond 6 months, patients who have not experienced rejection, poor graft function, or GVHD are generally given a lower dose of immunosuppressants and are thus at a lower risk for infectious complications. However, those who are maintained on high doses of immunosuppressant agent remain susceptible to many typical and opportunistic infections [47].

A CNS infection should be considered in any patient with headache, mental status changes, or seizure [47]. It is important to keep in mind that initial CSF studies may be underwhelming and even the imaging manifestations of a CNS infection may not be striking. Both the development of an inflammatory response in the CSF and formation of an abscess require a robust immune response; thus many of these patients may have only a mild CSF pleocytosis or a more phlegmon appearing lesion in their brain rather than an organized, diffusion restricting walled off fluid collection [47].

Bacterial infections account for a substantial proportion of infections in this population. Special consideration should be given to opportunistic infections such as Listeria and Nocardiosis. Nocardiosis presents as a pulmonary infection that is diagnosed with sputum, skin, or brain tissue and can present with a mass lesion. CNS involvement occurs in 50% of the cases and can present with fevers, meningismus, focal deficits, and seizures. It has been reported in <5% of renal transplant patients (1–6% of solid organ transplants [47–49]). Listeria presents with gastrointestinal symptoms, fevers, focal deficits, and seizures. Diagnosis is made by identification of gram positive bacilli in the CSF or blood.

Immunosuppressed patients are at high risk for opportunistic fungal infections such as aspergillosis, candidiasis, and cryptococcosis. All three of these fungal infections can present with disseminated pulmonary infiltrates and nodules while candida and cryptococcosis can also present in the lungs. These infections can manifest clinically as meningitis or with more focal symptoms suggestive of an abscess, both of which can lead to seizures [47]. Aspergillosis is unique in that it can present with septic and hemorrhagic infarctions. Presentation of fungal CNS infections includes encephalopathy (90%), focal neurological deficits (33%), seizures (40%), and meningeal signs (20%) [50]. Diagnosis depends on CSF and blood cultures and rarely, brain histology.

Opportunistic viral infections include herpes virus infections such as cytomegalovirus (CMV), Epstein–Barr virus (EBV), varicella-zoster virus (VZV), human herpes virus-6 (HHV-6), and herpes simplex virus (HSV) as well as JC virus induced progressive multifocal leukoencephalopathy (PML) [51]. These are generally the result of reactivation or primary infection and present with meningitis or limbic encephalitis. Mass lesions can be seen in the setting of EBV induced post-transplant lymphoproliferative disease (PTLD) as well as in the setting of JC induced PML [51]. These viral infections are diagnosed with CSF and blood culture as well as by identification of virus specific serologies or antibodies in the CSF. Treatments for herpes virus infections include acyclovir, ganciclovir or foscarnet, and cytarabine for PML. These infections are particularly a problem in HSCT recipients and can cause headache, confusion, and seizures several weeks after transplantation due to limbic encephalitis [51].

Other opportunistic infections that can affect organ transplant recipients include toxoplasmosis and tuberculosis. Toxoplasmosis can present with meningitis and abscess formation and is diagnosed with serology and CSF markers. Tuberculosis can present with basilar meningitis, abscess, "tuberculomas," and is diagnosed with CSF culture, smear, and serology [51].

One of the chief difficulties complicating the management of CNS infections is the interaction between many of the pharmacologic agents used to treat them with antirejection drugs and AEDs. For this reason, consulting a pharmacist and a careful risks/benefits may be helpful; however, adequate treatment of the infection must take priority over other considerations.

Post-transplant Malignancy

B-cell lymphoma and PTLD are the most common brain tumors seen in transplant recipients [52, 53]. These are most common after liver and small bowel transplants. PTLD is typically associated with EBV infection and should be considered in patients presenting with de novo seizures years following transplant (extreme cases 6 months posttransplantation have been reported. Lymphoma and PTLD in immunocompromised patients typically present with multiple periventricular ring enhancing lesions, similar to toxoplasmosis [52, 53]. Classically, increased uptake on SPECT or FDG/PET has been used to differentiate CNS lymphoma or PTLD from toxoplasmosis. In cases of high clinical suspicion, biopsy is recommended, followed by initiation of corticosteroids to reduce edema. In addition, reduction of immunosuppression therapy is advised [52, 53].

Posterior Reversible Encephalopathy Syndrome

PRES is a usually reversible neurologic syndrome of subcortical vasogenic brain edema in patients with acute neurologic symptoms (i.e., encephalopathy, headache, seizures, and visual disturbances) in the setting of renal failure, blood pressure fluctuations, autoimmune disorders, or cytotoxic drug administration (i.e., CNI therapy). PRES occurs in up to 2% of solid organ transplant recipients and up to 10% of patients receiving hematopoietic stem cell transplants [54, 55]. Most

cases of PRES occur within 30 days of transplant as it is during this time that derangements in drug levels, blood pressure, and other metabolic changes are most common [54–56]. However, late cases have been reported in renal transplant patients with malignant hypertension. Liver transplant patients are also at high risk of PRES due to blood–brain barrier disruption from hepatic encephalopathy [57]. Seizures occur in the majority of patients with PRES [54–56, 58]. One recent study demonstrated that up to half of seizures in heart transplants were attributable to PRES [59]. Seizures in the setting of PRES are typically generalized tonic-clonic seizures or less commonly, status epilepticus. EEG may show slowing, reflective of the encephalopathy, and periodic discharges, most frequently affecting the bioccipital regions. It is thought that a substantial proportion of CNI induced seizures are due to PRES [54, 55]. The diagnosis of PRES is generally made by a combination of both clinical and radiologic findings. Imaging is primarily useful to exclude alternative etiologies, but also often confirms the diagnosis. CT may show vasogenic primarily subcortical edema which is typically bilateral and asymmetric. MRI, particularly FLAIR/T2 sequences, is more sensitive for the demonstration of vasogenic edema (Fig. 15.1) and may also show areas of associated restricted diffusion. Associated intracranial hemorrhage is not incompatible with a diagnosis of PRES and is in fact present in 10–25% of cases. Kidney transplant patients tend to develop PRES later (>1 year) when compared with liver transplant patients [60]. Treatment of PRES is focused primarily on reversal of the underlying cause, whether that is CNI neurotoxicity, acute on chronic kidney injury, or hypertension [61]. The majority of cases resolve within 2 weeks.

Cerebrovascular Disease

Cerebrovascular diseases including ischemic infarctions and intracranial hemorrhages most commonly occur within the first month post-transplant. Because acute symptomatic seizures may complicate cerebrovascular events, prompt neuroimaging should be performed in all patients with new-onset seizure, especially those having focal neurological signs. Most studies quote a 2–4% incidence of these complications with higher rates in elderly patients and those with pretransplant diabetes. In cardiac and renal transplant recipients acute ischemic stroke can occur in up to 3–10%, and 8% of patients, respectively [62, 63]. In orthotopic heart transplant patients, 15% (12 of 82 consecutive patients) had seizures, with the most common etiology being postoperative stroke [64]. In kidney transplant patients, acute ischemic stroke tends to occur several years following transplant. Most poststroke seizures are focal and typically easily aborted with intravenous phenytoin, fosphenytoin, and valproic acid. However, status epilepticus can develop in 16–25% of all patients with poststroke seizures [65].

Acute hemorrhage is more common in patients who have undergone bone marrow or liver transplantation. Up to 7% of liver transplant patients suffer from acute cerebrovascular disease, a majority of which are hemorrhagic [66, 67]. There is often a concomitant coagulopathy due to the underlying liver disease. Hemorrhage typically occurs in the frontal and parietal lobes and less commonly in the subcortical areas. Intracranial hemorrhage secondary to thrombocytopenia and infarction or hemorrhage secondary to fungal infection can occur in up to 3% of BMT patients [65]. Cerebral venous thrombosis has also been reported in the HSCT population [68–70] and the most common presentation in those cases is seizures. The etiology and pathophysiology of this complication is unknown.

Seizures in Transplant Patients: Treatment

Goals of treatment in the acute setting were discussed previously and the management of status epilepticus is discussed in a separate chapter. Many of the etiologies discussed above are reversible upon cessation of the offending process (i.e., infection, hypertension, PRES, mass effect, etc.), and therefore do not require long-term AED therapy. However, there are some cases where long-term seizure control with AEDs is required. In patients who have recurrent seizures or a patient with a single seizure and a structural epileptogenic focus identified by neuroimaging, pharmacologic therapy should be initiated. Some patients can have their AEDs discontinued after 3 months without risk of recurrence, such as those with seizures in the setting of PRES. Patients with uncontrollable metabolic imbalances or structural CNS lesions may require even longer term AED therapy [5].

The primary considerations in selecting AEDs are efficacy and safety, in particular minimizing drug–drug interactions and effects on other organ systems. The pharmacokinetics and pharmacodynamics of AEDs and their effect on immunosuppressant agent metabolism need to be carefully considered. The ideal AEDs are those with minimal protein binding and minimal effects on induction or inhibition of drug metabolism pathways, especially among patients with liver transplants. For patients with renal transplants, AED agents may require dose adjustments due to variability in excretion. A number of AEDs have a more favorable profile in transplant patients with seizures and provide broad coverage in that they can treat both partial and generalized seizures.

Phenytoin and fosphenytoin are generally considered first line agents in the setting of recurrent seizures or status epilepticus. The benefit of these agents is that they are efficacious and can be loaded intravenously. Close blood pressure monitoring should be performed during administration of an IV load of these medications as they can cause hypotension. Also, it is important to consider that these agents can induce CNI metabolism which leads to lower doses of CNI and more vigilant titration of the agent is required to maintain therapeutic levels. Some transplant recipients may have hypoalbuminemia, and under those circumstances lower doses should be used as protein binding would be reduced. We advise that phenytoin levels be monitored by checking both free and total levels, as many of these patients have hypoalbuminemia and the total phenytoin level may not reflect the amount of free active drug.

Phenobarbital may be a good option in HSCT patients as it is one of a few AEDs that does not cause bone marrow suppression. Patients should be closely monitored during administration of a loading dose as it can be complicated by hypotension and respiratory depression. This agent can also interact with CNIs by inducing the CYP450 enzymes.

Valproate, which does not induce CYP450, was historically used to treat seizures in renal transplant patients, but is now discouraged due to the association with hepatic failure [5, 71]. This medication is also highly protein bound and lower doses should be considered in patients with reduced binding proteins. There have also been reports of valproic acid causing a coagulopathy by platelet dysfunction akin to von Willebrand disease and the drug should be avoided altogether in liver transplant recipients [72].

Levetiracetam has been gaining popularity for posttransplant seizures due to its broad spectrum efficacy and the fact that it is not extensively protein bound, or metabolized through the liver and lacks drug–drug interactions [71]. There is very sparse data on the efficacy of this medication in transplant recipients [73]. Levetiracetam can be taken orally or intravenously in patients of all ages and, when loaded, reaches therapeutic levels hours after the first dose. It does not affect CNI metabolism. Patients with impaired renal function may require a dosage decrease as it is primarily excreted through the urine [5]. It is also important to note that this medication is dialyzable and supplemental doses should be given after dialysis.

Lacosamide is another emerging option. It has been approved for refractory focal seizures and is available in both IV and oral formulations [74]. It has no known drug–drug interactions. It is primarily excreted in the urine and therefore must be renally dosed. Caution is advised in patients with severe cardiac disease or conduction defects and HSCT as it can cause PR prolongation, AV block, irregular atrial rhythms, and bone marrow suppression. Lacosamide has not been studied in the transplant patient population for monotherapy and its high cost may be preclusive in some patients (5).

If oral formulations are feasible, gabapentin and pregabalin may be considered. Similar to lacosamide these are approved for focal seizures and efficacy of monotherapy has not been established. The side effect profile is generally benign and does not cause any myelosuppression. They also require renal dosing as they are primarily excreted through urine. These agents do not have any known drug–drug interactions, are not heavily protein bound, and do not induce CYP450 enzymes.

Carbamazepine (CBZ) is generally not recommended as initial therapy. It can be used to treat focal seizures. It is heavily protein bound, and strongly induces CYP450 enzymes thereby lowering CNI levels. Close monitoring of CBZ levels should be considered in the first two weeks of administration as this agent has been known to undergo auto induction. Both 10,11 epoxide metabolite and CBZ levels should be performed in patients with liver failure if there is suspicion for medication toxicity as these patients can develop CBZ toxicity secondary to accumulation of the active metabolite despite normal CBZ levels. One of its notable side effects is hyponatremia secondary to SIADH which may be especially problematic in transplant recipients who are already pre-disposed to electrolyte disturbances. Oxcarbazepine is a structural derivative of carbamazepine and has similar indications as CBZ. It is a milder CYP450 inducer but has a higher risk of producing hyponatremia as compared with CBZ.

Topiramate, lamotrigine, and zonisamide may be considered in generalized and focal seizures. They all have hepatic metabolism. Topiramate has dose dependent liver enzyme inducing properties at doses above 200 mg. These agents should be used with caution given the potential for drug–drug interactions.

Seizures in Transplant Patients: Significance for Outcome

Although some studies suggest that seizures are associated with worse outcomes in HSCT and cardiac transplant recipients [3, 75, 76] one should consider that prognosis is dependent on a number of factors. Seizure duration, etiology, and failure to respond to the initial AED are each important factors impacting prognosis. A general principle is that patients with seizures resulting from CNS infection, cerebrovascular insults, or CNS malignancy will have worse outcomes than those with seizures resulting from drug toxicity or metabolic disturbances. This was demonstrated in previous studies on HSCT and liver recipients [77, 78]. Post-transplant seizures should be considered in context and rarely should influence decision about goals of care unless they are truly treatment refractory as can be the case with delayed onset idiopathic hyperammonemia.

References

1. Adams Jr HP et al. Stroke in renal transplant recipients. Arch Neurol. 1986;43(2):113–5.
2. Bhatt VR et al. Central nervous system complications and outcomes after allogeneic hematopoietic stem cell transplantation. Clin Lymphoma, Myeloma Leuk. 2015;15(10):606–11.
3. Zhang XH et al. Epileptic seizures in patients following allogeneic hematopoietic stem cell transplantation: a retrospective analysis of incidence, risk factors, and survival rates. Clin Transplant. 2013; 27(1):80–9.
4. Lowenstein DH, Alldredge BK. Status epilepticus. N Engl J Med. 1998;338(14):970–6.
5. Shepard PW, St Louis EK. Seizure treatment in transplant patients. Curr Treat Options Neurol. 2012;14(4):332–47.
6. Moini M, Schilsky ML, Tichy EM. Review on immunosuppression in liver transplantation. World J Hepatol. 2015;7(10):1355–68.
7. Zivkovic SA. Neurologic complications after liver transplantation. World J Hepatol. 2013;5(8):409–16.
8. Pless M, Zivkovic SA. Neurologic complications of transplantation. The Neurologist. 2002;8(2):107–20.
9. Dhar R, Human T. Central nervous system complications after transplantation. Neurol Clin. 2011;29(4):943–72.
10. Butterworth RF. Pathogenesis of hepatic encephalopathy and brain edema in acute liver failure. J Clin Exp Hepatol. 2015;5(Suppl 1):S96–S103.
11. Zivkovic SA, Abdel-Hamid H. Neurologic manifestations of transplant complications. Neurol Clin. 2010;28(1):235–51.
12. van Gelder T, van Schaik RH, Hesselink DA. Pharmacogenetics and immunosuppressive drugs in solid organ transplantation. Nat Rev Nephrol. 2014;10(12):725–31.
13. Wijdicks EF et al. FK506-induced neurotoxicity in liver transplantation. Ann Neurol. 1994;35(4):498–501.
14. Kelly PA, Burckart GJ, Venkataramanan R. Tacrolimus: a new immunosuppressive agent. Am J Health-System Pharm: AJHP: Off J Am Soc of Health-System Pharmacists. 1995;52(14):1521–35.
15. Moskowitz A et al. Posterior reversible encephalopathy syndrome due to sirolimus. Bone Marrow Transplant. 2007;39(10):653–4.
16. Qin W et al. Rapamycin-induced posterior reversible encephalopathy in a kidney transplantation patient. Int Urol Nephrol. 2011;43(3):913–6.
17. Small SL et al. Immunosuppression-induced leukoencephalopathy from tacrolimus (FK506). Ann Neurol. 1996;40(4):575–80.
18. Wijdicks EF, Wiesner RH, Krom RA. Neurotoxicity in liver transplant recipients with cyclosporine immunosuppression. Neurology. 1995;45(11):1962–4.
19. Jimenez-Perez M et al. Efficacy and safety of monotherapy with mycophenolate mofetil in liver transplantation. Transplant Proc. 2006;38(8):2480–1.
20. Martin MA et al. Nosocomial aseptic meningitis associated with administration of OKT3. JAMA. 1988;259(13):2002–5.
21. De La Camara R et al. High dose busulfan and seizures. Bone Marrow Transplant. 1991;7(5):363–4.
22. Murphy CP, Harden EA, Thompson JM. Generalized seizures secondary to high-dose busulfan therapy. Ann Pharmacother. 1992;26(1):30–1.
23. Snider S, Bashir R, Bierman P. Neurologic complications after high-dose chemotherapy and autologous bone marrow transplantation for Hodgkin's disease. Neurology. 1994;44(4):681–4.
24. Ferrucci PF et al. Evaluation of acute toxicities associated with autologous peripheral blood progenitor cell reinfusion in patients undergoing high-dose chemotherapy. Bone Marrow Transplant. 2000;25(2):173–7.
25. Melvin JJ, Huntley Hardison H. Immunomodulatory treatments in epilepsy. Semin Pediatr Neurol. 2014;21(3):232–7.
26. Vaughn BV et al. Seizures in lung transplant recipients. Epilepsia. 1996;37(12):1175–9.
27. Turhal NS. Cyclosporin A and imipenem associated seizure activity in allogeneic bone marrow transplantation patients. J Chemother. 1999;11(5):410–3.
28. Kushner JM, Peckman HJ, Snyder CR. Seizures associated with fluoroquinolones. Ann Pharmacother. 2001;35(10):1194–8.
29. Lee SH et al. Prospective, randomized study of ropivacaine wound infusion versus intrathecal morphine with intravenous fentanyl for analgesia in living donors for liver transplantation. Liver Transplant: Off Publ Am Assoc Study Liver Dis Int Liver Transplant Soc. 2013;19(9):1036–45.

30. Eker HE et al. Meperidine induced seizure in a patient with lyme borreliosis. J Clin Med Res. 2009;1(5):302–4.

31. Hocker S, Rabinstein AA, Wijdicks EF. Pearls & oy-sters: status epilepticus from hyperammonemia after lung transplant. Neurology. 2011;77(10):e54–6.

32. Drake K, Nehus E, Goebel J. Hyponatremia, hypo-osmolality, and seizures in children early post-kidney transplant. Pediatr Transplant. 2015;19(7):698–703.

33. Montas SM et al. More is not always better: a case postrenal transplant large volume diuresis, hyponatremia, and postoperative seizure. Transplant Int: Off J Eur Soc Organ Transplant. 2006;19(1):85–6.

34. Goldstein AB et al. Cystic fibrosis patients with and without central nervous system complications following lung transplantation. Pediatr Pulmonol. 2000;30(3):203–6.

35. Pinero F et al. Neurological events after liver transplantation: a single-center experience. Transplant Int: Off J Eur Soc Organ Transplant. 2014;27(12):1244–52.

36. Wszolek ZK et al. Pontine and extrapontine myelinolysis following liver transplantation. Relationship to serum sodium. Transplantation. 1989;48(6):1006–12.

37. Crivellin C et al. Risk factors for central pontine and extrapontine myelinolysis after liver transplantation: a single-center study. Transplantation. 2015;99(6):1257–64.

38. Philibert D et al. Incidence and severity of early electrolyte abnormalities following autologous haematopoietic stem cell transplantation. Nephrol Dial Transplant: Off Publ Eur Dial Transplant Assoc - Eur Renal Assoc. 2008;23(1):359–63.

39. Beier UH et al. Electrolyte imbalances in pediatric living related small bowel transplantation. Transplantation. 2008;85(2):217–23.

40. Al-Rasheed AK et al. Cyclosporine A neurotoxicity in a patient with idiopathic renal magnesium wasting. Pediatr Neurol. 2000;23(4):353–6.

41. Lee CH, Kim GH. Electrolyte and acid-base disturbances induced by clacineurin inhibitors. Electrolyte & Blood Pressure: E & BP. 2007;5(2):126–30.

42. Wijdicks EF. Neurotoxicity of immunosuppressive drugs. Liver Transplant: Off Publ Am Assoc Study Liver Dis Int Liver Transplant Soc. 2001;7(11):937–42.

43. Nobata H et al. Hypocalcemia immediately after renal transplantation. Clin Transplant. 2013;27(6):E644–8.

44. Gera DN et al. Posterior reversible encephalopathy syndrome in children with kidney disease. Indian J Nephrol. 2014;24(1):28–34.

45. Uygun V et al. Idiopathic hyperammonemia after hematopoietic stem cell transplantation: a case report. Pediatr Transplant. 2015;19(4):E104–5.

46. Matoori S, Leroux JC. Recent advances in the treatment of hyperammonemia. Adv Drug Delivery Rev. 2015;90:55–68.

47. Wright AJ, Fishman JA. Central nervous system syndromes in solid organ transplant recipients. Clin Infect Dis: Off Publ Infect Dis Soc Am. 2014;59(7):1001–11.

48. Chapman SW, Wilson JP. Nocardiosis in transplant recipients. Semin Respir infect. 1990;5(1):74–9.

49. Clark NM, Reid GE. Nocardia infections in solid organ transplantation. Am J Transplant: Off J Am Soc Transplant Am Soc Transplant Surg. 2013;13(Suppl 4):83–92.

50. Torre-Cisneros J et al. CNS aspergillosis in organ transplantation: a clinicopathological study. J Neurol Neurosurg Psychiatry. 1993;56(2):188–93.

51. Cohen BA, Stosor V. Opportunistic infections of the central nervous system in the transplant patient. Curr Neurol Neurosci Rep. 2013;13(9):376.

52. Al-Mansour Z, Nelson BP, Evens AM. Post-transplant lymphoproliferative disease (PTLD): risk factors, diagnosis, and current treatment strategies. Curr Hematol Malig Rep. 2013;8(3):173–83.

53. Korfel A, Schlegel U. Diagnosis and treatment of primary CNS lymphoma. Nat Rev Neurol. 2013;9(6):317–27.

54. Masetti R et al. PRES in children undergoing hematopoietic stem cell or solid organ transplantation. Pediatrics. 2015;135(5):890–901.

55. Potluri K, Holt D, Hou S. Neurologic complications in renal transplantation. Handb Clin Neurol. 2014;121:1245–55.

56. Heroux A, Pamboukian SV. Neurologic aspects of heart transplantation. Handb Clin Neurol. 2014;121:1229–36.

57. Chavarria L, Cordoba J. Encephalopathy and liver transplantation. Metab Brain Dis. 2013;28(2):285–92.

58. Cruz Jr RJ et al. Posterior reversible encephalopathy syndrome in liver transplant patients: clinical presentation, risk factors and initial management. Am J Transplant Off J Am Transplant Am Soc Transplant Surg. 2012;12(8):2228–36.

59. Navarro V et al. Incidence and risk factors for seizures after heart transplantation. J Neurol. 2010;257(4):563–8.

60. Bartynski WS et al. Posterior reversible encephalopathy syndrome after solid organ transplantation. AJNR Am J Neuroradiol. 2008;29(5):924–30.

61. Fugate JE, Rabinstein AA. Posterior reversible encephalopathy syndrome: clinical and radiological manifestations, pathophysiology, and outstanding questions. The Lancet Neurol. 2015;14(9):914–25.

62. Kim JM et al. Central nervous system complications after liver transplantation. J Clin Neurosci: Off J Neurosurg Soc Australas. 2015;22(8):1355–9.

63. Mour G, Wu C. Neurologic complications after kidney transplantation. Semin Nephrol. 2015;35(4):323–34.

64. Grigg MM et al. The etiology of seizures after cardiac transplantation. Transplant Proc. 1988;20(3 Suppl 3):937–44.

65. Coplin WM et al. Stroke after bone marrow transplantation: frequency, aetiology and outcome. Brain J Neurol. 2001;124(Pt 5):1043–51.

66. Wijdicks EF et al. Intracerebral hemorrhage in liver transplant recipients. Mayo Clin Proc. 1995;70(5):443–6.

67. Guarino M et al. EFNS guidelines on management of neurological problems in liver transplantation. Eur J Neurol: Off J Eur Fed Neurolog Soc. 2006;13(1):2–9.

68. Harvey CJ et al. MR angiographic diagnosis of cerebral venous sinus thrombosis following allogeneic bone marrow transplantation. Bone Marrow Transplant. 2000;25(7):791–5.

69. Motohashi K et al. Cerebral venous sinus thrombosis after allogeneic stem cell transplantation. Int J Hematol. 2010;91(1):154–6.

70. Bertz H et al. Sinus venous thrombosis: an unusual cause for neurologic symptoms after bone marrow transplantation under immunosuppression. Transplantation. 1998;66(2):241–4.

71. Chabolla DR, Wszolek ZK. Pharmacologic management of seizures in organ transplant. Neurology. 2006;67(12 Suppl 4):S34–8.

72. Kreuz W et al. Valproate therapy induces von Willebrand disease type I. Epilepsia. 1992;33(1):178–84.

73. Glass GA et al. Levetiracetam for seizures after liver transplantation. Neurology. 2005;64(6):1084–5.

74. Ben-Menachem E et al. Efficacy and safety of oral lacosamide as adjunctive therapy in adults with partial-onset seizures. Epilepsia. 2007;48(7):1308–17.

75. Cordelli DM et al. Etiology, characteristics and outcome of seizures after pediatric hematopoietic stem cell transplantation. Seizure. 2014;23(2):140–5.

76. van de Beek D et al. Effect of neurologic complications on outcome after heart transplant. Arch Neurol. 2008;65(2):226–31.

77. Wijdicks EF et al. Causes and outcome of seizures in liver transplant recipients. Neurology. 1996;47(6):1523–5.

78. Choi EJ et al. New-onset seizures after liver transplantation: clinical implications and prognosis in survivors. Eur Neurol. 2004;52(4):230–6.

79. Saner FH et al. Severe neurological events following liver transplantation. Arch Med Res. 2007;38(1):75–9.

80. Dhar R, Young GB, Marotta P. Perioperative neurological complications after liver transplantation are best predicted by pretransplant hepatic encephalopathy. Neurocrit care. 2008;8(2):253–8.

81. Bronster DJ et al. Central nervous system complications in liver transplant recipients–incidence, timing, and long-term follow-up. Clin Transplant. 2000;14(1):1–7.

82. Lewis MB, Howdle PD. Neurologic complications of liver transplantation in adults. Neurology. 2003;61(9):1174–8.

83. Denier C et al. Spectrum and prognosis of neurologic complications after hematopoietic transplantation. Neurology. 2006;67(11):1990–7.

84. Siegal D et al. Central nervous system complications after allogeneic hematopoietic stem cell transplantation: incidence, manifestations, and clinical significance. Biol Blood Marrow Transplant J Am Soc Blood Marrow Transplant. 2007;13(11):1369–79.

85. Sostak P et al. Prospective evaluation of neurological complications after allogeneic bone marrow transplantation. Neurology. 2003;60(5):842–8.

86. Munoz P et al. Infectious and non-infectious neurologic complications in heart transplant recipients. Medicine. 2010;89(3):166–75.

87. Mayer TO et al. Contrasting the neurologic complications of cardiac transplantation in adults and children. J Child Neurol. 2002;17(3):195–9.

88. Zierer A et al. Significance of neurologic complications in the modern era of cardiac transplantation. Ann Thorac Surg. 2007;83(5):1684–90.

89. Yardimci N et al. Neurologic complications after renal transplant. Exp Clin Transplant: Off J Middle East Soc Organ Transplant. 2008;6(3):224–8.

90. Mateen FJ et al. Neurological complications following adult lung transplantation. Am J Transplant. 2010;10(4):908–14.

91. Goldstein LS et al. Central nervous system complications after lung transplantation. J Heart Lung Transplant Off Publ Int Soc Heart Transplant. 1998;17(2):185–91.

92. Kiok MC. Neurologic complications of pancreas transplants. Neurol Clin. 1988;6(2):367–76.

93. Zivkovic SA et al. The clinical spectrum of neurologic disorders after intestinal and multivisceral transplantation. Clin Transplant. 2010;24(2):164–8.

Extreme Hypertension, Eclampsia, and Critical Care Seizures

16

Michel T. Torbey

Introduction

"Most physicians are familiar with the syndrome of a sudden elevation of blood pressure, preceded by a severe headache, and followed by convulsions, coma, or a variety of transitory cerebral phenomena. The pediatrician faces the problem with acute nephritis, the obstetrician with toxemia of pregnancy, and the internist with hypertensive vascular disease." [1]

Seizures have been reported in both chronic and acute hypertension [2]. The association between hypertension and seizure occurrence is unclear. In chronic hypertension, seizures may be secondary to the effect of blood pressure elevation on the cerebral blood vessels and its association with higher risk of stroke. In acute hypertension, seizures may be secondary to disruption of blood–brain barrier and secondary cerebral edema. In a population based study from Rochester, Minnesota, 195 patients ≥55 years old with first unprovoked seizures were matched on age, gender, and duration of follow-up with patients without seizures [3]. Blood pressure was obtained in the seizure patients before the first seizure occurrence. Overall, hypertension did not increase the risk of seizures, but the study found that a subgroup with left ventricular hypertrophy (LVH), a marker of severe, long standing hypertension, without diuretic treatment had an 11-fold increased risk of unprovoked seizures. Interestingly, those patients with LVH treated with diuretics did not have an increased risk. This chapter will review the different acute hypertensive syndromes encountered in the ICU and emphasize the specific management of seizures associated with these disorders.

M.T. Torbey (✉)
Neurology and Neurosurgery Department, Cerebrovascular and Neurocritical Care Division, The Ohio State University College of Medicine, 395 W. 12th Avenue, 7th Floor, Columbus, OH 43210, USA
e-mail: michel.torbey@osumc.edu

Hypertension and Pregnancy

Hypertensive disorders of pregnancy are common, affecting 7–15% of pregnant women [4]. In the UK, 18.6% of maternal deaths are caused by hypertensive diseases [5]. Four hypertensive disorders are commonly reported in pregnant women: (1) pre-eclampsia (PREC)—eclampsia (EC); (2) chronic hypertension (of any cause); (3) chronic hypertension with superimposed PREC; and (4) gestational hypertension [6]. Only PREC and EC are associated with seizures.

Pre-eclampsia and Eclampsia

Hippocrates was among the first to recognize fits occurring in pregnant women as early as the 4th century BC [7]. This condition was coined eclampsia—a Greek word meaning "shine forth"—implying a sudden development [8]. Pre-eclampsia and eclampsia are among the most common causes of maternal and fetal morbidity and mortality. In a retrospective review of 4024 pregnancy related deaths, 19.6% were related to PREC-EC [9].

According to the new American College of Obstetricians and Gynecologists (ACOG) guidelines the diagnosis of PREC no longer requires the detection of high levels of proteinuria. Pre-eclampsia is diagnosed as hypertension in association with thrombocytopenia, impaired liver function, the new development of renal insufficiency, pulmonary edema, or new-onset cerebral or visual disturbances [6]. Eclampsia is defined as the presence of new-onset grand mal in pre-eclamptic woman. Eclampsia can occur before, during, or after labor. Although EC is usually preceded by PREC, in up to 38% of cases it can occur without symptoms or signs of PREC [8]. Table 16.1 summarizes the definitions of both PREC and EC.

Table 16.1 Definition of PREC and EC

PREC defined as:
Blood pressure
Greater than or equal to 140 mmHg systolic or greater than or equal to 90 mmHg diastolic on two occasions at least 4 h apart after 20 weeks of gestation in a woman with previously normal blood pressure
Greater than or equal to 160 mmHg systolic or greater than or equal to 110 mmHg diastolic and
Proteinuria (>300 mg/24 h or 1+ in dipstick testing) or
Protein/creatinine ratio greater than or equal to 0.3
Dipstick reading of 1+
Or in the absence of proteinuria new-onset hypertension with the new onset of any of the following:
Thrombocytopenia: Platelet count less than 100,000/microliter
Renal insufficiency: Serum creatinine greater than 1.1 mg/dl or doubling of the serum creatinine concentration in the absence of other renal disease
Impaired liver function: elevated blood concentration of liver transaminases to twice normal concentration
Pulmonary edema
Cerebral or visula symptoms
<100,000/μL or increased aspartate or alanine transaminase
Eclampsia
Presence of seizures

Table 16.2 Specific causes of death among pre-eclampsia or eclampsia

Cause of Death	Pre-eclampsia(%)	Eclampsia (%)
Intracerebral hemorrhage	15.8	18.8
Cerebral edema	1.1	1.8
Cerebral embolism	0.4	0.8
Renal or hepatic Failure	7.2	5.4
HELLP Syndrome	4.8	2.3
Other	13.9	11.8

Adapted from [9]

placenta, kidneys, and brain [15]. A recent hypothesis by Odent [16] proposed that PREC could be the result of maternal-fetal conflict. The developing fetal brain requires EPA, a long chain n-3 polyunsaturated fatty acid. The theory suggests that the fetus need for EPA override the maternal need. A decrease in maternal EPA in PREC and EC women as compared to their normotensive counterparts appears to play a role in the development of this condition [16]. Other mechanisms suggested for eclamptic convulsions include cerebral vasospasm, hemorrhage or edema, metabolic or hypertensive encephalopathy [17].

Epidemiology

Pre-eclampsia affects up to 7% of pregnancies and <1% of these women develop EC [10]. Approximately 1 in 50 women experiencing eclamptic seizures will die annually from complications [11]. In a prospective survey of EC in the United Kingdom (UK), the incidence of EC was 4.9/1000 [12]. The leading cause of death with PREC-EC patients is cerebrovascular accidents particularly intracerebral hemorrhages. The mortality rate ranges from 2 to 24%. Table 16.2 summarizes the specific causes of death associated with EC and PREC. The case fatality in women with eclampsia is 71 per 10,000 [9]. Although the incidence of PREC has not changed significantly over the past 6 decades, the rate of major complications from the disease has been on a marked decline [13].

Several risk factors for EC have been identified. Those include prima gravidity, lack of prenatal care, urinary tract infections, family history, diabetes mellitus, multiple gestation, extremes of age, obesity, black ethnicity, preexisting hypertension, vascular renal disease, prolonged labor, and hydatidiform moles [10, 14].

Pathophysiology

To date, the underlying pathophysiology of EC is still not fully elucidated but vascular endothelial damage or dysfunction appears to be the common pathological feature in the

Clinical Presentation

By definition, EC is characterized by the presence of seizures. They can occur before, during, or after labor [18]. Antepartum EC refers to the onset of seizures before the start of labor. Intrapartum EC refers to seizures that occur during labor, and postpartum EC is the occurrence of seizures within 7 days of delivery of the fetus and placenta. Two percent of EC occur more than 7 days past delivery [19]. In some women seizures can occur as late as 11 days [20]. In the USA, 53% of women had antepartum seizures, 36% intrapartum seizures, and 11% postpartum seizures [19]. In the UK 38% had antepartum seizures, 18% intrapartum seizures, and 44% postpartum eclampsia [12].

The syndrome may also be associated with headaches, visual complaints, epigastric pain, oliguria, depression of consciousness, thrombocytopenia, fetal growth retardation, and elevated liver enzymes.

Electrographic and Radiographic Features

Abnormal EEGs are reported with PREC [21]. Diffuse slow activity (theta or delta waves) sometimes with focal slow activity is usually found on EEG [21]. Paroxysmal spike activity has been reported but this is not pathognomonic of PREC as similar patterns are found in other conditions [21]. No correlation was found between EEG abnormalities and the degree of maternal arterial blood pressure [21].

The radiological features found in EC patients are certainly not unique. Diffuse cerebral edema [22], hemorrhages [23], and infarcts [24] have been demonstrated in patients with EC using computed tomography (CT) scan. Magnetic resonance image (MRI) studies of brain of EC patients revealed focal changes characteristic of ischemia [25]. MRI features consistent with reversible posterior leukoencephalopathy have also been reported [26].

Management

Early detection remains the mainstay of treatment in EC patients. The best treatment for PREC and EC is delivery. If delivery is not possible, then management of the patient should include hospitalization, close observation, and seizure prophylaxis until delivery can safely be performed. In a review of obstetric patients admitted to a medical-surgical ICU in a large tertiary referral center over a 5-year period PREC was the single most common diagnosis representing 22 percent of all patients [27].

Over the last two decades magnesium has emerged as the drug of choice for preventing eclampsia. Large randomized trials and systematic reviews have shown the usefulness of magnesium sulfate in treating recurrent eclamptic seizures and in the prophylaxis of EC [28, 29].

In 1995 the Eclampsia Trial Collaborative Group showed unequivocally that magnesium given intramuscularly or intravenously is superior to phenytoin or diazepam in reducing recurrent eclamptic seizures [29]. This international multicenter randomized study included 1687 women with EC. The women allocated to magnesium sulfate therapy had a 52% (95% C.l. 64% to 37%) reduction in incidence of recurrent seizures compared to those given diazepam (13.2% vs. 27.9%). Maternal and perinatal morbidity were comparable between the two groups. In a second comparison between magnesium sulfate and phenytoin, the women randomized to receive magnesium sulfate had a 67% (95% C.I. 79–97%) reduced incidence of recurrent seizures (5.7% vs. 17.1%). Maternal mortality was non-significantly lower in the magnesium group compared with the phenytoin group [26]. Women who received magnesium were also less likely to be ventilated when compared to phenytoin (14.9% vs. 22.5%). The women in the magnesium group were also less likely to develop pneumonia (3.9% vs. 8.8%) and be less likely to be admitted to the ICU (16.7% vs. 25.1%) when compared to phenytoin.

The Magpie study, another randomized placebo-controlled trial, was designed to assess the value of magnesium for prophylaxis in EC [30]. The study included 10,000 women with PREC who were randomized to receive magnesium sulfate before or during labor, or after giving birth [30]. Magnesium was effective in reducing seizures 58% (95% C.I. 40–71%). Treatment was also safe for the neonate in this setting, and without any excess of serious maternal morbidity. Of the 5055 women who were randomized in the magnesium and the placebo groups 46 (0.9%) had respiratory depression and 5 (0.1%) had respiratory arrest in the magnesium group compared to 27 (0.5%) and 2 (0.04%) in the placebo group, respectively [30]. Respiratory arrest was responsible for one death in each group. 14 (0.3%) developed pneumonia in the magnesium group compared to 6 (0.1%) in the placebo group [30].

Another multicenter randomized unblinded study compared magnesium to calcium channel blocker nimodipine, a cerebral vasodilator to prevent EC [30]. PREC women who received nimodipine were more likely to have a seizure than those who received magnesium sulfate (2.6% vs. 0.8%, $p = 0.01$). The antepartum risk for EC did not differ between the two treatment arms, but the nimodipine arm had a higher risk of postpartum seizures (1.1% vs. 0%, $p = 0.01$). Neonatal outcomes did not differ between the two groups [30].

Similar results were reported in a Cochrane review analysis that included published randomized studies between magnesium and placebo or anti-epileptics [29]. The reviewers concluded from six studies that magnesium sulfate more than halves the risk of eclampsia, and probably reduces the risk of maternal death. A quarter of women had side effects, particularly flushing. Risk of placental abruption was reduced for women allocated magnesium sulfate (RR 0.64, 95% C.l. 0.5–0.8). Women allocated to magnesium sulfate had a small non-significant increase (5%) in the risk of caesarean section. Magnesium sulfate was better than phenytoin and nimodipine in reducing the risk of eclampsia, but with an increased risk of caesarean section (RR l.2, 95% C.I. 1.05–1.4). The summary of the Cochrane review is detailed in Table 16.3.

The most commonly used magnesium protocol in EC is 4–6 g IV bolus over 5 min, followed by 1–2 g/h IV infusion for at least 48 hours postpartum. If the treatment is used prophylactically in PREC, it can be stopped after 24 h [10]. Half this dose should be used in patients with serum creatinine more than 1.3 mg/dL [10].

Patients should be admitted to an intensive care unit and be monitored closely, particularly respirations, patellar reflexes, and urine output. Magnesium is known to affect the neuromuscular junction but it should not have any deleterious effect on a patient's mental status. If patellar reflexes are lost the next magnesium dose should be held and the magnesium level should be checked. It may be restarted at a lower dose

Table 16.3 Effect of magnesium on risk of eclampsia

Magnesium sulfate vs	Relative risk (95% CI)
Placebo [57]	0.41 (0.29–0.59)
Phenytoin [29]	0.05 (0–0.84)
Nimodipine [30]	0.33 (0.14–0.77)

when the reflexes return if still desired. If the urine output falls below 25 cc/hr., then the rate of infusion of magnesium or the IM dose should be cut into half. In case of respiratory depression or arrest the patient airway must be first secured (by endotracheal intubation if needed) and one gram of calcium gluconate (10% solution) should be administered IV.

In patients with refractory seizures several anticonvulsant regimens can be used. An additional dose 1–2 g IV of Mg can be given or a loading dose of phenytoin (18 mg/kg IV at a maximum rate of 50 mg/min) can be tried. A dark room with low noise, padded bed nails, and continuous fetal monitoring are additional measures.

HELLP Syndrome

Pritchard et al. first described the association between coagulation and liver enzymes abnormalities with PREC [31]. In 1982, Weinstein coined this syndrome of hemolysis (anemia, increase bilirubin schistocytes in blood smear), elevated liver enzymes, and a low platelet count (<100,000/mm³), as the HELLP syndrome [32]. It complicates up to 10% of eclamptic cases [17, 33]. Mortality resulting from HELLP syndrome ranges from 2 to 24% of cases [9]. Management of seizures in patients with HELLP syndrome is similar to EC patients. Magnesium should be initiated at seizure onset. Although no specific data exist regarding seizures, antepartum administration of corticosteroids (dexamethasone 10 mg every 13 h until delivery) has been shown in randomized trials to stabilize and improve the laboratory values and clinical status of the mother and potentially the fetus [34]. The increase in liver enzymes may limit the use of some anticonvulsants such as phenytoin, carbamazepine, and or valproic acid. Levetiracetam (Keppra©) may be used as a second line agent or as a second agent if magnesium failed to stop the seizures. Keppra can be started as 500 mg PO given every 12 h and may be increased to a maximum dose of 3000 mg/day. If patients develop status epilepticus, then phenobarbital or pentobarbital can be used as a therapeutic option. More details regarding treatment of seizures in patients with liver dysfunction can be found in the chapters on Treatment of Critical Care Seizures and SE.

Hypertensive Encephalopathy

Hypertensive encephalopathy (HE) is a complex cerebral disorder that is associated with a variety of conditions in which systemic BP rises acutely. The term was first coined by Oppenheimer and Fishberg in 1928 [35] and is defined as generalized or focal cerebral dysfunction that either partially or completely reverses with antihypertensive treatment [36].

Epidemiology

Hypertension is a prevalent disorder involving 20–30% of adults in developed countries [37]. The definition of hypertension remains controversial. In the UK, hypertension is defined as blood pressure more than 160/100 mmHg on two or more clinic readings whereas in the USA the cutoff is 140/90 mmHg. Although improved treatment of chronic hypertension has led to a reduction in the incidence of hypertensive emergencies [38], the recognition and treatment of hypertension in the general population are still not adequate [39].

Clinical Features

Hypertensive encephalopathy is characterized by acute or subacute onset of lethargy, confusion, visual disturbances, and seizures [2]. Other symptoms may include headache, stroke, and or papilledema [36]. Symptoms may or may not be associated with proteinuria or hypertensive retinopathy [2]. Seizures are often the initial presentation and they may be focal, generalized, or focal with secondary generalization [2]. Initially, it was thought that the cerebral dysfunction associated with elevated blood pressure was related to the uremia from kidney disease [40]. Table 16.4 summarizes the frequency of each of the presenting symptoms.

Pathophysiology

The endothelium plays an active role in controlling blood pressure by regulating the release of nitric oxide (NO) and other vasodilator molecules [2, 41]. Although the pathophysiology of HE is not fully understood, an initial abrupt rise in vascular resistance seems to be a necessary initiating step [2]. The sheer stress on the endothelial wall results in an initial burst of nitric oxide (NO) followed by steady release of NO promoting vasodilatation [2, 42]. If the blood pressure remains elevated the compensatory mechanism may fail

Table 16.4 Presenting symptoms of patients admitted with malignant hypertension

Symptoms	N (%)
Headache	10 (30)
Stroke	9 (27)
Cardiorespiratory	7 (21)
Altered mental status	4 (13)
Blurred vision	3 (9)
Seizures	3 (9)
Loss of consciousness	3 (9)
Dizziness	1 (3)
Asymptomatic	1 (3)

Adapted from reference [36]

causing more elevation in blood pressure and endothelial damage. A cascade follows which increases endothelial cell expression of adhesion molecules and makes the endothelium more permeable [2]. Ultimately, the endothelial fibrinolytic activity may be inhibited and the coagulation cascade activated.

Cerebral blood flow (CBF) is regulated through a homeostatic mechanism referred to as autoregulation. Normotensive individuals maintain persistent CBF when their mean arterial pressure (MAP) stays in a range of 60–120 [2]. Hyperperfusion of the cerebral vasculature is blunted by a compensatory vasoconstriction of the blood vessels. This compensatory mechanism is overwhelmed at MAP of 180 mmHg and cerebral autoregulation breaks down and vasodilatation occurs. This results in breakdown of the blood–brain barrier (BBB), which causes edema and possible microinfarcts. Previously normotensive patients can develop signs of HE at blood pressures as low as 160/100 mmHg, whereas individuals with chronic hypertension will tolerate pressure as high as 220/110 mmHg before signs of HE ensue.

Electrographic and Radiographic features

Currently, there is no known characteristic electroencephalographic feature of HE. Loss of posterior dominant alpha rhythm, generalized slowing, and posterior epileptiform discharges are seen on EEG. These findings usually resolve following the clinical improvement [43, 44].

Imaging of the brain in a hypertensive confused, lethargic patient who develops seizures in the ICU is crucial. Although the clinical presentation of HE is characteristic, the intensivist cannot exclude the presence of intracranial hemorrhage or other mass (especially if there are focal neurological signs present) which induces the elevation of systemic blood pressure as a compensatory mechanism for cerebral perfusion. This is indeed a very common situation with ischemic or hemorrhage stroke and many times it is unclear if it is the cause or the effect.

In uncomplicated cases cerebral imaging of individuals with HE shows edema in the cortex and sub-cortical white matter in the posterior areas of the brain, i.e., the occipital, the posterior parietal, and temporal lobes [45]. The predilection for involvement of posterior circulation may be due to paucity of sympathetic neural control in the posterior cerebral artery territory compared to the carotid artery territory [46]. Schwartz et al. findings of increased apparent diffusion coefficient (ADC) values and lack of high signal on the diffusion-weighted images support the theory that the edema associated with HE is vasogenic [45].

Management of Hypertensive Encephalopathy

Patients should be admitted to an intensive care unit (NICU) for treatment and monitoring. An arterial line for continuous pressure monitoring should be placed immediately. If cerebral edema was present on the initial head CT and the patient has a Glasgow coma score ≤8, an intracranial pressure monitoring device should be placed. It is important to obtain a thorough past medical history for previous CVAs and renal disease. One should also inquire about antihypertensive medications and compliance. It is also paramount to ask for over-the-counter medication use (i.e., sympathomimetics) and illicit drugs, such as cocaine (need to obtain a urine toxicology screen).

The goal of therapy in HE is to gradually decrease the MAP by approximately 25% or to reduce the diastolic BP to about 100 mmHg over a period of several minutes to hours. Precipitous reduction in BP to normotensive or hypotensive level should be avoided, as it may provoke cerebral hypoperfusion and ischemia. Sodium nitroprusside is the drug of choice for the initial treatment of HE. Due to the effect of nitroprusside on ICP, other agents such as beta-blockers or angiotensin converting enzyme (ACE) inhibitors should be used after the initial control of BP (Table 16.5). Hydralazine appears to be less effective in treating HE. Clonidine should be avoided because of its potential for CNS depression [45]. Bed rest, sedation, and analgesia may further help BP control. Table 16.5 summarizes the most common antihypertensives used and their side effects. Treatment of HE induced seizures is not different from the general treatment of ICU seizures, outlined in the chapter of Treatment of Critical Care Seizures and SE.

Posterior Leukoencephalopathy Syndrome

Posterior leukoencephalopathy (PLE) is a recently recognized neurological disorder. It is characterized by white matter edema in the posterior parietal and occipital lobes of the brain [47]. The term was first used by Hinchey et al. [47] when they described 15 patients admitted with a wide variety of medical illnesses. Of these, seven were receiving immunosuppressive therapy, four had HE, and three were not hypertensive at all. In all patients, the neurological abnormalities resolved within 2 weeks. This syndrome has also been reported with uremia, hemolytic uremic syndrome, thrombotic thrombocytopenia purpura, cyclosporine A use, cisplatin, interferon alpha, intrathecal methotrexate, severe hypercalcemia, and indinavir [48–50]. For those patients who do not exhibit hypertension (children or adult), the syndrome of posterior reversible leukoencephalopathy has been coined, also some believed that a term like reversible occipital-parietal encephalopathy is more appropriate since both gray and white matter are involved [17, 51].

Table 16.5 Commonly used parenteral antihypertensive drugs

Medication	Mechanism of action	Bolus dose	Infusion rate	Pros	Cons
Sodium nitroprusside	Vasodilator	No bolus dose	0.25–10.0 µg/kg/min	■ Short duration of action ■ Immediate onset of action	■ ↑CBF[a], ↑↑↑ ICP[b] ■ Cyanide toxicity
Nicardipine	Ca Channel blocker	No bolus dose	5–15 mg/h	■ Less variability in blood pressure ■ No risk of thiocyanate toxicity	
Clevidipine	Ca Channel blocker	No bolus dose	1–16 mg/h	■ Short acting	■ Should be avoided in aortic stenosis ■ Contraindicated in patients with egg product allergy.
Labetalol	$\alpha_1, \beta_1, \beta_2$ receptor antagonist	5–20 mg IV q 15 min for a total of 340 mg	0.5–2 mg/min	■ Rapid onset of action ■ No effect on ICP	■ CHF[c] ■ Bronchospasm ■ Bradycardia
Clonidine	α_2- agonist	0.1–0.2 mg PO	No drip	■ Might be helpful in alcohol withdrawal	■ ↓CBF
Enalaprilat	ACE[d] inhibitor	0.625–5 mg IV q6 hr	No drip	■ No effect on ICP or CBF	■ Could cause abrupt decrease in BP ■ Potential ↑ ICP in patients with poor compliance ■ Renal dysfunction

[a]*CBF* Cerebral Blood Flow
[b]*ICP* Intracranial Pressure
[c]*CHF* Congestive Heart Failure
[d]*ACE* Angiotensin Converting Enzyme

Clinical Features

The most common presenting signs and symptoms include lethargy, confusion, somnolence, paucity of speech, headaches, and visual complaints. Lethargy and somnolence are often the first signs noted. Memory difficulties are not uncommon. Visual disturbances range from blurred vision to hemianopsia [47].

Seizures are common at onset (11 out of 15 [73%] of the originally reported patients had one or more seizures). They are usually generalized but can also begin as focal. Multiple seizures are more common than single seizures. Status epilepticus has also been reported [47]. Seizures generally precede the manifestation of the syndrome. Visual aura or visual hallucinations also precede the tonic-clonic seizure or occipital seizures. Following a seizure patients usually have prolonged mental status changes and end up being in stupor or coma [52].

Pathophysiology

This syndrome shares similar pathophysiological mechanisms with HE and eclampsia. Two pathophysiological mechanisms for PLS have been proposed [53]. The first evokes cerebral vasospasm and cerebral ischemia as a cause to the changes seen on neuroimaging [54]. The second suggests a breakdown

in cerebrovascular autoregulation with secondary vasogenic edema. Recent MRI findings are in support of the autoregulation hypothesis [55]. The pathological process is characterized by cerebral edema and petechial hemorrhages especially in the parieto-occipital and occipital lobes. Microscopically, these petechiae are ring hemorrhages around capillaries and precapillaries that are occluded by fibrinoid materials [56].

Radiological Features

The most common neuroimaging abnormality on both MRI and CT is white mailer edema in the posterior areas of the cerebral hemispheres. These lesions are predominately symmetrical and involve specifically the occipital, parietal lobes, and posterior temporal lobes [47]. Other lesions are reported in the pons, thalamus, and the cerebellum. The gray matter is involved in some patients and hence the term leukoencephalopathy may not be the most appropriate [51, 55]. Individuals with predominate gray matter disease have a better course that individual with predominate white matter lesions. Brainstem lesions are found in 56% of patients [55]. On MR images, the high signal on diffusion-weighted imaging without the typical ADC dropout suggests vasogenic edema [45]. This is referred to as pseudonormalization. Some patients with pseudonormalization can progress to having an infarct.

Management

Patients may need to be monitored in the NICU. Indications for transfer to the NICU include cerebral edema with midline shift and seizures. Some of these patients may already be in an intensive care unit setting. If the cause of PLE is found to be acute hypertension, then aggressive blood pressure management should be initiated. Treatment paradigms are similar to HE. If a particular drug was thought to be the inciting agent, then discontinuing the drug should be seriously considered. If seizures are present, benzodiazepines are indicated as first choice agents. If seizures are refractory or recurrent, then an additional anticonvulsant is indicated. The choice of anticonvulsant will depend on the patient's general clinical condition and the associated renal or liver abnormalities. For more details regarding treatment of ICU seizures the reader should refer to the chapters on Treatment of Critical Care Seizures and SE.

Conclusion

The association between seizures and blood pressure elevation remains a common medical emergency encountered in an ICU setting. Fortunately, if treated immediately and aggressively, the pathophysiologic mechanism leading to seizures is reversible in most cases. Delayed treatment may result in irreversible brain injury.

References

1. Finnerty Jr FA. Hypertensive encephalopathy. Am Heart J. 1968;75(4):559–63.
2. Delanty N. Seizures: medical causes and management, Current clinical neurology. Totowa, N.J: Humana Press; 2002. p. 368.
3. Hesdorffer DC et al. Severe, uncontrolled hypertension and adult-onset seizures: a case-control study in Rochester, Minnesota. Epilepsia. 1996;37(8):736–41.
4. National High Blood Pressure Education Program Working Group Report on High Blood Pressure in Pregnancy. Am J Obstet Gynecol. 1990;163(5 Pt 1):1691–712.
5. Feinberg WM. Guidelines for the management of transient ischemic attacks. From the Ad Hoc committee on guidelines for the management of transient ischemic attacks of the stroke Council of the American Heart Association. Stroke. 1994;25(6):1320–35.
6. American College of Obstetricians and Gynecologists, Task Force on Hypertension in pregnancy. Report of the American college of obstetricians and gynecologists' task force on hypertension in pregnancy. Obstet Gynecol. 2013;122(5):1122–31.
7. O'Dowd MJ, Philipp EE. The history of obstetrics and gynecology. New York: Parthenon Publishing Group; 1994.
8. Mushambi MC, Halligan AW, Williamson K. Recent developments in the pathophysiology and management of pre-eclampsia. Br J Anaesth. 1996;76(1):133–48.
9. MacKay AP, Berg CJ, Atrash HK. Pregnancy-related mortality from preeclampsia and eclampsia. Obstet Gynecol. 2001;97(4):533–8.
10. Witlin AG et al. Cerebrovascular disorders complicating pregnancy--beyond eclampsia. Am J Obstet Gynecol. 1997;176(6):1139–45. discussion 1145-8
11. Munro PT. Management of eclampsia in the accident and emergency department. J Accid Emerg Med. 2000;17(1):7–11.
12. Douglas KA, Redman CW. Eclampsia in the United Kingdom. BMJ. 1994;309(6966):1395–400.
13. Leitch CR, Cameron AD, Walker JJ. The changing pattern of eclampsia over a 60-year period. Br J Obstet Gynaecol. 1997;104(8):917–22.
14. Ramin KD. The prevention and management of eclampsia. Obstet Gynecol Clin North Am. 1999;26(3):489–503. ix
15. Lyall F, Greer IA. Pre-eclampsia: a multifaceted vascular disorder of pregnancy. J Hypertens. 1994;12(12):1339–45.
16. Holtkamp M, Tong X, Walker MC. Propofol in subanesthetic doses terminates status epilepticus in a rodent model. Ann Neurol. 2001;49(2):260–3.
17. Usta IM, Sibai BM. Emergent management of puerperal eclampsia. Obstet Gynecol Clin North Am. 1995;22(2):315–35.
18. Lopez-Llera M. Main clinical types and subtypes of eclampsia. Am J Obstet Gynecol. 1992;166(1 Pt 1):4–9.
19. Katz VL, Farmer R, Kuller JA. Preeclampsia into eclampsia: toward a new paradigm. Am J Obstet Gynecol. 2000;182(6):1389–96.
20. Dziewas R et al. Late onset postpartum eclampsia: a rare and difficult diagnosis. J Neurol. 2002;249(9):1287–91.
21. Sibai BM et al. Effect of magnesium sulfate on electroencephalographic findings in preeclampsia-eclampsia. Obstet Gynecol. 1984;64(2):261–6.
22. Kirby JC, Jaindl JJ. Cerebral CT findings in toxemia of pregnancy. Radiology. 1984;151(1):114.
23. Milliez J, Dahoun A, Boudraa M. Computed tomography of the brain in eclampsia. Obstet Gynecol. 1990;75(6):975–80.
24. Gaitz JP, Bamford CR. Unusual computed tomographic scan in eclampsia. Arch Neurol. 1982;39(1):66.
25. Schwaighofer BW, Hesselink JR, Healy ME. MR demonstration of reversible brain abnormalities in eclampsia. J Comput Assist Tomogr. 1989;13(2):310–2.
26. Celik O, Hascalik S. Reversible posterior leukoencephalopathy in eclampsia. Int J Gynaecol Obstet. 2003;82(1):67–9.
27. Kilpatrick SJ, Matthay MA. Obstetric patients requiring critical care. A five-year review. Chest. 1992;101(5):1407–12.
28. American Heart Association issues management guidelines for acute ischemic stroke. Am Fam Physician. 1995;51(5):1301–4.
29. Duley L, Gulmezoglu AM, Henderson-Smart DJ. Magnesium sulphate and other anticonvulsants for women with pre-eclampsia. Cochrane Database Syst Rev. 2003;2:CD000025.
30. Belfort MA et al. A comparison of magnesium sulfate and nimodipine for the prevention of eclampsia. N Engl J Med. 2003;348(4):304–11.
31. Pritchard JA et al. Intravascular hemolysis, thrombocytopenia and other hematologic abnormalities associated with severe toxemia of pregnancy. N Engl J Med. 1954;250(3):89–98.
32. Weinstein L. Syndrome of hemolysis, elevated liver enzymes, and low platelet count: a severe consequence of hypertension in pregnancy. Am J Obstet Gynecol. 1982;142(2):159–67.
33. Haddad B et al. Risk factors for adverse maternal outcomes among women with HELLP (hemolysis, elevated liver enzymes, and low platelet count) syndrome. Am J Obstet Gynecol. 2000;183(2):444–8.
34. Magann EF et al. Antepartum corticosteroids: disease stabilization in patients with the syndrome of hemolysis, elevated liver enzymes, and low platelets (HELLP). Am J Obstet Gynecol. 1994;171(4):1148–53.
35. Oppenheimer BS. Hypertensive encephalopathy. Arch Intern Med. 1928;41:264–78.
36. Healton EB et al. Hypertensive encephalopathy and the neurologic manifestations of malignant hypertension. Neurology. 1982;32(2):127–32.

37. Cummins RO, Chamberlain D, Hazinski MF, Nadkarni V, Kloeck W, Kramer E, Becker L, Robertson C, Koster R, Zaritsky A, Bossaert L, Ornato JP, Callanan V, Allen M, Steen P, Connolly B, Sanders A, Idris A, Cobbe S. Recommended guidelines for reviewing, reporting, and conducting research on in-hospital resuscitation: the in-hospital "Utstein style". A statement for health care professionals from the American Heart Association, the European Resuscitation Council, the Heart and Stroke Foundation of Canada, the Australian Resuscitation Council, and the Resuscitation Councils of Southern Africa. Acad Emerg Med. 1997;4(6):603–27.

38. Bennett NM, Shea S. Hypertensive emergency: case criteria, sociodemographic profile, and previous care of 100 cases. Am J Public Health. 1988;78(6):636–40.

39. Berlowitz DR et al. Inadequate management of blood pressure in a hypertensive population. N Engl J Med. 1998;339(27):1957–63.

40. Auer LM. The pathogenesis of hypertensive encephalopathy. Experimental data and their clinical relevance with special reference to neurosurgical patients. Acta Neurochir Suppl (Wien). 1978;27:1–111.

41. Furchgott RF, Zawadzki JV. The obligatory role of endothelial cells in the relaxation of arterial smooth muscle by acetylcholine. Nature. 1980;288(5789):373–6.

42. Kuchan MJ, Frangos JA. Shear stress regulates endothelin-1 release via protein kinase C and cGMP in cultured endothelial cells. Am J Physiol. 1993;264(1 Pt 2):H150–6.

43. Torocsik HV et al. FK506-induced leukoencephalopathy in children with organ transplants. Neurology. 1999;52(7):1497–500.

44. Delanty N et al. Erythropoietin-associated hypertensive posterior leukoencephalopathy. Neurology. 1997;49(3):686–9.

45. Schwartz RB et al. Diffusion-weighted MR imaging in hypertensive encephalopathy: clues to pathogenesis. AJNR Am J Neuroradiol. 1998;19(5):859–62.

46. Vaughan CJ, Delanty N. Hypertensive emergencies. Lancet. 2000;356(9227):411–7.

47. Hinchey J et al. A reversible posterior leukoencephalopathy syndrome. N Engl J Med. 1996;334(8):494–500.

48. Covarrubias DJ, Luetmer PH, Campeau NG. Posterior reversible encephalopathy syndrome: prognostic utility of quantitative diffusion-weighted MR images. AJNR Am J Neuroradiol. 2002;23(6):1038–48.

49. Kastrup O et al. Posterior reversible encephalopathy syndrome due to severe hypercalcemia. J Neurol. 2002;249(11):1563–6.

50. Giner V et al. Reversible posterior leukoencephalopathy secondary to indinavir-induced hypertensive crisis: a case report. Am J Hypertens. 2002;15(5):465–7.

51. Pavlakis SG, Frank Y, Chusid R. Hypertensive encephalopathy, reversible occipitoparietal encephalopathy, or reversible posterior leukoencephalopathy: three names for an old syndrome. J Child Neurol. 1999;14(5):277–81.

52. Garg RK. Posterior leukoencephalopathy syndrome. Postgrad Med J. 2001;77(903):24–8.

53. Port JD, Beauchamp Jr NJ. Reversible intracerebral pathologic entities mediated by vascular autoregulatory dysfunction. Radiographics. 1998;18(2):353–67.

54. Trommer BL, Homer D, Mikhael MA. Cerebral vasospasm and eclampsia. Stroke. 1988;19(3):326–9.

55. Casey SO et al. Posterior reversible encephalopathy syndrome: utility of fluid-attenuated inversion recovery MR imaging in the detection of cortical and subcortical lesions. AJNR Am J Neuroradiol. 2000;21(7):1199–206.

56. Donaldson JO. Eclampsia. Adv Neurol. 1994;64:25–33.

57. Altman D, Carroli G, Duley L, Farrell B, Moodley J, Neilson J, Smith D, Magpie Trial Collaboration Group. Do women with pre-eclampsia, and their babies, benefit from magnesium sulphate? The Magpie Trial: a randomised placebo-controlled trial. Lancet. 2002;359(9321):1877–90.

Infection or Inflammation and Critical Care Seizures

Andrew C. Schomer, Wendy Ziai, Mohammed Rehman, and Barnett R. Nathan

Introduction

In the intensive care unit (ICU) setting, central nervous system (CNS) infection and inflammation are frequent precipitants of seizures. In critically ill patients seizures are significant independent contributors to patient morbidity and mortality [1]. Early recognition and treatment of seizures is associated with decreased mortality. In one series by Young et al. of patients with nonconvulsive seizures, a delay in recognition and duration of seizures was strongly associated with increased mortality [2]. Seizures are one of the most common sequelae of primary CNS infections, but are also frequently seen in patients admitted to the medical ICU as the sole neurologic manifestation of illness [3–5]. In ICU patients with an unexplained decrease in level of consciousness, nonconvulsive seizures are often responsible, and CNS infections are a common etiology [6]. Infectious causes of seizures are also a frequent cause of the most refractory seizures seen in the ICU. In patients with new onset refractory status epilepticus (NORSE), infectious causes are responsible for at least 18% of cases, and this likely underestimates the total given high number (52%) of cryptogenic cases [7].

There is a significant role for continuous electroencephalographic (EEG) monitoring (cEEG) in the ICU because it can detect purely electrographic seizure activity, including nonconvulsive status epilepticus (NCSE), in approximately 18–40% of patients presenting with an unexplained decreased level of consciousness or clinical seizures [8]. Moreover, electrographic seizures and other EEG findings such as periodic epileptiform discharges (PEDs) are associated with worse outcome in patients with acute neurological injuries, such as in the aftermath of convulsive status epilepticus and in those with intracerebral [9] or subarachnoid hemorrhages [10]. In patients with CNS infections, recent guidelines recommend cEEG for patients with bacterial meningitis with seizures or fluctuations in the level of consciousness [11]. In a retrospective cohort study by Carrera et al., it was noted that central nervous system infections undergoing cEEG monitoring, electrographic seizures, and/or PEDs were frequent, occurring in 48% of the cohort, with more than half showing no clinical correlate [12]. Additionally, for patients in the medical ICU (MICU) setting admitted with a diagnosis of sepsis but no primary neurologic injury, the presence of electrographic seizures (ESz) and PEDs was strongly associated with death or disability at time of discharge [13].

A.C. Schomer (✉)
Division of Neurocritical Care, Department of Neurology,
University of Virginia, 800394, Charlottesville, VA 22908, USA
e-mail: acs8bd@virginia.edu

W. Ziai
Neurosciences Critical Care Division, Departments of Neurology,
Neurosurgery, and Anesthesiology – Critical Care Medicine,
Johns Hopkins Hospital, Baltimore, MD, USA
e-mail: weziai@jhmi.edu

M. Rehman
Departments of Neurology and Neurosurgery, K-11 Henry Ford
Hospital, 2799 West Grand Blvd, Detroit, MI, USA
e-mail: Mrehman1@hfhs.org

B.R. Nathan
Division of Neurocritical Care, Department of Neurology,
University of Virginia, Charlottesville, VA, USA
e-mail: BRN3A@hscmail.mcc.virginia.edu

CNS Infectious Disorders

Meningitis

Meningitis is the inflammation of the pia and arachnoid membranes (leptomeninges) that surround the brain and spinal cord [14]. The classification of meningitis is based on its duration and recurrence and includes: acute (aseptic and septic) syndromes (<4 weeks duration), recurrent meningitis (multiple acute episodes of <4 weeks each), and chronic meningitis (>4 weeks duration).

© Springer International Publishing AG 2017
P.N. Varelas, J. Claassen (eds.), *Seizures in Critical Care*, Current Clinical Neurology, DOI 10.1007/978-3-319-49557-6_17

Acute aseptic meningitis, which is defined by negative routine screening cultures and stains of cerebrospinal fluid (CSF), is the most common form of meningitis [15]. The clinical syndrome starts with high-grade fever and severe headache associated with nausea, vomiting, pharyngitis, diarrhea, neck stiffness, and photophobia. Seizures are not a common manifestation. Rapid and complete recovery is the usual course. Viral infections are commonly the cause of aseptic meningitis, and the most common are the enteroviruses (echovirus, coxsackie A and B, poliovirus, and the numbered enteroviruses) [15, 16]. Other causes of aseptic meningitis include: Human immunodeficiency virus (HIV), parasites, rickettsiae and mycoplasma, and autoimmune diseases such as Behçet's disease, Kawasaki disease, and Vogt-Koyanagi-Harada disease [14]. Malignancies and drug reactions have also been implicated. In a population-based study, the 20-year risk for unprovoked seizures was 2.1% after aseptic meningitis, not higher than the general population risk for unprovoked seizures [17].

Acute septic meningitis is caused by a bacterial infection and inflammation of the meninges. It is a neurologic emergency with mortality rates as high as 15–33% even in hospitalized patients treated with antibiotics [18, 19]. The classic presentation of septic meningitis includes an acute onset over hours to days of a fever, headache, reduced alertness, and signs of meningeal irritation. The incidence of seizures in bacterial meningitis has been reported as 5–28% of cases, and often (76%) they occur within the first 24 h of presentation [20–23]. Seizures are an independent predictor of mortality (34% mortality in patients with seizures compared to 7% without seizures; odds ratio 17.6). Predictors of prognosis in bacterial meningitis include: age greater than 60 years, coma at onset or focal seizures within the first 24 h of admission (72% vs. 18% mortality among those with and without early onset seizures, respectively) [20]. In one retrospective study of 445 patients with acute bacterial meningitis, seizures had focal onset in 7%, generalized in 13%, and not characterized in 3% [20].

The effective evaluation and treatment of patients with bacterial meningitis involves early initiation of empiric antibiotics, collection of CSF to determine causative organism and antibiotic sensitivities, as well as adjunctive therapies (steroids) and additional evaluations (imaging, cEEG) in select patient populations. Delay in initiation of antibiotic therapy in patients who are septic has been shown to increase mortality by 7.6% for every hour of delay [24, 25]. Emergent treatment (<3 h from hospital admission) with empiric antibiotic therapy has been also been shown to reduce the risk of mortality at 3 months [19]. Although significant controversy exists as to the role of steroids, a recent Cochrane review supported the use of corticosteroids to reduce hearing loss and additional neurologic sequelae of bacterial meningitis [26]. The occurrence of seizures in patients with meningitis may indicate a cortically based complication (empyema, stroke, venous thrombosis), which merits neuroimaging studies (ideally a contrast enhanced CT scan or MRI). Cortical venous thrombosis usually presents with seizures and focal neurological signs albeit an uncommon event during bacterial meningitis (only 5.1% of autopsies of patients who died from meningitis had septic cortical vein thrombosis in a large series) [27]. Patients with persistent alteration in mental status or coma should undergo an EEG to rule out sub-clinical seizures. In one series continuous EEG (cEEG) was decisive or at least contributed to clinical decision-making in 12/13 patients with intracranial infection [28]. Since the widespread use of the vaccine for Haemophilus influenzae type B, *Streptococcus pneumoniae* has replaced it as the most common cause of acute community-acquired bacterial meningitis in industrialized countries. *S. pneumoniae* and *Neisseria meningitides* now account for the majority of cases of meningitis [25]. The rising incidence of beta-lactam-resistant pneumococci has to be considered when choosing a regimen for empiric antibiotic therapy [29]. Empiric antibiotic therapy for a suspected bacterial CNS infection should be given in consideration with the patient's age, competence of the immune system, and associated morbidities. An immune competent adult (ages 2–50) should be started on a third generation cephalosporin (ceftriaxone – 4 g/d or cefotaxime – 8–12 g/d) in addition to vancomycin (30–60 mg/kg per day (8–12 h) to achieve serum trough concentrations of 15–20 µg/mL), and the addition of ampicillin (12 g/d) for patients over age 50 who are more susceptible to *S. agalactiae* and *Listeria monocytogenes* [30]. An immune compromised adult should be treated with ampicillin, vancomycin (2–3 g/d), and a fourth generation cephalosporin such as cefepime (6 g/day), which has more stability against B-lactamase producing organisms and pseudomonas. Neurosurgical patients, including those with CSF shunts, and head trauma patients require both gram positive and negative coverage with a recommended combination of vancomycin and ceftazidime (6 g/d), cefepime (6 g/day) or meropenem (6 g/day) [30].

Recurrent meningitis can be due to infectious and non-infectious causes. Viruses are the most likely infectious agents. Mollaret's meningitis is a type of recurrent aseptic meningitis most frequently associated with herpes simplex type II virus. The clinical presentation may resemble aseptic meningitis, with headache (100%), photophobia (47%), self-reported fever (45%), meningismus (44%), and nausea and/or vomiting (29%) [31]. Seizures are part of the clinical presentation of Mollaret's meningitis [32].

Chronic meningitis has a non-specific presentation, with variable fever, headache, neck rigidity, and signs of parenchymal involvement, such as altered mental status, seizures, or focal neurologic deficits [14]. Infectious causes include: cryptococcus, coccidiomycosis, blastomycosis, histoplasmosis, aspergillosis, mycobacterial, and neurosyphilis [33].

Non-infectious causes include neoplasms, neurosarcoidosis, and CNS vasculitis [14]. Seizure treatment in the context of acute or chronic meningitis is not different from the treatment offered for other causes. Details can be found in the chapter "Management of Critical Care Seizures" and "Management of status epilepticus."

Encephalitis

Encephalitis is an acute infection of brain parenchyma and should be suspected in patients who present with altered mental status and signs of cerebral dysfunction, and often accompanied by a fever. There are numerous viral causes of encephalitis of which the most common are: Herpes simplex virus (HSV) (the most common sporadic viral cause of encephalitis), varicella zoster virus (VZV), cytomegalovirus (CMV), human herpesvirus 6, Epstein Barr virus (EBV), JC virus, enteroviruses, rabies as well as several arthropod-borne infections (Japanese encephalitis virus (the most common epidemic viral cause), West Nile virus, St. Louis encephalitis virus, La Crosse virus, Murray Valley encephalitis, Powassan virus, Tickborne encephalitis virus, Eastern equine encephalitis virus, Western equine encephalitis virus, Venezuelan equine encephalitis virus, and deer tick virus [34]. Specific viruses can have characteristic presentations, such as shingles associated with VZV, and several of these infections only present in patients who are immunocompromised (CMV, JC virus) [34]. The majority of patients with encephalitis have abnormal EEG findings, of which the most frequent EEG characteristics are uni- or bilateral periodic discharges, focal or generalized slow waves, and electrical seizures [35]. A normal EEG in acute encephalitis had a strong predictive value for a low relative risk of death in one series. Additionally, those patients with infectious causes of encephalitis were more likely to have nonreactive EEGs than those with an inflammatory or autoimmune etiology [35].

Seizures, both focal and generalized are a common manifestation of the viral encephalitides. These can be grouped as acute symptomatic seizures (those that occur within 7 days of an infection) and as unprovoked seizures (those that occur after 7 days). The estimated rate of seizures within the acute period is from 2 to –67%, however, this likely underestimates the total number given limited availability of EEG, subtle symptomatic seizures, and a high incidence of nonconvulsive seizures in comatose patients [36, 37]. For patients who have had viral encephalitis, there is thought to be 16 times the likelihood of developing unprovoked seizures later in life, and for those that have had seizures during the acute phase, the risk is 22 times that of the general population [36]. In another population-based study, Annegers et al. found that the risk of developing unprovoked seizures within 20 years was 22% in patients with viral encephalitis

and early seizures, 10% for those with viral encephalitis without early seizures, 13% in patients with bacterial meningitis and early seizures, and only 2.4% in patients with bacterial meningitis without early seizures [17]. Treatment of seizures with epilepsy surgery may be a better option in cases where there is a clearly localized focus. In a series of 38 patients who developed medically intractable partial seizures, Marks et al. found that 16 of them had a history of meningitis and 22 had encephalitis. Meningitis was pathologically associated with mesial temporal sclerosis and encephalitis with neocortical foci. However, in patients with encephalitis at less than 4 years of age, seizures were also associated with mesial temporal sclerosis [38].

Herpes Simplex Encephalitis

Herpes simplex virus (HSV) encephalitis is the most important form of treatable encephalitis and is the most common sporadic cause of viral encephalitis. It has an annual incidence of 1 in 250,000–500,000 [39, 40]. HSV encephalitis is a medical emergency with a mortality rate as high as 70% if left untreated [41]. Even with treatment, there is significant long-term morbidity in survivors including seizures, cognitive and behavioral disorders, and the prognosis often depends on the patient's condition once treatment is started [42]. A typical clinical presentation is often characterized by: fever (eventually in 100%), personality change (85%), dysphagia (76%), autonomic dysfunction (60%), ataxia (40%), hemiparesis (38%), seizures (38%), cranial nerve deficit (32%), visual field loss (14%), and papilledema (14%) [43].

Seizures can often be the presenting symptom and are thought to be common in the disease due to the predilection of the virus for the mesial temporal lobes and orbitofrontal cortices [36]. EEG findings in HSV encephalitis showed a significantly higher proportion of periodic discharges and focal slowing in the fronto-temporal and occipital regions as compared to encephalitis from other infectious or noninfectious causes [35]. Although no specific EEG patterns are pathognomonic of HSV encephalitis, focal or lateralized EEG abnormalities in the presence of encephalitis are highly suspicious [44]. Early changes in HSV encephalitis may be non-specific spike and slow wave activity, delta waves, or triphasic waves which can evolve into the typical 2–3 Hz unilateral periodic lateralized epileptiform discharges (PLEDs), originating from the temporal lobes, which are seen in 84% of the typical HSV encephalitis. Periodic discharges tend to occur only during the acute stage, and may disappear on the side of initial involvement before appearing on the newly involved side. When present bilaterally, they often occur in a time-locked relationship with each other [45]. The presence of bilateral epileptiform abnormalities was more common among those with poor outcome (0/18 with good outcome vs. 5/10 with poor outcome; $p < 0.01$) [42]. EEG should be performed when suspecting encephalitis to distinguish focal encephalitis from generalized encephalopathy and to look for abnormal findings of HSE. Diffuse, bi-hemispheric slow waves and triphasic waves as in hepatic failure may suggest encephalopathy. Their appearance later in the disease course may indicate a recurrence [46].

Examination of the cerebrospinal fluid (CSF) typically shows a lymphocytic pleocytosis, increased erythrocytes, and an elevated protein [47]. The gold standard diagnosis of HSV infection is through CSF polymerase chain reaction (PCR) to amplify viral DNA and has a sensitivity of 98% and a specificity of 94–100% [48]. MRI changes in the fluid-attenuated inversion recovery (FLAIR)/T2 signal are most often seen in the temporal lobe (87.5%), insula (70%), frontal lobe (67.5%), and thalamus (27.5%) [49]. Pathologically, HSV is an acute necrotizing encephalitis with preferential involvement of the inferior frontal, medial temporal, cingulate, and insular cortex [50]. Microscopically, there is evidence of necrosis and macrophage-rich inflammatory infiltrates with perivascular chronic infiltration and microglial nodules [51].

Specific treatment with acyclovir is indicated in HSV encephalitis, at a dosage of 10 mg/kg q8h (in adults) for 14 days (21 days in those that are immunocompromised). Additionally, new guidelines suggest that a repeat lumbar puncture should be performed after 14 days and if PCR remains positive, then acyclovir should be continued for an additional 7 days [52]. This additional duration of treatment is thought necessary due to the relatively high rate of relapse (5–26%) when the duration is insufficient [39, 43]. Supportive therapy also includes aggressive management of elevated intracranial pressure. If treated with acyclovir early on (<4 days from onset), treatment significantly increases the likelihood of survival from 65% to 100% [53]. Overall, even with treatment, there is approximately still a 20% mortality [41]. Cerebral edema, persistent vegetative state, and systemic infection are the usual predictors of a fatal outcome. Other risk factors for poor prognosis include MRI abnormalities, bilateral EEG abnormalities, and focal hyperperfusion on SPECT [54, 55].

Only half of patients return to their previous or similar level of productivity, and many patients have significant neurobehavioral problems (65) [56]. Some patients will go on to develop Kluver-Bucy syndrome, characterized by "psychic blindness," loss of normal anger and fear responses, and increased sexual activity [57]. Given the high incidence of seizures following an episode of encephalitis, especially in those that had seizures during the acute phase, seizure prophylaxis should be instituted. Surgical management is occasionally an option, but is thought to help only in a subgroup of patients suffering from unilateral mesio-temporal lobe epilepsy and congruent neuropsychological impairment [58].

Japanese Encephalitis

Japanese encephalitis (JE) is the most important epidemic viral encephalitis in the world, causing an estimated 70,000 cases annually and resulting in more than 14,000 deaths per year. Although JE virus is confined mainly to South East Asia, the virus is also endemic in the Western Pacific and Eastern Mediterranean. JE is an enzoonotic flavivirus transmitted by Culex mosquitoes; the main cycle of transmission is between wading birds and pigs, with the pigs acting as amplifying hosts [37]. JE virus is neurotropic and replicates rapidly in neurons, causing a perivascular inflammatory reaction, resulting in infection, neuronal dysfunction, and death [59]. In a prospective study of 144 patients infected with JE virus (134 children and 10 adults), 40 patients (28%) had a witnessed seizure during the admission; of these, the majority (62%) died or had a poor outcome compared to (14%) in the group with no witnessed seizure. The majority of patients who had a generalized tonic-clonic seizure or subtle clinical manifestations of seizures (twitching of a digit, eyebrow, nostrils, excess salivation, irregular breathing, eye deviation with or without nystagmus) were in status epilepticus [60].

EEG patterns during the acute period have also been associated with outcome in JE infection. Of 234 EEGs performed on 55 patients, poor outcome was associated with acute EEG findings of slow nonreactive, low amplitude, burst suppression, or isoelectric patterns in 16/19 patients (84%) compared with poor outcome in 14/36 patients (39%) with findings of slow reactive, or normal EEG patterns. Independent predictors of poor outcome were comatose state, more than one witnessed seizure, herniation syndrome, and illness for 7 days or more. Patients with seizures were more likely to have elevated opening pressure on lumbar puncture and to develop brainstem signs consistent with a herniation syndrome [60].

There is no specific treatment for Japanese Encephalitis, therefore therapeutic goals of seizure and ICP control are of critical importance. Prevention of illness through personal protective measures to limit mosquito bites in endemic areas is one of the major goals in limiting disease spread. An inactivated vaccine is also available for travelers who plan to spend time in endemic areas. A lack of resources has limited more widespread vaccination attempts [37].

Neurologic sequelae for Japanese Encephalitis include both neuropsychiatric symptoms and a "polio-like" illness. Many patients develop an acute flaccid paralysis following JE infection, and neurophysiologic studies of patients following a JE infection have shown varying degrees of anterior horn cell involvement [61, 62].

West Nile, La Crosse, Eastern Equine, and St. Louis Encephalitis

West Nile Virus (WNV) is a mosquito-born flavivirus first detected in North America in 1999 and now seen in all 48 contiguous states by 2012. As of 2015, over 41,000 cases of WNV have been reported in the USA. Most cases are either asymptomatic, or present with an influenza-like illness, but a small proportion (<1%) of cases will have neuroinvasive disease [63]. La Crosse Virus (LACV) is a mosquito-born bunyaviridae initially isolated from the brain of a young girl who died from encephalitis in La Crosse, Wisconsin. It primarily affects children under the age of 15 in the summer months in the Midwestern United States and through much of Appalachia (Tennessee, North Carolina, and West Virginia). There are approximately 42–174 cases reported per year in the USA. Infections often present as an uncomplicated fever (5%), meningitis (17%), meningoencephalitis (56%), and encephalitis (21%) [64]. Eastern Equine Encephalitis (EEEV) is an alphavirus first isolated from horses in Virginia and New Jersey in 1933. Most clinical cases of EEEV are reported from Massachusetts, Florida, Georgia, and New Jersey. From the period of 1964–2014 there were 220 confirmed cases. EEEV is the most virulent of the alphavirudae with a case fatality rate of 50–70% [65]. The majority of patients have a prodrome for several days, consistent with a viral illness. Neurologic symptoms typically follow and include: somnolence, focal weakness, seizures, and meningeal signs [66]. St. Louis Encephalitis (SLEV) is a flavivirus related to JEV and WNV thought to have been originally introduced from Africa to Argentina and Brazil but gradually dispersed into North America. It is thought to affect approximately 50 people per year in North America and has a case fatality rate of approximately 7%. Onset is characterized by a flu-like illness, occasionally with urinary tract symptoms [67].

The incidence of seizures, status epilepticus, and epilepsy in patients with arbovirus infections varies significantly in different series. Approximately 10% of patients with WNV will develop seizures during the acute illness [68]. The EEG was abnormal in 88% of patients with meningitis or meningoencephalitis and in 74% with any neurological involvement. EEG abnormalities were most frequently diffuse symmetric slowing with frontal predominance although temporal predominant slowing and asymmetric frontal slowing were seen in some cases [69]. The incidence of seizures in LACV is approximately 50%, with up to 10% of patients developing epilepsy long-term [64]. Similarly in EEEV, in one series in which 36 patients were followed, 18 of them had seizures, the majority of which were generalized tonic-clonic seizures. EEG in patients in that same series of EEEV patients showed generalized slowing and a disorganized background. One smaller study showed a distinctive pattern in EEEV of 0.25–0.5 Hz transients with lower voltages ($\sim$20–40 μV) than typically seen in herpes encephalitis. When paired with MRI findings of T2 hyperintensities in the lentiform nuclei, these findings were thought to be pathognomonic [66, 70].

Long-term sequelae of WNV infection include multiple physical and neuropsychiatric problems. The most common physical limitations following infection were muscle weakness (7–73%), fatigue (48–75%), and myalgias (19–49%). Memory loss (25–49%), depression (23–41%), and difficulty concentrating (34–48%) were the most frequent neuropsychiatric sequelae [63]. About 2% of LACV encephalitis cases develop persistent paresis, learning disabilities, or cognitive defects, as well as neurobehavioral sequelae such as attention deficits and hyperactivity [64]. In one series of EEEV patients, 13 of the 36 patients died (36%). Of the survivors, 1 recovered fully, 14 had mild impairments, three had moderate impairments, and five had severe impairments [66].

Human Immunodeficiency Virus infection and Seizures

Human Immunodeficiency Virus (HIV), a lentivirus which attacks the immune system and can lead to acquired immunodeficiency syndrome (AIDS), is estimated to affect 1.2 million persons living in the USA as of 2011 [71]. HIV poses a risk to patients for developing seizures for multiple reasons, including opportunistic infections, direct neurotropic effects of HIV, and the drugs that are used to treat the infection. New-onset seizures are common in HIV patients, occurring in 3–17% of patients [72]. Although most seizures are usually seen in the advanced stages of the disease, they may also occur early or as the presenting symptom of HIV infection [73].

In the majority of patients, seizures are associated with an underlying intracranial mass lesion, infection, or metabolic disturbance. Intracranial mass lesions, including opportunistic infections, neoplasms, and cerebrovascular disease make up almost half of neurological disorders in AIDS patients. These are all commonly associated with seizures. In one series of patients with new-onset seizures, generalized seizures occurred in 94% of patients, partial in 26%, and status epilepticus in 14%. An associated space occupying lesion or CNS infection was found in the majority of cases of patients who seized. The most common causes include: cerebral toxoplasmosis, CNS lymphoma, progressive multifocal leukoencephalopathy, cryptococcal meningitis, and infarction [72, 74]. Toxoplasmosis, the most common cause of intracranial mass lesions in AIDS, presents with seizures as an early manifestation in 15%–40% [75]. The second most common intracranial mass lesion producing seizures in AIDS patients is CNS lymphoma. Progressive multifocal leukoencephalopathy (PML), although a white matter disease without significant mass effect, can produce seizures, either partial or generalized. The highest risk factor for PML lesions to cause seizures was juxtacortical location (RR of 3.5) [76]. Meningitis and encephalitis are a frequent cause of seizures in HIV-infected patients, with cryptococcal meningitis being the most frequent meningo-encephalitis producing seizures [77]. There are several other less common causes for seizures in HIV-infected patients, including subacute sclerosing panencephalitis, aseptic meningitis, neurosyphilis, herpes zoster leukoencephalitis, and cytomegalovirus encephalitis. Other focal CNS lesions include brain abscess (tuberculous, cryptococcal, nocardial), tuberculomas, syphilitic gummas, and cerebrovascular diseases. [73, 78]

The pathophysiology of generalized seizures and status epilepticus in HIV-infected patients may be explained by lowered threshold for cortical excitability and impaired inhibitory mechanisms for terminating seizures once started. Specifically, HIV- or immune-related toxins produced by interactions between macrophages, microglia, monocytes, and astrocytes may injure or kill neurons [78]. Neurotoxic substances, including eicosanoids, platelet-activating factor, quinolate, cysteine, cytokines, and free radicals, increase glutamate release, activate voltage-dependent calcium channels and NMDA receptor-operated channels, leading to calcium influx and neuronal death. Postmortem neuropathological examination of the brain in 17 patients with HIV and otherwise unspecified etiologies for the seizures showed microglial nodules or multinucleated cells or both in six patients, suggesting that the HIV infection was the likely cause of the seizures. [74]

The medications used to treat HIV are also felt to be responsible for many cases of new-onset seizures. In one series it was found that 18% of patients with no identifiable etiology were taking foscarnet, which was postulated to be epileptogenic [73]. Additionally, drug–drug interactions often complicate the treatment of seizures in patients taking anti-retrovirals. As a result of hepatic enzyme induction and drug–disease interactions there is often a reduced concentration of protease inhibitors, which can lead to diminished antiviral efficacy. The choice of anticonvulsant is ideally one which has no effect on viral replication, has limited protein binding, and does not have effects on the cytochrome P450 system [79]. These include gabapentin, topiramate, levetiracetam, lacosamide, pregabalin, or lamotrigine, all of which have limited interactions with other drugs or no effect on the P450 system. Most nucleoside reverse transcriptase inhibitors are renally metabolized through glucuronidation by enzyme systems different than the cytochrome P450, thus not affecting the hepatically metabolized anti-epileptic drugs. On the other hand, the non-nucleoside reverse transcriptase inhibitors (like nevirapine, delaviradine, and efivanenz) use the cytochrome P450 system and may lead either to induction (efivarenz) or inhibition (nevirapine and delaviradine), affecting the anti-epileptics that use these systems.

It is critical to remember that the HIV-protease inhibitors decrease the functioning of the hepatic CYP3A enzyme system. In one study, carbamazepine dosed at 200 mg/day for post-zoster neuralgia, reached anti-epileptic therapeutic levels in an HIV patient receiving triple anti-retroviral therapy (indinavir, zidovudine, and lamivudine). Additionally complicating this picture, indinavir plasma concentrations decreased significantly and HIV-RNA became detectable during the period of carbamazepine treatment [80]. Hypoalbuminemia, a common situation in the ICU and in HIV seropositive patients should also be considered. Highly protein bound anti-epileptic (phenytoin, valproic acid, carbamazepine, clonazepam, diazepam) may displace highly protein bound anti-retroviral drugs (delaviradine, efivanez, saquinavir, vitonavir, nelfinavir, lopinavir, and ampenavir) or vice versa, leading to toxic free concentrations of either drug [81]. The HIV-induced hypergammaglobulinemia may also predispose patients to hypersensitivity reactions from anti-epileptics, especially phenytoin. In vitro studies have indicated that there may be stimulation of HIV replication when using valproic acid. In a retrospective study of manic HIV(+) patients who were taking divalproex sodium and anti-retrovirals, however, the HIV-1 viral load did not increase [82, 83].

Seizures are generally a poor prognostic indicator in HIV-infected patients and will likely recur. It is therefore recommended that patients experiencing a first seizure without a reversible cause be treated. The reported incidence of convulsive status epilepticus is 8–18% and is often associated with poor prognosis [72, 74, 84]. In one study of 42 patients with HIV infection and status epilepticus, the median duration of status was 2.0 ± 10 h. Most patients (88%) responded to IV benzodiazepine or phenytoin treatment. Nevertheless, (29%) patients died and (36%) developed new neurologic deficits [75]. The most common EEG finding is non-specific diffuse slowing, while focal slowing and epileptiform activity was infrequent. EEG showed generalized and diffuse slowing only in nine patients, regional slowing in 14 patients and regional slowing and epileptiform discharges in one patient. Only 14 of the patients had normal EEG [74, 77].

Brain Abscess

A brain abscess is a purulent infection of brain parenchyma that often occurs in patients with predisposing factors such as an immunocompromised state, disruption of natural protective barriers, or a systemic source of infection. The incidence of brain abscesses is thought to be 0.3–1.3 per 100,000 people per year, but is considerably higher in patients with HIV/AIDS. In one systematic review of the literature, the most commonly isolated species were Streptococcus (34%) and Staphylococcus (18%), however, numerous other organisms have been isolated including: gram-negative enteric species, pseudomonas, actinomycetales, parasites, and fungi [85]. The route of transmission is usually contiguous spread from a local primary focus such as paranasal sinusitis, otitis media, mastoiditis, or penetrating head trauma. Ten percent of cases spread hematogenously, usually from a pulmonary source such as bronchiectasis or lung abscess, but also from heart valves (infective endocarditis) or conditions causing a right to left shunt such as cyanotic heart disease in children [86].

The most common clinical presentation is a headache; fever and alterations in consciousness are uncommon. Focal deficits can also occur based on the site of the abscess [86]. In a review of the literature, seizure was the initial presentation of patients with brain abscesses approximately 25% of the time [85]. In one series in which 70 patients were followed after cerebral abscess, approximately 70% of patients developed seizures [87]. In a group of 205 patients enrolled in a 22-year retrospective study, 48 patients had seizures, 27 of whom had early seizures (those during the time of the bacterial infection), and 21 had late seizures. For those patients who developed seizures, the mortality rate was 23% [88].

Treatment of brain abscess requires antibiotic therapy, surgical intervention, and some authors have suggested the use of prophylactic anticonvulsants given the frequency of seizures [89]. Empiric antibiotic coverage with a third generation cephalosporin, vancomycin, and metronidazole is often appropriate for patients following neurosurgical procedures. For patients who have undergone organ transplantation, the addition of trimethoprim–sulfamethoxazole or sulfadiazine covers nocardia species, and voriconazole would cover fungal species, especially aspergillus. In the initial treatment of HIV-infected patients, coverage for toxoplasmosis (pyrimethamine plus sulfadiazine) is recommended, but only for those with positive test results for antitoxoplasma IgG antibodies. Treatment for tuberculosis (isoniazid, rifampin, pyrazinamide, and ethambutol) should be considered in those from endemic areas and in those with HIV infections [86]. It is recommended that anticonvulsants be continued for a period of 2 years after surgery and normalization of the EEG [90].

Intracranial Extra-axial Pyogenic Infections

Epidural abscesses and subdural empyemas are bacterial infections within the extra cerebral spaces. Epidural abscesses, typically present with headache, fever, and nausea. Neurological symptoms and complications are quite rare due to the protective effect of the tight adherence of dura to overlying skull. A subdural empyema, which is most commonly situated over the cerebral convexity, can cause altered level of consciousness, focal neurologic deficits, and seizures. The spread of infection through the subdural space can cause inflammation of the brain parenchyma and result in edema, elevated intracranial pressure, septic thrombophlebitis, venous infarction, or mass effect [91]. These extra-axial infections may result as a complication of trauma, neurosurgical procedures, meningitis, sinusitis, and other extracranial sources of infection. Subdural empyemas and epidural abscesses are commonly caused by staphylococcal species. Forty percent of cases can be polymicrobial. Streptococci, followed by staphylococcal organisms and anaerobes such as Propionebacterium and Peptostreptococcus are the most common causes [91].

Seizures are uncommon with epidural abscess and relatively common with subdural empyema. In a period of 14 years, 25 patients were retrospectively identified in a Taiwanese hospital (15 with subdural empyema and nine with epidural abscess). Seizures were found in 54% of patients; only in one patient with epidural abscess and in 12/15 (80%) patients with subdural empyema [92]. The same pattern of rarity of seizures with epidural abscess and relative frequency with subdural empyema is also encountered in children [93]. In a study reporting the incidence of early and late seizures after subdural empyema, early seizures occurred at a similar rate (62.5%) as that of late seizures (63%) in patients who survived. All patients received anticonvulsant prophylaxis, which was continued for 12–18 months. Early seizures were more common in cases with paranasal sinusitis, but did not correlate with occurrence of late epilepsy. Of those patients with follow-up, 29% who had early seizures had further attacks; of patients with no early seizures, 42% developed epilepsy during the follow-up period, most within the first 2 years. No factors predicting the occurrence of late seizures were identified [94].

Subdural empyema can be treated with intravenous antibiotic therapy, with a third-generation cephalosporin and metronidazole, followed by early surgical evacuation [95]. A prophylactic anticonvulsant is recommended. Craniotomy is generally preferred to multiple burr holes [94]. Antibiotics should be given intravenously for at least 2 weeks followed by oral therapy for up to a total of 6 weeks [95].

Ventriculitis

Ventriculitis is a pyogenic infection of the ventricular cavity. The ventricles may act as a reservoir for persistent inflammation, which may block the CSF outflow tracts and act as a brain abscess. The most common infecting organisms are Staphylococcal species. Thirty percent of all meningitis cases may be associated with ventriculitis while over 90% of neonatal meningitis is complicated by ventriculitis. Therefore, it should be considered in patients with meningitis who do not quickly respond to antibiotics. Ventriculitis is frequently (5%) associated with CSF shunts, intracranial devices, intrathecal chemotherapy, and rupture of a periventricular abscess [91, 96, 97].

The incidence of seizures in ventriculitis is not known although it is probably similar to meningitis due to the frequent co-occurrence of both conditions. Seizures are more frequent in ventriculitis following a shunt placement. In an older study, 18.2% of 99 patients with ventriculitis who were not shunted developed seizures vs. 65.4% of those receiving a shunt for hydrocephalus. EEG abnormalities were also more common in the shunted group (95%) vs. the non-shunted group (47%) [98]. In another study, 15.2% of children <1 year with ventricular shunts developed post-shunt epilepsy, in contrast with only 6.9% of patients >50 years old [99]. Most studies evaluating seizures and hydrocephalus are in children.

A large retrospective study of both children and adults from Oregon reported an increase in incidence of epilepsy (based on long-term administration of anti-epileptic drugs) from 12% before shunt insertion to 33% 10 years later. The hazard rate was 2% per year. The cause of hydrocephalus was a strong determinant of epilepsy (patients with post-hemorrhagic hydrocephalus had the highest risk and those with myelomeningocele the lowest). Interestingly, CSF shunt infection was not associated in this series with increased risk for epilepsy [100]. This finding was not confirmed in a later study in children shunted for hydrocephalus: children with shunt malfunction, infection, or a combination of these had higher incidence of epilepsy [101]. Thus, shunt-related ventriculitis may or may not increase the incidence of seizures, but the independent effect of infection compared to purely ventricular catheter or shunt placement (which is generally believed to increase incidence of seizures) has not been studied.

Treatment of ventriculitis generally requires externalization or removal and replacement of the infected intraventricular device. Vancomycin is preferred in acute gram-positive ventriculitis due to the increasing resistance patterns to beta-lactam antibiotics. Although Vancomycin adequately penetrates the blood brain barrier when the meninges are inflamed, CSF drug concentrations may be compromised in the case of ventriculitis or of an improving bacterial meningitis, where the meningeal inflammatory response may be less extensive. CSF penetration of vancomycin may be negligible under these conditions and intraventricular instillation of antibiotic may achieve adequate concentrations and be necessary for successful eradication. Treatment of gram-negative ventriculitis is more controversial as most studies show no significant clinical benefit with intrathecal administration of gentamicin or amikacin. The intrathecal or intraventricular instillation of anti-microbials may be a risk factor for seizures per se, although the risk may vary with the specific antibiotic (penicillins and cephalosporins are highly epileptogenic and never used). One should consider prophylactic anti-epileptic drug use in such cases, especially if there is cortical irritation by catheter associated hemorrhage [91, 102].

Inflammatory CNS Conditions

Vasculitides

Vasculitides comprise a heterogeneous group of multisystem disorders characterized by inflammation and necrosis of blood vessel walls, resulting in a variety of sequelae including aneurysms, vessel wall rupture with hemorrhage, and occlusion with infarction [103, 104]. Vasculitis affecting the central nervous system is both extremely variable and protean in presentation and challenging to be diagnosed, due to lack of specific signs and symptoms, and lack of non-invasive diagnostic tests. Vasculitis isolated to the CNS is referred to as primary CNS angiitis, whereas secondary vasculitis is associated with numerous conditions, including infections, lymphoproliferative disease (lymphoma), drug abuse (amphetamines), connective tissue disease, and other forms of systemic vasculitis [104]. In most cases, the diagnosis is made based on clinical presentation, presence of specific serum markers and confirmed by biopsy of lesions.

Necrotizing Vasculitides

This group of vasculitides thought of as necrotizing vasculitides includes: classic polyarteritis nodosa, granulomatosis with polyangitis, allergic angiitis and granulomatosis (Churg-Strauss—CS), necrotizing systemic vasculitis-overlap syndrome, and lymphomatoid granulomatosis [104].

Polyarteritis Nodosa

PAN is a necrotizing vasculitis, which targets medium-sized arteries and is not associated with glomerulonephritis or small vessel involvement [105]. CNS involvement in PAN ranges from 4 to 41% and is usually a late manifestation [103]. Peripheral nervous system damage is much more common (50–75% of cases). CNS lesions include focal lesions causing TIA, stroke (ischemic or hemorrhagic), seizures, and more commonly diffuse lesions causing multifocal neurologic findings and encephalopathy [103, 106]. Generalized or partial seizures have been described in 25–50% of patients with CNS complications and often occur together with acute disease such as headache, acute confusional state, and focal neurologic deficits [107]. Seizures in PAN do not usually require long-term treatment. CNS disease is usually associated with systemic features such as fevers, cutaneous involvement, and renal complications [108]. Elevated ESR, leukocytosis, anemia, thrombocytosis, hematuria, proteinuria, and circulating immune complexes may be found. Hepatitis B antigenemia is present in up to 30% of patients and their treatment and outcome may be different from those with idiopathic PAN [104, 108]. Angiography may demonstrate vasculitis as medium-sized vessels are involved. The presence of neurologic complications does not influence survival, which is significantly increased with treatment with corticosteroids and cytotoxic agents. Recommended treatment of seizures includes anticonvulsants as adjuncts to immunosuppressive therapy.

Granulomatosis with Polyangitis

Granulomatosis with polyangitis (formerly called Wegener's granulomatosis) is a necrotizing granulomatous vasculitis involving upper and lower respiratory tracts; three quarters of patients develop glomerulonephritis. Neurologic abnormalities are common and include cranial neuropathies, due to contiguous extension of granulomas from the nasopharynx, encephalopathy, seizures, pituitary abnormalities, and focal motor and sensory deficits due to small vessel vasculitis [109]. Peripheral neuropathies are also common. Little literature exists on the risk of seizures in this disease, though, when reported, they are usually a late complication.

Churg-Strauss Syndrome

CS syndrome can involve multiple organs, particularly pulmonary vessels causing asthma and pulmonary infiltrates along with eosinophilia [109]. Neurologic abnormalities are similar to PAN with early encephalopathy being frequent due to small vessel involvement. The CNS was involved in 62% of 47 cases from the Mayo Clinic. In this series, no patients had seizures [110].

Vasculitides Associated with Connective Tissue Disease

This group of vasculitides includes systemic lupus erythematosus (SLE), rheumatoid arthritis, scleroderma, Sjogren's syndrome, and mixed connective tissue disease (MCTD). Whereas CNS involvement is common in SLE and MCTD, occurring in 20–50% of patients, it is rare in scleroderma and rheumatoid arthritis [103].

Systemic Lupus Erythematosus

Systemic Lupus Erythematosus (SLE) is characterized by immunologic mediated damage to multiple organs, particularly skin, kidneys, and joints, secondary to generation of autoantibodies and immune complexes [104].

Seizures are a frequent complication of SLE, and occur unrelated to renal failure, hypertension, or medications in approximately 14–17% of patients. They are typically seen in the early phases of illness and most are non-recurrent [108]. In a large prospective cohort study of 1631 patients with lupus, 4.6% had one or more seizure during their disease course. Additionally, most seizures (76%) resolved in those affected without the need for anticonvulsant medications [111]. The presence of seizures does not alter mortality risk. However, during the terminal phases of disease, seizures may occur with increased frequency. Seizures commonly occur together with neuropsychiatric (NP) findings, thrombocytopenia, and cutaneous signs of vasculitis [108]. NP disturbances are common in SLE. They often occur in the first year of disease, but are rarely the presenting symptom [112]. Seizures were mostly generalized tonic-clonic. Serological and other clinical associations with NP syndromes in SLE patients include vasculitis, antiphospholipid antibodies and hematological complications (thrombocytopenia, leukopenia) [113, 114], higher risk of renal failure [115], and history of cyclophosphamide treatment [113].

The pathogenesis of seizures and other NP syndromes in SLE is not well understood. Antiphospholipid antibodies are more frequently found in patients with SLE and seizures than in patients with SLE without seizures. In a study of 221 unselected patients with SLE, 43.8% of patients with epilepsy had detectable lupus anticoagulant versus 20.8% of patients without. A significant association was found between moderate to high titers of IgG anti-cardiolipin antibodies and the presence of seizures [116]. One important mechanism is likely an occlusive vasculopathy, suggested by the strong association between antiphospholipid antibodies and NP symptoms [113, 114]. In a prospective study of 76 Indian women with SLE, a strong association was found between seizures and anti-cardiolipin and anti-beta 2 glycoprotein I antibodies [117]. Circulating anti-cardiolipin antibodies from SLE patients with seizures decreased GABA-mediated responses in snail neurons in vitro [118]. Pathologic studies of SLE patients with seizures have shown cerebral microinfarcts and subarachnoid hemorrhage [119].

True vasculitis is actually rare in SLE and frequent findings include hyalinization, perivascular inflammation, and endothelial proliferation [104, 119]. The most common pathological finding at autopsy is a noninflammatory small vessel vasculopathy [120]. In vitro and in vivo studies suggest that antiphospholipid antibodies may activate vascular endothelial cells, leading to expression of leukocyte adhesion molecules and generating a prothrombotic state on the endothelial cell surface [121, 122]. Evidence of disordered immune regulation is also present in the CNS in the form of immune complexes in the cerebrospinal fluid (CSF) [123] and choroid plexus [124], elevated IgG CSF/serum index, oligoclonal CSF IgG [125], and lymphocytotoxic antibodies that cross-react with brain [126]. More recently, autoantibodies to glutamate receptors, specifically NMDA NR2A or NR2B autoantibodies, some of which cross-react with double-stranded DNA, have been detected in 30% of SLE patients, with or without neuropsychiatric impairments [127]. Glutamate receptor autoantibodies are also found in many patients with epilepsy, and encephalitis, and may contribute to seizures and brain damage.

In patients with SLE who present with seizures, it is important to consider several possible etiologies for the seizures including infarction (cardioembolism from Libman-Sacks endocarditis, a mural thrombus, antibody-raised homocysteine levels, carotid dissection, and hypertensive small vessel disease), cerebral venous sinus thrombosis, encephalitis, and cerebral vasculitis. In patients on immunosuppressants, it is crucial to rule out infections, including intracranial abscess, and cryptococcal meningitis. Widespread vascular abnormalities on angiography should suggest a cause other than SLE for seizures due to lack of large vessel involvement by this disease [108]. EEG abnormalities are frequent, but non-specific findings [128]. One small study of brain pathology in SLE patients reported the strongest association between presence of cerebral microinfarcts and seizures (4/5 patients) [129]. Patients with SLE who are being treated with cytotoxic therapy have also been reported to develop reversible posterior leukoencephalopathy syndrome (RPLS) with resulting seizures and other typical clinical and radiological manifestations [130]. The etiology of RPLS in this context is believed to be dysfunction of the vascular endothelium secondary to several factors including hypertension, renal failure with fluid retention, and cytotoxic drugs. The condition is reversible with prompt antihypertensive, anticonvulsant, and correction of fluid overload management [130].

Treatment of seizures during a disease flare depends on frequency of attacks and etiology. Most CNS complications occur in untreated patients or those on low dose corticosteroids [108]. Single seizures occurring during disease flares may respond to corticosteroids alone, but recurrent attacks should be treated with anticonvulsants [108]. The risk of worsening disease with use of hydantoins, ethosuxamide, and trimethadione, causing drug-induced SLE is low and should not prevent the use of appropriate anticonvulsants [108]. The development of a rash during treatment should alert the clinician to the possibility of an allergic reaction, the unmasking of SLE by the drug or an anticonvulsant hypersensitivity syndrome. The latter is characterized by the triad of fever, rash, and internal organ involvement with incidence of 1:1000 to 1:10,000 exposures. Aromatic anti-epileptics (phenytoin, phenobarbital, carbamazepine) as well as lamotrigine, valproic acid, felbamate, primidone, and trimethadione have been implicated [131–134]. The reaction usually develops 1–12 weeks after initiation of therapy and is thought to be caused by insufficient detoxification of arene oxides (metabolites of aromatic anti-epileptics). Lymphadenopathy, hypothyroidism (even 2 months later), and multi-organ involvement (skin, liver, kidney, lungs, CNS) can lead to fatal complications. Cross-reactivity among aromatic anti-epileptics occurs in 75% of cases. Immediate discontinuation of the drug, hydration, antihistamines, topical, and systemic corticosteroids can be used. Because of genetic predisposition, siblings of patients may be at increased risk. Drug-induced SLE is much more frequent with distinct clinical and laboratory abnormalities. Drugs such as phenytoin, carbamazepine, ethosuxamide, trimethadione, primidone, and valproate have been implicated, but rarely phenobarbital and benzodiazepines [134]. The clinical presentation of drug-induced SLE is frequently abrupt onset of malaise and fever, but overall the disease is milder than idiopathic SLE and renal or neurological involvement is rare with pleuropulmonary and pericardial manifestations more common. The main difference between drug-induced SLE and hypersensitivity syndrome is the presence of autoantibodies in the former, including anti-histone, anti-nuclear antibodies, that may persist for months or years after discontinuation of the drug, as opposed to the symptoms that promptly remit.

Rheumatoid Arthritis, Scleroderma, Sjogren's syndrome, and Mixed Connective Tissue Disease

CNS involvement in rheumatoid arthritis, scleroderma, Sjogren's syndrome, and mixed connective tissue disease (MCTD) causing seizures is uncommon. In rheumatoid arthritis (RA) 20% of patients with CNS involvement have seizures [135] [136–139]. One report of RA of the CNS presenting with focal seizures was caused by a focal meningeal vasculitis [139]. The patient responded to etanercept, cochicine, and anticonvulsant therapy.

In scleroderma, neuropsychiatric symptoms have been reported in 5/32 (16%) patients with systemic sclerosis and secondary generalized or focal motor seizures were reported among them. EEG was normal in this series and primary CNS involvement could not be confirmed [140]. Simple partial motor seizures associated with fibrosis of cerebral arterioles and arteritis involving middle cerebral artery branches and vasa vasorum of the carotid artery have been reported in scleroderma patients [141]. These are thought to be the result of hypertension [104]. Sjogren's syndrome (SS), characterized by xerophthalmia and xerostomia, may also present with CNS involvement, either focal or diffuse in 25% of cases [103]. CNS manifestations include seizures as well as focal motor, sensory and speech deficits, movement disorders, brain stem syndromes, encephalopathy, dementia, and recurrent aseptic meningitis [103, 142]. Complex partial and simple partial motor seizures have been reported. Cerebral signs are associated with antineuronal antibodies, or an autoimmune inflammatory cerebral vasculopathy affecting predominantly small vessels, and multiple areas of increased signal intensity on T2 and proton-density weighted MRI [103, 143]. Other common findings are peripheral neuropathy, elevated erythrocyte sedimentation rate, cutaneous vasculitis, and renal tubular acidosis [142].

In MCTD, there have been reports of generalized motor seizures in association with ataxia, hemiparesis, meningeal signs, and psychiatric disturbances [144]. The neuropathology of these findings is not well understood. Intractable temporal lobe seizures have been reported in patients with ulcerative colitis. Steroid tapering and abdominal surgery led to status epilepticus [145].

Vasculitis Associated with Other Systemic Diseases

This group of vasculitides includes Behçet's disease, ulcerative colitis, sarcoidosis, relapsing polychondritis, and Kolmeier-Degos disease.

Behçet's Disease

Behçet's syndrome is a multisystem inflammatory disease of unknown cause, which involves the central nervous system in approximately 5% of patients [146]. Criteria for diagnosis (International Study Group for Behçet's syndrome) are recurrent oral ulceration plus two from recurrent genital ulceration, eye lesions, skin lesions, or positive pathery test (hypersensitivity of the skin to non-specific physiological insult [147]. Neurological involvement in Behçet's syndrome usually manifests as a subacute brainstem meningo-encephalitis, occasionally with hemispheric or spinal cord involvement, and MRI lesions in about 75% of cases [148]. Seizures are observed independently, but are an important indication of CNS involvement, or can accompany cerebral sinus thrombosis or may be related to interferon-A treatment [149–151]. In one review of 223 patients with neurologic Behçet's disease, seizures were observed in 10 (4.5%) of cases [149]. Seizures occurred during neurologic exacerbation in only five patients, making the prevalence of seizures due to Behçet's disease around 2%. In the other five patients, seizures were not related to neurologic Behçet's disease attacks. The most common seizure types were generalized tonic-clonic seizures and focal motor seizures, which were controllable in most cases. Seizures were associated with abnormal CSF findings (high protein, pleocytosis) in most cases, a poor prognostic factor in neuro-Behçet's disease, indicating parenchymal involvement [146]. It was postulated that seizure occurrence may indicate dissemination of the inflammatory process to involve the cortex. They may also be associated with cerebral hypoperfusion; in a study of seven patients with Behçet's disease evaluated by SPECT, three of them had seizures and hypoperfusion in the temporal lobe, including the mesial portion [152]. The occurrence of seizures also seemed to be associated with a high mortality rate, although they remain an unusual neurologic complication for this disease. Immunosuppressive therapy with intravenous steroids, and cyclophosphamide or chlorambucil may also help to control seizures [153].

Sarcoidosis

Sarcoidosis is affecting the central nervous system in 5–16% of the cases. Various neurological manifestations are observed, including: seizures in 5–10% of those with neuro-sarcoidosis [154], cognitive or psychic manifestations, hypothalamic and pituitary involvement, local pseudotumors, and hydrocephalus (very frequently associated with asymptomatic lymphocytic meningitis) and with cranial nerve palsy (particularly palsy of the seventh nerve) which occur less regularly. CNS localization is most often an early manifestation of the disease, unmasking sarcoidosis. It is often part of primary or secondary systemic polyvisceral sarcoidosis [155]. The diagnostic process should first confirm nervous system involvement and then provide supportive evidence for the underlying disease; in the absence of any positive tissue biopsy, the most useful diagnostic tests are gadolinium enhanced MRI of the brain and CSF analysis, although both are non-specific. The mainstay of treatment is corticosteroids, but these often have to be combined with other immunosuppressants such as methotrexate, hydroxychloroquine,

or cyclophosphamide. There is increasing evidence that infliximab is a safe treatment with good steroid sparing capacity [156]. Resection of the sarcoid lesion after intracranial mapping has been reported in a patient with neurosarcoidosis and super-refractory status epilepticus [157].

References

1. Wang K-W et al. The significance of seizures and other predictive factors during the acute illness for the long-term outcome after bacterial meningitis. Seizure. 2005;14:586–92.
2. Young BG, Jordan KG, Doig GS. An assessment of nonconvulsive seizures in the intensive care unit using continuous EEG monitoring: an investigation of variables associated with mortality. Neurology. 1996;47:83–9.
3. Bleck TP et al. Neurologic complications of critical medical illnesses. Crit Care Med. 1993;21:98–103.
4. Gans JD, Spanjaard L, Weisfelt M, Reitsma JB, Vermeulen M. Clinical features and prognostic factors in adults with bacterial meningitis. N Engl J Med. 2004;351:1849–59.
5. Sutter R, Stevens RD, Kaplan PW. Continuous electroencephalographic monitoring in critically ill patients. Crit Care Med. 2013;41:1124–32.
6. Claassen J, Mayer SA, Kowalski RG, Emerson RG, Hirsch LJ. Detection of electrographic seizures with continuous EEG monitoring in critically ill patients. Neurology. 2004;62:1743–8.
7. Gaspard N et al. New-onset refractory status epilepticus. Neurology. 2015;85:1604–13.
8. Claassen J, Mayer SA, Kowalski RG, Emerson RG, Hirsch LJ. Detection of electrographic seizures with continuous EEG monitoring in critically ill patients. Neurology. 2004;62:1743–8.
9. Claassen J et al. Electrographic seizures and periodic discharges after intracerebral hemorrhage. Neurology. 2007;69:1356–65.
10. Claassen J et al. Prognostic significance of continuous EEG monitoring in patients with poor-grade subarachnoid hemorrhage. Neurocrit Care. 2006;4:103–12.
11. van de Beek D, de Gans J, Tunkel AR, Wijdicks EFM. Community-acquired bacterial meningitis in adults. N Engl J Med. 2006;354:44–53.
12. Carrera E et al. Continuous electroencephalographic monitoring in critically ill patients with central nervous system infections. Arch Neurol. 2008;65:1612–8.
13. Oddo M, Carrera E, Claassen J, Mayer SA, Hirsch LJ. Continuous electroencephalography in the medical intensive care unit. Crit Care Med. 2009;37:2051–6.
14. Coyle P. Central nervous system infections. Neurol Clin. 1999;17:691–710.
15. Townsend GC, Scheld WM. Infections of the central nervous system. Adv Intern Med. 1998;43:403–47.
16. Rotbart HA. Enteroviral infections of the central nervous system. Clin Infect Dis. 1995;20:971–81.
17. Annegers JF, Hauser WA, Beghi E, Nicolosi A, Kurland LT. The risk of unprovoked seizures after encephalitis and meningitis. Neurology. 1988;38:1407–10.
18. Thigpen MC et al. Bacterial meningitis in the United States, 1998–2007. N Engl J Med. 2011;364:2016–25.
19. Auburtin M et al. Detrimental role of delayed antibiotic administration and penicillin-nonsusceptible strains in adult intensive care unit patients with pneumococcal meningitis: the PNEUMOREA prospective multicenter study. Crit Care Med. 2006;34:2758–65.
20. Durand ML et al. Acute bacterial meningitis in adults. A review of 493 episodes. N Engl J Med. 1993;328:21–8.

21. Pfister HW, Feiden W, Einhäupl KM. Spectrum of complications during bacterial meningitis in adults. Results of a prospective clinical study. Arch Neurol. 1993;50:575–81.

22. Sigurdardóttir B, Björnsson OM, Jónsdóttir KE, Erlendsdóttir H, Gudmundsson S. Acute bacterial meningitis in adults. A 20-year overview. Arch Intern Med. 1997;157:425–30.

23. Hussein AS, Shafran SD. Acute bacterial meningitis in adults. A 12-year review. Medicine (Baltimore). 2000;79:360–8.

24. Gaieski DF et al. Impact of time to antibiotics on survival in patients with severe sepsis or septic shock in whom early goal-directed therapy was initiated in the emergency department. Crit Care Med. 2010;38:1045–53.

25. Gaieski DF, Nathan BR, O'Brien NF. Emergency neurologic life support: meningitis and encephalitis. Neurocrit Care. 2015;23(Suppl 2):110–8.

26. Brouwer MC, McIntyre P, Prasad K, van de Beek D. Corticosteroids for acute bacterial meningitis. Cochrane Database Syst Rev. 2015;9:CD004405.

27. DiNubile MJ, Boom WH, Southwick FS. Septic cortical thrombophlebitis. J Infect Dis. 1990;161:1216–20.

28. Jordan KG. Continuous EEG monitoring in the neuroscience intensive care unit and emergency department. J Clin Neurophysiol. 1999;16:14–39.

29. Doern GV, Brueggemann A, Holley HP, Rauch AM. Antimicrobial resistance of Streptococcus pneumoniae recovered from outpatients in the United States during the winter months of 1994 to 1995: results of a 30-center national surveillance study. Antimicrob Agents Chemother. 1996;40:1208–13.

30. van de Beek D, Brouwer MC, Thwaites GE, Tunkel AR. Advances in treatment of bacterial meningitis. Lancet (London). 2012;380:1693–702.

31. Miller S, Mateen FJ, Aksamit AJ. Herpes simplex virus 2 meningitis: a retrospective cohort study. J Neurovirol. 2013;19:166–71.

32. Barontini F, Ghezzi M, Marconi GP. A case of benign recurrent meningitis of Mollaret. J Neurol. 1981;225:197–206.

33. Zunt JR, Baldwin KJ. Chronic and subacute meningitis. Continuum (Minneap Minn). 2012;18:1290–318.

34. Roos KL. Encephalitis. Handb Clin Neurol. 2014;121:1377–81.

35. Sutter R et al. Electroencephalography for diagnosis and prognosis of acute encephalitis. Clin Neurophysiol. 2015;126:1524–31.

36. Misra UK, Tan CT, Kalita J. Viral encephalitis and epilepsy. Epilepsia. 2008;49(Suppl 6):13–8.

37. Michael BD, Solomon T. Seizures and encephalitis: clinical features, management, and potential pathophysiologic mechanisms. Epilepsia. 2012;53(Suppl 4):63–71.

38. Marks DA, Kim J, Spencer DD, Spencer SS. Characteristics of intractable seizures following meningitis and encephalitis. Neurology. 1992;42:1513–8.

39. Solomon T, Hart IJ, Beeching NJ. Viral encephalitis: a clinician's guide. Pract Neurol. 2007;7:288–305.

40. Michael BD et al. Acute central nervous system infections in adults--a retrospective cohort study in the NHS North West region. QJM. 2010;103:749–58.

41. Hjalmarsson A, Blomqvist P, Sköldenberg B. Herpes simplex encephalitis in Sweden, 1990–2001: incidence, morbidity, and mortality. Clin Infect Dis. 2007;45:875–80.

42. McGrath N, Anderson NE, Croxson MC, Powell KF. Herpes simplex encephalitis treated with acyclovir: diagnosis and long term outcome. J Neurol Neurosurg Psychiatry. 1997;63:321–6.

43. Whitley RJ. Herpes simplex encephalitis: adolescents and adults. Antivir Res. 2006;71:141–8.

44. Lai CW, Gragasin ME. Electroencephalography in herpes simplex encephalitis. J Clin Neurophysiol. 1988;5:87–103.

45. Smith JB, Westmoreland BF, Reagan TJ, Sandok BA. A distinctive clinical EEG profile in herpes simplex encephalitis. Mayo Clin Proc. 1975;50:469–74.

46. Jha S, Patel R, Yadav RK, Kumar V. Clinical spectrum, pitfalls in diagnosis and therapeutic implications in herpes simplex encephalitis. J Assoc Physicians India. 2004;52:24–6.

47. Nahmias AJ, Whitley RJ, Visintine AN, Takei Y, Alford CA. Herpes simplex virus encephalitis: laboratory evaluations and their diagnostic significance. J. Infect. Dis. 1982;145:829–36.

48. Boivin G. Diagnosis of herpesvirus infections of the central nervous system. Herpes. 2004;11(Suppl 2):48A–56A.

49. Singh TD et al. Predictors of outcome in HSV encephalitis. J Neurol. 2015; doi:10.1007/s00415-015-7960-8.

50. Kennedy PG. A retrospective analysis of forty-six cases of herpes simplex encephalitis seen in Glasgow between 1962 and 1985. Q J Med. 1988;68:533–40.

51. Prayson R. Neuropathology Review. Neuropathol Rev. 2008; doi:10.1007/978-1-59745-219-9.

52. Solomon T et al. Management of suspected viral encephalitis in adults--Association of British Neurologists and British Infection Association National Guidelines. J Infect. 2012;64:347–73.

53. Whitley RJ, Gnann JW. Viral encephalitis: familiar infections and emerging pathogens. Lancet (London, England). 2002;359:507–13.

54. Hokkanen L, Salonen O, Launes J. Amnesia in acute herpetic and nonherpetic encephalitis. Arch Neurol. 1996;53:972–8.

55. Launes J et al. Unilateral hyperfusion in brain-perfusion SPECT predicts poor prognosis in acute encephalitis. Neurology. 1997;48:1347–51.

56. Arciniegas DB, Anderson CA. Viral encephalitis: neuropsychiatric and neurobehavioral aspects. Curr Psychiatry Rep. 2004;6:372–9.

57. Hart RP, Kwentus JA, Frazier RB, Hormel TL. Natural history of Klüver-Bucy syndrome after treated herpes encephalitis. South Med J. 1986;79:1376–8.

58. Sellner J, Trinka E. Seizures and epilepsy in herpes simplex virus encephalitis: current concepts and future directions of pathogenesis and management. J Neurol. 2012;259:2019–30.

59. Johnson RT et al. Japanese encephalitis: immunocytochemical studies of viral antigen and inflammatory cells in fatal cases. Ann Neurol. 1985;18:567–73.

60. Solomon T et al. Seizures and raised intracranial pressure in Vietnamese patients with Japanese encephalitis. Brain. 2002;125:1084–93.

61. Solomon T et al. Poliomyelitis-like illness due to Japanese encephalitis virus. Lancet (London, England). 1998;351:1094–7.

62. Misra UK, Kalita J. Anterior horn cells are also involved in Japanese encephalitis. Acta Neurol Scand. 1997;96:114–7.

63. Patel H, Sander B, Nelder MP. Long-term sequelae of West Nile virus-related illness: a systematic review. Lancet Infect Dis. 2015;15:951–9.

64. Hollidge BS, González-Scarano F, Soldan SS. Arboviral encephalitides: transmission, emergence, and pathogenesis. J NeuroImmune Pharmacol. 2010;5:428–42.

65. Zacks MA, Paessler S. Encephalitic alphaviruses. Vet Microbiol. 2010;140:281–6.

66. Deresiewicz RL, Thaler SJ, Hsu L, Zamani AA. Clinical and neuroradiographic manifestations of eastern equine encephalitis. N Engl J Med. 1997;336:1867–74.

67. Gould EA, Solomon T. Pathogenic flaviviruses. Lancet (London, England). 2008;371:500–9.

68. Kramer AH. Viral encephalitis in the ICU. Crit Care Clin. 2013;29:621–49.

69. Gandelman-Marton R et al. Electroencephalography findings in adult patients with West Nile virus-associated meningitis and meningoencephalitis. Clin Infect Dis. 2003;37:1573–8.

70. Babi M-A, Raleigh T, Shapiro RE, McSherry J, Applebee A. MRI and encephalography in fatal eastern equine encephalitis. Neurology. 2014;83:1483.

71. Hall HI et al. Prevalence of diagnosed and undiagnosed HIV infection–United States, 2008–2012. MMWR Morb Mortal Wkly Rep. 2015;64:657–62.

72. Kellinghaus C et al. Frequency of seizures and epilepsy in neurological HIV-infected patients. Seizure. 2008;17:27–33.

73. Dore GJ, Law MG, Brew BJ. Prospective analysis of seizures occurring in human immunodeficiency virus type-1 infection. J Neuro AIDS. 1996;1:59–69.

74. Wong MC, Suite ND, Labar DR. Seizures in human immunodeficiency virus infection. Arch Neurol. 1990;47:640–2.

75. Lee KC, Garcia PA, Alldredge BK. Clinical features of status epilepticus in patients with HIV infection. Neurology. 2005;65:314–6.

76. Miskin DP, Herman ST, Ngo LH, Koralnik IJ. Predictors and characteristics of seizures in survivors of progressive multifocal leukoencephalopathy. J. Neurovirol. 2015; doi:10.1007/s13365-015-0414-3.

77. Holtzman DM, Kaku DA, So YT. New-onset seizures associated with human immunodeficiency virus infection: causation and clinical features in 100 cases. Am J Med. 1989;87:173–7.

78. Garg RK. HIV infection and seizures. Postgrad Med J. 1999;75:387–90.

79. Barry M, Gibbons S, Back D, Mulcahy F. Protease inhibitors in patients with HIV disease. Clinically important pharmacokinetic considerations. Clin Pharmacokinet. 1997;32:194–209.

80. Hugen PW et al. Carbamazepine--indinavir interaction causes antiretroviral therapy failure. Ann Pharmacother. 2000;34:465–70.

81. Toler SM, Wilkerson MA, Porter WH, Smith AJ, Chandler MH. Severe phenytoin intoxication as a result of altered protein binding in AIDS. DICP. 24:698–700.

82. Moog C, Kuntz-Simon G, Caussin-Schwemling C, Obert G. Sodium valproate, an anticonvulsant drug, stimulates human immunodeficiency virus type 1 replication independently of glutathione levels. J Gen Virol. 1996;77(Pt 9):1993–9.

83. Maggi JD, Halman MH. The effect of divalproex sodium on viral load: a retrospective review of HIV-positive patients with manic syndromes. Can J Psychiatr. 2001;46:359–62.

84. Pesola GR, Westfal RE. New-onset generalized seizures in patients with AIDS presenting to an emergency department. Acad Emerg Med. 1998;5:905–11.

85. Brouwer MC, Coutinho JM, van de Beek D. Clinical characteristics and outcome of brain abscess: systematic review and meta-analysis. Neurology. 2014;82:806–13.

86. Brouwer MC, Tunkel AR, McKhann GM, van de Beek D. Brain abscess. N Engl J Med. 2014;371:447–56.

87. Legg NJ, Gupta PC, Scott DF. Epilepsy following cerebral abscess. A clinical and EEG study of 70 patients. Brain. 1973;96:259–68.

88. Chuang M-J et al. Predictors and long-term outcome of seizures after bacterial brain abscess. J Neurol Neurosurg Psychiatry. 2010;81:913–7.

89. Lu C-H, Chang W-N, Lui C-C. Strategies for the management of bacterial brain abscess. J Clin Neurosci. 2006;13:979–85.

90. Muzumdar D, Jhawar S, Goel A. Brain abscess: an overview. Int J Surg. 2011;9:136–44.

91. Scheld MW, Marra CM, Whitley RJ. Infections of the central nervous system. 4th ed. Philadelphia: Lippincott Williams & Wilkins; 2014.

92. Tsai Y-D et al. Intracranial suppuration: a clinical comparison of subdural empyemas and epidural abscesses. Surg Neurol. 2003;59:191–6. discussion 196

93. Smith HP, Hendrick EB. Subdural empyema and epidural abscess in children. J Neurosurg. 1983;58:392–7.

94. Bok AP, Peter JC. Subdural empyema: burr holes or craniotomy? A retrospective computerized tomography-era analysis of treatment in 90 cases. J Neurosurg. 1993;78:574–8.

95. Osborn MK, Steinberg JP. Subdural empyema and other suppurative complications of paranasal sinusitis. Lancet Infect Dis. 2007;7:62–7.

96. Humphreys H, Jenks PJ. Surveillance and management of ventriculitis following neurosurgery. J Hosp Infect. 2015;89:281–6.

97. Fried HI et al. The insertion and management of external ventricular drains: an evidence-based consensus statement: a statement for healthcare professionals from the neurocritical care society. Neurocrit Care. 2016;24:61–81.

98. Ines DF, Markand ON. Epileptic seizures and abnormal electroencephalographic findings in hydrocephalus and their relation to the shunting procedures. Electroencephalogr Clin Neurophysiol. 1977;42:761–8.

99. Dan NG, Wade MJ. The incidence of epilepsy after ventricular shunting procedures. J Neurosurg. 1986;65:19–21.

100. Piatt JH, Carlson CV. Hydrocephalus and epilepsy: an actuarial analysis. Neurosurgery. 1996;39:722–7. discussion 727–8

101. Bourgeois M et al. Epilepsy in children with shunted hydrocephalus. J Neurosurg. 1999;90:274–81.

102. Ng K, Mabasa VH, Chow I, Ensom MHH. Systematic review of efficacy, pharmacokinetics, and administration of intraventricular vancomycin in adults. Neurocrit Care. 2014;20:158–71.

103. Ferro JM. Vasculitis of the central nervous system. J Neurol. 1998;245:766–76.

104. Fieschi C, Rasura M, Anzini A, Beccia M. Central nervous system vasculitis. [Review] [76 refs]. J Neurol Sci. 1998;153:159–71.

105. Hernández-Rodríguez J, Alba MA, Prieto-González S, Cid MC. Diagnosis and classification of polyarteritis nodosa. J Autoimmun. 48–49:84–9.

106. Coblyn JS, McCluskey RT. Case records of the Massachusetts General Hospital. Weekly clinicopathological exercises. Case 3–2003. A 36-year-old man with renal failure, hypertension, and neurologic abnormalities. N Engl J Med. 2003;348:333–42.

107. Moore PM, Fauci AS. Neurologic manifestations of systemic vasculitis. A retrospective and prospective study of the clinicopathologic features and responses to therapy in 25 patients. Am J Med. 1981;71:517–24.

108. Messing RO, Simon RP. Seizures as a manifestation of systemic disease. Neurol Clin. 1986;4:563–84.

109. Ajmani A, Habte-Gabr E, Zarr M, Jayabalan V, Dandala S. Cerebral blood flow SPECT with Tc-99 m exametamine correlates in AIDS dementia complex stages. A preliminary report. Clin Nucl Med. 1991;16:656–9.

110. Sehgal M, Swanson JW, DeRemee RA, Colby TV. Neurologic manifestations of Churg-Strauss syndrome. Mayo Clin Proc. 1995;70:337–41.

111. Hanly JG et al. Seizure disorders in systemic lupus erythematosus results from an international, prospective, inception cohort study. Ann Rheum Dis. 2012;71:1502–9.

112. van Dam AP. Diagnosis and pathogenesis of CNS lupus. Rheumatol Int. 1991;11:1–11.

113. Mok CC, Lau CS, Wong RW. Neuropsychiatric manifestations and their clinical associations in southern Chinese patients with systemic lupus erythematosus. J Rheumatol. 2001;28:766–71.

114. Karassa FB, Ioannidis JP, Touloumi G, Boki KA, Moutsopoulos HM. Risk factors for central nervous system involvement in systemic lupus erythematosus. QJM. 2000;93:169–74.

115. Gibson T, Myers AR. Nervous system involvement in systemic lupus erythematosus. Ann Rheum Dis. 1975;35:398–406.

116. Herranz MT, Rivier G, Khamashta MA, Blaser KU, Hughes GR. Association between antiphospholipid antibodies and epilepsy in patients with systemic lupus erythematosus. Arthritis Rheum. 1994;37:568–71.

117. Shrivastava A, Dwivedi S, Aggarwal A, Misra R. Anti-cardiolipin and anti-beta2 glycoprotein I antibodies in Indian patients with systemic lupus erythematosus: association with the presence of seizures. Lupus. 2001;10:45–50.

118. Liou HH et al. Anticardiolipin antisera from lupus patients with seizures reduce a GABA receptor-mediated chloride current in snail neurons. Life Sci. 1994;54:1119–25.

119. Ellis SG, Verity MA. Central nervous system involvement in systemic lupus erythematosus: a review of neuropathologic findings in 57 cases, 1955--1977. Semin Arthritis Rheum. 1979;8:212–21.

120. West SG. Neuropsychiatric lupus. Rheum Dis Clin N Am. 1994;20:129–58.

121. Simantov R et al. Antiphospholipid antibodies activate vascular endothelial cells. Lupus. 1996;5:440–1.

122. Pierangeli SS et al. Antiphospholipid antibodies from antiphospholipid syndrome patients activate endothelial cells in vitro and in vivo. Circulation. 1999;99:1997–2002.

123. Seibold JR, Buckingham RB, Medsger TA, Kelly RH. Cerebrospinal fluid immune complexes in systemic lupus erythematosus involving the central nervous system. Semin Arthritis Rheum. 1982;12:68–76.

124. Atkins CJ, Kondon JJ, Quismorio FP, Friou GJ. The choroid plexus in systemic lupus erythematosus. Ann Intern Med. 1972;76:65–72.

125. Winfield JB et al. Intrathecal IgG synthesis and blood-brain barrier impairment in patients with systemic lupus erythematosus and central nervous system dysfunction. Am J Med. 1983;74:837–44.

126. Bluestein HG, Zvaifler NJ. Brain-reactive lymphocytotoxic antibodies in the serum of patients with systemic lupus erythematosus. J Clin Invest. 1976;57:509–16.

127. Levite M, Ganor Y. Autoantibodies to glutamate receptors can damage the brain in epilepsy, systemic lupus erythematosus and encephalitis. Expert Rev Neurother. 2008;8:1141–60.

128. Cohen SB, Hurd ER. Neurological complications of connective tissue and other 'collagen-vascular' diseases. Semin Arthritis Rheum. 1981;11:190–212.

129. Hanly JG, Walsh NM, Sangalang V. Brain pathology in systemic lupus erythematosus. J Rheumatol. 1992;19:732–41.

130. Primavera A, Audenino D, Mavilio N, Cocito L. Reversible posterior leucoencephalopathy syndrome in systemic lupus and vasculitis. Ann Rheum Dis. 2001;60:534–7.

131. Bessmertny O, Pham T. Antiepileptic hypersensitivity syndrome: clinicians beware and be aware. Curr Allergy Asthma Rep. 2002;2:34–9.

132. Knowles SR, Shapiro LE, Shear NH. Anticonvulsant hypersensitivity syndrome: incidence, prevention and management. Drug Saf. 1999;21:489–501.

133. Vittorio CC, Muglia JJ. Anticonvulsant hypersensitivity syndrome. Arch Intern Med. 1995;155:2285–90.

134. Drory VE, Korczyn AD. Hypersensitivity vasculitis and systemic lupus erythematosus induced by anticonvulsants. Clin Neuropharmacol. 1993;16:19–29.

135. Beck DO, Corbett JJ. Seizures due to central nervous system rheumatoid meningovasculitis. Neurology. 1983;33:1058–61.

136. Jan JE, Hill RH, Low MD. Cerebral complications in juvenile rheumatoid arthritis. Can Med Assoc J. 1972;107:623–5.

137. Makela A, Heikki L, Sillanpaa M. Neurological manifestations of rheumatoid arthritis. In: Vinken PJ, Bruyen GW, editors. Handbook of clinical neurology, vol. 38. Amsterdam: Elsevier North Holland; 1979. p. 479–503.

138. Mandybur TI. Cerebral amyloid angiopathy: possible relationship to rheumatoid vasculitis. Neurology. 1979;29:1336–40.

139. Neamtu L et al. Rheumatoid disease of the CNS with meningeal vasculitis presenting with a seizure. Neurology. 2001;56:814–5.

140. Hietaharju A, Jääskeläinen S, Hietarinta M, Frey H. Central nervous system involvement and psychiatric manifestations in systemic sclerosis (scleroderma): clinical and neurophysiological evaluation. Acta Neurol Scand. 1993;87:382–7.

141. Estey E, Lieberman A, Pinto R, Meltzer M, Ransohoff J. Cerebral arteritis in scleroderma. Stroke. 10:595–7.

142. Alexander E. Central nervous system disease in Sjögren's syndrome. New insights into immunopathogenesis. Rheum Dis Clin N Am. 1992;18:637–72.

143. Spezialetti R, Bluestein HG, Peter JB, Alexander EL. Neuropsychiatric disease in Sjögren's syndrome: anti-ribosomal P and anti-neuronal antibodies. Am J Med. 1993;95:153–60.

144. Bennett RM, Bong DM, Spargo BH. Neuropsychiatric problems in mixed connective tissue disease. Am J Med. 1978;65:955–62.

145. Akhan G, Andermann F, Gotman MJ. Ulcerative colitis, status epilepticus and intractable temporal seizures. Epileptic Disord. 2002;4:135–7.

146. Akman-Demir G, Serdaroglu P, Tasçi B. Clinical patterns of neurological involvement in Behçet's disease: evaluation of 200 patients. The Neuro-Behçet Study Group. Brain. 1999;122(Pt 1): 2171–82.

147. Criteria for diagnosis of Behçet's disease. International Study Group for Behçet's Disease. Lancet (London, England). 1990;335:1078–80.

148. Kidd D, Steuer A, Denman AM, Rudge P. Neurological complications in Behçet's syndrome. Brain. 1999;122(Pt 1):2183–94.

149. Aykutlu E, Baykan B, Serdaroglu P, Gökyigit A, Akman-Demir G. Epileptic seizures in Behçet disease. Epilepsia. 2002;43: 832–5.

150. Durán E, Chacón JR. Behçet's disease with atypical double neurological involvement. Rev Neurol. 33:333–4.

151. O'Duffy JD et al. Interferon-alpha treatment of Behçet's disease. J Rheumatol. 1998;25:1938–44.

152. Vignola S et al. Brain perfusion spect in juvenile neuro-Behçet's disease. J Nucl Med. 2001;42:1151–7.

153. Mead S, Kidd D, Good C, Plant G. Behçet's syndrome may present with partial seizures. J Neurol Neurosurg Psychiatry. 2000;68:392–3.

154. Krumholz A, Stern BJ. Neurologic manifestations of sarcoidosis. Handb Clin Neurol. 2014;119:305–33.

155. Valeyre D, Chapelon-Abric C, Belin C, Dumas JL. Sarcoidosis of the central nervous system. La Rev médecine interne/fondée … par la Société Natl Fr médecine interne. 1998;19:409–14.

156. Joseph FG, Scolding NJ. Sarcoidosis of the nervous system. Pract Neurol. 2007;7:234–44.

157. Varelas PN. How I treat status epilepticus in the Neuro-ICU. Neurocrit Care. 2008;9:153–7.

Electrolyte Disturbances and Critical Care Seizures

Claudine Sculier and Nicolas Gaspard

Introduction

Metabolic imbalances are a common issue in critically ill patients. Electrolyte disturbances are almost ubiquitous [1] and acid-base imbalances are seen in at least 10% of patients.

Metabolic disorders are a relatively uncommon cause of acute symptomatic seizures in the general population [2] but substantially contribute to the incidence of acute seizures in hospitalized patients, especially those admitted to an intensive care unit [3–5]. A recent retrospective study of 139 patients without history of seizures, who developed hospital-onset seizures, found that as many as 25% of seizures were related to an acute metabolic disturbance, mostly hyponatremia, hypoglycemia, and acute renal failure [4]. Similarly, acute metabolic disorders accounted for one third of new-onset generalized seizures observed in 55 patients admitted to a medical or surgical intensive care unit [3]. Electrolyte disorders, mostly hyponatremia, were the most common metabolic abnormalities. A strikingly identical proportion was reported in patients admitted to a neurological intensive care unit in India who presented with acute symptomatic seizures [5].

C. Sculier
Service de Neurologie–Centre de Référence pour le Traitement de l'Epilepsie Réfractaire, Université Libre de Bruxelles–Hôpital Erasme, Route de Lennik, 808 1070 Bruxelles, Belgium
e-mail: sculier.claudine@gmail.com

N. Gaspard (✉)
Service de Neurologie–Centre de Référence pour le Traitement de l'Epilepsie Réfractaire, Université Libre de Bruxelles–Hôpital Erasme, Route de Lennik, 808 1070 Bruxelles, Belgium

Department of Neurology, Comprehensive Epilepsy Center, Yale University School of Medicine, 15 York Street, New Haven, CT 06520, USA
e-mail: nicolas.gaspard@erasme.ulb.ac.be

Relationship Between Electrolytes, The Acid-Base Disequilibrium, and Neuronal Excitability

Transport of Water and Electrolytes Across the Blood–Brain Barrier and Regulation of Extracellular and Cellular Volumes

The BBB maintains the homeostasis of the cerebral environment. Except in a few areas devoid of BBB (area postrema, etc.) the presence of tight junctions between capillary endothelial cells effectively eliminates paracellular transport. Transcellular transport occurs through various mechanisms (Fig. 18.1). Small molecules that are soluble both in water and in the membrane lipid bilayer, such as O_2 and CO_2 gas molecules, ethanol or anesthetics, can passively diffuse through the cell membrane. Water and ions cross the blood–brain barrier by carrier-mediated transport. These carriers may be specific to one molecule (Na^+ channel) or allow several molecules to pass ($Na^+/K^+/Cl^-$ cotransport). Molecules can either passively diffuse through channels (e.g., water, small ions) or be transported by more complex systems that may require energy (e.g., the $Na^+–K^+$ ATPase) or the co-transport of another molecule ($Na^+–H^+$ carrier; $Na^+–$glutamate transporter).

Water readily crosses the BBB by diffusion, at least in part through aquaporin-4 channels, and moves freely in or out of the brain according to the osmotic gradient, whereas sodium and chloride ions depend on the combined action of an array of transporters (Fig. 18.1), with an exchange half-time of sodium ions of approximately 2 h. Thus, acute variations of plasma osmolality might cause a substantial shift of water across the BBB. When plasma osmolality decreases abruptly, as in acute hyponatremia, the movement of water driven by the osmotic gradient from the vascular compartment to the brain causes an expansion of the cerebral interstitial fluid. This leads to a decrease in extracellular tonicity and secondary swelling of neurons and astrocytes. The opposite phenomenon, shrinkage of interstitial and cellular volumes, occurs with an abrupt increase in plasma osmolality. Progressive changes in plasma osmolality do not have the

P.N. Varelas, J. Claassen (eds.), *Seizures in Critical Care*, Current Clinical Neurology, DOI 10.1007/978-3-319-49557-6_18

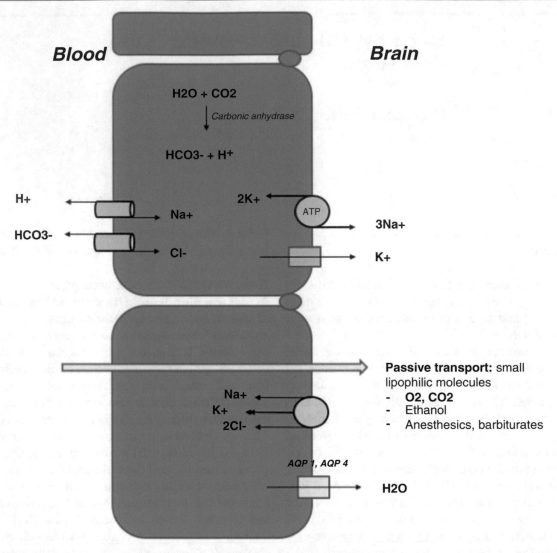

Fig. 18.1 Transport of water, gases, and electrolytes across the blood–brain barrier. Small lipophilic molecules passively diffuse through endothelial cells, while the transport of electrolytes and water is tightly regulated by transmembrane carriers

same consequences as cells are able to regulate their volume and osmolality. This regulation is based on the detection of volume changes and the activation of mechanisms of transport of electrolytes and organic osmoles, a process that can take 24–72 h. When a new equilibrium is reached, as in chronic hypernatremia, a rapid correction of plasma osmolality may thus be detrimental.

The BBB is impermeable to calcium, phosphorus, and magnesium ions . Their cerebrospinal fluid (CSF) levels (Table 18.1) are mostly determined by the secretion of a fluid of constant composition by the choroid plexus. CSF levels of calcium are approximately half of the plasma concentration and there is only a weak correlation between plasma and CSF levels. Magnesium is found in greater concentrations in the CSF than in the plasma and there is no clear correlation between CSF and plasma levels. Phosphorus levels in the CSF are approximately 60% of plasma levels. It should be noted that the immaturity of the blood–brain barrier in neonates allows calcium and magnesium ions to cross and their CSF levels correlate with their plasma levels [6].

The BBB is relatively impermeable to protons and bicarbonate ions, but it is very permeable to CO_2 gas molecules. CO_2 is also produced by neural cell metabolism. The pCO_2 is thus usually a few mm Hg higher and the pH slightly lower in the CSF than in the arterial blood. Changes in arterial pCO_2, by altering pH, activate homeostatic mechanisms that return the pH back toward normal. These mechanisms involve the adjustment of bicarbonate levels in the CSF and progressively take place over a period of several hours, whereas changes in CSF pCO_2 occur within minutes. Thus, compensation for changes in the pH of the CSF requires hours. Also, in a patient with an acute metabolic acidosis (decrease in plasma bicarbonate concentration) and a compensatory respiratory alkalosis (decrease in arterial pCO_2), the brain will be paradoxically alkalotic.

Neuronal Excitability: Membrane Potential, Ion Channels, Neurotransmitters, and Their Receptors

A seizure is the manifestation of the abnormal synchronous activation of a group of neurons. This is thought to be caused by an imbalance between neuronal excitation and inhibition. Recruitment of neurons during seizure can occur not only by excitatory glutamate-dependent synaptic transmission but also by extra-synaptic ephaptic coupling, a process during which local extracellular electrical fields generated by adjacent neurons feedback onto the electrical potential across the neuronal membrane. Inhibitory gamma-hydroxy-butyric acid (GABA)-dependent synaptic transmission represses seizure initiation and propagation (Fig. 18.2). Both synaptic and extra-synaptic transmission can be disrupted by changes in the electrolyte and acid-base composition of the extracellular fluid.

Extracellular low osmolality and hyponatremia increase neuronal excitability through various mechanisms [7–10]. To some extent, they enhance excitatory neurotransmission at the pre- and post-synaptic levels by facilitating calcium uptake [11, 12]. But the most important effect of low osmolality, whether it is caused or not by hyponatremia, occurs through cellular swelling, which enhances ephaptic coupling [7, 10, 13]. Additional effects of astrocytic swelling include the disruption of glutamate-glutamine metabolism and the release of excitatory amino acids by astrocytes [14, 15]. Low extracellular chloride concentrations also contribute to increase excitability by depressing GABA-dependent inhibitory currents [16]. Hyperosmolality has the reverse effect and decreases neuronal excitability [17].

Table 18.1 Electrolyte and acid-base composition of the CSF

	CSF	CSF/plasma ratio	Exchange half-time
Sodium	141.2 ± 6.0 (mmol/l)	0.95	1 h
Potassium	2.96 ± 0.45 (mmol/l)	0.70	24 h
Chloride	120.3 ± 3.3 (mmol/l)	1.10	
Osmolality	287.2 ± 5.5 (mOsm)	1.00	
Magnesium	2.71 ± 0.11 (mg/dL)	1.40	
Calcium	4.56 ± 0.32 (mg/dL)	0.50	
Phosphorus		0.60	
pH	7.32 ± 0.09	7.40 ± 0.06	
pCO$_2$	44 (mmHg)	40	Seconds
HCO_3^-	22 (mmol/l)	24	Hours to days
Water			12–25 s

Electrolytes and acid-base composition of the CSF compared to plasma values. Data from [193–197]

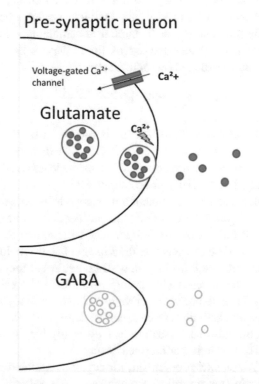
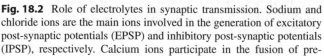
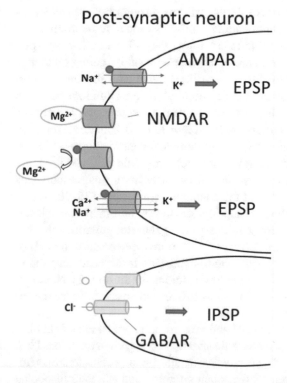

Fig. 18.2 Role of electrolytes in synaptic transmission. Sodium and chloride ions are the main ions involved in the generation of excitatory post-synaptic potentials (EPSP) and inhibitory post-synaptic potentials (IPSP), respectively. Calcium ions participate in the fusion of pre-synaptic vesicles and in neurotransmitter (both glutamate and GABA) release and contribute to the generation of EPSP, while magnesium ions limit the opening of glutamate NMDA channels

Calcium and magnesium ions both are voltage membrane stabilizers. They screen surface negative charges on neuronal membranes and regulate the activation of voltage-gated ion channels [9, 18]. There is an inverse correlation between extracellular calcium concentrations and neuronal excitability [19]. Immersing hippocampal slices in a low-calcium solution provokes the occurrence of spontaneous synchronized bursts similar to epileptiform discharges [20]. This is at least in part explained by an increase in resting membrane potential and a decrease of the firing threshold [21] and occurs even when excitatory neurotransmission is blocked [22]. Conversely, a high-calcium solution completely prevents seizure-like activity in hippocampal slices [23]. Similar findings are observed when manipulating extracellular magnesium concentrations in vitro. Sporadic epileptiform bursts followed by ictal discharges develop when hippocampal slices are bathed in a low-magnesium solution [23–26]. Calcium and magnesium ions act as antagonists at all chemical synapses. Calcium ions enter the pre-synaptic axon terminals through voltage-gated channels and bind to protein complexes, allowing the fusion of vesicles to the synaptic membrane and the release of neurotransmitters into the synaptic cleft (Fig. 18.2) [27–29]. Calcium entry through ligand-gated channels at the post-synaptic levels, such as the glutamate N-methyl-D-aspartate (NMDA) receptors, also contributes to excitatory neurotransmission. On the other hand, magnesium ions limit the influx of calcium ions through pre-synaptic voltage-dependent channels and thus modulate neurotransmitter release [25]. In addition, they also regulate synaptic transmission at the post-synaptic level by gating glutamate NMDA receptors in a voltage-dependent manner. At normal resting membrane potential, magnesium ions occupy a site inside the channel part of the receptor and prevent the influx of sodium and calcium ions. If synaptic excitation through other types of glutamate receptors (alpha-amino-3-hydroxy-5-methyl-4-isoxazolepropionic acid [AMPA] and kainate) causes sufficient depolarization, magnesium ions translocate out of the channels, which open [26, 30, 31].

While both synaptic potentiation and membrane destabilization are necessary to generate epileptiform discharges and seizures in the low-magnesium model of seizures [23], synaptic transmission is not necessary and in fact abolished in the low-calcium condition [32]. Neuronal synchronization thus has to occur in an ephaptic manner or through gap junctions.

The effect of pH and protons on neuronal excitability has received relatively little attention compared to other ions [33]. Current evidence indicates that the binding of protons to membrane proteins affects their conformation and their functional properties. Proteins whose activity is modulated by pH include voltage-gated ion channels, GABA receptors, NMDA receptors, gap junctions, calcium-sensing, and pH cation channels [16–24]. Acidosis has little influence on resting membrane potential [34] or axonal conduction [35] but decreases synaptic transmission by both pre- and post-synaptic mechanisms [34–36] and can suppress seizures [37, 38].

Water-Sodium Imbalance and Seizures

Epidemiology and Causes of Sodium and Osmotic Imbalance in Critically Ill Patients

Dysnatremia and water imbalance are frequent in critically ill patients. In a recent study on a large prospective cohort, dysnatremia was observed in 29% of patients [39]. Severe hyponatremia and hypernatremia are, however, much more rare, occurring in 1.2%, and 0.6% of patients, respectively, in another recent large survey [40].

Mechanisms of Sodium and Water Homeostasis

Body water content and sodium concentration are tightly regulated despite variable dietary intake, metabolic activity, and environmental factors. Total body water (TBW) is about 60% of body weight, two thirds of which are intracellular. Osmolarity is defined by the amount of solutes per liter of body fluid and is usually similar to osmolality, which is the amount of solutes per kg of fluid. Plasma osmolarity is mostly determined by sodium levels:

$$Osm = 2[serum\ Na^+] + \frac{[Glucose]}{18} + \frac{[BUN]}{2.8}$$

Fluid and sodium balance is preserved by the kidneys. Daily fluid intake is about 2–2.5 L, which is needed to replace losses from urine and insensible losses (sudation and perspiration). Daily urine output averages 1.5 L but adults with normal kidney function may excrete as little as the 200 mL of concentrated urines that are necessary to excrete the nitrogenous waste of cellular metabolism, and as much as 25 L in case of excessive fluid intake. Insensible losses represent 500–800 mL/day in a 70-kg adult, but they can substantially increase with fever (50–75 mL/day for each degree celsius of temperature elevation above normal), excessive muscular activity (exercise, convulsions), and heat exposure. Gastrointestinal losses are usually negligible, except when marked vomiting or diarrhea occurs.

Water excretion in the kidneys is regulated by vasopressin (antidiuretic hormone or ADH), which increases the expression of aquaporin channels and water reabsorption in the collecting ducts of the kidney. Vasopressin is produced by neurons in the supraoptic and paraventricular nuclei in the hypothalamus that project to the posterior pituitary gland. Its release is stimulated by increased plasma osmolality (through receptors in the hypothalamus), reduced blood volume (through baroreceptors in the carotid sinuses, veins and atria), angiotensin II (*see below*), and stress.

Water intake is regulated by thirst, which is triggered by receptors located in the anterolateral hypothalamus in response to increased plasma osmolality or decreased body fluid volume. Water ingestion decreases plasma osmolality, which in turn inhibits vasopressin secretion, allowing the kidneys to dilute urine. With dehydration, plasma osmolality rises, yielding the opposite effect. The system can also be activated by a loss of blood volume or a drop in blood pressure (such as in hemorrhage or extravasation).

The renin-angiotensin system provides an additional mechanism of water-sodium homeostasis. A drop in blood volume and pressure will decrease kidney perfusion, stimulating the release of renin by the juxtaglomerular cells. Renin cleaves angiotensinogen, an inactive propeptide, into angiotensin I, a minimally active peptide, which is then converted to angiotensin II by the angiotensin-converting enzyme (ACE) in lung capillaries. Angiotensin II acts by constricting afferent and efferent glomerular arterioles, effectively lowering glomerular blood flow and urine output while preserving glomerular filtration rate and facilitating water reabsorption. It also directly stimulates the reabsorption of sodium along the proximal tubule and loop of Henle. Finally, angiotensin II also causes the release of vasopressin by the pituitary and of aldosterone by the adrenal cortex. Aldosterone stimulates the reabsorption of sodium, in exchange for potassium, and of water from the urine by the distal tubules and collecting ducts. This increases blood volume and, therefore, blood pressure.

Angiotensin II and aldosterone thus act together to stimulate sodium and water reabsorption by the kidney and increase blood pressure. Their effects are opposed by natriuretic peptides (including the atrial natriuretic peptide [ANP] and the brain natriuretic peptide [BNP]), which are released by cardiomyocytes in response to high blood volume and excessive stretching [41, 42].

Hyponatremia

Hyponatremia is defined as plasma sodium concentration <135 mM/L. It may occur with low, normal, or high plasma tonicity (see Fig. 18.3).

Hyponatremia is the most common electrolyte disturbance and affects 12–38% patients admitted to a general ICU [39, 43, 44] and up to 50% of neurological and neurosurgical patients [45, 46]. Age, trauma, coma, and severity of illness are known risk factors. It is associated with increased in-hospital mortality, both if present on admission to the ICU [40] or if acquired during the ICU stay [47, 48], and particularly if corrected too fast or too slow. Even mild dysnatremia increases the risk of in-hospital mortality [40, 49]. Hyponatremia is also associated with longer ICU stay and a longer duration of mechanical ventilation [48, 50].

The most common causes of hyponatremia in critically ill patients are inappropriate fluid replacement and the syndrome of inappropriate antidiuretic hormone (SIADH). It is often the result of pneumonia [50] or of an acute brain injury, which itself can trigger seizures. In critically ill neurological patients, SIADH and the cerebral salt wasting syndrome (CSWS) are the two most common causes of hyponatremia [51]. Those that have been associated with acute seizures include SIADH, excessive fluid loading, extensive burns, vomiting and drugs [52], bowel preparation with polyethylene glycol, and bladder preparation for endoscopy [53]. There also rare reports of seizures due to water intoxication and exercise-induced hyponatremia [54], intoxication with 3,4-méthylènedioxy-méthamphétamine [55], and psychogenic polydipsia, which can be aggravated by the use of antipsychotic drugs [56].

CSWS has never clearly been identified as a cause of seizures and the underlying cerebral disorder is usually incriminated [57]. Some authors have also suggested that status epilepticus may be involved in the etiology of cerebral salt wasting, as natriuretic peptides levels increase during convulsions [58].

SIADH is the consequence of a direct lesion or dysfunction of the hypothalamus-pituitary axis or of the unregulated secretion of ADH or an ADH-related peptide by a malignancy. Frequent causes are listed in Table 18.2. The increase in ADH release results in excess water reabsorption and expansion of the extracellular fluid volume with hypotonic hyponatremia. Thus SIADH is a volume-expanded state although most patients do not show clinical signs of hypervolemia [51]. ANP is released due to vasopressin stimulation and due to overfilling of the plasma volume [59, 60].

Key features for the diagnosis of SIADH include low serum osmolality of <275 mOsm/kg, high urinary osmolality of >100 mOsm/kg, and persistent urine sodium excretion >20 meq/L. SIADH is associated with low uric acid levels (<4 mg/dL) and low blood urea nitrogen (BUN) concentrations (<5 mg/dL) (Table 18.3).

SIADH should be differentiated from the situation of non-osmotic appropriate release of ADH stimuli, as can be encountered with hypovolemia, hypotension, positive-pressure ventilation, pain, and stress.

Fig. 18.3 Diagnostic algorithm of hyponatremia

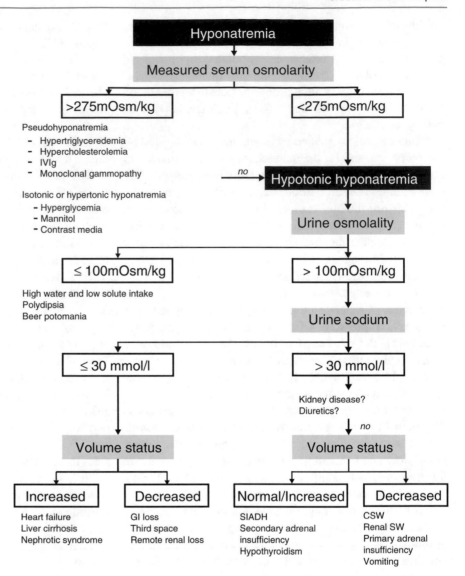

Another important of differential diagnosis to consider in patients who present with seizures and SIADH is limbic encephalitis, especially the type associated with antibodies to voltage-gated potassium channel complex [61].

CSWS is a hyponatremic and volume depleted state secondary to a renal loss of sodium and a decrease in extracellular fluid volume due to an intracranial disorder [62]. The mechanism by which cerebral disease results in renal sodium loss is still unclear. Two possible mechanisms have been suggested: impaired sympathetic neural input to the proximal tubule and direct release of natriuretic peptides. The resulting hypovolemia stimulates secondary ADH secretion. CSWS is typically encountered in neurosurgical patients or patients with intracranial disease or injury, especially SAH and meningitis [42, 63].

Hyponatremia is especially frequent after aneurysmal subarachnoid hemorrhage, occurring in approximately 30–56% cases, and is associated with a higher risk of delayed cerebral ischemia [64], but its etiology remains a matter of controversy [65]. SIADH is probably the main cause but CSWS, inadequate fluid replacement, and acute cortisol deficiency have also been implicated [65, 66].

The clinical expression of hyponatremia is related to the severity and acuteness of onset. Symptoms usually become manifest when serum concentrations fall suddenly (<48 h; rate of decrease > 0.5 meq/L/h) below 125 meq/L, as rapid changes of tonicity can exceed the capacity of the brain to adapt its solute content and regulate its volume (*see above*) [67]. Symptoms of hyponatremia include headache, nausea, vomiting, muscle cramps, and gait disturbance. Confusion and lethargy may ensue. With severe hyponatremia (≤120 meq/L), serious complications from cerebral edema can occur, including coma and eventually death from brain herniation [68].

Table 18.2 Causes of SIADH

CNS disorders	• Infections/inflammation (meningitis, encephalitis, AIDS, malaria) • Hemorrhage (SAH, subdural hematoma) • Traumatic brain injury • Guillain–Barre syndrome • Ischemic stroke • Shy–Drager syndrome
Pulmonary disorders	• Infections (bacterial viral, tuberculosis, aspergillosis) • Cystic fibrosis • Asthma
Malignancy	• CNS tumors (neuroblastoma) • Carcinoma (lung, gastrointestinal, genitourinary tract) • Lymphoma • Sarcoma (Ewing's sarcoma)
Medications stimulating the release of ADH	• SSRIs • Tricyclic antidepressants • Carbamazepine, oxcarbazepine • Phenytoin • Valproic acid • Lamotrigine • Cytotoxins (vincristine, cyclophosphamide, methotrexate, platinum compounds) • NSAIDs • Antipsychotics (phenothiazides, butyrophenones) • Opiates • MDMA • Interferon
Medications with ADH effects	• Desmopressin • Vasopressin • Oxytocin • Prostaglandins
Other causes	• Hereditary (mutation of V2 receptor) • Chronic inflammation • Prolonged exercise • Nausea • Pain, stress • Idiopathic • General anesthesia

Table 18.3 Comparison of SIADH and CSWS

	SIADH	CSW
Fluid balance	Positive	Negative
Sodium balance	Neutral or positive	Negative
Extracellular fluid volume	↑	↓
Clinical signs of dehydration	Absent	Present
Central venous pressure	↔ or ↑	↓
Weight	↔ or ↑	↓
Urine volume	↔ or ↓	↔ or ↑
Blood analysis • Sodium • Osmolality • Albumin • Bicarbonate • BUN • Hematocrit • Uric acid	 <135 mM/L <285 mOsm/L ↔ ↔ or ↓ ↔ or ↓ ↔ ↔ or ↓	 < 135 mM/L <285 mOsm/L ↑ ↑ ↑ ↑ ↔ or ↓
Urine analysis • Sodium • Osmolality	 ↑ >200	 ↑↑ >200

As previously mentioned, hyponatremia is one of the most common causes of new-onset seizures in hospitalized and critically ill patients [3–5].

The risk of seizures increases with decreasing sodium levels. In a single-center retrospective study of hospitalized patients with hyponatremia, the absolute risk of seizures was 0.7, 2.5, 5.3, and 10.8% for serum sodium values of 120–124, 115–119, 110–114, and <110 meq/L, respectively [52]. Another study found a 7% risk of seizure in patients with chronic hyponatremia and serum sodium level ≤110 meq/L but a 30% risk in patients with acute hyponatremia of this severity, highlighting the fact that not only the absolute value but also the rate at which sodium levels decrease is important [40, 69].

One should remember that mild hyponatremia in patients with chronic epilepsy might not be the cause of seizure but rather the simple consequence of anti-seizure treatment with drugs that cause SIADH, such as oxcarbazepine, carbamazepine, or valproic acid. However, this drug-induced hyponatremia can occasionally be severe enough to exacerbate epilepsy and precipitate seizures [70].

Hyponatremia-induced seizures are most commonly of the generalized tonic-clonic type [4, 52] but focal motor seizures, myoclonic seizures, complex partial seizures, and SE and absence SE have also been reported [4, 52, 71–73].

Seizures seem to be particularly common in children, with studies reporting a 27–66% seizure rate among children with hyponatremia [74, 75]. The majority of seizures in children present as SE. Water intoxication, associated with excessive sweating or gastroenteritis, is the most frequent cause [76, 77]. Severe respiratory syncytial virus infection may also be associated with hyponatremia and seizures [78]. Hyponatremia due to SIADH or CSW is an independent risk factor for post-neurosurgical seizures in children [79].

Management of Hyponatremia

The medical management of hyponatremia can be challenging.

The appropriate management of hyponatremia begins with a complete workup to determine the etiology (Fig. 18.3). Traditional algorithms rely on the clinical assessment of volume status, which can be difficult, and recent studies indicate that they allow physicians to reach a correct diagnosis in only a minority of cases [80]. Recent guidelines advocate the use of an alternative algorithm emphasizing urine electrolytes analysis [81]. It should be noted though that there are no gold standard cut-off values for urinary sodium and urine osmolality [46, 51, 60].

Another limitation of urine electrolytes analysis is that it cannot reliably differentiate SIADH and CSWS because both are characterized by elevated urine osmolality and sodium concentration. They are often difficult to distinguish as they have many features in common (Table 18.3). However, this distinction is important to make as their management strongly differs. It is mostly the presence of signs of volume depletion (hypotension, elevated hematocrit, and BUN/creatinine ratio) despite inappropriately high urine sodium concentration that suggests CSWS. When available, central venous pressure (CVP) (<5 mmHg) and pulmonary capillary wedge pressure (<8 mmHg) are good indicators of circulating blood volume. A negative sodium balance estimated over a period of one or several days supports the diagnosis of CSWS [68, 82]. When in doubt, the response to isotonic saline may also help distinguish between both entities. Restoration of euvolemia in CSWS should remove the stimulus to ADH release, resulting in a dilute urine and correction of the hyponatremia.

In contrast, isotonic saline often worsens the hyponatremia in SIADH as the salt is excreted and some of the water is retained.

Finally, it is important to remember that SIADH and CSWS sometimes succeed each other or occur simultaneously in the same patient and lack of urinary dilution upon isotonic saline administration does not necessarily exclude CSWS.

The correction method depends of the severity of hyponatremia. Treatment is indicated in the presence of acute symptomatic hyponatremia. The risks of hypotonicity should be balanced against those of therapy, as the correction of chronic hyponatremia can lead to neurological injury. Detailed recommendations on the treatment of hyponatremia have been recently published [81].

Severe symptomatic hyponatremia associated with alteration of consciousness or seizures should be quickly but cautiously managed with hypertonic saline solution, even before an etiological diagnosis is made. Intravenous infusion of 150 mL of NaCl 3% through a central venous line should be administered over 20 min in order to achieve an increase of 5 mM/L in serum sodium concentration. This can be repeated if needed. If symptoms improve, the patient can then be managed with isotonic saline until improvement or serum sodium concentration increases by 10 mM/L or reaches 130 mM/L. If symptoms do not improve, management is pursued with 3% hypertonic saline until improvement or serum sodium concentration increases by 10 mM/L reaches 130 mM/L. In both cases, the increase in serum sodium concentration should not exceed 10 mM/L during the first 24 h and 8 mM/L during the subsequent 24 h in order to avoid the risk of osmotic demyelination syndrome, which itself can cause seizures [83–85]. Close monitoring (every 4–6 h) of serum sodium levels is warranted. If over-rapid correction occurs, reversal using desmopressin and water is recommended [86].

Hyponatremia with mild or moderate symptoms can be managed less aggressively and should be guided by the cause. In the presence of moderate symptoms (nausea, headache, confusion) or if hyponatremia developed acutely, immediate administration of 3% saline is suggested.

Once symptoms improve or serum sodium concentration reaches 130 mM/L, management should focus on determining and treating the cause of the hyponatremia (Fig. 18.3). In addition, general measures such as avoiding hypotonic fluids, treating aggravating factors such as pain, nausea, and avoiding medications that can further decrease serum sodium concentration should be taken.

Hyponatremia with volume depletion should be treated by titration of isotonic saline solution with limited parallel free water intake.

Patients with CSWS need to receive isotonic or hypertonic saline to restore their intravascular volume, as long as sodium wasting persists. Colloids can be used when they have pronounced signs of volume contraction. Sodium chloride tablets and fludrocortisone may be helpful in less severe cases with adequate volume repletion [51]. Hypotonic fluids, free water, diuretics, and antidiuretic hormone therapy (vasopressin and desmopressin) should be avoided. Early use of fludrocortisone has been shown to reduce natriuresis [64] and the risk of vasospasm in hyponatremic SAH patients [46, 87].

On the other hand, free water restriction is required and often sufficient to treat SIADH and many patients have self-limiting disease. Identification and treatment of the underlying cause is an essential step. The volume of fluid restriction can be determined using the ratio of combined urinary sodium and potassium divided by serum sodium but patients are typically restricted to 1–1.5 L/day in clinical practice.

Some medications are effective as adjunct therapy to fluid restriction. A first choice is urea, an osmotic diuretic that enhances water flow from tissues into the interstitial fluid and plasma, thereby increasing serum osmolality. Demeclocycline, a tetracycline antibiotic, is also effective but can induce insipidus diabetes. More recently, vasopressin receptor antagonists (VRA) have emerged as a new class of drugs for the treatment of euvolemic and hypervolemic hyponatremia [88]. These molecules antagonize V2 receptors in the distal nephron, inducing then an aquaresis. Their optimal place in the treatment algorithm remains to be determined [51].

The treatment of hyponatremia-induced seizures and SE beyond correction of serum sodium levels has not been formally studied. Isolated seizures probably do not warrant any specific intervention but anti-seizure medications may be administered in case of SE. It is also probably reasonable to avoid medications that can aggravate hyponatremia, such as oxcarbazepine, carbamazepine, and valproic acid.

Hypernatremia

Hypernatremia is defined by a serum sodium concentration >145 mM/L. It is less frequent than hyponatremia with an incidence of 10% [89] of hospitalized patients.

Between 3.6 and 17% of critically ill patients experience hypernatremia with a sodium concentration >150 mM/L [39, 40, 43, 48, 90], most often during their first week in the ICU [40, 91].

It is often perceived as an indicator of the severity of the underlying disease and of the quality of care [92] and is associated with an increased risk of mortality [93].

Hypernatremia is invariably associated with hyperosmolality [94] but can result from a net loss of free water or an excess of sodium intake or retention, and thus can be either hypovolemic or hypervolemic, respectively (Table 18.4).

Hypovolemic hypernatremia is most often due to water deficiency or inadequate water supplementation. It is most common in young children, the elderly, and critically ill individuals who rely on others for their water intake. Fever, GI losses, and the use of diuretics are common precipitants.

Diabetes insipidus (DI) is defined by an inappropriate free water outflow with polyuria. It is the consequence of the failure of release of ADH (central DI) or of the resistance of the kidney to ADH (nephrogenic DI). The impermeability of the collecting ducts to water due to the lack of ADH activity results in urine dilution (<100 mOsm/kg), while plasma osmolality rises as a consequence of the progressive dehydration. Causes of DI are listed in Table 18.5. The severity of DI depends of the rate of residual ADH secretion. It is particularly dangerous if the thirst mechanism is impaired too, which can occur with central DI due to a cerebral mass in the hypothalamus-pituitary region. Central diabetes insipidus occurred in 3.7% patients in a neurosurgical intensive care unit [42].

Critically ill patients receiving mechanical ventilation are inclined to develop hypernatremia. Iatrogenic sodium gain occurs quickly with hypertonic perfusions but isotonic solutions can also lead to hypernatremia in the presence of diluted urines [95]. Potassium-rich solutions can also trigger

Table 18.4 Cause of hypernatremia

Hypovolemia	• Altered thirst mechanism • No access to water • Intra-renal water loss: central or nephrogenic diabetes insipidus, osmotic diuresis, diuretics • Extra-renal water loss: respiratory or GI losses, fever
Hypervolemia	• Iatrogenic: administration of large amounts of fluids to avoid hypovolemia • Mineralocorticoid excess: primary hyperaldosteronism, Cushing syndrome

Table 18.5 Causes of diabetes insipidus

Primary polydipsia (psychogenic polydipsia)
Central (neurogenic) diabetes insipidus
• Idiopathic, possibly autoimmune
• Pituitary surgery
• Traumatic brain injury
• Anoxic encephalopathy
• Death by neurological criteria (brain death)
• Hereditary
Nephrogenic diabetes insipidus
• Hereditary (ADH receptor V2 mutation)
• Lithium
• Hypercalcemia

sodium accumulation [91]. Diuretics, and in particular loop diuretics, hyperglycemia, osmotic diuresis, acute and chronic renal dysfunction, nasogastric drainage, diarrhea, and fever are all common in critical care patients. They induce the loss of free water and can further aggravate the hypernatremia.

Symptoms and signs of hypernatremia include nausea, headache, lethargy, and ultimately coma. Seizures are infrequent but can occasionally be seen in the setting of extra-pontine demyelination, which occurs with acute severe hypernatremia [96, 97].

Given the rarity of seizures attributable to hypernatremia, alternate causes should be actively sought, such as cerebral sinus or cortical vein thrombosis [98, 99]. In fact, seizures are much more likely to occur as the consequence of the aggressive treatment of chronic hypernatremia than as the consequence of hypernatremia itself [100, 101]. It is important to remember that it is the rate of decrease in serum sodium concentration itself rather than the absolute value that determines the risk of seizure.

Another factor confounding the relationship between hypernatremia and seizures is that generalized tonic-clonic seizures are accompanied by water shift into the intracellular space and can cause transient hypernatremia [102].

Management of Hypernatremia

The etiology of hypernatremia can usually be determined by concomitant measurement of serum and urine osmolality. The diagnosis of central DI is suggested by the presence of hypotonic urine (<300 mM/kg) in the setting of an elevated serum osmolality (>295 mM/kg). Central DI can be distinguished from nephrogenic DI by fluid restriction and desmopressin response tests. A magnetic resonance imaging is indicated to identify the underlying etiology of central DI.

Urine osmolality >600 mM/kg indicates intact ADH secretion and action and suggests either dehydration from renal, GI or insensible loss, or sodium overload. These causes can be further discriminated by measuring the urine sodium concentration, which is typically <25 meq/L in case of volume depletion and >100 meq/L in case of sodium overload.

Symptomatic management of hypernatremia begins by assessing the degree of water deficit and determining the appropriate rate of correction. Water deficit can be estimated using the following formula:

$$Water\ deficit = current\ total\ bodyweight \times$$
$$(serum[Na]/140 - 1).$$

In patients with chronic hypernatremia (present for longer than 48 h), the goal is to lower the serum sodium by 10 meq/L in 24 h, since lowering the plasma sodium concentration too rapidly can lead to cerebral edema and seizures. There is also evidence that excessively slow correction (lower than 6 meq/L in 24 h) is detrimental as well, since untreated severe hypernatremia can cause permanent brain injury.

The amount of water to be replaced in the first 24 h is limited and can thus be estimated as:

$$Desired\ water\ replacement = Water\ deficit \times$$
$$(10)/(Serum[Na] - 140).$$

In patients with known acute hypernatremia (present for 48 h or less), correction can occur faster and the entire water deficit can be corrected in 24 h.

These methods only measure the current deficit. The fluid repletion regimen should also take into account any ongoing losses; otherwise the correction rate will be substantially lower than expected.

Serum sodium has to be measured 2–4 h after initiation of the repletion regimen and the correction rate adjusted accordingly. Once a serum sodium concentration of 145 meq/L is reached, the infusion rate can be decreased to 1 mL/kg/h until normonatremia is reached.

Free water is usually provided as an intravenous solution of 5% dextrose in water. In patients who can drink or have nasogastric tubes, free water can be administered enterally every 4–6 h. Many hypernatremic patients have concurrent volume depletion and will require fluid resuscitation with 0.45% or 0.225% saline solution, which provide only one half or three-quarters, respectively, of free water, compared to dextrose solution. This needs to be taken into account when estimating the required volume of fluid needed to correct serum sodium levels.

Similarly, many patients also have hypokalemia. Potassium can be added to the administered fluids but thus will also decrease the amount of free water being given.

The rapid administration of 5% dextrose solution can lead to hyperglycemia, especially in patients with diabetes mellitus or a physiological stress. In order to avoid increased water losses from glycosuria, a 2.5% dextrose solution may be preferred in patients who develop hyperglycemia.

In addition to symptomatic management, patients with DI require desmopressin therapy.

Calcium and Seizures

Calcium Homeostasis

Serum calcium plays an essential role in skeletal mineralization, neuromuscular excitability, and coagulation. Intracellular calcium is involved in muscular contraction, hormone secretion, nerve conduction, and cell proliferation.

Approximately 90% of total body calcium is stored in bones. Calcium in the blood is bound to proteins, mainly albumin, and small anions such as phosphate and citrate. The active fraction is extracellular ionized calcium that represents only 1 mM. Intracellular calcium is mainly bound to proteins or sequestered in organelles.

Calcium balance is regulated mainly by the interplay between parathyroid hormone (PTH) and calcitonin, secreted by parafollicular cells in the thyroid. Ionized serum calcium exerts a feedback control on the parathyroid gland and parafollicular cells through calcium-sensing receptors so that PTH is released and calcitonin secretion is inhibited when serum calcium level decreases and PTH release is inhibited and calcitonin is released when calcium level increases.

PTH increases calcium concentration by reducing urinary calcium and phosphate excretion, increasing bone resorption and stimulating the synthesis of calcitriol (1,25 dihydroxyvitamin D3), the activated form of vitamin D3, in the kidney. Calcitriol stimulates calcium resorption by the gut. Calcitonin decreases calcium levels by stimulating bone mineralization.

Hypocalcemia

The most common cause of hypocalcemia is renal failure. (Table 18.6). The gastrointestinal absorption is reduced because of decreased renal production of calcitriol and because of increased serum phosphorus.

Hypoparathyroidism is the second most important cause of hypocalcemia and can be the consequence of surgery, an autoimmune disease (autoimmune polyglandular syndromes), hypomagnesemia, radiation, infiltrative diseases, or a genetic disorder. Up to 54% patients with hypoparathyroidism may present with seizures [103, 104].

Hypocalcemia is common in critically ill patients [105]. Sepsis and severe illness can lead to hypocalcemia by several mechanisms: hypomagnesemia, serial blood transfusions, acute renal failure from inflammation, and kidney injury [106]. The prevalence is variable but can reach 55–85% [107–109]. Hypocalcemia correlates with disease severity and is associated with an increased mortality in many studies [106–111]. Iatrogenic hypocalcemia can be accompanied by seizures.

Table 18.6 Causes of hypocalcemia

Etiologies
Renal failure
Hypoparathyroidism or pseudohypoparathyroidism (PTH resistance)
Magnesium deficiency
Pancreatitis
Osteoblastic metastasis
Tumor lysis syndrome
Sepsis
Vitamin D deficiency or receptor defects (nutritional deficiency, malabsorption)
Calcium-sensing receptor mutations
Drugs: bisphosphonates, anticonvulsants, calcitonin, phosphate, tyrosine kinase inhibitors (Imatinib)
Hypoalbuminemia (pseudohypocalcemia)
Transfusion of citrated blood products
Hyperphosphatemia

Drugs that have been implicated include proton-pump inhibitors [112, 113], bisphosphonates [114, 115], calcitonin, and tyrosine kinase inhibitors (imatinib). Proton-pump inhibitors reduce magnesium absorption by the gut and may lead to hypomagnesemia and secondary hypocalcemia. Accidental parathyroidectomy during thyroidectomy can result in unexpected and untreated hypocalcemia and seizures, sometimes years after the surgery [116–118].

Hypocalcemia-related seizures are well documented in children with congenital or idiopathic hypoparathyroidism [119–122], celiac disease [123], and rickets [124].

Neonates are at particular risk of hypocalcemia, either during the first 3 days after birth, when it is associated with premature birth, hypoxic-ischemic encephalopathy and maternal diabetes, or after the first week, when it is caused by vitamin D deficiency, dietary phosphate overload, and endocrine disorders [125]. Neonates born from mothers with asymptomatic hyperparathyroidism may develop impaired parathyroid responsiveness to hypocalcemia and seizures [126]. Hypocalcemia-related neonatal seizures used to be frequent [127] but their incidence has steadily decreased, owing to better screening and prevention of hypocalcemia in high-risk neonates.

Finally, the anticonvulsant phenytoin may increase the metabolism of vitamin D, leading to hypocalcemia and occasionally to hypocalcemia-related seizures [128]. Therefore, clinicians are advised to check calcium in cases of antiepileptic drug refractory seizures.

Normal total serum calcium ranges between 8.5 and 10.2 mg/dL and ionized calcium between 4.4 and 5.4 mg/dL (1.1 and 1.35 mM/l).

In case of protein depletion, total calcium decreases but the ionized calcium, which is metabolically active, is normal because it is still hormonally regulated. This situation is called pseudohypocalcemia. Corrected serum calcium levels can be estimated using the following formula:

$$Corrected[Ca] = Measured[Ca] + 0.8 \times (4 - [albumin]).$$

Similarly, ionized calcium levels can be estimated from total calcium levels:

$$[Ca^{2+}] = Total[Ca] - 0.8 \times [protein].$$

However, the binding of the albumin-calcium complex is influenced by pH, which renders the estimate inaccurate in most critically ill patients where direct measure of ionized calcium should be preferred. For instance, a study in trauma patients compared 22 methods to estimate corrected total serum calcium and serum ionized calcium and found that they had an average sensitivity of 25% for the detection of hypocalcemia [129]. However, a marked serum hypocalcemia with less than 7 mg/dL total calcium levels is generally a good marker of ionized hypocalcemia in critically ill patients [130].

Manifestations of hypocalcemia are explained by the hyperexcitability of the peripheral and central nervous system. Tetany is the hallmark of acute hypocalcemia, mostly occurring with ionized calcium below 4.3 mg/dL and total serum calcium below 7.5 mg/dL [131]. Patients first complain of paresthesias around the mouth and in the extremities and of muscle spasms. The Chvostek and Trousseau signs can be observed. Gastrointestinal symptoms can occur because of the stimulation of the vagal nerve system, with dysphagia, nausea, biliary colic, abdominal pain, or cramping [19, 132]. Lethargy, stupor, and finally coma occur. Laryngospasm and bronchospasm are potential and severe complications.

Chronic hypocalcemia, mostly seen in patients with hypoparathyroidism, leads to skin and dental changes, basal ganglia calcifications, extrapyramidal signs (parkinsonism or choreo-athetosis), and cataract.

Seizures are most commonly of the generalized tonic-clonic type but nonconvulsive status epilepticus can occur [133]. Patients often exhibit symptoms and signs of neuromuscular hyperexcitability but isolated seizures have been reported [134].

Management of Hypocalcemia

Symptomatic patients with tetany or seizures and patients with prolonged QT interval or with calcium below 7.5 mg/dL should receive intravenous calcium. Otherwise, oral supplementation can be used.

Calcium gluconate is generally given diluted at a dose of 1 or 2 g over 10–20 min and not faster because of the risk of cardiac dysfunction. The supplementation is continued with an intravenous drip of 10% calcium gluconate or calcium chloride. Calcium gluconate is usually preferred, as it carries a lower risk of tissue necrosis in case of accidental extravasation. The infusion rate is guided by improvement of symptoms and ionized serum calcium monitoring every hour.

The underlying cause should be identified, by measuring PTH, magnesium, creatinine, phosphate, and vitamin D levels, and treated. Concurrent hypomagnesemia should be corrected.

Hypercalcemia

The most frequent causes of hypercalcemia are primary hyperparathyroidism, due to parathyroid adenoma, and malignancy. Rare causes include granulomatous diseases, such as sarcoidosis or tuberculosis, drugs, and genetic disorders. A mild chronic hypercalcemia is typical of primary hyperparathyroidism and is often asymptomatic while the hypercalcemia associated with malignancy is usually more severe (>13 mg/dL), develops more rapidly and is thus more often symptomatic.

Primary hyperparathyroidism is usually caused by a PTH-secreting parathyroid adenoma. The incidence reaches 1/1000 in postmenopausal women. Patients with secondary hyperparathyroidism due to severe chronic renal disease or tertiary hyperparathyroidism can also develop hypercalcemia. Familial hypocalciuric hypercalcemia is a rare genetic disorder in which higher than normal serum calcium concentrations are required to suppress PTH release due to a loss-of-function mutation in the calcium-sensing receptors.

Hypercalcemia can complicate malignancy, mainly lung, breast, and hematological cancers. In lung and breast carcinomas, there is secretion of an active PTH-related protein (PTH-RP) that acts as PTH and activates the renal and intestinal absorption of calcium and its mobilization from the bones. In turn, serum levels of PTH are very low, as its secretion by the parathyroid glands is inhibited [135].

In granulomatous disorders, calcitriol is synthesized from 25-OH vitamin D by activated macrophages independently of PTH, leading to uncontrolled intestinal absorption of calcium.

Drugs such as lithium, thiazides, and theophylline can interfere with calcium homeostasis and lead to hypercalcemia.

Most often, hypercalcemia is part of the reason for the admission of patient in the ICU but it sometimes can develop as a consequence of critical illness. Patients with prolonged immobilization, extensive burns or rhabdomyolysis, and acute renal failure are at risk.

Other causes of hypercalcemia are summarized in Table 18.7.

Mild hypercalcemia is often asymptomatic but severe hypercalcemia causes nausea, vomiting, polyuria, constipation, headache, lethargy, and ultimately coma. Chronic hypercalcemia can lead to nephrolithiasis. Hypercalcemia causes afferent arteriolar vasoconstriction, which may lead to renal failure.

Seizures due to hypercalcemia are probably very rare. Only a handful of cases have been described in the literature [136–138]. Two cases of milk-alkali syndrome with hypercalcemia and status epilepticus have been reported but both

Table 18.7 Causes of hypercalcemia

Primary hyperparathyroidism	
Malignancy-associated hypercalcemia	
Granulomatous disease	Sarcoidosis Tuberculosis Candidiasis Leprosy
Familial hypocalciuric hypercalcemia	
Milk-alkali syndrome	
Endocrine associated hypercalcemia	Adrenal insufficiency Hyperthyroidism
Immobilization	
Drugs	Lithium Vit D Vit A Estrogen Theophylline Thiazide diuretics

patients were later found to have mesial temporal sclerosis [139]. Whether it was a cause or a consequence of the episode of status epilepticus is unclear. Another case of milk-alkali syndrome was complicated by status epilepticus but the patient also had acute renal failure and metabolic alkalosis which may both have contributed to seizures [140].

The fact that hypercalcemia can lead to seizures may indeed appear paradoxical as extracellular calcium plays a stabilizing role on neuronal membranes and reduces epileptiform discharges in vitro (see above). One possible explanation is that hypercalcemia may cause reversible vasoconstriction (RCVS) and posterior reversible encephalopathy syndromes (PRES), which themselves are often complicated by seizures. Several cases have been described, usually without significant renal failure or hypertension [141–144].

Management of Hypercalcemia

In the absence of an obvious cause to the hypercalcemia, PTH should be measured to rule out primary hypoparathyroidism. If PTH levels are normal or low, PTH-RP levels and vitamin D metabolites are measured.

When hypercalcemia is mild and not symptomatic, the treatment is the treatment of the underlying cause. In addition, all calcium-containing medications should be discontinued and aggravating factors, including thiazide diuretics, dehydration, and prolonged bed rest, should be avoided.

When hypercalcemia is >14 mg/dL or symptomatic, supportive management should be initiated.

The concurrent administration of massive saline infusion and loop diuretics that used to be recommended in the past is now discouraged due to the high rate of electrolyte complications (hypokalemia, hypomagnesemia) and volume depletion, and the availability of drugs that inhibit bone resorption, such as calcitonin and bisphosphonates.

Hydration with isotonic saline is still recommended but only to correct possible volume depletion due to hypercalcemia-induced polyuria. Patients should concurrently receive calcitonin (4 IU/kg SC). The response to calcitonin occurs within 12–24 h and should be monitored. If the patient responds, the administration can be repeated, up to 8 IU/kg every 6–8 h. Bisphosphonates (zoledronic acid 4 mg IV) should be administered as well and will contribute to the long-term control of normocalcemia.

Hemodialysis can be considered in patients with serum calcium concentrations >18 mg/dL and neurologic symptoms or in those with renal failure [135].

The treatment of the underlying cause also should be initiated. High dose glucocorticoids are effective in patients with vitamin D dependent hypercalcemia as in sarcoidosis, T-cell lymphomas, or multiple myeloma.

Magnesium and Seizures

Magnesium (Mg) plays an essential role in many physiological processes, including as a cofactor in key enzymatic reactions and as a stabilizer of cellular membranes [145]. Low Mg is known to be associated with poor clinical outcome in hospitalized patients, especially when ionized Mg is decreased, and is correlates with a higher mortality in the intensive care unit [146]. High ionized Mg (>0.6 mM/L) is also associated with higher mortality in critical care units [146].

Magnesium Homeostasis

Magnesium homeostasis is entirely dependent on dietary intake. One third of the ingested magnesium (around 360 mg daily) is absorbed in the small bowel and balance is regulated by urinary excretion and reabsorption. This regulation is not under hormonal regulation, in contrast to other ions, but is driven by sodium and water reabsorption in the proximal tubules.

Magnesium is stored almost entirely intracellularly, mainly in bones. It is the second intracellular cation after potassium. The extracellular magnesium is largely bound to anions or protein. Normal serum Mg concentration ranges from 0.7 to 1 mM/L (1.7–2.2 mg/dL) and ionized magnesium from 0.45 to 0.6 mM/L [147]. In case of decreased dietary intake or renal loss, Mg is mobilized from bones, but this is a slow process that takes weeks.

Hypomagnesemia

Hypomagnesemia is a frequent electrolyte disturbance. It occurs in approximately 12% hospitalized patients and up to 50–60% ICU patients [148, 149].

Causes of hypomagnesemia are detailed in Table 18.8 and be subdivided in decreased dietary intake and abnormal gastrointestinal or renal loss [150]. Patients with chronic alcoholism are at high risk of hypomagnesemia, due to poor diet and increased renal loss. The effect of diuretics is usually mild but can be potentiated by the co-administration of proton-pump inhibitors.

Hypomagnesemia presents with signs of neuromuscular hyperexcitability (tremor, fasciculations, tetany with positive Trousseau and Chvostek signs, hyperreflexia) but the frequently associated hypocalcemia also contributes to these clinical features. Nonspecific signs of CNS dysfunction such as fatigue and lethargy might occur. Vertical nystagmus is a rare but alarming sign of severe hypomagnesemia [151].

Magnesium ions play a role in Na^+/K^+ ATPase pump function and calcium channel blockade. If magnesium levels decrease, intracellular calcium concentration increases, which can induce vasoconstriction and increased blood pressure [152]. Cardiac arrhythmias and electrocardiographic changes include intractable ventricular tachycardia and fibrillation, *torsades de pointes*, multifocal atrial tachycardia, and digitalis-toxic ventricular tachyarrhythmia [150]. High blood pressure induces dilatation of the myogenic vasoconstriction of cerebral arteries and arterioles, increases BBB permeability, and causes edema formation [153].

Table 18.8 Causes of hypomagnesemia

Decreased nutritional intake	• Alcohol (also in part due to renal loss) • Parenteral feeding
Gastrointestinal loss	• Malabsorption, chronic diarrhea, small bowel bypass surgery, acute pancreatitis [14], PPI
Bone redistribution in hyperparathyroidism and hungry bone syndrome	
Renal loss	• Polyuria (diabetes, osmotic, recovery from AKI, obstruction, and transplantation) • Hypercalcemia < metastases (inhibits reabsorption) but not hyperPTH • Tubular dysfunction • Extracellular fluid expansion (nephrotic syndrome, liver failure, cardiac failure) • Iatrogenic renal wasting • Thiazides and loop diuretics • Nephrotoxic drugs (platinum-based agents, epithelial growth factor (EGF) receptor-blockers, amphothericin B, aminoglycosides, foscarnet, cyclosporine/tacrolimus) • Genetic disorders: familial renal magnesium wasting (diagnosis of exclusion) • Most frequent is Gitelman syndrome, Bartter's syndrome
Cutaneous loss	Extensive burn injuries

Chronic hypomagnesemia leads to dysregulation of calcium homeostasis with hypocalcemia, hypoparathyroidism, vitamin D deficiency, and osteoporosis [154], and to refractory hypokalemia, due to renal potassium wasting.

The relationship between hypomagnesemia and seizures is unclear.

There is weak evidence that people with epilepsy are more likely to have chronic magnesium deficiency [155, 156] and a small uncontrolled study suggested that magnesium supplementation might improve seizure control in patients with refractory epilepsy [157]. High dose intravenous magnesium infusion has been used to treat super-refractory status in children with mitochondrial disorder due to mutation in the *polg1* gene [158]. Magnesium is also the favored agent for seizure prophylaxis in women with pre-eclampsia [159, 160].

Altogether, these findings might suggest a direct anticonvulsant effect of magnesium and an increased risk for seizures with hypomagnesemia.

However, magnesium barely crosses the BBB and reports of seizures due to hypomagnesemia are scarce. In the few reported adult cases, other potential causes of seizures were present [161–164]. In neonates with primary hypomagnesemia, seizures are frequently reported but severe hypocalcemia is also often present and might at least in part be responsible for the seizures [127, 165].

The anti-seizure effect of magnesium in pre-eclampsia might also relate more to its vasodilating and hypotensive effects [166–168].

Lastly, another confounding factor is that generalized tonic-clonic seizures are accompanied by catecholamine release that can aggravate hypomagnesemia caused by an intracellular magnesium shift [169, 170].

Management of Hypomagnesemia

Total serum and ionized magnesium levels have to be measured together with calcium, potassium, albumin, and creatinine levels. If the cause is not obvious, the urine excreted fraction should be measured. If the excreted fraction is <5%, GI loss or cellular uptake should be suspected. An excreted fraction >5% indicates renal loss [171].

The best technic to measure magnesium status is still discussed [147]. Routine laboratory tests assess total Mg serum levels, but only the ionized fraction is physiologically active. Both fractions may vary independently in magnesium dysregulation. A study found that half of the patients with ionized hypomagnesemia had normal total magnesium concentration [146] and reliable concentrations of serum ionized magnesium can be obtained only by direct measurement [149].

The treatment of Mg depletion depends on its severity and on the presence of clinical manifestations. The deficiency should be corrected if symptomatic or if the levels are persistently <0.5 mM/L.

Patients with arrhythmias, tetany, or seizures should receive 1–2 g intravenous magnesium sulfate over 2–15 min, if the patient is hemodynamically unstable or over 60 min, if stable. This initial dose is followed by an infusion of 4–8 g over 12–24 h during 3 or 5 days. Magnesium uptake by the cell is slow and a large part infused will be excreted in urines (around 50%). This treatment has to be adapted in case of renal dysfunction. The serum concentration should be monitored frequently particularly with renal insufficiency.

Oral Mg replacement therapy should be given to asymptomatic patients. The underlying disease should be diagnosed and treated. Amiloride could also be used for its ability to increase Mg reabsorption and prevent hypomagnesemia in patients with renal failure or receiving thiazide or loop diuretics.

Acid-Base Disorders and Seizures

Although acid-base disorders are common in the critically ill but they do not appear to be a major precipitant of acute seizures. These disturbances can, however, be severe and are often associated with worse outcome, especially metabolic acidosis [172, 173]. The point prevalence of severe metabolic or mixed acidemia (pH < 7.20) in critically ill patients was 6% in a recent prospective multi-center study and it was associated with an ICU mortality rate of 57%, but other studies have not found such an association [174]. A metabolic alkalemia with a pH of 7.55 is associated with increased mortality [175].

The most frequent cause of acidosis is septic shock. Other causes of acidosis and alkalosis are presented in Table 18.9.

The acid-base balance is finely controlled by different mechanisms to keep the blood pH within a between 7.35 and 7.45. The Henderson–Hasselbach equation

$$pH = 6.4 + \log 10 \left(\frac{HCO_3^-}{0.0307 \times pCO_2} \right)$$

determines that blood pH is set by the ratio of the serum bicarbonate concentration and the $PaCO_2$.

Any acid-base disturbance leads to a compensatory respiratory and renal response. The respiratory compensation is fast, acting within minutes, and is triggered by pH-sensitive neurons in respiratory center of the central nervous system. When blood pH decreases, ventilation increases, and more carbon dioxide is released by the lungs, effectively lowering $PaCO_2$ and bringing back pH to normal values. On the contrary, when pH increases, ventilation rate decreases, $PaCO_2$ increases, and pH decreases back. The kidneys also play a central role in acid-base balance by excreting excess acids or bases but these adjustments are slower than lungs and take several days. Additionally, pairs

Table 18.9 Causes of acidosis and alkalosis

Metabolic acidosis	• Diabetic ketoacidosis • Drugs: acetazolamide, alcohol, aspirin, iron • Poisons: carbon monoxide, cyanide, ethylene glycol, methanol • Lactic acidosis • Loss of bases (bicarbonate) through the digestive tract (diarrhea, colostomy, etc.) • Advanced kidney disease • Renal tubular acidosis
Metabolic alkalosis	• Loss of hydrogen from vomiting, stomach drainage, congenital chloride diarrhea • Mineralocorticoid excess (Cushing syndrome, adrenal tumors) • Bartter or Gitelman syndrome • Diuretics (thiazides, furosemide) • Hypercalcemia and the milk-alkali syndrome • Hypokalemia • Alkali administration
Respiratory acidosis	• Lung disorders (chronic bronchitis, severe asthma, pneumonia, etc.) • Sleep disorders breathing • Disorders of the nerves or muscles of the chest (Guillain–Barre syndrome, amyotrophic lateral sclerosis) • Drugs: alcohol, opioids, strong sedatives
Respiratory alkalosis	• Anxiety • Aspirin overdose (early stage) • Fever • Low levels of oxygen • Pain

of weak acids and bases, such as carbonic acid and bicarbonate ions, and inorganic phosphate ions, also act as fast buffers to maintain control blood pH.

Acid-base disturbances cause potassium to shift into and out of the cells. In metabolic acidosis, hydrogen ions excess is buffered into the cells and to preserve the electro neutrality, potassium ions move from the intracellular to the extracellular fluid. Hyperkalemia is thus commonly seen in diabetic ketoacidosis. pH also modifies the binding equilibrium of calcium with small inorganic ions. Ionized calcium levels decrease when pH increases, which contributes to some of the symptoms and signs of alkalosis.

Metabolic acidosis causes nausea, vomiting, fatigue, and if severe, encephalopathy. Patients typically have a deep and rapid breathing (Kussmaul breathing). An inability to generate the respiratory response to acidosis should raise the question of a respiratory or neurologic disease. Respiratory acidosis manifestations are headache, confusion, lethargy and breathing is typically slow.

Metabolic alkalosis is often asymptomatic or symptoms are related to the hypokalemia or the underlying cause but acute respiratory alkalosis may be spectacular. Patients with alkalosis present with irritability, paresthesias, muscle twitching or cramps, and muscle spasms, a clinical picture very similar to hypocalcemia and hypomagnesemia.

Sudden changes in PCO_2 can provoke severe neurologic manifestations with seizures and coma [176, 177], especially in patients with chronic liver disease because the alkaline pH favors the ammonia entrance into the central nervous system [178, 179].

It should be first mentioned that metabolic (lactic) and respiratory acidosis are often the transient consequence of seizures, especially of generalized tonic-clonic type [22, 23]. In fact, lactic acidosis is a good indicator of seizures in patients who present with a first episode of loss of consciousness. Seizures also directly acidify the cerebral extracellular fluid, which can reduce neuronal excitability and is thought to contribute to seizure arrest and postictal refractoriness [180].

Some anti-seizure medications, including topiramate, zonisamide and acetazolamide, slightly acidify the blood through inhibition of the carbonic anhydrase. The role of this induced non-anion gap metabolic acidosis in seizure control in this setting is unclear. Conversely, voluntary hyperventilation is used during routine electroencephalography to reveal epileptiform discharges [181, 182]. It will trigger a seizure in virtually all children with absence epilepsy. It is somewhat less helpful in other situations, but may nonetheless increase the frequency, and thus the chance to observe, of interictal discharges [183, 184].

Hyperthermia-induced hyperventilation and alkalosis are associated with febrile seizures in children [185, 186], although a causal relationship is still not clearly demonstrated.

A few cases of severe metabolic alkalosis and seizures have been reported in relationship with the ingestion of large quantities of sodium bicarbonate (baking soda), as an over-the-counter antacid medication. Other cases occurred in the setting of Gitelman syndrome, an autosomal recessive kidney disorder caused by loss of function mutations of the thiazide sensitive sodium chloride symporter. The role of alkalosis in inducing seizures is unclear as these patients also had other electrolyte disturbances, including hypomagnesemia.

On the other hand, respiratory acidosis is a potent antiseizure agent. Inhalation of 5% CO_2 has been successfully used to abort seizures in animals [187] and in children with absence epilepsy [188] and has been proposed as a treatment for prolonged febrile seizures.

In critically ill patients, seizures have been reported in association with metabolic acidosis. The role of acidosis is unclear, though, as almost all cases were confounded by the presence of intoxication (non-steroidal anti-inflammatory drugs intoxication, alpha-lipoic acid, neem oil, margosa oil, citalopram, isoniazid, paracetamol, 5-FU, cocaine/amphetamines, cyanide, strychnine, ethanol, propylene glycol, ethylene glycol, methanol), an underlying inborn error of metabolism, an associated electrolyte imbalance, renal failure, Wernicke encephalopathy, or PRES. In fact, the association of acidosis, encephalopathy and seizures should strongly suggest the possibility of an acute intoxication or metabolic disturbance. Also, while blood pH decreases with metabolic acidosis, brain pH may in fact increase as the BBB is relatively impermeable to bicarbonate ions but not to CO_2 gas molecules, whose concentration decreases due to the compensatory respiratory mechanism [189]. Thus, it is possible that acute metabolic acidosis may trigger seizures in part due to secondary brain alkalosis.

Recent studies in neonates have demonstrated that post-asphyxia seizures are attributable to brain alkalosis due to an enhanced extrusion of H^+ ions across the blood–brain barrier in the recovery phase from asphyxia-induced acidosis [190].

Management of Acid-Base Disorders

The acid-base disorders are categorized as metabolic or respiratory to choose effective therapeutic strategies. The diagnosis requires the measurement of arterial blood gases, electrolyte lactate and glucose levels, and renal function. The treatment focuses on correcting the underlying etiology [191]. The correction of acidemia by itself with the administration of intravenous buffers (sodium bicarbonate) remains controversial [192].

References

1. Barron R, Freebairn R. Electrolyte disorders in the critically ill. Anaesth Intensive Care Med. 2010;11:523–8. doi:10.1016/j.mpaic.2010.09.010.
2. Annegers JF, Hauser WA, Lee JR, Rocca WA. Incidence of acute symptomatic seizures in Rochester, Minnesota, 1935–1984. Epilepsia. 1995;36:327–33.
3. Wijdicks EF, Sharbrough FW. New-onset seizures in critically ill patients. Neurology. 1993;43:1042–4.
4. Fields MC, Labovitz DL, French JA. Hospital-onset seizures: an inpatient study. JAMA Neurol. 2013;70:360–4. doi:10.1001/2013.jamaneurol.337.
5. Narayanan JT, Murthy JMK. New-onset acute symptomatic seizure in a neurological intensive care unit. Neurol India. 2007;55:136–40.
6. Sandler DL, Burchfield DJ, Riley WJ, Drummond WH. A comparison of CSF and serum magnesium levels in new born NICU infants. Seattle: Society for Pediatric Research; 1995.
7. Pasantes-Morales H, Tuz K. Volume changes in neurons: hyperexcitability and neuronal death. Contrib Nephrol. 2006;152:221–40. doi:10.1159/000096326.
8. Rosen AS, Andrew RD. Osmotic effects upon excitability in rat neocortical slices. Neuroscience. 1990;38:579–90.
9. Somjen GG. Ions in the brain: normal function, seizures, and stroke. New York: OUP; 2004.
10. Schwartzkroin PA, Baraban SC, Hochman DW. Osmolarity, ionic flux, and changes in brain excitability. Epilepsy Res. 1998;32:275–85.
11. Somjen GG. Low external NaCl concentration and low osmolarity enhance voltage-gated Ca currents but depress K currents in freshly isolated rat hippocampal neurons. Brain Res. 1999;851:189–97.
12. Chebabo SR, Hester MA, Aitken PG, Somjen GG. Hypotonic exposure enhances synaptic transmission and triggers spreading depression in rat hippocampal tissue slices. Brain Res. 1995;695:203–16.
13. Andrew RD, Fagan M, Ballyk BA, Rosen AS. Seizure susceptibility and the osmotic state. Brain Res. 1989;498:175–80.
14. Arundine M, Tymianski M. Molecular mechanisms of glutamate-dependent neurodegeneration in ischemia and traumatic brain injury. Cell Mol Life Sci. 2004;61:657–68. doi:10.1007/s00018-003-3319-x.
15. Hyzinski-García MC, Vincent MY, Haskew-Layton RE, et al. Hypo-osmotic swelling modifies glutamate-glutamine cycle in the cerebral cortex and in astrocyte cultures. J Neurochem. 2011;118:140–52. doi:10.1111/j.1471-4159.2011.07289.x.
16. Avoli M, Drapeau C, Perreault P, et al. Epileptiform activity induced by low chloride medium in the CA1 subfield of the hippocampal slice. J Neurophysiol. 1990;64:1747–57.
17. Huang R, Somjen GG. Effects of hypertonia on voltage-gated ion currents in freshly isolated hippocampal neurons, and on synaptic currents in neurons in hippocampal slices. Brain Res. 1997;748:157–67.
18. Hille B, Woodhull AM, Shapiro BI. Negative surface charge near sodium channels of nerve: divalent ions, monovalent ions, and pH. Philos Trans R Soc Lond Ser B Biol Sci. 1975;270:301–18.
19. Han P, Trinidad BJ, Shi J. Hypocalcemia-induced seizure: demystifying the calcium paradox. ASN Neuro. 2015; doi:10.1177/1759091415578050.
20. Agopyan N, Avoli M. Synaptic and non-synaptic mechanisms underlying low calcium bursts in the in vitro hippocampal slice. Exp Brain Res. 1988;73:533–40.
21. Han P, Trinidad BJ, Shi J. Hypocalcemia-induced seizure: demystifying the calcium paradox. ASN Neuro. 2015;7 doi:10.1177/1759091415578050.
22. Roper SN, Obenaus A, Dudek FE. Increased propensity for non-synaptic epileptiform activity in immature rat hippocampus and dentate gyrus. J Neurophysiol. 1993;70:857–62.
23. Isaev D, Ivanchick G, Khmyz V, et al. Surface charge impact in low-magnesium model of seizure in rat hippocampus. J Neurophysiol. 2012;107:417–23. doi:10.1152/jn.00574.2011.
24. Tancredi V, Avoli M, Hwa GG. Low-magnesium epilepsy in rat hippocampal slices: inhibitory postsynaptic potentials in the CA1 subfield. Neurosci Lett. 1988;89:293–8.
25. Anderson WW, Lewis DV, Swartzwelder HS, Wilson WA. Magnesium-free medium activates seizure-like events in the rat hippocampal slice. Brain Res. 1986;398:215–9.
26. Hallak M. Effect of parenteral magnesium sulfate administration on excitatory amino acid receptors in the rat brain. Magnese Res Off Organ Int Soc Dev Res Magnes. 1998;11:117–31.
27. Del Castillo J, Engbaek L. The nature of the neuromuscular block produced by magnesium. J Physiol. 1954;124:370–84.
28. Katz B. Nerve, muscle, and synapse. New York: McGraw-Hill; 1966.
29. Somjen GG. Ions in the brain: normal function, seizures, and stroke. New York: Oxford University Press; 2004.
30. Hille B. Ionic channels in excitable membranes. Current problems and biophysical approaches. Biophys J. 1978;22:283–94. doi:10.1016/S0006-3495(78)85489-7.
31. Zito K, Scheuss V, Knott G, et al. Rapid functional maturation of nascent dendritic spines. Neuron. 2009;61:247–58. doi:10.1016/j.neuron.2008.10.054.
32. Feng Z, Durand DM. Suppression of excitatory synaptic transmission can facilitate low-calcium epileptiform activity in the hippocampus in vivo. Brain Res. 2004;1030:57–65. doi:10.1016/j.brainres.2004.09.063.
33. Ruusuvuori E, Kaila K. Carbonic anhydrases and brain pH in the control of neuronal excitability. Subcell Biochem. 2014;75:271–90. doi:10.1007/978-94-007-7359-2_14.

34. Hsu KS, Liang YC, Huang CC. Influence of an extracellular aci-dosis on excitatory synaptic transmission and long-term potentia-tion in the CA1 region of rat hippocampal slices. J Neurosci Res. 2000;62:403–15.

35. Walz W, Harold DE. Brain lactic acidosis and synaptic function. Can J Physiol Pharmacol. 1990;68:164–9.

36. Velísek L. Extracellular acidosis and high levels of carbon dioxide suppress synaptic transmission and prevent the induc-tion of long-term potentiation in the CA1 region of rat hip-pocampal slices. Hippocampus. 1998;8:24–32. doi:10.1002/(sici)1098-1063(1998)8:1<24::aid-hipo3>3.3.co;2-2.

37. de Curtis M, Manfridi A, Biella G. Activity-dependent pH shifts and periodic recurrence of spontaneous interictal spikes in a model of focal epileptogenesis. J Neurosci. 1998;18:7543–51.

38. Pavlov I, Kaila K, Kullmann DM, Miles R. Cortical inhibition, pH and cell excitability in epilepsy: what are optimal targets for anti-epileptic interventions? J Physiol. 2013;591:765–74. doi:10.1113/jphysiol.2012.237958.

39. Vandergheynst F, Sakr Y, Felleiter P, et al. Incidence and prognosis of dysnatraemia in critically ill patients: analysis of a large preva-lence study. Eur J Clin Investig. 2013;43:933–48. doi:10.1111/eci.12123.

40. Funk G-C, Lindner G, Druml W, et al. Incidence and prognosis of dysnatremias present on ICU admission. Intensive Care Med. 2010;36:304–11. doi:10.1007/s00134-009-1692-0.

41. Pollock AS, Arieff AI. Abnormalities of cell volume regulation and their functional consequences. Am J Phys. 1980;239:F195–205.

42. Tisdall M, Crocker M, Watkiss J, Smith M. Disturbances of sodium in critically ill adult neurologic patients: a clinical review. J Neurosurg Anesthesiol. 2006;18:57–63.

43. Sakr Y, Rother S, Ferreira AMP, et al. Fluctuations in serum sodium level are associated with an increased risk of death in sur-gical ICU patients. Crit Care Med. 2013;41:133–42. doi:10.1097/CCM.0b013e318265f576.

44. Laville M, Burst V, Peri A, Verbalis JG. Hyponatremia second-ary to the syndrome of inappropriate secretion of antidiuretic hor-mone (SIADH): therapeutic decision-making in real-life cases. Clin Kidney J. 2013;6:i1–i20. doi:10.1093/ckj/sft113.

45. Sherlock M, O'Sullivan E, Agha A, et al. Incidence and patho-physiology of severe hyponatraemia in neurosurgical patients. Postgrad Med J. 2009;85:171–5. doi:10.1136/pgmj.2008.072819.

46. Kirkman MA, Albert AF, Ibrahim A, Doberenz D. Hyponatremia and brain injury: historical and contemporary perspectives. Neurocrit Care. 2013;18:406–16. doi:10.1007/s12028-012-9805-y.

47. Darmon M, Diconne E, Souweine B, et al. Prognostic conse-quences of borderline dysnatremia: pay attention to minimal serum sodium change. Crit Care Lond Engl. 2013;17:R12. doi:10.1186/cc11937.

48. Stelfox HT, Ahmed SB, Khandwala F, et al. The epidemiology of intensive care unit-acquired hyponatraemia and hypernatrae-mia in medical-surgical intensive care units. Crit Care Lond Engl. 2008;12:R162. doi:10.1186/cc7162.

49. Kovesdy CP, Lott EH, Lu JL, et al. Hyponatremia, hypernatremia, and mortality in patients with chronic kidney disease with and without congestive heart failure. Circulation. 2012;125:677–84. doi:10.1161/CIRCULATIONAHA.111.065391.

50. Padhi R, Panda BN, Jagati S, Patra SC. Hyponatremia in critically ill patients. Indian J Crit Care Med. 2014;18:83–7. doi:10.4103/0972-5229.126077.

51. Sodium disorders in critically ill neurologic patients: a focus on pharmacologic management. OA Critical Care. http://www.oapublishinglondon.com/article/1300. Accessed 20 Jul 2015

52. Halawa I, Andersson T, Tomson T. Hyponatremia and risk of seizures: a retrospective cross-sectional study. Epilepsia. 2011;52:410–3. doi:10.1111/j.1528-1167.2010.02939.x.

53. Ko S-H, Lim C-H, Kim J-Y, et al. Case of inappropriate ADH syn-drome: hyponatremia due to polyethylene glycol bowel prepara-tion. World J Gastroenterol WJG. 2014;20:12350–4. doi:10.3748/wjg.v20.i34.12350.

54. Richter S, Betz C, Geiger H. Severe hyponatremia with pulmo-nary and cerebral edema in an Ironman triathlete. Dtsch Med Wochenschr. 2007;132:1829–32. doi:10.1055/s-2007-984973.

55. Sue Y-M, Lee Y-L, Huang J-J. Acute hyponatremia, seizure, and rhabdomyolysis after ecstasy use. J Toxicol Clin Toxicol. 2002;40:931–2.

56. Gill M, McCauley M. Psychogenic polydipsia: the result, or cause of, deteriorating psychotic symptoms? A case report of the consequences of water intoxication. Case Rep Psychiatry. 2015;2015:846459. doi:10.1155/2015/846459.

57. Ganong CA, Kappy MS. Cerebral salt wasting in children. The need for recognition and treatment. Am J Dis Child. 1960;147:167–9.

58. Çelik T, Tolunay O, Tolunay İ, Çelik Ü. Cerebral salt wasting in status epilepticus: two cases and review of the literature. Pediatr Neurol. 2014;50:397–9. doi:10.1016/j.pediatrneurol.2013.11.019.

59. Peri A, Pirozzi N, Parenti G, et al. Hyponatremia and the syn-drome of inappropriate secretion of antidiuretic hormone (SIADH). J Endocrinol Investig. 2010;33:671–82. doi:10.1007/BF03346668.

60. Oh JY, Shin JI. Syndrome of inappropriate antidiuretic hor-mone secretion and cerebral/renal salt wasting syndrome: simi-larities and differences. Front Pediatr. 2014;2:146. doi:10.3389/fped.2014.00146.

61. Vincent A, Buckley C, Schott JM, et al. Potassium chan-nel antibody-associated encephalopathy: a potentially immunotherapy-responsive form of limbic encephalitis. Brain J Neurol. 2004;127:701–12. doi:10.1093/brain/awh077.

62. Cerdà-Esteve M, Cuadrado-Godia E, Chillaron JJ, et al. Cerebral salt wasting syndrome: review. Eur J Intern Med. 2008;19:249–54. doi:10.1016/j.ejim.2007.06.019.

63. Betjes MGH. Hyponatremia in acute brain disease: the cerebral salt wasting syndrome. Eur J Intern Med. 2002;13:9–14.

64. Diringer MN, Wu KC, Verbalis JG, Hanley DF. Hypervolemic therapy prevents volume contraction but not hyponatremia fol-lowing subarachnoid hemorrhage. Ann Neurol. 1992;31:543–50. doi:10.1002/ana.410310513.

65. Marupudi NI, Mittal S. Diagnosis and management of hyponatre-mia in patients with aneurysmal subarachnoid hemorrhage. J Clin Med. 2015;4:756–67. doi:10.3390/jcm4040756.

66. Hasan D, Wijdicks EF, Vermeulen M. Hyponatremia is associ-ated with cerebral ischemia in patients with aneurysmal sub-arachnoid hemorrhage. Ann Neurol. 1990;27:106–8. doi:10.1002/ana.410270118.

67. Verbalis JG. Control of brain volume during hypoosmolality and hyperosmolality. Adv Exp Med Biol. 2006;576:113–29. discus-sion 361–363 doi:10.1007/0-387-30172-0_8.

68. Rabinstein AA, Wijdicks EFM. Hyponatremia in critically ill neu-rological patients. Neurologist. 2003;9:290–300. doi:10.1097/01.nrl.0000095258.07720.89.

69. Sterns RH, Thomas DJ, Herndon RM. Brain dehydration and neurologic deterioration after rapid correction of hyponatremia. Kidney Int. 1989;35:69–75.

70. Van Amelsvoort T, Bakshi R, Devaux CB, Schwabe S. Hyponatremia associated with carbamazepine and oxcarbaze-pine therapy: a review. Epilepsia. 1994;35:181–8.

71. Azuma H, Akechi T, Furukawa TA. Absence status associ-ated with focal activity and polydipsia-induced hyponatremia. Neuropsychiatr Dis Treat. 2008;4:495–8.

72. Primavera A, Fonti A, Giberti L, Cocito L. Recurrent absence status epilepticus and hyponatremia in a patient

with polydipsia. Biol Psychiatry. 1995;38:189–91. doi:10.1016/0006-3223(95)00145-7.

73. Barolomei F, Gastaut JL. Complex partial status epilepticus provoked by hyponatremia. Eur Neurol. 1998;40:53–4.

74. Sarnaik AP, Meert K, Hackbarth R, Fleischmann L. Management of hyponatremic seizures in children with hypertonic saline: a safe and effective strategy. Crit Care Med. 1991;19:758–62.

75. Sharf RE. Seizure from hyponatremia in infants. Early recognition and treatment. Arch Fam Med. 1993;2:647–52.

76. Bruce RC, Kliegman RM. Hyponatremic seizures secondary to oral water intoxication in infancy: association with commercial bottled drinking water. Pediatrics. 1997;100:E4.

77. Farrar HC, Chande VT, Fitzpatrick DF, Shema SJ. Hyponatremia as the cause of seizures in infants: a retrospective analysis of incidence, severity, and clinical predictors. Ann Emerg Med. 1995;26:42–8. doi:10.1016/S0196-0644(95)70236-9.

78. Hanna S, Tibby SM, Durward A, Murdoch IA. Incidence of hyponatraemia and hyponatraemic seizures in severe respiratory syncytial virus bronchiolitis. Acta Paediatr Oslo Nor. 2007;92:430–4.

79. Hardesty DA, Kilbaugh TJ, Storm PB. Cerebral salt wasting syndrome in post-operative pediatric brain tumor patients. Neurocrit Care. 2012;17:382–7. doi:10.1007/s12028-011-9618-4.

80. Hoorn EJ, Halperin ML, Zietse R. Diagnostic approach to a patient with hyponatraemia: traditional versus physiology-based options. QJM Mon J Assoc Physicians. 2005;98:529–40. doi:10.1093/qjmed/hci081.

81. Spasovski G, Vanholder R, Allolio B, et al. Clinical practice guideline on diagnosis and treatment of hyponatraemia. Intensive Care Med. 2014;40:320–31. doi:10.1007/s00134-014-3210-2.

82. Carlotti AP, Bohn D, Rutka JT, et al. A method to estimate urinary electrolyte excretion in patients at risk for developing cerebral salt wasting. J Neurosurg. 2001;95:420–4. doi:10.3171/jns.2001.95.3.0420.

83. Sterns RH, Cappuccio JD, Silver SM, Cohen EP. Neurologic sequelae after treatment of severe hyponatremia: a multicenter perspective. J Am Soc Nephrol JASN. 1994;4:1522–30.

84. Sterns RH, Riggs JE, Schochet SS. Osmotic demyelination syndrome following correction of hyponatremia. N Engl J Med. 1986;314:1535–42. doi:10.1056/NEJM198606123142402.

85. Karp BI, Laureno R. Pontine and extrapontine myelinolysis: a neurologic disorder following rapid correction of hyponatremia. Medicine (Baltimore). 1993;72:359–73.

86. Sterns RH, Hix JK. Overcorrection of hyponatremia is a medical emergency. Kidney Int. 2009;76:587–9. doi:10.1038/ki.2009.251.

87. Mori T, Katayama Y, Kawamata T, Hirayama T. Improved efficiency of hypervolemic therapy with inhibition of natriuresis by fludrocortisone in patients with aneurysmal subarachnoid hemorrhage. J Neurosurg. 1999;91:947–52. doi:10.3171/jns.1999.91.6.0947.

88. Decaux G. SIADH and vaptans. Ann Endocrinol. 2012;73:130–4. doi:10.1016/j.ando.2012.04.005.

89. Palevsky PM, Bhagrath R, Greenberg A. Hypernatremia in hospitalized patients. Ann Intern Med. 1996;124:197–203.

90. Overgaard-Steensen C, Ring T. Clinical review: practical approach to hyponatraemia and hypernatraemia in critically ill patients. Crit Care Lond Engl. 2013;17:206. doi:10.1186/cc11805.

91. Lindner G, Funk G-C. Hypernatremia in critically ill patients. J Crit Care. 2013;28:216.e11–20. doi:10.1016/j.jcrc.2012.05.001.

92. Polderman KH, Schreuder WO, Strack van Schijndel RJ, Thijs LG. Hypernatremia in the intensive care unit: an indicator of quality of care? Crit Care Med. 1999;27:1105–8.

93. Waite MD, Fuhrman SA, Badawi O, et al. Intensive care unit-acquired hypernatremia is an independent predictor of increased mortality and length of stay. J Crit Care. 2013;28:405–12. doi:10.1016/j.jcrc.2012.11.013.

94. Kumar S, Berl T. Sodium. Lancet Lond Engl. 1998;352:220–8. doi:10.1016/S0140-6736(97)12169-9.

95. Hoorn EJ, Betjes MGH, Weigel J, Zietse R. Hypernatraemia in critically ill patients: too little water and too much salt. Nephrol Dial Transplant. 2008;23:1562–8. doi:10.1093/ndt/gfm831.

96. Odier C, Nguyen DK, Panisset M. Central pontine and extrapontine myelinolysis: from epileptic and other manifestations to cognitive prognosis. J Neurol. 2010;257:1176–80. doi:10.1007/s00415-010-5486-7.

97. Brown WD, Caruso JM. Extrapontine myelinolysis with involvement of the hippocampus in three children with severe hypernatremia. J Child Neurol. 1999;14:428–33.

98. Hbibi M, Abourazzak S, Babakhouya A, et al. Severe hypernatremic dehydration associated with cerebral venous and aortic thrombosis in the neonatal period. BMJ Case Rep. 2012; doi:10.1136/bcr.07.2011.4426.

99. Fleischer LM, Wilson TA, Parker MM. Hypernatremic dehydration, diabetes insipidus, and cerebral venous sinus thrombosis in a neonate: a case report. J Med Case Rep. 2007;1:66. doi:10.1186/1752-1947-1-66.

100. Castilla-Guerra L, del Carmen Fernández-Moreno M, López-Chozas JM, Fernández-Bolaños R. Electrolytes disturbances and seizures. Epilepsia. 2006;47:1990–8. doi:10.1111/j.1528-1167.2006.00861.x.

101. Andreoli TE, Reeves WB, Bichet DG. Endocrine control of water balance. Compr Physiol. 2010; doi:10.1002/cphy.cp070314.

102. Welt LG, Orloff J, Kydd DM, Oltman JE. An example of cellular hyperosmolarity. J Clin Invest. 1950;29:935–9. doi:10.1172/JCI102328.

103. Gupta MM. Calcium imbalance in hypoparathyroidism. J Assoc Physicians India. 1991;39:616–8.

104. Bhadada SK, Bhansali A, Upreti V, et al. Spectrum of neurological manifestations of idiopathic hypoparathyroidism and pseudohypoparathyroidism. Neurol India. 2011;59:586–9. doi:10.4103/0028-3886.84342.

105. Kelly A, Levine MA. Hypocalcemia in the critically ill patient. J Intensive Care Med. 2013;28:166–77. doi:10.1177/0885066611411543.

106. Zivin JR, Gooley T, Zager RA, Ryan MJ. Hypocalcemia: a pervasive metabolic abnormality in the critically ill. Am J Kidney Dis Off J Natl Kidney Found. 2001;37:689–98.

107. Steele T, Kolamunnage-Dona R, Downey C, et al. Assessment and clinical course of hypocalcemia in critical illness. Crit Care Lond Engl. 2013;17:R106. doi:10.1186/cc12756.

108. Zhang Z, Xu X, Ni H, Deng H. Predictive value of ionized calcium in critically ill patients: an analysis of a large clinical database MIMIC II. PLoS One. 2014;9:e95204. doi:10.1371/journal.pone.0095204.

109. Hästbacka J, Pettilä V. Prevalence and predictive value of ionized hypocalcemia among critically ill patients. Acta Anaesthesiol Scand. 2003;47:1264–9.

110. Chernow B, Zaloga G, McFadden E, et al. Hypocalcemia in critically ill patients. Crit Care Med. 1982;10:848–51.

111. Carlstedt F, Lind L, Rastad J, et al. Parathyroid hormone and ionized calcium levels are related to the severity of illness and survival in critically ill patients. Eur J Clin Investig. 1998;28:898–903.

112. Milman S, Epstein E. Proton pump inhibitor-induced hypocalcemic seizure in a patient with hypoparathyroidism. Endocr Pract. 2010;17:104–7. doi:10.4158/EP10241.CR.

113. Deroux A, Khouri C, Chabre O, et al. Severe acute neurological symptoms related to proton pump inhibitors induced hypomagnesemia responsible for profound hypoparathyroidism with hypocalcemia. Clin Res Hepatol Gastroenterol. 2014;38:e103–5. doi:10.1016/j.clinre.2014.03.005.

114. Maclsaac RJ, Seeman E, Jerums G. Seizures after alendronate. J R Soc Med. 2002;95:615–6.

115. Tsourdi E, Rachner TD, Gruber M, et al. Seizures associated with zoledronic acid for osteoporosis. J Clin Endocrinol Metab. 2011;96:1955–9. doi:10.1210/jc.2011-0418.

116. Cox RE. Hypoparathyroidism: an unusual cause of seizures. Ann Emerg Med. 1983;12:314–5.

117. Mrowka M, Knake S, Klinge H, et al. Hypocalcemic generalised seizures as a manifestation of iatrogenic hypoparathyroidism months to years after thyroid surgery. Epileptic Disord Int Epilepsy J Videotape. 2004;6:85–7.

118. Fonseca OA, Calverley JR. Neurological manifestations of hypoparathyroidism. Arch Intern Med. 1967;120:202–6.

119. Tsai P-L, Lian L-M, Chen W-H. Hypocalcemic seizure mistaken for idiopathic epilepsy in two cases of DiGeorge syndrome (chromosome 22q11 deletion syndrome). Acta Neurol Taiwanica. 2009;18:272–5.

120. Bindu M, Harinarayana CV. Hypoparathyroidism: a rare treatable cause of epilepsy–report of two cases. Eur J Neurol Off J Eur Fed NeurolSoc.2006;13:786–8.doi:10.1111/j.1468-1331.2006.01287.x.

121. Kinoshita H, Kokudo T, Ide T, et al. A patient with DiGeorge syndrome with spina bifida and sacral myelomeningocele, who developed both hypocalcemia-induced seizure and epilepsy. Seizure. 2010;19:303–5. doi:10.1016/j.seizure.2010.04.005.

122. Cheung ENM, George SR, Andrade DM, et al. Neonatal hypocalcemia, neonatal seizures, and intellectual disability in 22q11.2 deletion syndrome. Genet Med Off J Am Coll Med Genet. 2014;16:40–4. doi:10.1038/gim.2013.71.

123. Korkmaz HA, Dizdarer C, Ecevit CO. Hypocalcemic seizure in an adolescent with down syndrome: a manifestation of unrecognized celiac disease. Turk J Pediatr. 2013;55:536–8.

124. Erdeve O, Atasay B, Arsan S, et al. Hypocalcemic seizure due to congenital rickets in the first day of life. Turk J Pediatr. 2007;49:301–3.

125. Kossoff EH, Silvia MT, Maret A, et al. Neonatal hypocalcemic seizures: case report and literature review. J Child Neurol. 2002;17:236–9.

126. Korkmaz HA, Özkan B, Terek D, et al. Neonatal seizure as a manifestation of unrecognized maternal hyperparathyroidism. J Clin Res Pediatr Endocrinol. 2013;5:206–8. doi:10.4274/Jcrpe.1037.

127. Clarke PC, Carré IJ. Hypocalcemic, hypomagnesemic convulsions. J Pediatr. 1967;70:806–9.

128. Ali FE, Al-Bustan MA, Al-Busairi WA, Al-Mulla FA. Loss of seizure control due to anticonvulsant-induced hypocalcemia. Ann Pharmacother. 2004;38:1002–5. doi:10.1345/aph.1D467.

129. Dickerson RN, Alexander KH, Minard G, et al. Accuracy of methods to estimate ionized and "corrected" serum calcium concentrations in critically ill multiple trauma patients receiving specialized nutrition support. JPEN J Parenter Enteral Nutr. 2004;28:133–41.

130. Dickerson RN, Henry NY, Miller PL, et al. Low serum total calcium concentration as a marker of low serum ionized calcium concentration in critically ill patients receiving specialized nutrition support. Nutr Clin Pract. 2007;22:323–8.

131. Tartaglia F, Giuliani A, Sgueglia M, et al. Randomized study on oral administration of calcitriol to prevent symptomatic hypocalcemia after total thyroidectomy. Am J Surg. 2005;190:424–9. doi:10.1016/j.amjsurg.2005.04.017.

132. Biller J, Ferro JM. In: Aminoff J, Boller F, Swaab DF, editors. Neurologic aspects of systemic disease part II: handbook of clinical neurology: Newnes; 2014. Neurologic disorders of mineral metabolism and parathyroid disease. Agrawal L, Habib Z, Emanuele NV. Neurologic disorders of mineral metabolism and parathyroid disease. Handb Clin Neurol. 2014;120:737–48. doi: 10.1016/B978-0-7020-4087-0.00049-8.

133. Kline CA, Esekogwu VI, Henderson SO, Newton KI. Nonconvulsive status epilepticus in a patient with hypocalcemia. J Emerg Med. 1998;16:715–8.

134. Zuckermann EC, Glaser GH. Anticonvulsive action of increased calcium concentration in cerebrospinal fluid. Arch Neurol. 1973;29:245–52.

135. Hariri A, Mount DB, Rastegar A. Disorders of calcium, phosphate, and magnesium metabolism. In: Mount DB, Sayegh MH, Singh AK, Core concepts in the disorders of fluid, electrolytes and acid-base balance. New York: Springer, 2013. P. 103–146.

136. TAD C, Kauffman RP, Myles TD. Primary hyperparathyroidism, hypercalcemic crisis and subsequent seizures occurring during pregnancy: a case report. J Matern-Fetal Neonatal Med. 2002;12:349–52. doi:10.1080/jmf.12.5.349.352.

137. Hauser GJ, Gale AD, Fields AI. Immobilization hypercalcemia: unusual presentation with seizures. Pediatr Emerg Care. 1989;5:105–7.

138. Nordt SP, Williams SR, Clark RF. Pharmacologic misadventure resulting in hypercalcemia from vitamin D intoxication. J Emerg Med. 2002;22:302–3.

139. Dinnerstein E, McDonald BC, Cleavinger HB, et al. Mesial temporal sclerosis after status epilepticus due to milk alkali syndrome. Seizure. 2008;17:292–5. doi:10.1016/j.seizure.2007.07.013.

140. Kashouty R, Yono N, Al Samara M. Status epilepticus secondary to milk-alkali syndrome induced by hypercalcemia (oral antacids). Seizure. 2011;20:659–61. doi:10.1016/j.seizure.2011.03.011.

141. Chen T-H, Huang C-C, Chang Y-Y, et al. Vasoconstriction as the etiology of hypercalcemia-induced seizures. Epilepsia. 2004;45:551–4. doi:10.1111/j.0013-9580.2004.57003.x.

142. Kastrup O, Maschke M, Wanke I, Diener HC. Posterior reversible encephalopathy syndrome due to severe hypercalcemia. J Neurol. 2002;249:1563–6. doi:10.1007/s00415-002-0895-x.

143. Kaplan PW. Reversible hypercalcemic cerebral vasoconstriction with seizures and blindness: a paradigm for eclampsia? Clin EEG Electroencephalogr. 1998;29:120–3.

144. Demir BC, Ozerkan K, Ozbek SE, et al. Comparison of magnesium sulfate and mannitol in treatment of eclamptic women with posterior reversible encephalopathy syndrome. Arch Gynecol Obstet. 2012;286:287–93. doi:10.1007/s00404-012-2268-8.

145. Fawcett WJ, Haxby EJ, Male DA. Magnesium: physiology and pharmacology. Br J Anaesth. 1999;83:302–20.

146. Soliman HM, Mercan D, Lobo SSM, et al. Development of ionized hypomagnesemia is associated with higher mortality rates. Crit Care Med. 2003;31:1082–7. Springer, New York 2013 doi:10.1097/01.CCM.0000060867.17556.A0.

147. Fairley J, Glassford NJ, Zhang L, Bellomo R. Magnesium status and magnesium therapy in critically ill patients: a systematic review. J Crit Care. 2015;30:1349. doi:10.1016/j.jcrc.2015.07.029.

148. Tong GM, Rude RK. Magnesium deficiency in critical illness. JIntensiveCareMed.2005;20:3–17.doi:10.1177/0885066604271539.

149. Huijgen HJ, Soesan M, Sanders R, et al. Magnesium levels in critically ill patients. What should we measure? Am J Clin Pathol. 2000;114:688–95. doi:10.1309/0Q7F-QTGM-6DPD-TLGY.

150. Iseri LT, Allen BJ, Brodsky MA. Magnesium therapy of cardiac arrhythmias in critical-care medicine. Magnesium. 1989;8:299–306.

151. Saul RF, Selhorst JB. Downbeat nystagmus with magnesium depletion. Arch Neurol. 1981;38:650–2.

152. Kass L, Weekes J, Carpenter L. Effect of magnesium supplementation on blood pressure: a meta-analysis. Eur J Clin Nutr. 2012;66:411–8. doi:10.1038/ejcn.2012.4.

153. Schwartz RB, Feske SK, Polak JF, et al. Preeclampsia-eclampsia: clinical and neuroradiographic correlates and insights into the pathogenesis of hypertensive encephalopathy. Radiology. 2000;217:371–6. doi:10.1148/radiology.217.2.r00nv44371.

154. Rude RK, Gruber HE, Norton HJ, et al. Reduction of dietary magnesium by only 50% in the rat disrupts bone and mineral metabolism. Osteoporos Int. 2006;17:1022–32. doi:10.1007/s00198-006-0104-3.

155. Sinert R, Zehtabchi S, Desai S, et al. Serum ionized magnesium and calcium levels in adult patients with seizures. Scand J Clin Lab Invest. 2007;67:317–26. doi:10.1080/00365510601051441.

156. Sood AK, Handa R, Malhotra RC, Gupta BS. Serum, CSF, RBC and urinary levels of magnesium and calcium in idiopathic generalised tonic clonic seizures. Indian J Med Res. 1993;98:152–4.

157. Abdelmalik PA, Politzer N, Carlen PL. Magnesium as an effective adjunct therapy for drug resistant seizures. Can J Neurol Sci J Can Sci Neurol. 2012;39:323–7.

158. Visser NA, Braun KPJ, Leijten FSS, et al. Magnesium treatment for patients with refractory status epilepticus due to POLG1-mutations. J Neurol. 2011;258:218–22. doi:10.1007/s00415-010-5721-2.

159. Lucas MJ, Leveno KJ, Cunningham FG. A comparison of magnesium sulfate with phenytoin for the prevention of eclampsia. N Engl J Med. 1995;333:201–5. doi:10.1056/NEJM199507273330401.

160. Duley L, Henderson-Smart DJ, Walker GJ, Chou D. Magnesium sulphate versus diazepam for eclampsia. Cochrane Database Syst Rev. 2010:CD000127. doi:10.1002/14651858.CD000127.pub2.

161. Pande SD, Wee CK, Maw NN. Unusual case of hypomagnesaemia induced seizures. BMJ Case Rep. 2009;2009:bcr0620091933. doi:10.1136/bcr.06.2009.1933.

162. Matthey F, Gelder CM, Schon FE. Isolated hypomagnesaemia presenting as focal seizures in diabetes mellitus. Br Med J (Clin Res Ed). 1986;293:1409.

163. Fagan C, Phelan D. Severe convulsant hypomagnesaemia and short bowel syndrome. Anaesth Intensive Care. 2001;29:281–3.

164. Gandhi NY, Sharif WK, Chadha S, Shakher J. A patient on long-term proton pump inhibitors develops sudden seizures and encephalopathy: an unusual presentation of hypomagnesaemia. Case Rep Gastrointest Med. 2012;2012:632721. doi:10.1155/2012/632721.

165. Visudhiphan P, Visudtibhan A, Chiemchanya S, Khongkhatithum C. Neonatal seizures and familial hypomagnesemia with secondary hypocalcemia. Pediatr Neurol. 2005;33:202–5. doi:10.1016/j.pediatrneurol.2005.03.009.

166. Viveros H, Somjen GG. Magnesium-calcium antagonism in the contraction of arterioles. Experientia. 1968;24:457–9.

167. Euser AG, Cipolla MJ. Magnesium sulfate for the treatment of eclampsia: a brief review. Stroke J Cereb Circ. 2009;40:1169–75. doi:10.1161/STROKEAHA.108.527788.

168. Efstratiadis G, Sarigianni M, Gougourelas I. Hypomagnesemia and cardiovascular system. Hippokratia. 2006;10:147–52.

169. Swaminathan R. Magnesium metabolism and its disorders. Clin Biochem Rev. 2003;24:47–66.

170. Shorvon SD, Andermann F, Guerrini R. The causes of epilepsy: common and uncommon causes in adults and children. Cambridge: Cambridge University Press; 2011.

171. Reddi PAS. Disorders of magnesium: hypomagnesemia. In: Fluid electrolyte acid-base disorders. New York, NY: Springer; 2014. p. 271–83.

172. Gunnerson KJ, Kellum JA. Acid-base and electrolyte analysis in critically ill patients: are we ready for the new millennium? Curr Opin Crit Care. 2003;9:468–73.

173. Mallat J, Barrailler S, Lemyze M, et al. Use of sodium-chloride difference and corrected anion gap as surrogates of Stewart variables in critically ill patients. PLoS One. 2013;8:e56635. doi:10.1371/journal.pone.0056635.

174. Paz Y, Zegerman A, Sorkine P, Matot I. Severe acidosis does not predict fatal outcomes in intensive care unit patients: a retrospective analysis. J Crit Care. 2014;29:210–3. doi:10.1016/j.jcrc.2013.11.007.

175. Anderson LE, Henrich WL. Alkalemia-associated morbidity and mortality in medical and surgical patients. South Med J. 1987;80:729–33.

176. Fitzgibbons LJ, Snoey ER. Severe metabolic alkalosis due to baking soda ingestion: case reports of two patients with unsuspected antacid overdose. J Emerg Med. 1999;17:57–61.

177. Stephani J, Wagner M, Breining T, et al. Metabolic alkalosis, acute renal failure and epileptic seizures as unusual manifestations of an upside-down stomach. Case Rep Gastroenterol. 2012;6:452–8. doi:10.1159/000341509.

178. Perez GO, Oster JR, Rogers A. Acid-base disturbances in gastrointestinal disease. Dig Dis Sci. 1987;32:1033–43.

179. Kramer L, Tribl B, Gendo A, et al. Partial pressure of ammonia versus ammonia in hepatic encephalopathy. Hepatol Baltim Md. 2000;31:30–4. doi:10.1002/hep.510310107.

180. During MJ, Fried I, Leone P, et al. Direct measurement of extracellular lactate in the human hippocampus during spontaneous seizures. J Neurochem. 1994;62:2356–61.

181. Holmes MD, Dewaraja AS, Vanhatalo S. Does hyperventilation elicit epileptic seizures? Epilepsia. 2004;45:618–20. doi:10.1111/j.0013-9580.2004.63803.x.

182. Raybarman C. Is hyperventilation an effective activating procedure in routine clinical EEG studies in children? J Child Neurol. 2009;24:1294–5. doi:10.1177/0883073809334383.

183. Ahdab R, Riachi N. Reexamining the added value of intermittent photic stimulation and hyperventilation in routine EEG practice. Eur Neurol. 2014;71:93–8. doi:10.1159/000353650.

184. Assenza G, Mecarelli O, Tombini M, et al. Hyperventilation induces sympathetic overactivation in mesial temporal epilepsy. Epilepsy Res. 2015;110:221–7. doi:10.1016/j.eplepsyres.2014.12.003.

185. Hirabayashi Y, Okumura A, Kondo T, et al. Efficacy of a diazepam suppository at preventing febrile seizure recurrence during a single febrile illness. Brain Dev. 2009;31:414–8. doi:10.1016/j.braindev.2008.07.010.

186. Schuchmann S, Hauck S, Henning S, et al. Respiratory alkalosis in children with febrile seizures. Epilepsia. 2011;52:1949–55. doi:10.1111/j.1528-1167.2011.03259.x.

187. Schuchmann S, Schmitz D, Rivera C, et al. Experimental febrile seizures are precipitated by a hyperthermia-induced respiratory alkalosis. Nat Med. 2006;12:817–23. doi:10.1038/nm1422.

188. Tolner EA, Hochman DW, Hassinen P, et al. Five percent CO2 is a potent, fast-acting inhalation anticonvulsant. Epilepsia. 2011;52:104–14. doi:10.1111/j.1528-1167.2010.02731.x.

189. Somjen GG, editor. Ions in the brain: normal function, seizures, and stroke. Oxford, NY: Oxford University Press; 2004. p. 432.

190. Helmy MM, Ruusuvuori E, Watkins PV, et al. Acid extrusion via blood-brain barrier causes brain alkalosis and seizures after neonatal asphyxia. Brain J Neurol. 2012;135:3311–9. doi:10.1093/brain/aws257.

191. Kaplan LJ, Frangos S. Clinical review: acid-base abnormalities in the intensive care unit–part II. Crit Care Lond Engl. 2005;9:198–203. doi:10.1186/cc2912.

192. Jung B, Rimmele T, Le Goff C, et al. Severe metabolic or mixed acidemia on intensive care unit admission: incidence, prognosis and administration of buffer therapy. A prospective, multiple-center study. Crit Care Lond Engl. 2011;15:R238. doi:10.1186/cc10487.

193. Cooper ES, Lechner E, Bellet S. Relation between serum and cerebrospinal fluid electrolytes under normal and abnormal conditions. Am J Med. 1955;18(4):613–21.

194. Hunter G, Smith HV. Calcium and magnesium in human cerebrospinal fluid. Nature. 1960;186:161–2.

195. Sambrook MA. The relationship between cerebrospinal fluid and plasma electrolytes in patients with meningitis. J Neurol Sci. 1974;23(2):265–73.

196. Woodbury J, Lyons K, Carretta R, Hahn A, Sullivan JF. Cerebrospinal fluid and serum levels of magnesium, zinc, and calcium in man. Neurology. 1968;18(7):700–5.

197. Bradbury MW, Sarna GS. Homeostasis of the ionic composition of the cerebrospinal fluid. Exp Eye Res. 1977;25(Suppl):249–57.

Alcohol-Related Seizures in the Intensive Care Unit

Chandan Mehta, Mohammed Rehman, and Panayiotis N. Varelas

Introduction

Alcohol use disorders have become fairly common in the general population, and are quite frequently under-addressed in the inpatient setting. In 2010, 17.9 million Americans were identified as alcohol-dependent or abusers. An estimated 10–33% of patients in the critical care setting carry the diagnosis of alcohol use or dependence [1]. Rates are higher in adult men (12.4%) than adult women (4.9%). The DSM-5 estimates that 1 in 5 ICU admissions in some urban hospitals may be related to alcohol, and that at least 20% of ER visits by adult patients may be related to alcohol abuse or withdrawal [2, 3]. Diagnostic criteria for alcohol abuse and dependence disorders have now been unified into a spectrum of qualifying characteristics which help providers delineate the appropriate diagnosis to guide management [2]. Before discussing management of alcohol-related seizures within the intensive care unit (ICU), it is necessary to familiarize oneself with the revised diagnostic criteria for abuse and dependence disorders, and to acknowledge the multiple confounding medical comorbidities that patients with alcohol withdrawal syndromes often present with.

This chapter will review the definition of alcohol use disorders, pathophysiology of alcohol withdrawal and alcohol-related seizures, associated electrographic findings, treatment of alcohol-related seizures, and management of other comorbid medical conditions and other critical care dilemmas,

which may arise while treating these patients for seizures in the ICU; including delirium, agitation, and the need for mechanical ventilation.

Definition and Diagnosis of Alcohol Spectrum Disorders

The DSM-5 characterizes the severity of alcohol use on a spectrum of mild to severe based on the number of symptoms the patient exhibits. Mild use is characterized by the presence of 2–3 symptoms, moderate use as 4–5 symptoms, and severe use by the presence of 6 or more symptoms. Presence of two of these symptoms indicates an Alcohol Use Disorder (AUD). Qualifying symptoms include: (1) Use in larger amounts or over a longer period than intended. (2) Persistent desire or unsuccessful efforts to cut down or control use. (3) Excessive amounts of time spent in the procurement, usage, or recovery from its effects. (4) Craving, or a strong desire or urge to use alcohol. (5) Recurrent use resulting in a failure to fulfill major role obligations at work, school, or home. (6) Continued use despite having persistent or recurrent social or interpersonal problems caused or exacerbated by the effects of alcohol. (7) Reduction or cessation of important social, occupational, or recreational activities because of use. (8) Recurrent use in situations in which are physically hazardous. (9) Continued alcohol use despite knowledge of having a persistent or recurrent physical or psychological problem caused or exacerbated it. Additional qualifying characteristics may include presence of tolerance and or a withdrawal syndrome.

Tolerance is defined as either an increased amount of alcohol necessary to achieve intoxication or desired effect, or a diminished effect with ingestion of the same amount of alcohol [2]. Blood alcohol concentration (BAL) is the most objective test to judge tolerance to alcohol. An individual who has a BAL of 150 mg of ethanol per deciliter who demonstrates no signs of intoxication should be considered as having some tolerance to alcohol. In the non-tolerant individual, a BAL of 200 mg of ethanol/deciliter ingestion

C. Mehta • M. Rehman
Departments of Neurology and Neurosurgery, K-11 Henry Ford Hospital, 2799 West Grand Blvd, Detroit, MI, USA
e-mail: cmehta1@hfhs.org; Mrehman1@hfhs.org

P.N. Varelas (✉)
Departments of Neurology and Neurosurgery, Henry Ford Hospital, 2799 West Grand Blvd, Detroit, MI 48202, USA

Department of Neurology, Wayne State University, Detroit, MI, USA
e-mail: varelas@neuro.hfh.edu

© Springer International Publishing AG 2017
P.N. Varelas, J. Claassen (eds.), *Seizures in Critical Care*, Current Clinical Neurology, DOI 10.1007/978-3-319-49557-6_19

should lead to severe intoxication. BAL of 400 mg/dL may lead to coma and death [4].

Elevated serum gamma glutamyl transferase (γ-GT) levels (>35 units) may also be indicative of heavy chronic drinking. Elevated levels may be present in up to 70% of chronic drinkers. Carbohydrate-deficient transferrin (CDT) levels may also be elevated (>20 units), and may be helpful in identifying heavy alcohol users. As these levels return to normal during periods of abstinence, it is crucial to obtain a clear history of alcohol use in order to define where an individual may fall on the diagnostic spectrum in order to predict whether they are likely to withdrawal [2, 5–8].

The genetic profile of the individual may also play a role in alcohol consumption. A three to fourfold increase in risk of alcohol use disorders has been observed in children of individuals with preexisting alcohol use disorders, whether they are raised by them or adoptive parents. There are additionally significantly higher rates of dysfunctional use in monozygotic versus dizygotic twins when one twin has a diagnosis of an alcohol use disorder [2].

Table 19.1 Signs and symptoms of alcohol withdrawal syndrome, from last alcohol consumption presented by time-degree (modified from Mirijello et al. [3]). There is overlap between the degrees

Degree	Time from last ethanol consumption (hours)	Presenting clinical signs and symptoms
A. Mild sympathomimetic symptoms	6–12	Tremors, diaphoresis, hyperthermia, nausea/vomiting, hypertension, tachycardia, tachypnea, mydriasis
B. Alcoholic hallucinosis (25%)	12–24	Visual, auditory and tactile altered perceptions, with patient recognizing them as unreal
C. Alcohol withdrawal seizures (10%)	24–48	Generalized tonic-clonic seizures (with short or no postictal period), rarely partial onset seizures
D. Delirium tremens (5%)	48–72	Delirium (hyperactive, hypoactive, or mixed type), disorientation, psychosis, hallucinations, hyperthermia, malignant hypertension, insomnia, seizures, tremors, asterixis, coma

Alcohol Withdrawal Syndrome

Withdrawal symptoms may develop anywhere between 4 and 24 h after heavy ingestion [3]. One must take care to delineate true withdrawal symptoms from manifestations of alternative disease processes; for example, tremors from hypoglycemia or drug effect and psychomotor agitation or seizures from street or prescription drug withdrawal. It is often difficult to isolate true withdrawal symptoms as many patients have overlapping comorbidities with similar presentation. Alcohol withdrawal symptoms may range from mild to severe. The risk of developing alcohol withdrawal symptoms increases with quantity of intake and chronicity of alcohol use [9]. Habitual consumption of greater than eight drinks per day may predispose individuals to withdrawal symptoms [2]. As the effects of alcohol withdrawal may be deleterious, individuals may choose to continue to self-medicate with alcohol or other drugs to avoid developing symptoms.

Criteria have been established to define the syndrome of alcohol withdrawal. These include abrupt cessation or reduction in prolonged, heavy alcohol intake accompanied by two or more of the following: (1) autonomic hyperactivity (sweating, heart rates greater than 100 bpm), (2) hand tremors, (3) insomnia, (4) nausea or vomiting, (5) transient tactile, visual, or auditory hallucinations (delirium tremens), (6) psychomotor agitation, (7) anxiety, (8) generalized tonic-clonic seizures [2, 10].

These symptoms and signs must cause significant distress and impairment in functioning, and may not be attributable to other comorbid medical conditions, including psychiatric conditions or drug intoxication [2]. Symptoms may be relieved by alcohol or benzodiazepine administration, and evolve in time after the last drink (Table 19.1), usually peaking in intensity during day two of cessation, with improvement usually by days four or five. Anxiety, tremors, and insomnia may persist for 3–6 months. Less than 10–20% of chronic abusers will suffer from severe withdrawal symptoms (delirium tremens), and 3–10% of abusers will suffer from alcohol withdrawal seizures in the outpatient setting [3, 8, 9].

Due to essentially enforced abstention from alcohol use in the critical care setting during hospital admission, up to 30% of patients may develop symptoms associated with complicated (severe) alcohol withdrawal syndrome, including delirium tremens (24–33%) [11] and alcohol withdrawal seizures (5–17%) [12]. Mortality from delirium tremens may be as high as 8% in some patient populations, and may often be related secondarily to concurrent comorbid problems, such as infection leading sepsis or cardiac death.

Consideration for hospital admission includes presence of alcohol withdrawal symptoms as defined above, fever, encephalopathy, symptoms or objective laboratory data suggestive of infection or other systemic processes which may be secondary to alcohol use, or alcohol-related seizures, such as trauma.

Approximately 70% of patients admitted and treated in the ICU for severe alcohol withdrawal symptoms are intubated and mechanically ventilated during their stay [11]. The majority of patients, however, may only suffer from mild to moderate withdrawal symptoms, and overuse of medication triggered by scoring scales for treatment of withdrawal symptoms may have deleterious effects such as over sedation and respiratory depression [12].

Scales for Monitoring Withdrawal Symptoms

Multiple assessment scales have been devised for evaluation of withdrawal symptoms [3, 5, 12]. The most commonly utilized scale to quantify the severity of alcohol withdrawal is the Clinical Institute Withdrawal Assessment of Alcohol Scale, Revised (CIWA-Ar). The CIWA-Ar is a ten item questionnaire, which scores withdrawal severity in a range of 0–67. Scores 0–8 indicate *absent to minimal withdrawal*, 9–15 *moderate withdrawal*, and scores greater than 16 demonstrate *severe withdrawal* [8].

Most patients require ICU care for symptomatic treatment for scores greater than 15–20 [12, 13]. Use of the CIWA-Ar scale for symptomatic guidance of therapy in the critical care setting may be difficult in mechanically ventilated patients not able to verbalize responses appropriately. This may potentially lead to falsely inflated scores and subsequent medication over-administration, as symptoms of comorbid critical illness may be erroneously misinterpreted as withdrawal symptoms; or to delay in appropriate critical care, as symptoms and signs are attributed to alcohol withdrawal [5].

The Prediction of Alcohol Withdrawal Severity Scale (PAWSS) has also been developed and utilized in conjunction with the CIWA-Ar scale as a clinical prediction scale to define patients which are more likely to suffer from complicated alcohol withdrawal syndrome. The questionnaire has threshold criteria of alcohol use within 30 days; if patients meet this requirement they are screened into receiving the questionnaire; and are given points for previous episodes of severe intoxication, blackouts, delirium tremens, seizures, comorbid substance use, and previous alcohol rehabilitation treatment. Points are also given for meeting clinical criteria of BAL>200 mg ethanol/deciliter, or evidence of autonomic hyperactivity.

Patients with PAWSS< 4 are considered at low risk for complicated alcohol withdrawal syndrome; scores of PAWSS ≥4 are considered at high risk for complicated alcohol withdrawal syndrome. The study by Maldonado et al. suggested that using a PAWSS cutoff score of 4 led the scale to have a sensitivity for identifying complicated alcohol withdrawal syndrome of 93.1%, specificity of 99.5%, positive predictive value of 93.1%, and negative predictive value of 99.5% [12].

Incidence and Timeline of Alcohol-Related Seizures

Alcohol-related seizures (ARS) are a frequent occurrence in the critical care setting, and appropriate recognition and management may help decrease length of stay and improve morbidity and mortality outcomes in that patient population. Seizures are found to occur predominately in the setting of alcohol withdrawal due to the neurochemical adaptive changes, which manifest secondary to chronic alcohol usage

[5, 6, 8, 14, 15]. Seizures related to alcohol withdrawal usually occur prior to the onset of delirium tremens, (i.e., at onset of admission up to 72 h, and usually within a 5 day period of admission). In previous literature reviews, questions have been raised as to whether there is an actual association between alcohol withdrawal seizures and delirium tremens; or if these are of overlapping, but independent pathologies [5, 11].

Seizures may also occur during episodes of severe intoxication. While this may be less commonly encountered, this must remain in the differential diagnosis of the severely intoxicated patient who remains unarousable, or has focality in their neurologic exam. Patients with history of previous head trauma or previous intracranial pathology, toxometabolic abnormalities, renal or hepatic dysfunction, increased age (>60), or history of epilepsy may be more prone to seizures during acute alcohol intoxication. Cerebral atrophy combined with coagulopathy secondary to bone marrow suppression and hepatic dysfunction occurring with severe, prolonged alcohol use may lead to predisposition to development of subdural or epidural hematomas, leaving one vulnerable to alcohol-related seizures. Acute hepatic failure due to severe alcohol intoxication may also result in seizures, cerebral edema, coma, and death. Profound hyponatremia associated with chronic alcohol use may also lead to seizures during severe intoxication. Thorough laboratory workup including biochemical profile, blood counts, coagulation profile, liver profile, ammonia level, blood glucose levels, along with blood alcohol level, and arterial blood gases may be key in directing and predicting risk of seizures.

Pathophysiology of Alcohol Withdrawal and Alcohol-Related Seizures

In the normal brain, there exists a carefully orchestrated balance between excitatory and inhibitory neurotransmission. Alcohol withdrawal produces not only changes in the autonomic system (which may result in hypertension, tachycardia, or psychomotor agitation), but also changes which may lead to seizures and coma. Alcohol acts as a central nervous system depressant. Acute alcohol ingestion causes up regulation and potentiation of the inhibitory γ-aminobutyric acid (GABA) pathway on efferent neurons and inhibition of the excitatory N-methyl-D-aspartate (NMDA) receptors, resulting in significant CNS sedation [3]. As an adaptive mechanism, chronic use of alcohol results in down regulation of the GABA pathway, causing a decrease in the number and sensitivity of GABA receptors as well as reduction in endogenous levels of GABA [16].

Over time, in order to produce the same levels of CNS sedation, an increased concentration of alcohol is needed (usually resulting in increased amounts of alcohol ingestion). This phenomenon is known as tolerance [8, 11]. In parallel, compensatory increases in the activation of the excitatory glutamate pathways also occur, resulting in up regulation of NMDA receptors and increased levels of glutamate [3, 5, 8, 16, 17].

Abrupt cessation or reduction in chronic alcohol intake in a patient who has become physiologically dependent on alcohol creates an imbalance in the CNS, with unopposed excitation resulting in hyperactivity of the autonomic system, leading to withdrawal symptoms, and potentially to alcohol withdrawal seizures [8]. All of these changes over time lead to neuroplastic changes in the mesocorticolimbic system and the extended amygdala, which result in the strengthening of the compulsivity and relapse behaviors present during withdrawal phases in order to avoid manifestation of withdrawal symptoms [16].

Alcohol withdrawal in itself can also potentiate hippocampal neuronal loss and can lead to a kindling effect which may lead to increased severity of future episodes of alcohol withdrawal, ultimately negative impacting memory and cognitive functioning [12].

In individuals where there is a suspected history of chronic alcohol use and impending withdrawal is predicted to occur, coverage with oral or IV benzodiazepines should be utilized to prevent withdrawal symptoms and ultimately seizures for at least a 7 day course. Patients may be considered for therapy, if daily consumption reaches ten beverages in a female or 15 beverages in a male (with each beverage containing ~8 g of ethanol), history of recent withdrawal symptoms or history of withdrawal seizures, recent heavy binge drinking (greater than 20 drinks or 160 g of ethanol daily for longer than 7 days) [15].

Genetic Influence

Genetic predisposition to alcohol intolerance may self-select some individuals from engaging in ingestion of excessive amounts of alcohol or vice versa.

Genetic polymorphisms of alcohol dehydrogenase (ADH) and aldehyde dehydrogenase (ALDH), two enzymes involved in alcohol metabolism may contribute to the variability in tolerance and abuse of alcohol in different patient populations across the world [15]. Most often seen in Asian populations, individuals with these variants (specifically in ALDH2*2 allele (Glu504Lys)) often have low alcohol tolerance and experience a flushing syndrome and palpitations [18]. This may affect up to 40% of Chinese, Korean, and Japanese populations, and may result in lower levels of alcohol abuse, withdrawal, and presence of alcohol-related seizures, which, if they occur, may be secondary to comparatively lower consumption amounts.

Polymorphisms in ALDH1A1 and ALDH1B1 enzymes have been associated with alcohol consumption in Finnish and Danish populations, respectively [18]. There have been a significant number of genes, and gene polymorphisms which have been implicated in the development of alcohol dependence, predisposition for withdrawal symptoms and alcohol-related seizures.

A specific cluster of 58 genes has been identified by Morozova et al. in networks that were significantly enriched for alcohol metabolism and biotransformation. Some of these genes include GRIA1 and GRIA4, which encode ionotropic AMPA 1 and 4 glutamate receptors, and GRIN1, GRIN2B, and GRIN2C, which encode NMDA ionotropic glutamate receptor subunits 1, 2B, and 2C, indicating the importance of glutamatergic transmission as a central role in alcohol abuse, dependence, and withdrawal. Further studies need to be conducted in order to develop genetically tailored therapies, or at least genetic mapping to identify individuals likely to engage in alcohol abuse behaviors [18].

Multiple additional genetic factors regarding predisposition to dependence and withdrawal have been studied in rats and other small animals. In rats, low levels or pharmacological blockade of mGluR2 mRNA were found to increase alcohol intake, and alcohol seeking behavior. In post-mortem evaluation of frontal cortex samples of alcohol-dependent patients, presence of decreased expression of metabotropic glutamate receptor mGluR2 mRNA was found to be prevalent, which may act as a marker of alcohol dependence [16]. In the complex environment of the ICU, how much these and additional genes, interacting with each other and with the medications administered, lead to seizure development, is unknown.

Comorbidities in the Alcoholic Patient with Seizures Admitted to an ICU

Based on the aforementioned, seizures in the alcoholic patient may be multifactorial. As noted previously, patients admitted and found to have severe alcohol withdrawal symptoms may suffer from alcohol withdrawal seizures at a rate of 5–17%. Alcohol abusers may ultimately also suffer from a significant number of medical comorbidities which may leave them prone to having seizures for other reasons. Often times, these individuals may concurrently suffer from anxiety, depression, or other psychiatric disorders. They may be prescribed anxiolytics, opioids, and antipsychotics, and may additionally be abusing other substances. An emergency toxicology screen and STAT CT head as well as EKG, and lab work including complete blood count, biochemical profile, electrolytes, ammonia, troponin, lipase, amylase, blood glucose, and infectious workup should always be obtained. Consideration should additionally be made for lumbar puncture, if the clinical picture and patient history indicate a diagnosis of meningitis, which should be treated without delay.

Acute systemic comorbidities, such as electrolyte disturbances (hypomagnesemia, hyponatremia, hypoglycemia), diabetic ketoacidosis, uncontrolled hypertension, myocardial infarction, immunosuppression leading to infectious processes (bacteremia, urinary tract infections, pneumonia), and respiratory depression or insufficiency or central nervous system comorbidities, such as infections (including meningitis, encephalitis, brain abscess), previous or concurrent ischemic or hemorrhagic strokes, traumatic brain injury, tumors and other intracranial pathologies, may all lead to decrease the threshold for seizures in the context of alcohol withdrawal.

Chronic alcohol abuse may lead to a host of systemic medical issues. Neurologic manifestations of major concern may include Wernicke's encephalopathy (triad of ataxia, confusion, and ophthalmoplegia), secondary to thiamine deficiency, which may progress to Wernicke-Korsakoff syndrome, a later manifestation which further includes confabulation and memory loss. Prophylactic treatment with IV thiamine and folic acid should be administered on admission, and prior to administration of any dextrose containing solution, as glucose oxidation is dependent on thiamine, and in case of thiamine deficiency may lead to worsening of neurologic injury. Treatment of hypomagnesemia which usually accompanies low thiamine levels is necessary, as low magnesium levels may hinder thiamine absorption.

Additional neurologic manifestations may include profound neuropathy, burning mouth syndrome (from thiamine deficiency), myopathy, severe memory impairment, difficulty with executive decision processes, insomnia, tremors, and profound ataxia from cerebellar degeneration.

Cardiac abnormalities include development of alcohol-related cardiomyopathy, electrolyte disturbances resulting in arrhythmias (from profound hypokalemia and hypomagnesemia), or elevated risk for cardiovascular disease including hypertension, hypertriglyceridemia, and myocardial infarction.

Gastrointestinal disturbances may include gastric or duodenal ulcers, alcoholic hepatitis, cirrhosis, fulminant liver failure leading to death, coagulopathies, pancreatitis, esophagitis, esophageal varices, as well as esophageal, pancreatic, and liver cancers. Risk of re-feeding syndrome due to malnutrition (which may also be suggested by hypomagnesemia, hypokalemia, and hypophosphatemia) must be considered.

Bone marrow suppression or hypersplenism from cirrhosis may be prominent in these patients, and caution should be taken to evaluate for thrombocytopenia prior to performing any procedures. By the same token, if there is concern for infectious process, consideration should be made to provide broad spectrum coverage with antibiotics.

Changes in hormonal balance may also occur, and males may suffer from low testosterone, gynecomastia, and erectile dysfunction. Females may suffer from irregular menses, spontaneous abortions, and births of infants with risk of fetal alcohol syndrome, if alcohol use is continued during pregnancy.

Alcohol-Related Seizures

Some studies have proposed that ARS are more common in patients that have been repeatedly detoxified from alcohol, as opposed to chronic abusers with abrupt cessation. Postulation of increased rate of withdrawal seizures in repeatedly detoxified patient relies on the kindling model of seizure activity in alcoholic individuals [19]. Individuals who imbibe greater than 50 g of ethanol daily are at higher risk of developing alcohol withdrawal seizures [15]. Patients with history of repeated binge drinking are at less of a risk of developing ARS than the above two groups, unless they have a history of previous post-traumatic epilepsy or idiopathic epilepsy, which may make even moderate amounts of alcohol intoxication lower the seizure threshold, and may increase the ability for these patients to seize.

Previous reviews have identified clinical predictors of those more likely to suffer from severe alcohol withdrawal syndrome and ARS. These include having had previous documented episodes of delirium tremens; previous documented ARS; higher ALT on admission (clinical predictor of severe alcohol withdrawal), higher γ-GT (clinical predictor for ARS), hypokalemia, and or thrombocytopenia on admission [11]. ARS usually precede delirium tremens. Seizures after the 5–7 day post-withdrawal period should be investigated for alternative comorbidities, including intracranial pathology, infection, hypoxemia, metabolic disturbance (electrolyte or blood glucose), or drugs which may decrease the threshold for seizures.

Most ARS are of generalized onset (80%), and manifest as generalized tonic-clonic seizures, with some studies reporting partial onset seizures in 8.3–22%. Some of these patients may have overlapping underlying localization related epilepsy, idiopathic generalized epilepsy, or post-traumatic epilepsy. MRI brain with and without gadolinium and with epilepsy protocol should be obtained on patients with any focality found on the clinical examination or the EEG to help differentiate whether there is an underlying organic pathology, which may have been exacerbated by alcohol withdrawal [20–27].

Rarely, ARS progresses into status epilepticus. Patients should be placed on continuous EEG monitoring, and consideration should be made for airway protection with intubation if seizures persist. Evaluation for underlying pathology (infectious or intracranial pathology) via imaging and CSF analysis should be obtained. Rare cases of non-convulsive status epilepticus (NCSE) have also been reported. If obtundation persists despite normalization of BAL and correction of toxometabolic abnormalities, consideration for NCSE should be made. Continuous EEG should be initiated and AED treatment administered if findings are indicative of seizure activity.

A proposed condition of subacute encephalopathy with seizures in alcoholics (SESA) has been recognized in rare cases, and has been proposed as a new subset of NCSE. Less than ten cases have been reported. First described in the 1980s, case reports describe chronic alcoholics presenting with confusion, persistent encephalopathy despite toxometabolic workup, intermittent unilateral weakness or jerking (in some cases) and presence of persistent ictal activity on EEG, or presence of periodic lateralized epileptiform discharges (PLEDS). SESA has been postulated as a variant of NSCE which has gone unrecognized in the alcohol population thought of to have had a single seizure with prolonged post-ictal state (which may have been NCSE, just not recorded on EEG). MRI findings may demonstrate T2 hyperintensities on FLAIR, and DWI changes which may resolve. It has been postulated that the pathophysiology of SESA is similar to that of PRES, as FLAIR and DWI changes have been shown to resolve in some case reports, with resolution of ictal activity. While only a few cases have been reported; if this indeed is responsible for the suspected "prolonged post ictal state" found in many alcoholics with seizures, SESA NCSE may responsible for a larger number of cases of unexplained prolonged encephalopathy than previously thought.

Electrographic Findings on EEG Monitoring of Patients with Alcohol Abuse and or Alcohol-Related Seizures

EEG in abstinent individuals with a history of alcohol use is generally normal. In chronic habitual alcohol users there may be more prominent amounts of theta (slower) and beta (faster) activity, which may overall be of lower voltage. The prominence and amplitude of alpha range activity may be reduced. It has been proposed that increased beta activity may also be related to administration of benzodiazepines in the withdrawing patient [22]. Additionally, non-focal slowing may also occur in early abstinence [22, 24, 28, 29].

In the subgroup analysis of known epileptic patients versus patients with known ARS by Sand et al., quantitative EEG analysis of both groups post-seizure demonstrated a statistically significant lower amount of slow wave (delta) activity in the alcohol-related seizures group, as compared to EEG delta wave activity post-seizure in the known epileptic group. Reduced alpha amplitudes on quantitative EEG also supported a clinical diagnosis of ARS [22].

In comparing occipital photic driving response to 18 Hz and 24 Hz stimulation, Sand et al. also found a statistically significant variation in response in alcoholics who presented with ARS as compared to epileptic or control patients. A diminished photic driving response was witnessed in patients with known ARS. There was also significant correlation between high AUDIT scores, and severity of alcohol abuse, and diminished response to 24 Hz photic stimulation.

The authors proposed that this may be used as a marker of alcohol abuse severity [30].

In a study by Coutin-Churchman et al., 191 male alcoholics, with average ethanol consumption of 100 g daily, were admitted for detoxification and had electroencephalography performed at least 1 week post-admittance/alcohol abstention. Only 7 out of 191 patients had no abnormality on EEG. 42.4% showed decreased delta–theta power and increased beta power, 17.3% showed only decreased delta–theta power, 15.2% had only increased beta power, 14.7% had decreased delta–theta–alpha power, and the remaining abnormal EEGs demonstrated combinations of the above. [23]

Valladeres et al. demonstrated that delta slow wave sleep is attenuated in patients with alcohol dependence, along with decrease in vagal tone and sympathetic hyperactivity as compared to controls abstinent to alcohol [31].

EEG in patients admitted for alcohol withdrawal, but with seizures from alternative etiologies may reveal electroencephalographic changes that may potentially reflect an underlying organic pathology which may be contributing to the current event. Focal slow waves may be seen in areas of cortical damage, and sharp and spike waves may be visualized in areas of cortical irritability. Generalized spike wave patterns may be seen in patients with primary generalized epilepsy, or focal spike wave patterns may be seen in patients with localization related epilepsy. EEG findings of sharply contoured waves with triphasic morphology may be indicative of an underlying toxometabolic pathology, which may be contributing to a patient's unresponsive state.

Alcohol-related seizures may infrequently reveal an underlying diagnosis of idiopathic generalized epilepsy (IGE), which may have an underlying genetic component, or post-traumatic epilepsy which may have been triggered by alcohol use, particularly in young adults. These underlying diagnoses must be considered in the differential diagnosis of new onset seizures in the patient with alcohol abuse. Less than 1% of patients who seize within 6 h of alcohol use, but present with no symptoms of alcohol withdrawal, were noted to have idiopathic generalized epilepsy (IGE) in one study and were found to have electrographic patterns on EEG, indicative of such. These patients had lower mean alcohol intake, and had lower alcohol use disorders identification test (AUDIT) scores than patients with ARS [20]. This underscores the importance of a precise clinical history obtained either from the patient, family, or from other medical documentation, as patients with underlying epilepsy may require long term antiepileptic drug therapy.

Therefore, one should not forget that treatment of seizures related to these conditions is ultimately reliant on addressing the underlying disease process, and associated alcohol-related seizures may be treated first by standard ICU protocol for management of seizures or status epilepticus, rather than simple measures against the latter.

Medications Used in the Treatment of Alcohol-Related Seizures

Benzodiazepines

Treatment of ARS should begin with benzodiazepines (BZD) as first line agents. These are most often already in use to treat withdrawal symptoms, and can be utilized in either oral or IV scheduled and triggered formulations. BZD are GABA-ergic and cross tolerant with alcohol, and not only play a role in membrane stabilization, but also additionally function efficaciously in controlling withdrawal symptoms, including agitation, tachycardia, anxiety, and progression to full delirium tremens.

Choice or availability of BZD may be institution dependent. Consideration should be made in drug choice with multiple variables in mind, including age of the patient, metabolic clearance, and respiratory function. Shorter acting agents, such as midazolam or lorazepam, should be considered in the elderly; otherwise agents such as diazepam and chlordiazepoxide may be considered, as the longer half-life of diazepam and chlordiazepoxide may allow for a smoother detoxification process [5, 8, 32]. Patients who have significant hepatic dysfunction should avoid diazepam or chlordiazepoxide, as these are mainly hepatically metabolized. Length of therapy may be dependent on recurrence of seizure activity and or withdrawal symptoms. Traditionally symptom and seizure triggered therapy is initiated, and then maintenance therapy is utilized, with additional seizure or withdrawal triggered therapy available on an as needed basis. In the ICU setting, midazolam is commonly used as a first line infusion choice, and oral lorazepam may be added on a scheduled basis. Lorazepam infusions are generally avoided due to risk of propylene glycol toxicity associated with prolonged infusions. Monitoring of respiratory function is imperative in nonintubated and mechanically ventilated patients. Previously, clobazam has also been used as an adjunct agent to deal with withdrawal symptoms, however, it also may be effective in seizure control. As this medication must be titrated slowly, it may not be an optimal first line choice in the ICU setting for control of ARS. It also has not been clearly studied as an agent to control ARS).

Propofol

Escalation of therapy should be considered if the patient continues to convulse, using either propofol or barbiturates. Propofol is a short acting, lipid-soluble, IV infusion, administered in the ICU setting on mechanically ventilated patients. In BZD-refractory seizures, propofol may be added with success, based on the notion that GABA receptor saturation may occur, and the additional inhibitory effects on the NMDA subtype of glutamate receptors may be responsible for controlling both seizures and withdrawal symptoms [9, 15, 21, 33–36].

Risk of propofol infusion syndrome [37] may occur with prolonged infusions or high rates of infusion. Serial creatine phosphokinase, triglyceride levels, and liver function panels should be obtained. Enteral nutrition may also need to be reduced on the intubated patient receiving tube feeds, as the propofol infusion is similar in composition to a 10% parenteral lipid emulsion, which provides 1.1 kcals/mL as fat.

Barbiturates

If patient does not respond to BZDs and continues exhibiting ARS, escalation to phenobarbital administration is a reasonable option, as a synergistic effect of the drug to BZD is believed to exist. Loading doses of 15–20 mg/kg IV x1 may be utilized, followed with maintenance dosing of 1–3 mg/kg total daily dosing administered IV or PO in divided doses ever 8 or 12 h, 12 h after administration of the phenobarbital loading dose. Care should be taken in administration of phenobarbital in the elderly population due to significant sedative effects and longer half-life.

Carbamazepine

Carbamazepine has been successful in the treatment of ARS due to its agonistic GABA-ergic and antagonistic NMDA receptor effects. It has been reported to be more effective than placebo, and at least as effective as BZD in treatment of ARS. Doses should start at 600–800 mg/day in divided doses, which should be tapered to 200 mg daily by days 5–7. A disadvantage is that there is so far no IV formulation in the USA, therefore enteric administration may lead to erratic absorption in ICU patients. Care should be taken to monitor for hyponatremia and agranulocytosis [3, 38, 39].

Valproic Acid

Commonly used in doses from 500 mg every 8–12 hours, valproic acid is a GABA-ergic antiepileptic, which may also have antagonistic properties against NMDA receptors. Valproic acid has been proven to be successful in control of ARS, as well as alcohol withdrawal symptoms, and mood stabilization. Careful monitoring of liver function tests, complete blood counts, and ammonia levels is required in the ICU. As it is hepatically metabolized and may interact with several other ICU medications through inhibition of cytochrome P-450, valproic acid may not be the drug of choice in patients with preexisting hepatic dysfunction [3].

Topiramate

Topiramate works on multiple receptors. It has $GABA_A$-ergic effects and is antagonistic at the AMPA and kainate glutamate receptors. This inherently leads to reduced dopamine release in the nucleus accumbens, and via effects on multiple other receptors may contribute in reduction of autonomic hyperactivity and alcohol withdrawal symptoms, in addition to quelling ARS. Use of 50 mg daily or 50 mg twice per day has been demonstrated to reduce incidence of ARS. Like carbamazepine, there is no IV topiramate formulation [3, 38].

Pregabalin

In mouse models, pregabalin has been found to work effectively in prevention of ARS. Pregabalin binds to the alpha-2-delta subunit of voltage gated calcium channels, which inhibits activity dependent calcium influx in nerve terminals, thus reducing release of glutamate, norepinephrine, and Substance P. It has anticonvulsant, anxiolytic, and analgesic properties. It does not bind to plasma proteins, and is excreted in the urine, which may prove to be a viable alternative to hepatically metabolized medications. In rat models of alcohol withdrawal, it has been shown to reduce alcohol withdrawal seizures on EEG, as well as reduce alcohol withdrawal symptoms [28].

Gabapentin

Gabapentin has been showed to have modest effects of alcohol withdrawal symptoms and minimal effect on ARS. There have been no studies showing usefulness of gabapentin as first line agent in ARS, but it may be used as an adjunct agent. It has been speculated that dose titration, and the fact that one must titrate from low doses due to sedative effects, may be part of the reason as to the lower response rates of ARS to gabapentin as first line therapy [3].

Treatment of Alcohol Withdrawal and Related Agitation and Delirium

Benzodiazepines have long been a mainstay in alcohol withdrawal treatment as well as in the treatment of ARS. They may be used in oral, intravenous, or intramuscular injection forms. If patients are actively being detoxified, a 7 day course of BZD should be pursued, with oversight by a physician or other skilled provider, due to abuse potential [40]. Treatment paradigms for management of alcohol withdrawal patients vary significantly in the literature, which reflects variability in institution policies [3, 6, 8–10, 14, 15, 17, 41–45].

Most institutions rely on symptom-triggered scales like CIWA-Ar, or derivatives of this, however, this scale has not been validated in the critical care setting where most patients are intubated, and likely sedated. While most retrospective studies have evaluated use of continuous as well as intermittent BZD administration for symptom control in intubated patients, one observational study of 188 patients by Stewart et al. used high dose BZD in alcohol withdrawal patients, who were not intubated, unless they developed signs of aspiration or significant cardiopulmonary depression. They found that there was no significant increase in morbidity or mortality associated with not intubating these patients. They did, however, demonstrate a statistically significant increase in length of hospitalization in intubated versus non-intubated patients (15 days vs 6 days, respectively) [14].

In the ICU setting, concurrent use of dexmedetomidine has been shown to be a very successful treatment in maintaining control of agitation and delirium in the critically ill, alcohol withdrawing patient, without the additive risk of significant respiratory depression. Dexmedetomidine is a selective $\alpha2$-agonist, which acts in the locus ceruleus and spinal cord. It may be utilized in a continuous IV formulation as an adjunct therapy to BZD in patients not able to tolerate oral medications or patients who are intubated [1, 40, 46]. Dexmedetomidine provides reduction in severity of symptoms of autonomic hyperactivity, but does not cause respiratory depression or profound sedation that BZD may exhibit at higher doses. It may, however, cause as side effects bradycardia and hypotension, and patients receiving this medication need to be monitored in a telemetry unit [46].

A retrospective controlled cohort study by VanderWeide et al. showed that use of dexmedetomidine in critically ill patients withdrawing from alcohol may decrease BZD usage in dexmedetomidine versus control groups to a statistically significant amount at 12 h (on the average minus 20 mg of BZD use in the dexmedetomidine group compared to minus 8.3 mg BZD use in the control group) and with a trend towards benefit in reduction of BZD usage at 24 h (average minus 29.7 mg BZD use in dexmedetomidine group compared to minus 11 mg BZD use in the control group) at 24 h. There were no statistically significant differences in either group in length of ICU stay, hospital stay or length of mechanical intubation [1].

As well as for control of ARS, propofol has also been used for control of alcohol withdrawal. A retrospective review by Sorhaby et al. showed that use of BZD infusions versus propofol infusions for control of alcohol withdrawal syndrome showed no difference in intubated days, length of stay, length of ICU stay, or days of mechanical ventilation. However, patients utilizing BZD infusions required a significantly larger number of BZD symptom-triggered IV boluses of medication as compared to the propofol infusion group [44].

Use of typical and atypical antipsychotics, such as haloperidol, quetiapine, and risperidone in low doses, has been shown to control agitation, confusion, and hallucinations, which may occur in the acute and subacute state in the ICU. Care must be checked to evaluate for QTc prolongation, and these drugs should not be administered in these patients due to the risk for torsades de pointes. Generally, once the patient leaves the ICU setting, these medications can be tapered or eliminated completely.

Conclusion

Treatment for alcohol withdrawal syndrome and ARS is still broadly undefined due to the limitations in current clinical research. Most data are retrospective, and most studies have confounding variables, as alcoholic patients commonly have multiple medical problems affecting the risk for seizures in multiple ways. Clinical history is of utmost importance in order to help delineate timeline and causation of ARS or alcohol withdrawal symptoms and expedite appropriate therapy.

References

1. VanderWeide LA, Foster CJ, MacLaren R, Kiser TH, Fish DN, Mueller SW. Evaluation of early dexmedetomidine addition to the standard of care for severe alcohol withdrawal in the icu: a retrospective controlled Cohort study. J Intensive Care Med. 2016;31(3):198–204.
2. American Psychiatric Association Publishing. Substance-related and addictive disorders. In:Diagnostic and statistical manual of mental disorders. 5th ed: American Psychiatric Association Publishing; 2013.
3. Mirijello A, D'Angelo C, Ferrulli A, et al. Identification and management of alcohol withdrawal syndrome. Drugs. 2015;75(4): 353–65.
4. Welch KA. Neurological complications of alcohol and misuse of drugs. Pract Neurol. 2011;11(4):206–19.
5. Sutton LJ, Jutel A. Alcohol withdrawal syndrome in critically ill patients: identification, assessment, and management. Crit Care Nurse. 2016;36(1):28–38.
6. Mehta AJ. Alcoholism and critical illness: A review. World J Crit Care Med. 2016;5(1):27–35.
7. Burnett EJ, Chandler LJ, Trantham-Davidson H. Glutamatergic plasticity and alcohol dependence-induced alterations in reward, affect and cognition. Prog Neuro-Psychopharmacol Biol Psychiatry. 2016;65:309–20.
8. Sachdeva A, Choudhary M, Chandra M. Alcohol Withdrawal Syndrome: Benzodiazepines and Beyond. J Clin Diagn Res. 2015;9(9):VE01–7.
9. Kim DW, Kim HK, Bae EK, Park SH, Kim KK. Clinical predictors for delirium tremens in patients with alcohol withdrawal seizures. Am J Emerg Med. 2015;33(5):701–4.
10. Schuckit MA. Recognition and management of withdrawal delirium (delirium tremens). N Engl J Med. 2014;371(22):2109–13.
11. Goodson CM, Clark BJ, Douglas IS. Predictors of severe alcohol withdrawal syndrome: a systematic review and meta-analysis. Alcohol Clin Exp Res. 2014;38(10):2664–77.
12. Maldonado JR, Sher Y, Das S, et al. Prospective validation study of the prediction of alcohol withdrawal severity scale (PAWSS) in medically ill inpatients: a new scale for the prediction of complicated alcohol withdrawal syndrome. Alcohol. 2015;50(5):509–18.
13. Yousuf T, Brinton T, Kramer J, et al. Correlation between partial pressure of arterial carbon dioxide and end tidal carbon dioxide in patients with severe alcohol withdrawal. Ochsner J. 2015;15(4):418–22.
14. Stewart R, Perez R, Musial B, Lukens C, Adjepong YA, Manthous CA. Outcomes of patients with alcohol withdrawal syndrome treated with high-dose sedatives and deferred intubation. Ann Am Thorac Soc. 2016;13(2):248–52.
15. Visée H. The relationship between alcohol and seizures: an overview of the major data. Int J Neurorehabilitation. 2015;2(1):1000141.
16. Rao PS, Bell RL, Engleman EA, Sari Y. Targeting glutamate uptake to treat alcohol use disorders. Front Neurosci. 2015;9:144.
17. Wong A, Benedict NJ, Armahizer MJ, Kane-Gill SL. Evaluation of adjunctive ketamine to benzodiazepines for management of alcohol withdrawal syndrome. Ann Pharmacother. 2015;49(1):14–9.
18. Morozova TV, Mackay TF, Anholt RR. Genetics and genomics of alcohol sensitivity. Mol Gen Genomics. 2014;289(3):253–69.
19. Lechtenberg R, Worner TM. Seizure risk with recurrent alcohol detoxification. Arch Neurol. 1990;47(5):535–8.
20. Sandeep P, Cherian A, Iype T, Chitra P, Suresh MK, Ajitha KC. Clinical profile of patients with nascent alcohol related seizures. Ann Indian Acad Neurol. 2013;16(4):530–3.
21. LaRoche SM, Shivdat-Nanhoe R. Subacute encephalopathy and seizures in alcoholics (SESA) presenting with non-convulsive status epilepticus. Seizure. 2011;20(6):505–8.
22. Sand T, Bjork M, Brathen G, Michler RP, Brodtkorb E, Bovim G. Quantitative EEG in patients with alcohol-related seizures. Alcohol Clin Exp Res. 2010;34(10):1751–8.
23. Coutin-Churchman P, Moreno R, Anez Y, Vergara F. Clinical correlates of quantitative EEG alterations in alcoholic patients. Clin Neurophysiol. 2006;117(4):740–51.
24. Sand T, Brathen G, Michler R, Brodtkorb E, Helde G, Bovim G. Clinical utility of EEG in alcohol-related seizures. Acta Neurol Scand. 2002;105(1):18–24.
25. Stratone A, Topoliceanu F, Driga O, et al. EEG patterns in alcohol withdrawal syndrome. Rev Med Chir Soc Med Nat Iasi. 2000;104(4):71–4.
26. Alldredge BK, Lowenstein DH. Status epilepticus related to alcohol abuse. Epilepsia. 1993;34(6):1033–7.
27. Krauss GL, Niedermeyer E. Electroencephalogram and seizures in chronic alcoholism. Electroencephalogr Clin Neurophysiol. 1991;78(2):97–104.
28. Becker HC, Myrick H, Veatch LM. Pregabalin is effective against behavioral and electrographic seizures during alcohol withdrawal. Alcohol Alcohol. 2006;41(4):399–406.
29. Veatch LM, Becker HC. Electrographic and behavioral indices of ethanol withdrawal sensitization. Brain Res. 2002;946(2):272–82.
30. Sand T, Bjork M, Brathen G, Brodtkorb E, Michler RP, Bovim G. The EEG response to photic stimulation is not increased in alcohol-related seizures. Clin Neurophysiol. 2010;121(11):1810–5.
31. Valladares EM, Eljammal SM, Iyer AV, Irwin MR. EEG and vagal tone degradation during nocturnal sleep in abstinent alcohol dependence. Sleep Med. 2007;8(3):284–5.
32. Rathlev NK, Ulrich AS, Delanty N, D'Onofrio G. Alcohol-related seizures. J Emerg Med. 2006;31(2):157–63.
33. Riegle MA, Masicampo ML, Shan HQ, Xu V, Godwin DW. Ethosuximide reduces mortality and seizure severity in response to pentylenetetrazole treatment during ethanol withdrawal. Alcohol Alcohol. 2015;50(5):501–8.
34. Riegle MA, Masicampo ML, Caulder EH, Godwin DW. Ethosuximide reduces electrographical and behavioral correlates of alcohol withdrawal seizure in DBA/2 J mice. Alcohol. 2014;48(5): 445–53.

35. McMicken D, Liss JL. Alcohol-related seizures. Emerg Med Clin North Am. 2011;29(1):117–24.

36. Orser BA, Bertlik M, Wang LY, MacDonald JF. Inhibition by propofol (2,6 di-isopropylphenol) of the N-methyl-D-aspartate subtype of glutamate receptor in cultured hippocampal neurones. Br J Pharmacol. 1995;116(2):1761–8.

37. Smith H, Sinson G, Varelas P. Vasopressors and propofol infusion syndrome in severe head trauma. Neurocrit Care. 2009;10(2): 166–72.

38. Minozzi S, Amato L, Vecchi S, Davoli M. Anticonvulsants for alcohol withdrawal. Cochrane Database Syst Rev. 2010;3:CD005064.

39. Perry EC. Inpatient management of acute alcohol withdrawal syndrome. CNS Drugs. 2014;28(5):401–10.

40. Pandharipande PP, Pun BT, Herr DL, et al. Effect of sedation with dexmedetomidine vs lorazepam on acute brain dysfunction in mechanically ventilated patients: the MENDS randomized controlled trial. JAMA. 2007;298(22):2644–53.

41. Wong A, Benedict NJ, Kane-Gill SL. Multicenter evaluation of pharmacologic management and outcomes associated with severe resistant alcohol withdrawal. J Crit Care. 2015;30(2):405–9.

42. Linn DD, Loeser KC. Dexmedetomidine for alcohol withdrawal syndrome. Ann Pharmacother. 2015;49(12):1336–42.

43. Feeney C, Alter HJ, Jacobsen E, et al. A simplified protocol for the treatment of alcohol withdrawal. J Addict Med. 2015;9(6):485–90.

44. Sohraby R, Attridge RL, Hughes DW. Use of propofol-containing versus benzodiazepine regimens for alcohol withdrawal requiring mechanical ventilation. Ann Pharmacother. 2014;48(4):456–61.

45. Skinner RT. Symptom-triggered vs. fixed-dosing management of alcohol withdrawal syndrome. Medsurg Nurs. 2014;23(5):307–15.

46. MacLaren R, Preslaski CR, Mueller SW, et al. A randomized, double-blind pilot study of dexmedetomidine versus midazolam for intensive care unit sedation: patient recall of their experiences and short-term psychological outcomes. J Intensive Care Med. 2015;30(3):167–75.

Drug-Induced Seizures in Critically Ill Patients

Denise H. Rhoney and Greene Shepherd

Introduction

Detection and prevention of drug related problems during hospitalization are a focus area for many clinicians. Adverse drug events, many of which are preventable, account for greater than 100,000 deaths annually in hospitalized patients [1]. In addition it is estimated that adverse drug events extend the hospital length of stay by 2 days subsequently resulting in increased costs ranging from $2500 to $5500 per patient [2–4]. The intensive care unit has the highest incidence of adverse drug events and the greatest severity risk compared to other areas of the hospital [4, 5]. Drug-induced seizures represent a potentially serious adverse drug event. Critically ill patients with and without neurologic disease may develop seizures during their hospitalization. Bleck et al. [6] reported that over a 2-year observation period of patients without neurologic problems admitted to large university medical center intensive care units (ICU), 12.3% experienced neurologic complications during their stay. Of the patients who developed these complications, 28% experienced seizures. Importantly patients who developed these neurologic complications demonstrated increased risk of in-hospital mortality and experienced two-fold longer lengths of stay compared to those patients who did not develop these complications [6]. Many complications may arise as a result of drug related seizures including hypoxemia, shock, hyperthermia, rhabdomyolysis, metabolic acidosis, status epilepticus, respiratory failure, and other drug specific complications. Assessment of complications of patients presenting to the emergency department (ED) with drug-induced seizure shows that this complication rate is relatively high (60%) with three factors predicting these complications (hyperglycemia, stimulant exposure, initial acidosis) [7]. Therefore it is essential that all clinicians have increased vigilance towards recognition of iatrogenic seizures and associated causes.

Epidemiology

The true incidence of drug-induced seizures is currently unknown. The Food and Drug Administration relies upon voluntary reporting of adverse drug events, including drug related seizures, which impacts the ability to acquire true estimates. Additionally many patients are receiving polypharmacy complicating the ability to make an accurate association to the offending agent. Therefore most of the information that is available is based upon data from experimental studies and case reports/case series.

The Drug Abuse Warning Network (DAWN) estimated that of the total 108 million ED visits in 2005, 14% of visits were a result of drug misuse and abuse (31% illicit drugs and 27% prescription drugs) [8]. Seizures appear to be a rare effect associated with drug administration although the DAWN estimates do not report data on specific complications such as seizures. The Boston Collaborative Drug Surveillance Program evaluated over 32,000 inpatient records and found that drug related seizures occurred in 0.08% of the group [9]. More recent studies have estimated that 6.1–9% of new-onset seizures and status epilepticus is drug related [10, 11]. Thundiyil et al. [12] assessed 386 cases drug related seizures reported to a poison control center and found the leading causes of seizures to be bupropion (23%), diphenhydramine (8.3%), tricyclic antidepressants (7.7%), tramadol (7.5%), amphetamines (6.9%), isoniazid (5.9%), and venlafaxine (5.9%). In the majority of these patients (68.6%) only one seizure was reported while 3.6% experi-

D.H. Rhoney (✉)
Division of Practice Advancement and Clinical Education, UNC Eshelman School of Pharmacy, 115 Beard Hall, Campus Box 7574, Chapel Hill, NC 27599-7574, USA
e-mail: drhoney@unc.edu

G. Shepherd
Division of Practice Advancement and Clinical Education, UNC Eshelman School of Pharmacy, One University Heights, CPO 2125, Asheville, NC 28804, USA
e-mail: greene_shepherd@unc.edu

© Springer International Publishing AG 2017
P.N. Varelas, J. Claassen (eds.), *Seizures in Critical Care*, Current Clinical Neurology, DOI 10.1007/978-3-319-49557-6_20

enced status epilepticus as a result. When compared to data published 10 years prior, there was a statistically significant increase in newer antidepressant related seizures (bupropion and venlafaxine), but a decrease in tricyclic antidepressant (TCA) and cocaine-associated seizures [13]. Other older reports in hospitalized patients found the most common drugs associated with seizures were penicillins, isoniazid, insulin, lidocaine, and psychotropic agents (including tricyclic antidepressants and antipsychotics) [9, 14]. Wijdicks and Sharbrough [15] found that 15% of their cohort of new-onset seizures in the ICU was related to drug toxicity (antibiotics and antiarrhythmics). Drug-induced seizures are associated with poor outcome and increased risk of aspiration pneumonitis [16] along with 15% of drug-associated seizures presenting as status epilepticus [14]. Recently Finkelstein et al. [17] found about 5% of pediatric patients presenting to ED for medical toxicology consult had a drug-induced seizure. The majority were teenagers in whom the ingestion was intentional with antidepressants (bupropion being most common). The second most common drug class leading to pediatric seizures was over-the-counter anticholinergics/antihistamines [17].

Risk Factors

Patients with a pre-existing seizure disorder have an increased propensity to develop seizures during critical illness; however, all critically ill patients have the ability to experience seizures while hospitalized. Outside of neurological causes, other risk factors that may lower seizure threshold in critically ill patients include electrolyte imbalance, medications, medication withdrawal, medication overdose, organ failure, extremes of ages (elderly and infants), glucose abnormalities, infections, alterations in volume of distribution due to post-operative fluid shifts or dialysis/continuous veno-venous hemofiltration, and ischemic-hypoxic encephalopathy [18]. Many medications used routinely in critically ill patients have been associated with drug-induced seizures at both therapeutic and toxic concentrations [19, 20]. Patients with critical illness have several factors that may increase their vulnerability to drug-induced seizures including altered pharmacokinetics especially reduced drug elimination due to end organ damage and the use of multiple drug regimens that could result in drug interactions. Most drug-induced seizures are concentration dependent, therefore anything that could result in increased central nervous system (CNS) concentrations of the drug would place the patient at risk. There are a wide spectrum of drug related risk factors for induction of seizures including the intrinsic epileptogenicity of the agent, factors that increase serum concentrations (dose, route schedule, route of elimination, drug interactions) and factors enhancing CNS concentrations (alterations in blood-brain-barrier permeability, lipid

solubility, molecular weight, ionization, protein binding, transport by endogenous systems) [21]. Due to the complex nature of medication regimens in critically ill patients, drug interactions, especially with the cytochrome P450 (CYP450) drug metabolizing enzymes, may represent a significant risk for patients in the ICU. The CYP3A4 isoenzyme subfamily accounts for metabolism of approximately 60% of all drugs used today. In addition there are patient-related risk factors including the presence of a seizure disorder, neurologic abnormality, reduced drug elimination, and conditions that disrupt the blood-brain barrier [21].

The contribution of genetics to variability in drug metabolism is now well recognized and will determine drug exposure in individuals. Approximately 60% of adverse effects are believed to be associated with drugs metabolized by polymorphic phase 1 drug metabolizing enzyme [22]. Four major metabolic phenotypes have been characterized; poor metabolizer (PM), intermediate metabolizer (IM), extensive metabolizer (EM), and ultrarapid metabolizer (UM). PM that either have no or reduced enzyme activity would be predicted to accumulate high drug concentrations due to decreased metabolism [23]. While drug-induced seizure activity has not been directly attributed to pharmacogenomics, it is important to consider this as an important risk factor. For example, in recent years there have been several reports of near fatal outcomes associated with opioids due to CYP2D6 genotypes [24, 25]. Please refer to other more extensive publications on pharmacogenomic alterations as a cause of adverse drug reactions [23, 26, 27].

When clinicians suspect a drug related seizure in patients who are critically ill there are important questions that should be evaluated:

Is there a temporal relationship between the initiation of the drug or dosage titration and seizure?
What was the dose prescribed compared to recommended doses?
Was the dose appropriately adjusted for organ function?
Was there an administration error?
Are there any possible drug interactions?
Does the patient have any other possible cause of a seizure like electrolyte disturbance?

Prevention

The best treatment for drug-induced seizures is prevention. Increased awareness and monitoring will often identify potential problems before they occur. General principles of drug use, particularly those that have been associated with an increased seizure risk, should be to use the minimally effective dose, avoid polypharmacy, and avoid abrupt discontinuation. To assist in prevention the clinician should consider the following points especially in patients who are considered to be at increased risk for seizures, as described previously:

What is the patient age? Is there a need to adjust the dose or use smaller doses?
Is there a need for the prescribed agent?
Is there an alternative agent that may have lower potential for seizures?
Are you using the smallest, effective dose?
Is there a need to taper an agent to avoid withdrawal?
What is the appropriate titration schedule?
Is there a possibility of drug interactions with the medication regimen?

Causative Agents

There have been many agents that critically ill patients are exposed to that have been reported to cause seizures. Table 20.1 contains a list of these agents along with possible mechanisms for the seizure in addition to a previously published mnemonic [28] (Otis Campbell – the town drunk from the Andy Griffith show) that has to be adapted to apply more specifically to critically ill patients. Overall the primary mechanism by which drugs induce seizures is related to some interference with neurotransmitters in the CNS. In most instances, drugs with epileptogenic potential have a dose-related risk. However, as denoted in the table, some agents may have a seizure inducing risk even at therapeutic concentrations. Since most seizures are dose-related the importance of optimized drug dosing in critically ill patients becomes essential, especially given the potential for significant pharmacokinetic alterations due to drug interactions, pharmacogenomics, protein binding alterations, CNS uptake, and dynamic alterations in drug clearance Overall, there is a lack of high-quality clinical data assessing seizure risk and most of these associations are based upon case-reports or small case series data.

Analgesics

Opioids

In animals opioids are associated with electroencephalogram (EEG) proven seizure activity; however, the dose required to replicate this in the clinical setting is far greater that what is administered with either analgesia or anesthesia. On the other hand, focal neuroexcitation on the EEG occasionally occurs in humans after large doses of fentanyl, alfentanil, sufentanil, and remifentanil [29–32]. In animal studies midazolam, naloxone, and phenytoin have been shown to prevent seizure activity on the EEG where seizure activity was induced by large doses of fentanyl [33]. All strong mu agonists can cause

myoclonus after an IV bolus with some of the more rapid-onset agents more likely the culprits [34]. However, the relationship between myoclonus or rigidity, subcortical seizure activity and cortical seizures is unclear. The postulated neuronal mechanisms of seizure induction include opioid induced disinhibition of GABAergic interneurons and inhibition of hyperpolarization-activated potassium currents [35, 36]. It is important to note that epidural and intrathecal administration of opioids has also been linked to seizure activity [37–39]. The most common reason for seizures due to opioids is linked to opioid withdrawal and use of agents with a higher risk for causing seizures (meperidine and tramadol).

Meperidine is metabolized via N-demethylation to an active metabolite normeperidine, which is then renally excreted. Accumulation of this metabolite is associated with seizure activity and patients with renal impairment or receiving large doses are at risk [40, 41]. Oral administration of meperidine will result in increased concentrations of normeperidine due to extensive first-pass metabolism, thus having increased risk for seizures at therapeutic dosing [42]. The elimination half-life is approximately five times as long as the parent compound (3–6 h versus 15–40 h), thus the toxic metabolite can quickly accumulate. Typically normeperidine toxicity develops at concentrations greater than 0.8 mg/dL. EEG changes associated with normeperidine include slow wave activity and epileptiform discharges that will resolve once normeperidine is eliminated [43]. Normeperidine induced seizures often begin after the onset of other clinical sequelae such as delirium, tremors, or myoclonus. Seizures that develop are usually generalized tonic-clonic. Naloxone does not reverse the toxicity and could exacerbate the seizure activity. Treatment includes supportive measures and withdrawal of meperidine. Treatment with traditional antiepileptic drugs (AEDs) should be avoided as they have been shown to accelerate the conversion of meperidine to normeperidine potentially worsening the seizures [44]. Return to baseline neurologic functioning is dependent upon removal of the parent compound and the toxic metabolite so it would not be anticipated until a few days after meperidine discontinuation.

Morphine can induce seizures at high doses in neonates with immature blood-brain barriers but has never been shown to be associated with seizures in adults [45]. There have been some reports of seizure activity with fentanyl, alfentanil, and sufentanil [46–50], which have not been confirmed with EEG findings of seizure activity [51, 52]. Surface EEG recordings are characterized by high-voltage slow delta waves following administration of these agents [44]. It has been postulated that the tonic-clonic movements originally reported is somatic muscle rigidity or subcortical seizure activity and not true seizure activity.

Tramadol is a weak mu-receptor agonist with other pharmacological properties including inhibition of serotonin and norepinephrine reuptake. Tramadol has been reported to cause

Table 20.1 Drug related seizures in critically ill patients and associated mechanisms

Agent	Proposed mechanism
High risk agents	
Antipsychotics[a]	D1 agonists and D2 antagonists are proconvulsant. Antagonism of α_1-receptors, agonism of α_2-receptors, and inhibition of histamine-1 receptors may promote seizure activity
Flumazenil[a]	Not a direct effect of the drug rather the resultant effects of benzodiazepine reversal
Meperidine[a]	Mediated through normeperidine, a toxic metabolite that is proconvulsant
Theophylline[b]	Lowers seizure threshold by elevating cyclic GMP levels in brain and antagonizes the depressant effects of adenosine on cerebral cortex (other actions include pyridoxine depletion and inhibition of GABA)
Penicillins[b]	GABA antagonists by blocking $GABA_A$ Cl^- channels and prevent GABA binding to $GABA_A$ receptors
Carbapenems[b]	Prevent GABA binding to $GABA_A$ receptors
Medium risk agents	
Bupropion	Inhibition of dopamine reuptake
Fluoroquinolones	Prevent GABA binding to $GABA_A$ receptors
Cephalosporins[b]	Prevent GABA binding to $GABA_A$ receptors
Isoniazid[b]	↓ brain levels of GABA via inhibitory action of glutamic acid decarboxylase
Tramadol	Inhibition of monoamine (serotonin, norepinephrine) reuptake rather than to opioid effects
Tricyclic antidepressants	Inhibition of reuptake of norepinephrine or serotonin in the brain. Overdose produces anticholinergic toxidrome (hypotension, QRS interval prolongations, ventricular arrhythmias, and seizures)
Withdrawal alcohol benzodiazepines Barbiturates opioids	Disinhibition syndrome (loss of inhibitory control leading to excess stimulation and release of glutamate, NMDA, norepinephrine, and serotonin). Opioids may possess mu-receptor anticonvulsant properties that can precipitate seizures upon withdrawal
Low risk agents	
Other antidepressants	Inhibition of reuptake of norepinephrine or serotonin in the brain
Local anesthetics	Antagonism of Na^+ channel
Volatile general anesthetics[b]	Activation of NMDA receptors (enflurane and sevoflurane)
Other opioids	Unknown; likely mediated by selective stimulation of opioid receptors
Antihistamines	Histamine may be anticonvulsive via central H_1 receptors
Metronidazole	Unknown
Baclofen	Inhibition of presynaptic or postsynaptic inhibitory neurons
Beta blockers	Nonspecific action on centrally located neurons (membrane-stabilizing effects)
Cyclosporine	Structural damage to central nervous system
Cocaine	Augments the effects of catecholamines by blocking the reuptake at the synaptic junction and lowers seizure threshold
Stimulants	Augments the effects of catecholamines by blocking the reuptake at the synaptic junction
Antivirals	May be the result of inhibition of mitochondrial DNA polymerase and altered mitochondrial cell function
Antiepileptic drugs	AED in high concentrations may have depressant effect on inhibitory interneurons resulting in disinhibition of excitatory neurons and facilitation of epileptic discharges. Absence seizures may be induced by facilitating synchronization of the firing neurons in the thalamocortical network
Aspirin	Depletion of brain glucose

Mnemonic for drug related seizures in critically ill (Otis Campbell) [28]
GABA gamma aminobutyric acid,
O Opioid withdrawal oral hypoglycemics
T Tricyclic antidepressants, theophylline
I Isoniazid, insulin
S Sympathomimetics, salicylates
C Cocaine, carbapenems, cyclosporine
A Amphetamines, antibiotics, antidepressants, antipsychotics, anesthetics
M Meperidine, Methyl xanthines
P PCP. Propoxyphene
B Benzodiazepine withdrawal
E Ethanol withdrawal
L Lithium
L Lidocaine
[a]Seizures commonly occur at therapeutic doses
[b]Seizures occasionally occur at therapeutic doses

seizures following overdose and also with therapeutic dosing (primarily with chronic dosing) [53]. The lowest dose associated with seizures was 200 mg with the seizure occurring within 6 h of administration [54]. The incidence of seizures following overdose has been reported to be around 8% and the risk of a recurrent seizure is low (7%) [55–57]. Subsequently during the second year the agent was on the market a warning letter was issued by the Food and Drug Administration to all healthcare practitioners based upon the increased number of reports of seizures they had received. In most of the cases, patients were receiving other agents that were known to increase the risk of seizures and many were overdoses [58]. In a post-marketing surveillance case-controlled study in over 10,000 patients the risk of seizures with tramadol was similar to other analgesic agents [59]. The use of naloxone and risk of inducing a seizure in tramadol poisonings is controversial with some studies showing improvement in brain waves [60], others showing increased clonic seizures [61], and others showing no benefit [62]. Tapentadol is an orally active, central synthetic analgesic that acts via the mu-opioid receptor and inhibition of norepinephrine reuptake. The seizure rate of tapentadol reported to the National Poison Data System is 1.8% which was less than that associated with tramadol (13.7%) [63].

Seizures can also be the result of opioid withdrawal. Interestingly, Wijdicks and Sharbrough [15] attributed one-third of new-onset seizures in the critically ill patients in their cohort to opioid withdrawal. In this cohort, all patients who experienced new-onset seizures received at least 7 days of repeated intramuscular injections. Seizures related to drug withdrawal typically occur 2–4 days after last ingestion depending on the pharmacokinetic profile of the offending agent. Gradual tapering of agents that are associated with drug withdrawal, including opioids, is optimal in preventing seizures.

Salicylates

Salicylate toxicity primarily mediated through salicylic acid clinically presents with neurologic abnormalities including seizures. Most seizures are generalized and related to the depletion of brain glucose and increased CNS oxygen consumption even with normal blood glucose. First-line treatment for salicylate induced seizures is benzodiazepines followed by barbiturates as second-line agents. Since seizure is the most important symptom of severe salicylate toxicity other treatment should include gastrointestinal decontamination, urine alkalinization, and hemodialysis [19].

Anesthetics

General Anesthetics

Seizure activity associated with general anesthetic agents is largely thought to be an uncommon event. Nonetheless seizure activity has been reported with both volatile and nonvolatile agents. These agents are commonly used in the operating or procedure rooms and rarely in the ICUs. Therefore, their potential epileptogenic effects may be encountered in critically ill patients only in cases of immediate post-op transfer to an ICU bed without passing through the recovery room.

The most widely reported volatile anesthetic agent associated with seizures is enflurane [64]. This agent produces high amplitude spikes and periods of electrical silence on the EEG with the hyperexcitability originating in the limbic system and then spreading to other areas [65]. Most seizures reportedly occur during recovery from anesthesia [66, 67]. Interestingly, delayed seizures have also been reported up to eight postoperative days even with an initial normal EEG [68–70]. The occurrence of seizures can be minimized by using lower concentrations (less than 1.5 minimum alveolar concentration) and avoiding hypocapnia [71]. However others have reported seizure activity with enflurane even with normocapnia in patients with seizure disorders [72]. No specific recommendations are available regarding the use of these agents. With the availability of other volatile agents, however, that have less seizure risk, it is best to avoid enflurane in patients with a pre-existing seizure disorder or is at risk of seizures.

There have also been a couple reports of isoflurane-associated seizures [73, 74]. In these reports, myoclonic seizures occurred 2 h after induction and progressed to generalized seizures with sustained myoclonus during recovery. However the bulk of information in humans suggests that isoflurane has anticonvulsant properties [75, 76].

Sevoflurane has a reported incidence of seizures up to 12% in clinical trials conducted in children, healthy adults, and elective gynecological surgery [77–83]. Most of the seizures were reported within 90 min of sevoflurane administration and epileptiform EEG activity was seen in over 70% of the cases. A case report also described seizure activity with emergence from sevoflurane anesthesia [82]. When compared to isoflurane, sevoflurane has stronger epileptogenic property. Recently postulated risk factors for epileptiform activity include high alveolar sevoflurane concentration (greater than 2.0 MAC), more rapid anesthetic induction, hyperventilation, history of epilepsy, and female gender [84]. The concomitant use of nitrous oxide, benzodiazepine, or opioid seems to counteract the epileptogenic property of sevoflurane [81, 85]. The postulated mechanism is via NMDA receptor activation, similar to that observed with enflurane, since both agents have a similar molecular structure with seven fluoride atoms [86].

The seizure potential of the nonvolatile agents appears to be negligible. Some of the agents have been used intraoperatively, however, to activate epileptogenic foci during epilepsy surgery. There have been some reports of seizures associated with ketamine anesthesia [87, 88], although EEG recordings have not revealed seizure activity in patients without a seizure disorder. However, it is well described that ketamine can activate epileptogenic foci, primarily subcortical seizure activity originating in the thalamic and limbic areas, in patients with a known seizure disorder [89, 90]. There is no evidence of seizure activity in cortical regions. Ketamine does possess anticonvulsant properties and has received attention as an intervention for patients with refractory status epilepticus [91].

During induction and maintenance of anesthesia, etomidate is associated with involuntary myoclonic movements, which may simulate a tonic seizure but not correlated with any epileptogenic activity [92, 93]. It is also possible that this represents subcortical seizure activity [44]. In patients with a history of seizure disorders, surface EEG recordings have documented proconvulsant activity of etomidate at lower concentrations [94, 95]. Further studies are necessary to further evaluate the proconvulsant nature of these agents.

There have been several types of CNS reactions to propofol including twitching, hypertonia, myoclonus, and seizure activity [96]. Propofol has been used in the treatment of status epilepticus; however, there are some reports correlating propofol to seizure activity in patients without a seizure disorder history [97]. The seizure activity described in these reports primarily occurred during induction and emergence of anesthesia with induction doses of 0.5–5.2 mg/kg with 34% of the patients having associated EEG abnormal tracings [97]. The Committee on the Safety of Medicines in the United Kingdom estimated the seizure incidence as 1 in 47,000 [98]. However it is uncertain if the reports are simply "abnormal movements" or seizure activity since there is very little EEG epileptiform activity reported.

Local Anesthetics

Local anesthetics are known to be associated with both neurotoxicity and cardiotoxicity, especially following overdose in patients with and without a seizure disorder. The most commonly cited local anesthetic agents associated with seizures are lidocaine and bupivacaine.

Lidocaine can be administered to critically ill patients by a variety of different dosing routes, including topical, subcutaneous, intravenous, and intraspinal/epidural and seizures (clonic and tonic/clonic) following each route of administration has been reported. The greatest risk for neurotoxicity is following intravenous administration and when the drug is inadvertently injected directly into the blood vessel. Lidocaine is metabolized to monoethylglycinexylidide (MEGX), which can also contribute to its toxicity by lowering the seizure threshold [99]. The risk of seizures is correlated to serum concentration with seizures commonly reported with lidocaine concentrations of 8–12 mg/dL. Seizures are usually short lived ranging from a few seconds to a few minutes. At concentrations between 0.5 and 5 mg/dL, lidocaine can suppress the clinical and EEG manifestations of seizures in experimental models and has been used to treat status epilepticus in the clinical setting [100, 101]. There are several factors that can affect serum concentrations of local anesthetics including site and rate of injection, concentration, total dose administered, use of a concomitant vasoconstrictor, degree of

ionization, degree of plasma and tissue binding, age, weight, and rate of metabolism and excretion [102]. Bupivacaine is similar to lidocaine in epileptogenic potential. This agent is approximately 7 times more potent than lidocaine so toxicity can develop at doses as low as 2–3 mg/kg [103].

Patients who are at the greatest risk for local anesthetic induced seizures are those with a history of renal or hepatic failure, older age, congestive heart failure, and/or septic shock [20]. In addition toxicity has been reported as a result of drug interactions with cimetidine and propranolol [104, 105]. Clinicians should utilize the lowest effective dose, follow serum concentrations, and avoid long-term infusions. Treatment for seizures associated with local anesthetics should include benzodiazepines and supportive care.

Antiepileptic Agents

The concept of antiepileptic drugs (AED) inducing seizures is controversial and many times overlooked by clinicians. The difficulty lies in differentiating between drug effect and natural course of the disease. Seizure disorders, in and of themselves, are usually infrequent and unpredictable with swings between periods of seizure control success and failure. There are several conditions that have been identified that are associated with increased risk of seizures from these agents. These conditions include: (1) paradoxical reaction of the drug; (2) toxic concentrations of the AED; (3) result of AED-induced encephalopathy; (4) incorrect choice of AED in treatment of an epileptic syndrome or seizure type; (5) patients with mixed seizure types; and (6) AED withdrawal or regimen change [106]. Before concluding that an increase in seizures after the introduction of a new AED is associated with that agent, alternative explanations should be explored. These include spontaneous fluctuation of seizure frequency, the presence of known seizure aggravators (such as sleep deprivation, alcohol, and electrolyte abnormality), drug interactions, concurrent use of other epileptogenic inducing drugs, progression of epilepsy, and the development of drug resistance [107].

Even when AED drugs are chosen correctly for a clinical seizure type, they may provoke an increase in seizures. This usually occurs early after a patient is started on the AED and serum concentrations are within the normal range. Paradoxical seizures appear to be more common in children compared to adults. Both carbamazepine and phenytoin have been shown to provoke complex partial seizures [106]. Tonic-clonic seizures have been exacerbated by carbamazepine, gabapentin, lamotrigine, and benzodiazepines, while absence or absence status has been provoked by phenobarbital, oxcarbazepine, valproate, clonazepam with valproate and myoclonic seizures are increased with lamotrigine or oxcarbazepine [106–108].

Increased seizures may occur as a result of toxic AED serum concentrations. A neurotoxicity syndrome associated with AED overdose has been described and includes seizure exacerbation and coma [106, 107]. The AEDs, which are best described to cause seizures with intoxication, include phenytoin, carbamazepine, and valproate [106]. Carbamazepine has been associated with seizures following overdose or in the setting of increased carbamazepine-10,11-epoxide (active metabolite) concentrations [109, 110]. Therefore drug interactions that can increase the concentration of this active metabolite increase the risk of seizure exacerbation.

Several AEDS have been associated with development of encephalopathy. Encephalopathy presents clinically as coma, asterixis, fever, aggravation of pre-existing neurological deficits, and seizures. Agents that have been reported to cause encephalopathy include valproate, carbamazepine, and phenytoin [107]. Encephalopathy due to phenytoin is not commonly associated with an increase in seizure activity. On the other hand, an increase in seizure frequency due to valproate-induced encephalopathy is common. This is generally seen within the first week of treatment but can develop within the first 9 months of initiation [107]. Benzodiazepines are usually ineffective in treating these seizures, therefore the best treatment is to remove the offending agent [106, 107].

Incorrect selection of AED for a given seizure type may not only be ineffective but may provoke a seizure. For example, phenytoin, gabapentin, and carbamazepine may increase the frequency of primary generalized seizures, especially absence seizures, when incorrectly prescribed for this seizure type [20]. Carbamazepine and phenytoin have been shown to provoke or intensify generalized spike and wave discharges on EEG [111, 112]. In addition, myoclonic and atonic seizures are provoked by carbamazepine, lamotrigine, and gabapentin [106].

Seizure syndromes, such as West syndrome or Lennox Gastaut syndrome, consist of heterogeneous seizure types, with the EEG showing continuous abnormal patterns of diffuse slowing and generalized spike and wave activity [106]. Seizure exacerbation from AED is frequently reported, especially in children. The application of an AED to treat a seizure may actually unmask a second seizure component of an epilepsy syndrome, leading to an apparent increase in seizure frequency, when in fact the second seizure had been present all along. Agents that have increased seizure frequency in Lennox-Gastaut syndrome include phenytoin, carbamazepine, and benzodiazepines, while provocation of tonic seizures in West syndrome has been reported with benzodiazepines [106, 107].

In epileptic patients on antiepileptic polytherapy, seizure worsening is not easy to appreciate since worsening may be due to the withdrawal of an AED that was beneficial, rather than the introduction of a new one. An increase in seizures associated with withdrawal of the AED is expected by the decrease of seizure control resulting from the falling AED serum level. One must be watchful not only for the obvious actual removal of the medication, but also for the more insidious effective removal of the AED through the addition or withdrawal of an interacting medication. It appears that the rate of withdrawal of the AED influences the patient's susceptibility to the subsequent onset of seizures. In patients, where the drug is quickly discontinued, there appears to be an increase in post-withdrawal seizures, as compared to the cohort of patients where a gradual decrease in AED dose [113].

Just as the addition or deletion of medications must be carefully monitored to prevent AED toxicity, vigilance must also be maintained with respect to lowering therapeutic AED levels by new pharmacologic therapies, a very common situation in the ICU. The addition of an enzyme inducing medication may speed the metabolism of an AED, causing an iatrogenic AED withdrawal when, in fact, the AED dose has remained constant. The addition of a second or third AED may have this property and can cause this effect on the first AED's level. Table 20.2 presents common interactions between AEDs.

Finally, one must consider the protein binding of several ICU drugs. Many AEDs are heavily protein bound and free drug is the active moiety and is associated with toxicity. Not uncommonly, ICU patients have low serum albumin and protein levels, leading to a higher or even toxic free AED levels; this may pass unnoticed, if not specifically checked. In addition, competition for protein binding between the

Table 20.2 Effect on present AED plasma levels with addition of new AED [103, 244]

Added AED	Present AED							
	PHT	TPM	PHB	CBZ	VPA	LEV	BDZ	LAM
Phenytoin (PHT)	…	↓	↔	↓	↓	↔	↔	↓
Phenobarbital (PHB)	↑ then ↓	↔	…	↔	↓	↔	↓	↓
Carbamazepine (CBZ)	↔	↓	↔	…	↓	↔	↓	↑
Valproic acid (VPA)	↓/[a]	↓	↑	↔/[b]	…	↔	↑	↔
Levetiracetam (LEV)	↔	↔	↔	↔	↔	…	↔	↔
Benzodiazepines (BZD)	↓	↔	↔	↔	↔	↔	…	↔
Lamotrigine (LAM)	↔	↑	↔	[b]	↔	↔	↔	…
Topiramate (TPM)	↑	…	↔	↔	↓	↔	↔	↔[c]

[a]Increases free PHT levels
[b]Increases active epoxide metabolite
[c]No change at doses up to 400 mg/day

Table 20.3 Relative protein binding affinities for commonly used ICU Drugs and AEDs

Drug	% bound
Amiodarone	96
Digoxin	20–30
Nitroglycerin	60
Atracurium	82
Vecuronium	60–90
Propofol	>95
Phenytoin	90
Valproic Acid	90
Carbamazepine	75–90
Phenobarbital	20–45
Lamotrigine	55
Felbamate	25
Oxcarbazepine (MHD)	38
Topiramate	15
Zonisamide	40
Tiagabine	95
Leviracetam	<10
Vigabatrin	–
Gabapentin	–

various highly bound ICU medications (AEDs or others) may also lead to higher than expected active free levels of individual drugs accounting for signs of toxicity. Therefore, it is imperative in critical care that the clinician measure both total and free levels of drugs whenever possible. Table 20.3 illustrates the wide variety of protein binding that may occur with several common medications, and emphasizes the need to look at more discreet pharmacologic interactions in these medically complex patients.

Antimicrobial Agents

Antibiotics, especially beta-lactams, have often been linked to seizures in critically ill patients. The critically ill patient typically develops severe infections often requiring aggressive antibiotic dosing. In addition when a seizure occurs in an infected patient, additional work-up is required to exclude the co-existence of a CNS infection as a cause of the seizure. Many of the antibiotics act by antagonizing the action of GABA by various different mechanisms (See Table 20.1). Renal insufficiency is a well-documented risk factor for antibiotic, particularly β-lactam, toxicity. The most appropriate therapy for most antibiotic associated seizures is withdrawal of the agent and administration of benzodiazepines.

Beta-lactams

Seizure activity has been most commonly described with the penicillin class dating back to 1945 where myoclonic twitching was described in a toddler following intraventricular administration of benzylpenicillin [114]. Since that time, beta-lactams have been associated with neurotoxicity to

varying degrees. Penicillin consistently produces seizures via any route of administration, although more common after intrathecal administration [115, 116]. The most frequently reported seizure types are myoclonus and generalized tonic-clonic seizures occurring 23 to 72 h after initiation of antibiotic therapy [117, 118]. Risk factors for seizures are those associated with increasing CNS concentrations and include older age, infants, renal impairment, history of meningitis, past history of central nervous system abnormality, administration of intraventricular antibiotics, continuous infusion administration, and history of seizures [119]. Penicillin brain toxicity is also due to a decrease in active transport out of CNS, when co-administered with other drugs, including anesthetics and probenecid, leading to an accumulation in the CNS at a higher concentration than in the blood [120]. Neurotoxicity has not been shown to correlate to CSF or serum concentrations of the antibiotic while brain tissue concentration is a better indicator [120]. The convulsive activity following semisynthetic penicillins has been described; however, their proconvulsant potency is lower than what is observed for benzylpenicillin [121].

Cephalosporins have a similar risk of inducing seizures in experimental models yet in clinical practice cephalosporins rarely produce seizures unless given in high doses or in patients with renal impairment [122]. In a recent systematic review of cephalosporin-induced neurotoxicity more than 10% of the cases evaluated reported overt seizures and similar proportion had EEG-confirmed nonconvulsive status epilepticus [123]. Essentially, all generations of cephalosporins are reported to cause seizures, but approximately 50% of reported cases have renal insufficiency and/or elderly patients with pre-existing neurological disease [123]. There have been several reports of nonconvulsive status epilepticus in patients with renal dysfunction who were being treated with cefepime [124, 125]. Naeije et al. [126] evaluated patients with normal renal function who underwent continuous EEG monitoring and also received cefepime or meropenem. They found that 1.25% of patients who were receiving cefepime with normal renal function showed epileptiform discharges compared to 0.19% of those patients receiving meropenem. If one considers, however, those patients with concomitant to the administration of the antibiotic EEG testing, the percentages are quite different: 23.7% of those with cefepime infusion had continuous epileptiform discharges versus 3.75% of those with meropenem [126]. This study suggests that cefepime may be an independent risk factor for periodic epileptiform discharges so clinicians should be cognizant of this potential. Most patients develop seizure 1–5 days after starting the agent. Treatment of beta-lactam associated seizures includes benzodiazepines and barbiturates.

Carbapenems

Carbapenems are synthetic beta-lactam agents that are typically used for treating serious infections in hospitalized patients. The postulated mechanism of seizure induction is via binding to the GABAA receptor [127]. The traditional carbapenem, imipenem/cilastatin, has been associated with seizures at lower concentrations than other antibiotic agents and has a reported incidence of seizures ranging from 1.8–6% [120, 127]. Experimental studies suggest that imipenem is 10 times more neurotoxic than benzylpenicillin [128]. The toxicity associated with imipenem is due to accumulation of an open lactam metabolite of imipenem with cilastatin having no role alone in increasing seizure risk. Risk factors for seizures associated with imipenem include high dose, renal impairment, elderly, pre-existing neurologic abnormality, and *Pseudomonas aeruginosa* infection [129]. Seizures typically occur within 3–7 days of treatment initiation and are generalized or focal [129, 130]. The average daily dose of imipenem-cilastatin in those patients who experienced seizures ranged between 13 mg/kg to 4 g of imipenem [130]. As with other beta-lactam agents the treatment of choice for seizure activity is removal of the agent and administration of benzodiazepines. Phenytoin and other sodium channel blockers should be avoided. The newer carbapenems (e.g., meropenem) have a lower affinity for GABA$_A$ receptor and have a reduced incidence of seizures (0.8%) [131]. Patients whose medical course is complicated by hydrocephalus show a marked decrease in the elimination rate of meropenem from the CSF as compared to that from the serum [127].

Fluoroquinolones

Fluoroquinolone agents are associated with seizures in animals; however in the clinical setting, seizures are rare and generally associated with overdoses or in patients who are susceptible to seizures [132]. The mechanism of seizures is similar to that of beta-lactams. Receptor binding affinity is likely secondary to the similarities between the chemical structures of GABA and the antibiotics [133]. The incidence of CNS toxicity of fluoroquinolones was originally thought to be associated with lipophilicity of the agent although that theory has since been disproven [132]. There does appear to be varying degrees of binding to the GABA receptor, which may result in inhibiting or displacing GABA from the receptors. Animal studies also suggest that these agents have an agonist effect on the glutamate receptor NMDA [134]. The most epileptogenic agent is trovafloxacin followed by enoxacin, moxifloxacin, ciprofloxacin, ofloxacin, and gatifloxacin, which is equivalent in epileptogenicity to levofloxacin [132, 135]. The estimated incidence in humans of seizure activity is 1% or less [136]. The seizures that have been described include tonic-clonic and generalized myoclonic activity occurring anywhere from 8 h to 12 days after initiation of therapy, although seizures have been reported up to a week following discontinuation of therapy [109, 137, 138]. Additionally seizures have been reported when fluoroquinolones are co-administered with theophylline and nonsteroidal anti-inflammatory drugs [20].

Isoniazid

Isoniazid (INH) remains one of the most common agents for drug-induced seizures in the USA [13]. INH has a 1–3% risk for development of seizures. The epileptogenic potential results from INH being metabolized to hydrazines, resulting in a pyridoxine (vitamin B6) deficiency via inhibition of pyridoxine phosphokinase (the enzyme transforming pyridoxine to pyridoxal phosphate). Pyridoxal phosphate (activated B6) is required by glutamic acid decarboxylase to convert glutamic acid to GABA thus leading to decreased levels of GABA [139]. Mortality associated with INH is reported as high as 19%, particularly after ingestion of 10–15 g of INH [139]. An overdose of INH is very frequently associated with seizures, although therapeutic doses have also been linked to seizure activity primarily in elderly patients [140, 141]. Serum INH concentrations greater than 10 mg/L on presentation, greater than 3.2 mg/L 2 h after ingestions or greater than 0.2 mg/L 6 h after ingestion are associated with severe toxicity [142]. Seizures associated with INH may occur without warning usually 1–3 h after ingestion, frequently as generalized tonic-clonic seizures, which are prolonged and difficult to treat [143]. Other symptoms that accompany seizures include coma and metabolic acidosis. Phenytoin is ineffective in treating seizures associated with INH. Benzodiazepines are considered first-line agents; however, patients may be refractory since the agents require the presence of GABA for their therapeutic effects. Therefore, primary treatment includes intravenous administration of pyridoxine in amounts equivalent to ingested INH dose (1 g IV pyridoxine for each gram of INH ingested [144, 145]. If unknown quantities are ingested, then the dose of pyridoxine should be 5 g IV. This dose may be repeated on five to 20 min intervals until control of seizures has been obtained [20, 120]. A low threshold should be used for pyridoxine administration in the setting of INH toxicity. One study reported the absence of adverse effects with pyridoxine doses of up to 357 mg/kg [145].

Isoniazid remains less likely than other antibiotics to cause seizures within the hospital or the ICU, as most cases of INH-induced seizure result from acute, accidental, or intentional overdose. In this case, the presence of an unexplained anion-gap metabolic acidosis with high lactate level in the presence of no seizures or after a brief seizure should alert the intensivist for the possibility of INH overdose. Damaging neurologic sequelae have resulted from exposures as low as 20 mg/kg [120]. This is striking, as the recommended dosage for children requiring therapy runs from 10–15 mg/kg [120]. Clear understanding of dosage regimens must be carefully communicated, not only to the health care team, but also to patients or parents of patients on INH.

Metronidazole

Experimental evidence and scattered case reports suggest that metronidazole has proconvulsant activity [146–149]. The mechanism of action by which metronidazole induces epileptogenicity is largely unknown [120]. It is known that seizures seem to develop approximately seven to 10 days following the initiation of high dose therapy (5–6 g/day) in susceptible patients [120]. Patients witnessed to have seizures on metronidazole therapy were also afflicted with metastatic cancers (metronidazole was used as a radiation sensitizer) and were also treated with other medications with known pro-convulsant actions (for example, phenothiazines, cefamandole, ciprofloxacin, and theophylline) [120]. Based on these rare human reports and some limited evidence from animal experiments, metronidazole use should be considered safe, if not used in high doses or in combination with other epileptogenic drugs.

Antiviral Agents

Antiviral agents rarely produce seizures except when given at high doses or to patients with a seizure disorder. Ganciclovir, foscarnet, and zidovudine have been reported to cause seizures in human immunodeficiency virus (HIV)-infected patients; however, these patients have multiple reasons for seizures so it is hard to establish the causal relationship [20]. Risk factors for foscarnet-related seizures include the presence of toxoplasmosis with CNS involvement and a decrease in creatinine clearance [150]. Without the presence of these risk factors and in the absence of any electrolyte abnormalities, there have been no reported seizures in the foscarnet-treated population [150].

Neurologic sequelae (vomiting hallucinations and confusion or coma, rarely seizures) as a result of acyclovir dosing have been reported in the literature, although mostly through case reports [151]. Often, this comes as a consequence of intravenous administration, but it has also been found to occur in patients receiving oral therapy. While patients with pre-existing renal dysfunction, the elderly or those patients with overdose may be most susceptible to adverse neurological events [151], seizures cannot be entirely attributed to the drug, but instead to the primary CNS insult by herpes simplex virus or varicella zoster virus. Nevertheless, acyclovir neurotoxicity is distinguished from viral encephalitis by its sudden onset, absence of fever or headache, lack of focal neurologic findings and normal cerebrospinal fluid [152]. Discontinuation of the drug and hemodialysis should be considered in case of suspicion of neurotoxicity leading to seizures from this drug.

Ganciclovir administration has been associated with seizures after the first month of administration in patients infected with the HIV. Seizures worsened with increased dosing and the seizures did not respond to phenytoin administration and stopped when ganciclovir was discontinued [153].

The incidence of seizures occurring in patients infected with HIV is higher than in the general population [154, 155] The question yet to be definitively answered is if this increased seizure risk is secondary to the disease progression itself, complicated by the many medications required to prolong life, especially in advanced disease, or it is a manifestation of the anti-viral medications required for the prevention of this progression. In a study that followed 550 patients for 1 year and monitored for seizure incidence, only one patient (0.018%) had a seizure attributed to the toxic effects of anti-retroviral (zidovudine) therapy when taken in overdose with sulfonamides [154]. Because of the difficulty in assessing the cause-effect relationship with these agents and seizure activity, it is accepted that AED therapy should be initiated in patients infected with HIV after their initial seizure [155]. Selection of AED agent is crucial in this population, as many drug interactions and disease interactions exist. Valproate, for example, can increase viral reproduction of both the HIV virus in addition to cytomegalovirus, while phenytoin, phenobarbital, and carbamazepine may increase the metabolism of protease inhibitors via the CYP450 system [155]. For more information on these interactions, the interested reader should refer to the Chapter Seizures and Infection in the ICU.

Bronchodilators

Seizures are a frequent adverse sequela of theophylline and aminophylline toxicity mediated primarily through the antagonism of adenosine receptors, the inhibition of phosphodiesterase, and the increase in cAMP; however, some have suggested other mechanisms including depletion of pyridoxine and inhibition of GABA [28]. The incidence of theophylline-associated seizures is 8–14% with mortality reported as high as 50% [156]. The associated EEG findings include periodic lateralized epileptiform discharges, generalized epileptiform discharges, and generalized slowing and focal status epilepticus [157]. Generalized seizures occur in 33% and secondarily generalized seizures occur in 30% of patients. Almost half of patients have ≥3 seizures with status epilepticus occurring in 29% of them, usually without permanent neurologic sequelae [113].

Serum theophylline concentrations do not always correlate well to the risk of seizures, particularly in chronic toxicity since serum and CNS theophylline concentrations are poorly correlated [158, 159], although many reports suggest that seizures less likely occur with serum concentrations of less than 60 mg/dL [160]. Some authors suggest that patients who are at increased risk of seizures be maintained with theophylline concentrations at 10–15 mg/dL [157]) Serum concentrations of >21 mg/dL are commonly associated with drug-induced seizures in acute toxicity and in one study seizures were seen in two out of three cases reaching this concentration [113]. Serum concentrations do not correlate with the number of seizure a patient may develop. Nonetheless clinicians should be aware of the risk, as other reports have also seen seizure activity in therapeutic or mildly elevated concentrations [157].

Several risk factors for seizures have been reported in patients on long-term treatment including advanced age, previous seizure history, encephalitis, cerebral vascular insufficiency, alcohol withdrawal, and other brain anomalies [161]. In addition the potential for drug interactions may increase risk of toxicity as seizures with theophylline have been described in patients concurrently receiving theophylline along with metronidazole, ciprofloxacin, gatifloxacin, moxifloxacin, or imipenem [149]. The addition of a quinolone can increase theophylline serum concentrations through inhibition of theophylline metabolism. Also, theophylline has been shown to increase the antagonism of the GABAA receptor achieved by the fluoroquinolones, thus increasing the epileptogenicity of the antibiotic [120].

Seizures due to theophylline are known to be prolonged and difficult to treat. The general principle in management is to stop the seizure as soon as possible (within 5–6 h of ingestion) as a correlation exists between morbidity and mortality and the duration of seizures. Barbiturates and benzodiazepines are the cornerstone of management (phenytoin is ineffective), although many cases may require general anesthesia and aggressive gastrointestinal decontamination and hemodialysis [162]. Hemodialysis and hemoperfusion is commonly used when serum theophylline concentrations are greater than 100 mg/dL following acute toxicity and greater than 60 mg/dL with chronic toxicity [163]. Midazolam has been reported to be effective against refractory seizures caused by theophylline toxicity [164].

Immunosuppressive Agents

Seizure etiology in the post transplant patient population may be the most difficult to assess, given the level of medical complexity that these patients possess. Metabolic abnormalities, including non-ketotic hyperosmolar hyperglycemia, weakened immune systems, polypharmacy, and potential coagulopathies all pose as possible instigators of neurologic toxicity. Before the intensivist attributes seizures to a metabolic or drug cause, an extensive work-up to exclude infectious agents invading the CNS should be completed.

The most common immunosuppressive agent associated with seizures is cyclosporine. The overall incidence of CNS toxicity with cyclosporin is 10% and includes cerebellar disorders, neuropathies, and seizures [165]. The incidence of seizures is approximately 3% in bone marrow transplant patients and around 1% in solid-organ transplants [165]. Of solid organ transplants, cyclosporine induced seizures are more commonly reported after liver transplant compared to renal transplant. Patients with the highest risk for seizure during cyclosporine therapy include those on simultaneous high-dose steroids, children, and those with hypertension, hypomagnesemia, and/or hypoalbuminemia [166]. The onset of seizures ranges from 2 to 180 days of treatment initiation (usually early during aggressive dose escalation) even in patients without risk factors for seizures. The highest risk for seizures was in patients with cyclosporine concentrations above 250 mcg/mL. Cyclosporin produces structural injury to the CNS [167]. White matter is particularly susceptible to toxicity, manifested by characteristic focal lesions on magnetic resonance imaging. The brain contains high concentrations of the cytosolic-binding protein cyclophilin, which suggests increased cellular uptake of cyclosporin [165]. Calcineurin inhibitors may also exacerbate an underlying seizure focus by enhancing neuronal excitability. The EEG in patients with cyclosporine neurotoxicity consists of diffuse slowing [165].

Cyclosporine's metabolic pathway may be induced by phenytoin, phenobarbital, and carbamazepine [166]. Careful monitoring of cyclosporine serum concentrations is imperative in the patient who must be maintained on one of these AEDs. Valproic acid is one AED, which has failed to show any impact on the metabolism of cyclosporine [166]. For that reason it may be recommended as a possible therapeutic option, although its use should be avoided in patients less than 2 years old who have undergone liver transplantation as it has had reported deleterious effects on the liver itself [166]. Newer AEDs, which are non-hepatic enzyme inducers, like gabapentin, oxcarbazepine, or levetiracetam may also be considered to control seizures [168]) Calcineurin inhibitor-sparing regimens with mycophenolate mofetil and corticosteroids may be useful in reducing the incidence of neurotoxicity [169]. Calcineurin inhibitors can then be started when encephalopathy and electrolyte shifts have resolved, usually within 48 hours. Please refer to the ICU Seizures in Organ Transplantation Recipients Chapter for more information.

Other immunosuppressing agents used after organ transplantation, increasing the risk for seizures includes tacrolimus (FK506) and OKT3. Since tacrolimus is also a calcineurin inhibitor it has a similar risk for neurotoxicity to cyclosporine. Sirolimus is a newer agent related to tacrolimus, but its mechanism of action differs where it does not inhibit calcineurin. No evidence of neurotoxicity with sirolimus therapy for up to 18 months has been found [170]. In renal transplant patients, OKT3 caused seizures in 6%

(8/122) of cases, all with non-functioning grafts, due to tubular necrosis [171].

Chemotherapeutic Agents

Chemotherapeutic agents may also be associated with seizures, including alkylating agents (chlorambucil and busulfan) cisplatinum, 5-fluorouracil, high dose methotrexate, vincristine, etoposide, and ifosfamide [20, 172–174]. The greatest risk of seizures from chemotherapeutic agents is after excessive doses such as the regimens used for myeloablative treatment in preparation for bone marrow transplant. Children also seem to be susceptible to seizures especially with chlorambucil and vincristine. Seizures occur within hours or days of drug administration, but can be delayed in patients with impaired renal or hepatic clearance.

Psychotropic Agents

Psychotropic drugs have been implicated in drug-induced seizures for many years. The San Francisco General study noted that psychotropic drugs accounted for 34% of all witnessed drug-induced seizures occurring in hospital [14]. This is not surprising given the potential of these agents through their pharmacologic activity to lower the seizure threshold and through drug interactions with other medications to either result in toxicity or result in lowering of concurrent AEDs. Most of these agents utilize the CYP450 hepatic enzyme system for elimination, thus co-administration with other agents that inhibit this system may inadvertently lead to toxicity and increase risk of seizures. The epileptogenic potential of the agents varies and data is limited regarding the impact of these agents on seizure threshold in epileptic versus non-epileptic brains. In general it is recommended to use the less epileptogenic agent in patients with a history of seizures at the lowest effective dose. The risk factors for antipsychotic-induced seizures include: history or epilepsy, electroconvulsive therapy, abnormal EEG, history of drug-induced seizures, neurodegenerative disorder, head injury, insulin shock therapy, larger doses of antipsychotics, polypharmacy with multiple antipsychotics, and sudden changes in the dose [175]. The intensivist should be aware of the seizure potential and maintain a conservative approach to managing critically ill patients, balancing the risk and benefit in each individual patient.

Antipsychotic Agents

Seizures associated with psychotropic agents are often the cause for ICU admission, particularly as a result of overdose. Even though all patients receiving antipsychotic agents are at risk for drug-induced seizures, the most common time for seizures to develop is upon initiation or during dosage titration particularly rapid titration schedules. The epileptogenic

Table 20.4 Risk of seizures associated with antipsychotics [176]

Low risk agents	Medium risk agents	High-risk agents
Fluphenazine	Olanzapine	Clozapine
Haloperidol	Quetiapine	Chlorpromazine
Molindone	Thioridazine	
Risperidone		
Trifluoperazine		

potential of antipsychotics depends somewhat on the ratio of dopamine-1 (D1) to dopamine-2 (D2) blockade, as well as the balance of glutamate and GABA activity. D1 agonists and D2 antagonists are proconvulsant. Also antagonism of α_1-receptors, agonism of α_2-receptors, and inhibition of histamine-1 receptors may promote seizure activity. Another potential mechanism is via influence of neurosteroid sex hormones produced in the brain [176]. Traditionally the low potency agents were thought to possess the highest risk of seizure activity (see Table 20.4).

The literature suggests that chlorpromazine and other aliphatic phenothiazines (promazine and trifluoperazine) are commonly associated with seizures (1.2% overall incidence) [177, 178], while piperazine phenothiazines (fluphenazine, perphenazine, prochlorperazine, trifluoperazine) are less associated with seizures (0.3–0.9% overall incidence with therapeutic dosing) [177–179]. Doses exceeding 1000 mg per day of chlorpromazine have a 9% incidence of seizures. Seizures most commonly occur at the onset of treatment or after a rapid dose increase with other associated risk factors including an abnormal EEG tracing or evidence of a brain abnormality. Phenothiazines induce diffuse, paroxysmal EEG changes [20]. In addition the phenothiazines can interact with phenytoin and phenobarbital resulting in reduced concentrations of these AEDs placing patients at increased risk of seizures [20]. Butyrophenones (haloperidol and droperidol) have been associated with seizures although this class of drugs may carry a lower risk than other antipsychotic agents [179, 180].

The atypical antipsychotic, clozapine, has a 2.8% risk of seizures with the risk higher in patients receiving doses >600 mg/day (risk = 4.4–14%) or with the use of a rapid titration schedule [181, 182]. Status epilepticus following clozapine administration has also been reported [183]. Seizures occurring during clozapine therapy do not necessarily lead to discontinuation of therapy, especially since clozapine is held for refractory patients. Administration of seizure prophylaxis with valproic acid, phenytoin, or topiramate is often considered [184, 185]. The risk of seizures for the remainder of newer, atypical antipsychotic agents is not well defined and appears to be low. Outside of olanzapine, none of the other second-generation antipsychotics induce EEG changes [186]. Olanzapine is associated with EEG slowing and epileptiform abnormalities [186, 187]. The consensus is that risperidone (0.34% incidence), olanzapine (0.9% incidence), ziprasidone (0.4% incidence), aripiprazole (0.1% incidence), quetiapine

(0.8% incidence) are not associated with an increased risk of seizures [188–192]. The agent with the most concern is olanzapine since it is structurally related to clozapine and there are isolated cases of seizures and status epilepticus reported at therapeutic doses [186, 193–195]. The case reports of the other agents were in patients receiving polytherapy with agents that are associated with seizure activity. It should be considered that all patients who are predisposed to seizures are at increased risk when prescribed any antipsychotic agent. When using these agents, it is best to use the lowest effective dose with slow dosage titration and avoid using them with other agents that may lower the seizure threshold.

If patients experience an antipsychotic-associated seizure and there is a need to continue therapy, then agents with the lowest potential to lower seizure threshold should be used (e.g., risperidone, haloperidol, fluphenazine, pimozide, molindone, trifluoperazine, thioridazine) [175]. Phenothiazines are more likely to lower seizure threshold than butyrophenones. Therefore, haloperidol would be the agent of choice for treating delirium in the intensive care unit in patients at risk of seizures. The agents with the highest risk potential for seizures are clozapine and chlorpromazine [194, 196, 197] and in this case should be avoided in the ICU.

Antidepressants

Antidepressant drugs have both convulsant and anticonvulsant properties. The convulsant properties are more prominent at higher concentrations and particularly prevalent in overdose cases. The propensity of antidepressant agents to cause seizures varies from 0.1 to 20% (see Table 20.5) [198–200]. Since these agents are used for a variety of indications clinically ranging from depression to smoking cessation the exposure to these agents has increased so it is essential to understand their seizure risk profile. It is important for the intensivist to evaluate this data (See Table 20.5) and then extrapolate to decision-making on initiating or continuing these agents in the ICU patient.

Tricyclic Antidepressants

The first report of seizures associated with tricyclic antidepressants (TCA) occurred not long after the introduction of the first agent to the market (imipramine) [201]. Since that time, the overall incidence of TCA-induced seizure ranged from 4 to 20%, primarily in acute overdose [199, 200]. Not all of the TCAs share the same potential for seizures at therapeutic doses. Agents that have been reported to most commonly be associated with seizures are amoxapine, amitriptyline, imipramine, nortriptyline, desipramine, doxepin, and protriptyline. Clomipramine is associated with increased risk of seizures at doses greater than 300 mg/day [202]. Seizures generally occur within three to 6 h post ingestion and are uncommon after 24 h [176]. It has been suggested that the risk of seizures could be reduced by monitoring plasma concentrations since the isoenzymes responsible for TCA metabolism are known to be subject to genetic polymorphisms that could result in toxic concentrations in the small percentage of patients who may be lacking this isoenzyme [203]. However, there is a lack of consensus on the utility of serum concentration monitoring, since the incidence of seizures in patients treated with "low dose" TCA does not differ significantly from that of the general population, implying that it is not the medication itself, but rather the brain insult that is causing the seizure [176].

Maprotiline is a semi-TCA but has a higher risk for seizures compared to other TCA, potentially related to a toxic metabolite. The risk of seizures is increased at doses above 225 mg/day. The pharmacologic action of these agents includes inhibition of serotonin and norepinephrine reuptake, histamine (H1) antagonism and alpha-1 receptor antagonism. The exact mechanism by which these agents induce seizures has not been elucidated since many studies have found varying effects of these agents on the seizure threshold. Seizures generally occur within a few days of initiation of therapy or when changing to higher doses.

In overdose, TCA produce an anticholinergic toxidrome that includes hypotension, QRS interval prolongation, ventricular arrhythmias, and seizures. Mortality is significantly increased with the presence of seizures [204]. TCA-induced seizures, with the exception of amoxapine, is generally accompanied by a widened QRS duration on electrocardiogram [205]. A QRS duration of 0.10 s or longer was moderately predictive of seizures while durations of 0.16 s or longer was highly predictive of seizures [206]. Seizures associated with TCA are more likely to be prolonged and multiple and associated with increased risk of medical complications (hypotension, coma, other cardiovascular compli-

Table 20.5 Risk of Seizures Associated with Antidepressants [176, 245]

Minimal risk agents	Low risk agents	Medium risk agents	High-risk agents
Phenelzine	SSRI	Amitriptyline	Maprotiline
Tranylcypromine	Trazodone	Imipramine	Amoxapine
	Mirtazapine	Desipramine	Clomipramine
	Nefazodone	Nortriptyline	Bupropion
		Protriptyline	Citalopram
		Doxepin	
		Venlafaxine	

SSRI selective serotonin reuptake inhibitors

cations) and death [13, 207]. Treatment of TCA overdose includes supportive care, benzodiazepines for seizures, and sodium bicarbonate for cardiac toxicity.

Selective Serotonin Reuptake Inhibitors

The selective serotonin reuptake inhibitors (SSRI) administered alone have been reported to have anticonvulsant effects [208]. In overdosage situations, however, fluoxetine, sertraline, citalopram, escitalopram, and fluvoxamine have been reported to cause seizures [176, 209, 210]. In overdose situations, citalopram was reported to more likely cause seizures than escitalopram at comparable doses [211]. Accumulating data suggest that at therapeutic doses the incidence of seizures with fluoxetine is 0.2%; however, these agents appear to be less epileptogenic than TCA [196]. Another important consideration is possible drug interactions through CYP450 since SSRI are both inhibitors and substrates for this enzyme system. It is important that clinicians carefully review all medication regimens in patients in the ICU to assess for potentially serious drug interactions. When these agents are co-administered with other agents that mimic serotonin or with monoamine oxidase inhibitors, "serotonin syndrome" may develop. This syndrome is associated with seizures, delirium, myoclonus, and autonomic instability [212, 213].

Monoamine Oxidase Inhibitors

Monoamine oxidase inhibitors occasionally are associated with seizure activity in patients suffering from hypertensive crisis as part of tyramine ingestion [214]. In general when these agents are used in the recommended doses and without external interacting factors, there is very little risk of drug-induced seizures.

Bupropion

Bupropion is a unique agent that works pharmacologically by inhibiting the reuptake of dopamine, norepinephrine, and serotonin. Bupropion displays similar characteristics to TCA in overdose, although they are not structurally similar, with conduction delays on ECG reported in 2–3% of overdose cases [215]. Initially the maximum recommended doses were 450–900 mg/day and the overall incidence of seizures was 2–5.4% leading to the drug being withdrawn from the market in 1986 [216]. It was later re-introduced to the market with a maximum recommended dose of 450 mg/day. The incidence of seizures at doses greater than 450 mg/day has been reported to be as high as 2.2% compared to maximal doses less than 450 mg/day, which conferred a 0.44% seizure incidence [216]. Seizure risk is increased in patients with the following: history of seizures, head trauma, anorexia/bulimia, CNS tumor, severe hepatic cirrhosis, and use with other medications that lower the seizure threshold. Bupropion was also reported to be an important cause of drug-related new-onset generalized seizures presenting to the emergency department

[11]. The sustained release formulation is hypothesized to have a lower epileptogenic potential since it produces lower peak concentrations compared to the immediate release product; however, there have been reports of tonic clonic seizures associated with the use of the sustained release product [216, 217]. In a recent cohort of patients, seizures with bupropion XL overdoses (doses of 600 mg in adults and 16 mg/kg in children) developed in 32% of patients, with the onset of seizures ranging from 0.5 h up to 24 h (mean 7.3 h) after ingestion [218]. This data would suggest an observational period of at least 24 h for patients who ingest the XL formulation. In general, bupropion is thought to have a higher risk of seizures compared to other antidepressant agents and should be used with caution in patients with a seizure disorder [219, 220].

Miscellaneous Antidepressants

Both trazodone and nefazodone have a very low risk for new-onset seizures and are probably safe in patients with seizure disorders. Venlafaxine is another agent pharmacologically similar to bupropion, but with lesser effect on dopamine reuptake inhibition. Cardiotoxicity with QRS interval widening and arrhythmias have been reported with venlafaxine overdose, but to a lesser extent than that experienced with TCA, although the reported incidence of seizures is also high and ranges from 8 to 14% [221].

Lithium

Lithium is well known to be associated with serious neurological side effects, especially seizures. There is very limited information describing lithium's pharmacologic effects, but these are likely mediated through effects on neuronal ion transport and inhibition of norepinephrine and serotonin reuptake. The EEG changes seen after lithium is generalized slowing and paroxysmal diffuse alpha activity, which typically develop within one to 2 weeks of therapy onset and are reversible with elimination of the drug [222]. Seizures associated with lithium generally occur with supratherapeutic concentrations (>3 mEq/L); however, seizures have been reported in patients with therapeutic concentrations and upon drug withdrawal. Therefore it is imperative that the clinical presentation of the patient is treated instead of treating a laboratory value. Except in chronic overdosing, serum concentration correlates with severity of toxicity symptoms [223, 224]. Risk factors for lithium-associated seizures include pre-existing EEG abnormality, clinical seizure disorder (including childhood febrile seizures), decreased renal function, and acute psychotic symptoms [20]. Because the combination of lithium and carbamazepine has been implicated in acute neurotoxicity even with "therapeutic" concentrations of both agents, the intensivist should be aware and use alternative AED or mood stabilizing agents [225, 226]. Treatment of lithium toxicity includes supportive care, gastrointestinal decontamination, enhanced elimination with hemodialysis and benzodiazepines.

Stimulants

Psychostimulants such as caffeine, amphetamines, methylphenidate, and modafinil are gaining increasing popularity in the treatment of diseases such as attention deficit-hyperactivity disorder (ADHD), narcolepsy, and obesity [227]. Due to their diffuse action within the CNS, one would imagine the risk for seizures induced by this class of medications to be high. Studies have shown, however, that the relative epileptogenicity of these medications is quite low [228]. There are no data available regarding the seizure risk with their anecdotal use in ICU comatose patients.

While caffeine is certainly the most widely used medication in this class, methylphenidate remains the most widely prescribed for the aforementioned disease states. Overall, this stimulant has proven to be quite safe with regard to seizure induction. In fact, methylphenidate has actually been shown to decrease the incidence of seizure in patients with acute brain trauma [229]. When this stimulant is used in patients with seizure disorders that are well controlled on AEDs, there is very minimal risk of seizure exacerbation or prolongation [230]. In fact, methylphenidate may increase the serum concentrations of some AEDs, including phenobarbital and primidone [228]. Again, the importance of careful monitoring of serum concentrations of medications with the addition or removal of any medical therapy cannot be understated.

For patients without a previous history of seizures, if the luxury of a pre-treatment EEG is available, it may well prove beneficial in determining a patient's potential risk for developing seizures while on stimulant therapy. In one study of pediatric patients started on stimulants for ADHD, the risk for seizure in patients with a normal EEG prior to therapy was 0.6%, while for patients presenting with epileptiform abnormalities on the EEG prior to the beginning of therapy the risk was 10% ($P < 0.003$). In both groups the seizures occurred during treatment with methylphenidate, except for one patient with previous history of seizures, who had one event after discontinuing the drug [230].

Modafinil is an alerting agent approved for the treatment of narcolepsy in adults. It has been also used in children with excessive daytime somnolence. In a small case series of children with these disorders, exacerbation of seizures and psychotic symptoms was reported with modafinil therapy in 2/13 children [231].

Drug Withdrawal

Literature has suggested that 45% of seizures in the hospital or ICU are the result of alcohol or drug toxicity and drug withdrawal [103]. Drug withdrawal may occur at several different times during the patient's hospitalization. Early withdrawal related to agents the patient ingested prior to admission might occur as patients are moved from the emergency department to the ward or the ICU or when medications are changed or abruptly stopped. Early withdrawal seizures can be attributed to many agents and may be predictable and preventable by assessment of the admission toxicology screen. More information regarding ICU seizures related to withdrawal from legal or illegal drugs can be found in a separate chapter.

Miscellaneous Agents

Baclofen is a centrally acting muscle relaxant administered either orally or intrathecally. Withdrawal from baclofen, a GABA_B agonist, has been reported to be similar to ethanol and sedative withdrawal and may include seizures. Both abrupt discontinuation of oral therapy and intrathecal pump failure have been associated with seizures [232–234]. The treatment of these seizures includes benzodiazepines and the readministration of oral therapy. However oral replacement therapy may not reach sufficient CSF concentrations to be effective in patients with intrathecal pump failure [234].

Diphenhydramine is the most common antihistamine agent associated with seizures and was recently reported as the second most common agent associated with drug-induced seizures reported to a poison control center [12]. Seizures associated with diphenhydramine appear to be most common in overdose situations (~5% of cases) and are generally brief and self-limited within 2–3 h of ingestion [235]. Children have an increased susceptibility to the convulsive effects of these agents with fatality being reported after ingesting less than 150 mg [236].

Intravenous contrast media have been associated with tonic-clonic and partial seizures within 10 min of administration. The risk is generally low (0.2–0.5%) except in patients with metastatic cancer to the brain where the incidence increased to 15% [237, 238]. In animal models, the use of iodinated contrast triggered seizures when given by various routes of administration including intravenous, intra-arterial, intracerebral, and subarachnoid. Seizures are usually self-limiting occurring within 30 min of infusion with status epilepticus rarely occurring. The risk factors include dose administered, speed of administration, use of ionic agents, osmolarity, history of seizure disorder, and structural brain abnormality [237].

Beta-adrenergic blocking agents can cause seizures in overdose with the majority of cases involving propranolol [239]. The cardioselective agents and ones with lower lipid solubility seem to be less epileptogenic but still can result in seizures [240].

Other agents that have been associated with seizures include exogenous administration of thyroid hormone, hypoglycemic agents, and electrolyte derangements. These areas are specifically covered in individual chapters in this book.

Treatment

Overall the management strategy involves supportive care, removal of offending agent (if possible), and administration of an antiseizure agent with benzodiazepines as first-line agents followed by phenobarbital [241]. The specific approach for managing drug-related seizures is covered within another chapter of this text. For other detailed information on managing seizures in the intensive care unit, please refer to previously published comprehensive reviews [242, 243].

Summary

While the overall incidence of drug-induced seizures appears to be relatively low, critically ill patients may be more vulnerable to the epileptogenicity of drugs. Unfortunately, the occurrence of drug-related seizures in critically ill patients is often difficult to assess and is dependent upon certain patient and drug attributes that would place the patients at increased risk. The complexity of the illness and delivery of care in critically ill patients certainly contribute to the risk. Numerous drugs have been implicated as a cause of seizures but to varying degrees. The true incidence and causality is difficult to assess as most of the data is from published case reports or post-marketing surveillance programs. Therefore, clinicians should report any drug related seizures to appropriate formulary committees or databases in order to further clarify any relationships between the drug and this adverse consequence. Prevention is the key treatment for drug-induced seizures with the first step being familiarity with the agents that may cause seizures followed by prospective assessment of drug regimens. Critically ill patients possess many of the risk factors for drug related adverse events so recognition and vigilance is essential by all clinicians. In addition since most drug-induced seizures are dose-related, it is important to use the lowest effective dose adjusted for end organ function in an effort to minimize this potentially serious adverse effect. Treatment of seizures is usually symptomatic and includes, when possible, discontinuing the offending agent. In general the first-line agents for treating drug-induced seizures are benzodiazepines, which should be initiated promptly in an effort to minimize the morbidity and mortality associated with this adverse effect of drugs.

References

1. Lazarou J, Pomeranz BH, Corey PN. Incidence of adverse drug reactions in hospitalized patients: a meta-analysis of prospective studies. JAMA. 1998;279:1200–5.
2. Suh DC, Woodall BS, Shin SK, Hermes-De Santis ER. Clinical and economic impact of adverse drug reactions in hospitalized patients. Ann Pharmacother. 2000;34:1373–9.
3. Classen DC, Pestotnik SL, Evans RS, Lloyd JF, Burke JP. Adverse drug events in hospitalized patients. Excess length of stay, extra costs, and attributable mortality. JAMA. 1997;277:301–6.
4. Bates DW, Spell N, Cullen DJ, et al. The costs of adverse drug events in hospitalized patients. Adverse Drug Events Prevention Study Group. JAMA. 1997;277:307–11.
5. Smith KM, Jeske CS, Young B, Hatton J. Prevalence and characteristics of adverse drug reactions in neurosurgical intensive care patients. Neurosurgery. 2006;58:426–33. discussion -33
6. Bleck TP, Smith MC, Pierre-Louis SJ, Jares JJ, Murray J, Hansen CA. Neurologic complications of critical medical illnesses. Crit Care Med. 1993;21:98–103.
7. Thundiyil JG, Rowley F, Papa L, Olson KR, Kearney TE. Risk factors for complications of drug-induced seizures. J Med Toxicol. 2011;7:16–23.
8. Drug Abuse Warning Network, 2005:National Estimates of Drug-Related Emergency Department Visits. Substance Abuse and Mental Health Services Administration, 2007. (Accessed. October 15, 2015)
9. Drug-induced convulsions. Report from Boston collaborative drug surveillance program. Lancet. 1972;2:677–9.
10. Lowenstein DH, Alldredge BK. Status epilepticus at an urban public hospital in the 1980s. Neurology. 1993;43:483–8.
11. Pesola GR, Avasarala J. Bupropion seizure proportion among new-onset generalized seizures and drug related seizures presenting to an emergency department. J Emerg Med. 2002;22:235–9.
12. Thundiyil JG, Kearney TE, Olson KR. Evolving epidemiology of drug-induced seizures reported to a Poison Control Center System. J Med Toxicol. 2007;3:15–9.
13. Olson KR, Kearney TE, Dyer JE, Benowitz NL, Blanc PD. Seizures associated with poisoning and drug overdose. Am J Emerg Med. 1994;12:392–5.
14. Messing RO, Closson RG, Simon RP. Drug-induced seizures: a 10-year experience. Neurology. 1984;34:1582–6.
15. Wijdicks EF, Sharbrough FW. New-onset seizures in critically ill patients. Neurology. 1993;43:1042–4.
16. Isbister GK, Downes F, Sibbritt D, Dawson AH, Whyte IM. Aspiration pneumonitis in an overdose population: frequency, predictors, and outcomes. Crit Care Med. 2004;32:88–93.
17. Finkelstein Y, Hutson JR, Freedman SB, Wax P, Brent J, Toxicology Investigators Consortium Case R. Drug-induced seizures in children and adolescents presenting for emergency care: current and emerging trends. Clin Toxicol. 2013;51:761–6.
18. Delanty N, Vaughan CJ, French JA. Medical causes of seizures. Lancet. 1998;352:383–90.
19. Kunisaki TA, Augenstein WL. Drug- and toxin-induced seizures. Emerg Med Clin North Am. 1994;12:1027–56.
20. Garcia PA, Alldredge BK. Drug-induced seizures. Neurol Clin. 1994;12:85–99.
21. Alldredge BK. Drug-induced seizures: controversies in their identification and management. Pharmacotherapy. 1997;17:857–60.
22. Phillips KA, Veenstra DL, Oren E, Lee JK, Sadee W. Potential role of pharmacogenomics in reducing adverse drug reactions: a systematic review. JAMA. 2001;286:2270–9.
23. Vuilleumier PH, Stamer UM, Landau R. Pharmacogenomic considerations in opioid analgesia. Pharmacogen Personal Med. 2012;5:73–87.
24. Gasche Y, Daali Y, Fathi M, et al. Codeine intoxication associated with ultrarapid CYP2D6 metabolism. N Engl J Med. 2004;351: 2827–31.
25. Stamer UM, Stuber F. Codeine induced respiratory depression in a child. Paediatr Anaesth. 2008;18:272–3. author reply 5-6
26. Allen JM, Gelot S. Pharmacogenomics in the intensive care unit: focus on potential implications for clinical practice. Recent Patents Biotechnol. 2014;8:116–22.
27. Yip VL, Hawcutt DB, Pirmohamed M. Pharmacogenetic Markers of Drug Efficacy and Toxicity. Clin Pharmacol Ther. 2015;98:61–70.

28. Wills B, Erickson T. Chemically induced seizures. Clin Lab Med. 2006;26:185–209. ix
29. Haber GW, Litman RS. Generalized tonic-clonic activity after remifentanil administration. Anesth Analg. 2001;93:1532–3. table of contents
30. Ross J, Kearse Jr LA, Barlow MK, Houghton KJ, Cosgrove GR. Alfentanil-induced epileptiform activity: a simultaneous surface and depth electroencephalographic study in complex partial epilepsy. Epilepsia. 2001;42:220–5.
31. Sprung J, Schedewie HK. Apparent focal motor seizure with a jacksonian march induced by fentanyl: a case report and review of the literature. J Clin Anesth. 1992;4:139–43.
32. Tempelhoff R, Modica PA, Bernardo KL, Edwards I. Fentanyl-induced electrocorticographic seizures in patients with complex partial epilepsy. J Neurosurg. 1992;77:201–8.
33. Sinz EH, Kofke WA, Garman RH. Phenytoin, midazolam, and naloxone protect against fentanyl-induced brain damage in rats. Anesth Analg. 2000;91:1443–9.
34. Smith NT, Benthuysen JL, Bickford RG, et al. Seizures during opioid anesthetic induction--are they opioid-induced rigidity? Anesthesiology. 1989;71:852–62.
35. Lupica CR. Delta and mu enkephalins inhibit spontaneous GABA-mediated IPSCs via a cyclic AMP-independent mechanism in the rat hippocampus. J Neurosci Off J Soc Neurosci. 1995;15:737–49.
36. Svoboda KR, Lupica CR. Opioid inhibition of hippocampal interneurons via modulation of potassium and hyperpolarization-activated cation (Ih) currents. J Neurosci Off J Soc Neurosci. 1998;18:7084–98.
37. Parkinson SK, Bailey SL, Little WL, Mueller JB. Myoclonic seizure activity with chronic high-dose spinal opioid administration. Anesthesiology. 1990;72:743–5.
38. Shih CJ, Doufas AG, Chang HC, Lin CM. Recurrent seizure activity after epidural morphine in a post-partum woman. Can J Anaesth. 2005;52:727–9.
39. Gozdemir M, Muslu B, Usta B, Sert H, Demircioglu RI, Gumus II. Generalized seizure in patient receiving epidural meperidine during cesarean section. Ann Pharmacother. 2008;42:1145.
40. Armstrong PJ, Bersten A. Normeperidine toxicity. Anesth Analg. 1986;65:536–8.
41. Knight B, Thomson N, Perry G. Seizures due to norpethidine toxicity. Aust NZ J Med. 2000;30:513.
42. Mather LE, Tucker GT. Systemic availability of orally administered meperidine. Clin Pharmacol Ther. 1976;20:535–40.
43. Kaiko RF, Foley KM, Grabinski PY, et al. Central nervous system excitatory effects of meperidine in cancer patients. Ann Neurol. 1983;13:180–5.
44. Modica PA, Tempelhoff R, White PF. Pro- and anticonvulsant effects of anesthetics (Part I). Anesth Analg. 1990;70:303–15.
45. Koren G, Butt W, Chinyanga H, Soldin S, Tan YK, Pape K. Postoperative morphine infusion in newborn infants: assessment of disposition characteristics and safety. J Pediatr. 1985;107:963–7.
46. Brian Jr JE, Seifen AB. Tonic-clonic activity after sufentanil. Anesth Analg. 1987;66:481.
47. Katz RI, Eide TR, Hartman A, Poppers PJ. Two instances of seizure-like activity in the same patient associated with two different narcotics. Anesth Analg. 1988;67:289–90.
48. Rao TL, Mummaneni N, El-Etr AA. Convulsions: an unusual response to intravenous fentanyl administration. Anesth Analg. 1982;61:1020–1.
49. Safwat AM, Daniel D. Grand mal seizure after fentanyl administration. Anesthesiology. 1983;59:78.
50. Strong WE, Matson M. Probable seizure after alfentanil. Anesth Analg. 1989;68:692–3.
51. Murkin JM, Moldenhauer CC, Hug Jr CC, Epstein CM. Absence of seizures during induction of anesthesia with high-dose fentanyl. Anesth Analg. 1984;63:489–94.
52. Sebel PS, Bovill JG, Wauquier A, Rog P. Effects of high-dose fentanyl anesthesia on the electroencephalogram. Anesthesiology. 1981;55:203–11.
53. Gardner JS, Blough D, Drinkard CR, et al. Tramadol and seizures: a surveillance study in a managed care population. Pharmacotherapy. 2000;20:1423–31.
54. Marquardt KA, Alsop JA, Albertson TE. Tramadol exposures reported to statewide poison control system. Ann Pharmacother. 2005;39:1039–44.
55. Spiller HA, Gorman SE, Villalobos D, et al. Prospective multicenter evaluation of tramadol exposure. Journal of. toxicology. 1997;35:361–4.
56. Talaie H, Panahandeh R, Fayaznouri M, Asadi Z, Abdollahi M. Dose-independent occurrence of seizure with tramadol. J Med Toxicol. 2009;5:63–7.
57. Shadnia S, Brent J, Mousavi-Fatemi K, Hafezi P, Soltaninejad K. Recurrent seizures in tramadol intoxication: implications for therapy based on 100 patients. Basic Clin Pharmacol Toxicol. 2012;111:133–6.
58. Kahn LH, Alderfer RJ, Graham DJ. Seizures reported with tramadol. JAMA. 1997;278:1661.
59. Gasse C, Derby L, Vasilakis-Scaramozza C, Jick H. Incidence of first-time idiopathic seizures in users of tramadol. Pharmacotherapy. 2000;20:629–34.
60. Saidi H, Ghadiri M, Abbasi S, Ahmadi SF. Efficacy and safety of naloxone in the management of postseizure complaints of tramadol intoxicated patients: a self-controlled study. Emerg Med J EMJ. 2010;27:928–30.
61. Smolen A, Smolen TN, van de Kamp JL. The effect of naloxone administration on pregnancy-associated seizures. Life Sci. 1986;38:1899–905.
62. Eizadi-Mood N, Ozcan D, Sabzghabaee AM, Mirmoghtadaee P, Hedaiaty M. Does naloxone prevent seizure in tramadol intoxicated patients? Int J Prev Med. 2014;5:302–7.
63. Tsutaoka BT, Ho RY, Fung SM, Kearney TE. Comparative toxicity of tapentadol and tramadol utilizing data reported to the national poison data system. Ann Pharmacother. 2015;49:1311–6.
64. Quail AW. Modern inhalational anaesthetic agents. A review of halothane, isoflurane and enflurane. Med J Aust. 1989;150:95–102.
65. Julien RM, Kavan EM, Elliott HW. Effects of volatile anaesthetic agents on EEG activity recorded in limbic and sensory systems. Can Anaes Soc J. 1972;19:263–9.
66. Jenkins J, Milne AC. Convulsive reaction following enflurane anaesthesia. Anaesthesia. 1984;39:44–5.
67. Rosen I, Soderberg M. Electroencephalographic activity in children under enflurane anesthesia. Acta Anaesthesiol Scand. 1975;19:361–9.
68. Ohm WW, Cullen BF, Amory DW, Kennedy RD. Delayed seizure activity following enflurane anaesthesia. Anesthesiology. 1975;42:367–8.
69. Kruczek M, Albin MS, Wolf S, Bertoni JM. Postoperative seizure activity following enflurane anaesthesia. Anesthesiology. 1980;53:175–6.
70. Burchiel KJ, Stockard JJ, Calverley RK, Smith NT. Relationship of pre- and postanesthetic EEG abnormalities to enflurane-induced seizure activity. Anesth Analg. 1977;56:509–14.
71. Michenfelder JD, Cucchiara RF. Canine cerebral oxygen consumption during enflurane anesthesia and its modification during induced seizures. Anesthesiology. 1974;40:575–80.
72. Yamashiro M, Sumitomo M, Furuya H. Paroxysmal electroencephalographic discharges during enflurane anaesthesia in patients with a history of cerebral convulsions. Br J Anaesth. 1985;57:1029–37.
73. Hymes JA. Seizure activity during isoflurane anesthesia. Anesth Analg. 1985;64:367–8.
74. Harrison JL. Postoperative seizures after isoflurane anesthesia. Anesth Analg. 1986;65:1235–6.

75. Kofke WA, Young RS, Davis P, et al. Isoflurane for refractory status epilepticus: a clinical series. Anesthesiology. 1989;71:653–9.

76. Kofke WA, Snider MT, Young RS, Ramer JC. Prolonged low flow isoflurane anesthesia for status epilepticus. Anesthesiology. 1985;62:653–6.

77. Yli-Hankala A, Vakkuri A, Sarkela M, Lindgren L, Korttila K, Jantti V. Epileptiform electroencephalogram during mask induction of anesthesia with sevoflurane. Anesthesiology. 1999;91:1596–603.

78. Jantti V, Yli-Hankala A, Vakkuri A. The epileptogenic property of sevoflurane and in patients without epilepsy. Anesth Analg. 2001;92:1359.

79. Vakkuri A, Yli-Hankala A, Sarkela M, et al. Sevoflurane mask induction of anaesthesia is associated with epileptiform EEG in children. Acta Anaesthesiol Scand. 2001;45:805–11.

80. Jaaskelainen SK, Kaisti K, Suni L, Hinkka S, Scheinin H. Sevoflurane is epileptogenic in healthy subjects at surgical levels of anesthesia. Neurology. 2003;61:1073–8.

81. Constant I, Seeman R, Murat I. Sevoflurane and epileptiform EEG changes. Paediatr Anaesth. 2005;15:266–74.

82. Mohanram A, Kumar V, Iqbal Z, Markan S, Pagel PS. Repetitive generalized seizure-like activity during emergence from sevoflurane anesthesia. Can J Anaesth. 2007;54:657–61.

83. Woodforth IJ, Hicks RG, Crawford MR, Stephen JP, Burke DJ. Electroencephalographic evidence of seizure activity under deep sevoflurane anesthesia in a nonepileptic patient. Anesthesiology. 1997;87:1579–82.

84. Julliac B, Guehl D, Chopin F, et al. Risk factors for the occurrence of electroencephalogram abnormalities during induction of anesthesia with sevoflurane in nonepileptic patients. Anesthesiology. 2007;106:243–51.

85. Iijima T, Nakamura Z, Iwao Y, Sankawa H. The epileptogenic properties of the volatile anesthetics sevoflurane and isoflurane in patients with epilepsy. Anesth Analg. 2000;91:989–95.

86. Rudo FG, Krantz Jr JC. Anaesthetic molecules. Br J Anaesth. 1974;46:181–9.

87. Corssen G, Little SC, Tavakoli M. Ketamine and epilepsy. Anesth Analg. 1974;53:319–35.

88. Steen PA, Michenfelder JD. Neurotoxicity of anesthetics. Anesthesiology. 1979;50:437–53.

89. Ferrer-Allado T, Brechner VL, Dymond A, Cozen H, Crandall P. Ketamine-induced electroconvulsive phenomena in the human limbic and thalamic regions. Anesthesiology. 1973;38:333–44.

90. Bennett DR, Madsen JA, Jordan WS, Wiser WC. Ketamine anesthesia in brain-damaged epileptics. Electroencephalographic and clinical observations. Neurology. 1973;23:449–60.

91. Sheth RD, Gidal BE. Refractory status epilepticus: response to ketamine. Neurology. 1998;51:1765–6.

92. Laughlin TP, Newberg LA. Prolonged myoclonus after etomidate anesthesia. Anesth Analg. 1985;64:80–2.

93. Ghoneim MM, Yamada T. Etomidate: a clinical and electroencephalographic comparison with thiopental. Anesth Analg. 1977;56:479–85.

94. Krieger W, Copperman J, Laxer KD. Seizures with etomidate anesthesia. Anesth Analg. 1985;64:1226–7.

95. Ebrahim ZY, DeBoer GE, Luders H, Hahn JF, Lesser RP. Effect of etomidate on the electroencephalogram of patients with epilepsy. Anesth Analg. 1986;65:1004–6.

96. Sutherland MJ, Burt P. Propofol and seizures. Anaesth Intensive Care. 1994;22:733–7.

97. Walder B, Tramer MR, Seeck M. Seizure-like phenomena and propofol: a systematic review. Neurology. 2002;58:1327–32.

98. Bevan JC. Propofol-related convulsions. Can J Anaesth. 1993;40:805–9.

99. Blumer J, Strong JM, Atkinson Jr AJ. The convulsant potency of lidocaine and its N-dealkylated metabolites. J Pharmacol Exp Ther. 1973;186:31–6.

100. Lemmen LJ, Klassen M, Duiser B. Intravenous lidocaine in the treatment of convulsions. JAMA. 1978;239:2025.

101. Bernhard CG, Bohm E. On the effects of xylocain on the central nervous system with special reference to its influence on epileptic phenomena. Experientia. 1954;10:474–6.

102. Reynolds F. Adverse effects of local anaesthetics. Br J Anaesth. 1987;59:78–95.

103. Varelas PN, Mirski MA. Seizures in the adult intensive care unit. J Neurosurg Anesthesiol. 2001;13:163–75.

104. Ochs HR, Carstens G, Greenblatt DJ. Reduction in lidocaine clearance during continuous infusion and by coadministration of propranolol. N Engl J Med. 1980;303:373–7.

105. Feely J, Wilkinson GR, McAllister CB, Wood AJ. Increased toxicity and reduced clearance of lidocaine by cimetidine. Ann Intern Med. 1982;96:592–4.

106. Bauer J. Seizure-inducing effects of antiepileptic drugs: a review. Acta Neurol Scand. 1996;94:367–77.

107. Gayatri NA, Livingston JH. Aggravation of epilepsy by antiepileptic drugs. Dev Med Child Neurol. 2006;48:394–8.

108. Gelisse P, Genton P, Kuate C, Pesenti A, Baldy-Moulinier M, Crespel A. Worsening of seizures by oxcarbazepine in juvenile idiopathic generalized epilepsies. Epilepsia. 2004;45:1282–6.

109. Fink MP, Snydman DR, Niederman MS, et al. Treatment of severe pneumonia in hospitalized patients: results of a multicenter, randomized, double-blind trial comparing intravenous ciprofloxacin with imipenem-cilastatin. The Severe Pneumonia Study Group. Antimicrob Agents Chemother. 1994;38:547–57.

110. Weaver DF, Camfield P, Fraser A. Massive carbamazepine overdose: clinical and pharmacologic observations in five episodes. Neurology. 1988;38:755–9.

111. Wilkus RJ, Dodrill CB, Troupin AS. Carbamazepine and the electroencephalogram of epileptics: a double blind study in comparison to phenytoin. Epilepsia. 1978;19:283–91.

112. Milligan N, Oxley J, Richens A. Acute effects of intravenous phenytoin on the frequency of inter-ictal spikes in man. Br J Clin Pharmacol. 1983;16:285–9.

113. Schachter SC. Iatrogenic seizures. Neurol Clin. 1998;16: 157–70.

114. Walker AE, Johnson HC. Convulsive factor in commercial penicillin. Arch Surg. 1945;50:69–73.

115. Porter J, Jick H. Drug-induced anaphylaxis, convulsions, deafness, and extrapyramidal symptoms. Lancet. 1977;1:587–8.

116. Gutnick MJ, Van Duijn H, Citri N. Relative convulsant potencies of structural analogues of penicillin. Brain Res. 1976;114: 139–43.

117. Fossieck Jr B, Parker RH. Neurotoxicity during intravenous infusion of penicillin. A review. J Clin Pharmacol. 1974;14:504–12.

118. Nicholls PJ. Neurotoxicity of penicillin. J Antimicrob Chemother. 1980;6:161–5.

119. Barrons RW, Murray KM, Richey RM. Populations at risk for penicillin-induced seizures. Ann Pharmacother. 1992;26:26–9.

120. Wallace KL. Antibiotic-induced convulsions. Crit Care Clin. 1997;13:741–62.

121. De Sarro A, De Sarro GB, Ascioti C, Nistico G. Epileptogenic activity of some beta-lactam derivatives: structure-activity relationship. Neuropharmacology. 1989;28:359–65.

122. Bechtel TP, Slaughter RL, Moore TD. Seizures associated with high cerebrospinal fluid concentrations of cefazolin. Am J Hosp Pharm. 1980;37:271–3.

123. Grill MF, Maganti R. Cephalosporin-induced neurotoxicity: clinical manifestations, potential pathogenic mechanisms, and the role of electroencephalographic monitoring. Ann Pharmacother. 2008;42:1843–50.

124. Dakdouki GK, Al-Awar GN. Cefepime-induced encephalopathy. Int J Infect Dis: IJID. 2004;8:59–61.

125. Fernandez-Torre JL, Martinez-Martinez M, Gonzalez-Rato J, et al. Cephalosporin-induced nonconvulsive status epilepticus:

clinical and electroencephalographic features. Epilepsia. 2005;46:1550–2.

126. Naeije G, Lorent S, Vincent JL, Legros B. Continuous epileptiform discharges in patients treated with cefepime or meropenem. Arch Neurol. 2011;68:1303–7.

127. Norrby SR. Neurotoxicity of carbapenem antibacterials. Drug Saf. 1996;15:87–90.

128. Schliamser SE, Broholm KA, Liljedahl AL, Norrby SR. Comparative neurotoxicity of benzylpenicillin, imipenem/cilastatin and FCE 22101, a new injectible penem. J Antimicrob Chemother. 1988;22:687–95.

129. Calandra G, Lydick E, Carrigan J, Weiss L, Guess H. Factors predisposing to seizures in seriously ill infected patients receiving antibiotics: experience with imipenem/cilastatin. Am J Med. 1988;84:911–8.

130. Pestotnik SL, Classen DC, Evans RS, Stevens LE, Burke JP. Prospective surveillance of imipenem/cilastatin use and associated seizures using a hospital information system. Ann Pharmacother. 1993;27:497–501.

131. Norrby SR, Gildon KM. Safety profile of meropenem: a review of nearly 5, 000 patients treated with meropenem. Scand J Infect Dis. 1999;31:3–10.

132. Christ W. Central nervous system toxicity of quinolones: human and animal findings. J Antimicrob Chemother. 1990;26(Suppl B):219–25.

133. Akahane K, Sekiguchi M, Une T, Osada Y. Structure-epileptogenicity relationship of quinolones with special reference to their interaction with gamma-aminobutyric acid receptor sites. Antimicrob Agents Chemother. 1989;33:1704–8.

134. Christie MJ, Wong K, Ting RH, Tam PY, Sikaneta TG. Generalized seizure and toxic epidermal necrolysis following levofloxacin exposure. Ann Pharmacother. 2005;39:953–5.

135. O'Donnell JA, Gelone SP. Fluoroquinolones. Infect Dis Clin N Am. 2000;14:489–513. xi

136. Lietman PS. Fluoroquinolone toxicities. An update. Drugs. 1995;49(Suppl 2):159–63.

137. Schwartz MT, Calvert JF. Potential neurologic toxicity related to ciprofloxacin. DICP. 1990;24:138–40.

138. Slavich IL, Gleffe RF, Haas EJ. Grand mal epileptic seizures during ciprofloxacin therapy. JAMA. 1989;261:558–9.

139. Coyer JR, Nicholson DP. Isoniazid-induced convulsions. South Med J. 1976;69:294–7.

140. Devadatta S. Isoniazid-induced encephalopathy. Lancet. 1965;2:440.

141. Mahler ME. Seizures: common causes and treatment in the elderly. Geriatrics. 1987;42:73–8.

142. Orlowski JP, Paganini EP, Pippenger CE. Treatment of a potentially lethal dose isoniazid ingestion. Ann Emerg Med. 1988;17:73–6.

143. Nelson LG. Grand mal seizures following overdose of isoniazid. a report of four cases. Am Rev Respir Dis. 1965;91:600–4.

144. Alvarez FG, Guntupalli KK. Isoniazid overdose: four case reports and review of the literature. Intensive Care Med. 1995;21:641–4.

145. Wason S, Lacouture PG, Lovejoy Jr FH. Single high-dose pyridoxine treatment for isoniazid overdose. JAMA. 1981;246:1102–4.

146. Frytak S, Moertel CH, Childs DS. Neurologic toxicity associated with high-dose metronidazole therapy. Ann Intern Med. 1978;88:361–2.

147. Kusumi RK, Plouffe JF, Wyatt RH, Fass RJ. Central nervous system toxicity associated with metronidazole therapy. Ann Intern Med. 1980;93:59–60.

148. Bailes J, Willis J, Priebe C, Strub R. Encephalopathy with metronidazole in a child. Am J Dis child (1960). 1983;137:290–1.

149. Semel JD, Allen N. Seizures in patients simultaneously receiving theophylline and imipenem or ciprofloxacin or metronidazole. South Med J. 1991;84:465–8.

150. Jayaweera DT. Minimising the dosage-limiting toxicities of foscarnet induction therapy. Drug Saf. 1997;16:258–66.

151. Kitching AR, Fagg D, Hay NM, Hatfield PJ, Macdonald A. Neurotoxicity associated with acyclovir in end stage renal failure. New Zealand Med J. 1997;110:167–9.

152. Rashiq S, Briewa L, Mooney M, Giancarlo T, Khatib R, Wilson FM. Distinguishing acyclovir neurotoxicity from encephalomyelitis. J Intern Med. 1993;234:507–11.

153. Barton TL, Roush MK, Dever LL. Seizures associated with ganciclovir therapy. Pharmacotherapy. 1992;12:413–5.

154. Pascual-Sedano B, Iranzo A, Marti-Fabregas J, et al. Prospective study of new-onset seizures in patients with human immunodeficiency virus infection: etiologic and clinical aspects. Arch Neurol. 1999;56:609–12.

155. Romanelli F, Jennings HR, Nath A, Ryan M, Berger J. Therapeutic dilemma: the use of anticonvulsants in HIV-positive individuals. Neurology. 2000;54:1404–7.

156. Zwillich CW, Sutton FD, Neff TA, Cohn WM, Matthay RA, Weinberger MM. Theophylline-induced seizures in adults. Correlation with serum concentrations. Ann Intern Med. 1975;82:784–7.

157. Bahls FH, Ma KK, Bird TD. Theophylline-associated seizures with "therapeutic" or low toxic serum concentrations: risk factors for serious outcome in adults. Neurology. 1991;41:1309–12.

158. Gaudreault P, Guay J. Theophylline poisoning. Pharmacological considerations and clinical management. Med Toxicol. 1986;1:169–91.

159. Aitken ML, Martin TR. Life-threatening theophylline toxicity is not predictable by serum levels. Chest. 1987;91:10–4.

160. Paloucek FP, Rodvold KA. Evaluation of theophylline overdoses and toxicities. Ann Emerg Med. 1988;17:135–44.

161. Zaccara G, Muscas GC, Messori A. Clinical features, pathogenesis and management of drug-induced seizures. Drug Saf. 1990;5:109–51.

162. Henderson A, Wright DM, Pond SM. Management of theophylline overdose patients in the intensive care unit. Anaesth Intensive Care. 1992;20:56–62.

163. Olson KR, Benowitz NL, Woo OF, Pond SM. Theophylline overdose: acute single ingestion versus chronic repeated overmedication. Am J Emerg Med. 1985;3:386–94.

164. Kumar A, Bleck TP. Intravenous midazolam for the treatment of refractory status epilepticus. Crit Care Med. 1992;20:483–8.

165. Scott JP, Higenbottam TW. Adverse reactions and interactions of cyclosporin. Med Toxicol Adv Drug Exp. 1988;3:107–27.

166. Gilmore RL. Seizures and antiepileptic drug use in transplant patients. Neurol Clin. 1988;6:279–96.

167. Truwit CL, Denaro CP, Lake JR, DeMarco T. MR imaging of reversible cyclosporin A-induced neurotoxicity. AJNR. 1991;12:651–9.

168. Glass GA, Stankiewicz J, Mithoefer A, Freeman R, Bergethon PR. Levetiracetam for seizures after liver transplantation. Neurology. 2005;64:1084–5.

169. Ekberg H, Grinyo J, Nashan B, et al. Cyclosporine sparing with mycophenolate mofetil, daclizumab and corticosteroids in renal allograft recipients: the CAESAR Study. Am J Transplant. 2007;7:560–70.

170. Maramattom BV, Wijdicks EF. Sirolimus may not cause neurotoxicity in kidney and liver transplant recipients. Neurology. 2004;63:1958–9.

171. Thistlethwaite Jr JR, Stuart JK, Mayes JT, et al. Complications and monitoring of OKT3 therapy. Am J Kidney Dis. 1988;11:112–9.

172. Kay HE, Knapton PJ, O'Sullivan JP, et al. Encephalopathy in acute leukaemia associated with methotrexate therapy. Arch Dis Child. 1972;47:344–54.

173. Johnson FL, Bernstein ID, Hartmann JR, Chard Jr RL. Seizures associated with vincristine sulfate therapy. J Pediatr. 1973;82:699–702.

174. Singh G, Rees JH, Sander JW. Seizures and epilepsy in oncological practice: causes, course, mechanisms and treatment. J Neurol Neurosurg Psychiatry. 2007;78:342–9.

175. Pisani F, Oteri G, Costa C, Di Raimondo G, Di Perri R. Effects of psychotropic drugs on seizure threshold. Drug Saf. 2002;25:91–110.

176. Alldredge BK. Seizure risk associated with psychotropic drugs: clinical and pharmacokinetic considerations. Neurology. 1999;53:S68–75.

177. Logothetis J. Spontaneous epileptic seizures and electroencephalographic changes in the course of phenothiazine therapy. Neurology. 1967;17:869–77.

178. Cold JA, Wells BG, Froemming JH. Seizure activity associated with antipsychotic therapy. DICP. 1990;24:601–6.

179. Remick RA, Fine SH. Antipsychotic drugs and seizures. The Journal of clinical psychiatry. 1979;40:78–80.

180. Chase PB, Biros MH. A retrospective review of the use and safety of droperidol in a large, high-risk, inner-city emergency department patient population. Acad Emerg Med Off J Soc Acad Emerg Med. 2002;9:1402–10.

181. Devinsky O, Honigfeld G, Patin J. Clozapine-related seizures. Neurology. 1991;41:369–71.

182. Ereshefsky L, Watanabe MD, Tran-Johnson TK. Clozapine: an atypical antipsychotic agent. Clin Pharm. 1989;8:691–709.

183. Wilson WH, Claussen AM. Seizures associated with clozapine treatment in a state hospital. The Journal of clinical psychiatry. 1994;55:184–8.

184. Toth P, Frankenburg FR. Clozapine and seizures: a review. Can J Psychiatr. 1994;39:236–8.

185. Navarro V, Pons A, Romero A, Bernardo M. Topiramate for clozapine-induced seizures. Am J Psychiatry. 2001;158:968–9.

186. Centorrino F, Price BH, Tuttle M, et al. EEG abnormalities during treatment with typical and atypical antipsychotics. Am J Psychiatry. 2002;159:109–15.

187. Amann BL, Pogarell O, Mergl R, et al. EEG abnormalities associated with antipsychotics: a comparison of quetiapine, olanzapine, haloperidol and healthy subjects. Human Psychopharmacol. 2003;18:641–6.

188. Barnes TR, McPhillips MA. Critical analysis and comparison of the side-effect and safety profiles of the new antipsychotics. Br J Psychiatry. 1999;34-43

189. Citrome L. New antipsychotic medications: what advantages do they offer? Postgrad Med. 1997;101:207–10. 13-4

190. Casey DE. The relationship of pharmacology to side effects. The Journal of clinical psychiatry. 1997;58(Suppl 10):55–62.

191. Hedges D, Jeppson K, Whitehead P. Antipsychotic medication and seizures: a review. Drugs Today (Barc). 2003;39:551–7.

192. Alper K, Schwartz KA, Kolts RL, Khan A. Seizure incidence in psychopharmacological clinical trials: an analysis of Food and Drug Administration (FDA) summary basis of approval reports. Biol Psychiatry. 2007;62:345–54.

193. Wyderski RJ, Starrett WG, Abou-Saif A. Fatal status epilepticus associated with olanzapine therapy. Ann Pharmacother. 1999;33:787–9.

194. Lee JW, Crismon ML, Dorson PG. Seizure associated with olanzapine. Ann Pharmacother. 1999;33:554–6.

195. Pillmann F, Schlote K, Broich K, Marneros A. Electroencephalogram alterations during treatment with olanzapine. Psychopharmacology. 2000;150:216–9.

196. Lee KC, Finley PR, Alldredge BK. Risk of seizures associated with psychotropic medications: emphasis on new drugs and new findings. Expert Opin Drug Saf. 2003;2:233–47.

197. Woolley J, Smith S. Lowered seizure threshold on olanzapine. Br J Psychiatry. 2001;178:85–6.

198. Rosenstein DL, Nelson JC, Jacobs SC. Seizures associated with antidepressants: a review. The Journal of clinical psychiatry. 1993;54:289–99.

199. Wedin GP, Oderda GM, Klein-Schwartz W, Gorman RL. Relative toxicity of cyclic antidepressants. Ann Emerg Med. 1986;15:797–804.

200. Starkey IR, Lawson AA. Poisoning with tricyclic and related antidepressants--a ten-year review. The Quarterly journal of medicine. 1980;49:33–49.

201. Brooke G, Weatherly JR. Imipramine. Lancet. 1959;2:568–9.

202. DeVeaugh-Geiss J, Landau P, Katz R. Preliminary results from a multicenter trial of clomipramine in obsessive-compulsive disorder. Psychopharmacol Bull. 1989;25:36–40.

203. Preskorn SH, Fast GA. Tricyclic antidepressant-induced seizures and plasma drug concentration. J Clin Psy. 1992;53:160–2.

204. Lowry MR, Dunner FJ. Seizures during tricyclic therapy. Am J Psychiatry. 1980;137:1461–2.

205. Kulig K, Rumack BH, Sullivan Jr JB, et al. Amoxapine overdose. Coma and seizures without cardiotoxic effects. JAMA. 1982;248:1092–4.

206. Boehnert MT, Lovejoy Jr FH. Value of the QRS duration versus the serum drug level in predicting seizures and ventricular arrhythmias after an acute overdose of tricyclic antidepressants. N Engl J Med. 1985;313:474–9.

207. Ellison DW, Pentel PR. Clinical features and consequences of seizures due to cyclic antidepressant overdose. Am J Emerg Med. 1989;7:5–10.

208. Favale E, Rubino V, Mainardi P, Lunardi G, Albano C. Anticonvulsant effect of fluoxetine in humans. Neurology. 1995;45:1926–7.

209. Braitberg G, Curry SC. Seizure after isolated fluoxetine overdose. Ann Emerg Med. 1995;26:234–7.

210. Kelly CA, Dhaun N, Laing WJ, Strachan FE, Good AM, Bateman DN. Comparative toxicity of citalopram and the newer antidepressants after overdose. J Toxicol. 2004;42:67–71.

211. Akcan A, Sozuer E, Akyildiz H, Ozturk A, Atalay A, Yilmaz Z. Predisposing factors and surgical outcome of complicated liver hydatid cysts. World J Gastroenterol WJG. 2010;16:3040–8.

212. Bodner RA, Lynch T, Lewis L, Kahn D. Serotonin syndrome. Neurology. 1995;45:219–23.

213. Carbone JR. The neuroleptic malignant and serotonin syndromes. Emerg Med Clin North Am. 2000;18:317–25. x

214. Lieberman JA, Kane JM, Reife R. Neuromuscular effects of monoamine oxidase inhibitors. J Clin Psychopharmacol. 1985;5:221–8.

215. Belson MG, Kelley TR. Bupropion exposures: clinical manifestations and medical outcome. J Emerg Med. 2002;23:223–30.

216. Davidson J. Seizures and bupropion: a review. The Journal of clinical psychiatry. 1989;50:256–61.

217. Rissmiller DJ, Campo T. Extended-release bupropion induced grand mal seizures. J Am Osteopathic Assoc. 2007;107:441–2.

218. Starr PA, Martin AJ, Larson PS. Implantation of deep brain stimulator electrodes using interventional MRI. Neurosurg Clin N Am. 2009;20:193–203.

219. Nierenberg AA, Cole JO. Antidepressant adverse drug reactions. The Journal of clinical psychiatry. 1991;52(Suppl):40–7.

220. Johnston JA, Lineberry CG, Ascher JA, et al. A 102-center prospective study of seizure in association with bupropion. The Journal of clinical psychiatry. 1991;52:450–6.

221. Whyte IM, Dawson AH, Buckley NA. Relative toxicity of venlafaxine and selective serotonin reuptake inhibitors in overdose compared to tricyclic antidepressants. QJM. 2003;96:369–74.

222. Struve FA. Lithium-specific pathological electroencephalographic changes: a successful replication of earlier investigative results. Clin EEG (electroencephalography). 1987;18:46–53.

223. Hansen HE, Amdisen A. Lithium intoxication. (Report of 23 cases and review of 100 cases from the literature). Q J Med. 1978;47:123–44.

224. Okusa MD, Crystal LJ. Clinical manifestations and management of acute lithium intoxication. Am J Med. 1994;97:383–9.

225. Mayan H, Golubev N, Dinour D, Farfel Z. Lithium intoxication due to carbamazepine-induced renal failure. Ann Pharmacother. 2001;35:560–2.

226. Shukla S, Godwin CD, Long LE, Miller MG. Lithium-carbamazepine neurotoxicity and risk factors. Am J Psychiatry. 1984;141:1604–6.

227. Happe S. Excessive daytime sleepiness and sleep disturbances in patients with neurological diseases: epidemiology and management. Drugs. 2003;63:2725–37.

228. Zagnoni PG, Albano C. Psychostimulants and epilepsy. Epilepsia. 2002;43(Suppl 2):28–31.

229. Thomas S, Upadhyaya H. Adderall and seizures. J Am Acad Child Adolesc Psychiatry. 2002;41:365.

230. Hemmer SA, Pasternak JF, Zecker SG, Trommer BL. Stimulant therapy and seizure risk in children with ADHD. Pediatr Neurol. 2001;24:99–102.

231. Ivanenko A, Tauman R, Gozal D. Modafinil in the treatment of excessive daytime sleepiness in children. Sleep Med. 2003;4:579–82.

232. Green LB, Nelson VS. Death after acute withdrawal of intrathecal baclofen: case report and literature review. Arch Phys Med Rehabil. 1999;80:1600–4.

233. Kofler M, Arturo LA. Prolonged seizure activity after baclofen withdrawal. Neurology. 1992;42:697–8.

234. Greenberg MI, Hendrickson RG. Baclofen withdrawal following removal of an intrathecal baclofen pump despite oral baclofen replacement. Journal of. toxicology. 2003;41:83–5.

235. Koppel C, Ibe K, Tenczer J. Clinical symptomatology of diphenhydramine overdose: an evaluation of 136 cases in 1982 to 1985. Journal of. toxicology. 1987;25:53–70.

236. Magera BE, Betlach CJ, Sweatt AP, Derrick Jr CW. Hydroxyzine intoxication in a 13-month-old child. Pediatrics. 1981;67:280–3.

237. Nelson M, Bartlett RJ, Lamb JT. Seizures after intravenous contrast media for cranial computed tomography. J Neurol Neurosurg Psychiatry. 1989;52:1170–5.

238. Avrahami E, Weiss-Peretz J, Cohn DF. Focal epileptic activity following intravenous contrast material injection in patients with metastatic brain disease. J Neurol Neurosurg Psychiatry. 1987;50:221–3.

239. Weinstein RS. Recognition and management of poisoning with beta-adrenergic blocking agents. Ann Emerg Med. 1984;13:1123–31.

240. Das G, Ferris JC. Generalized convulsions in a patient receiving ultrashort-acting beta-blocker infusion. Drug Intell Clin Pharm. 1988;22:484–5.

241. Shah AS, Eddleston M. Should phenytoin or barbiturates be used as second-line anticonvulsant therapy for toxicological seizures? Clin Toxicol. 2010;48:800–5.

242. Varelas PN, Spanaki MV, Mirski MA. Seizures and the neurosurgical intensive care unit. Neurosurg Clin N Am. 2013;24:393–406.

243. Ziai WC, Kaplan PW. Seizures and status epilepticus in the intensive care unit. Semin Neurol. 2008;28:668–81.

244. Sabers A, Gram L. Newer anticonvulsants: comparative review of drug interactions and adverse effects. Drugs. 2000;60:23–33.

245. Franson KL, Hay DP, Neppe V, et al. Drug-induced seizures in the elderly. Causative agents and optimal management. Drugs Aging. 1995;7:38–48.

Illicit Drugs and Toxins and Critical Care Seizures

Maggie L. McNulty, Andreas Luft, and Thomas P. Bleck

Introduction

Seizures due to toxins and illicit drugs are usually related to an imbalance in the cerebral equilibrium of excitation and inhibition. Neuronal excitation is a result of an influx of sodium and calcium, or a decrease in chloride influx or potassium efflux. In contrast, neuronal inhibition is facilitated by a decrease in sodium influx or an augmentation of chloride influx or potassium efflux. Several pathways trigger seizures, including drugs that block adenosine, histamine, and GABA receptors as well as substances that stimulate cholinergic and glutamate receptors [1] (see Table 21.1). Toxins such as cocaine or soman (a nerve agent) cause seizures in part by increasing excitatory amino acids, as opposed to flumazenil, lindane, or pentylenetetrazole, which have proconvulsant effects due to their effect on GABA receptors. Adenosine is an endogenous neurotransmitter that may be responsible for interictal cessation of seizures, since adenosine release is associated with brief periods of postictal electrical silence. Adenosine antagonists such as theophylline in toxic doses have been associated with status epilepticus (SE) with as high as a 23% incidence of death [2].

A variety of drugs and toxins cause seizures or SE requiring ICU admission. Increased morbidity has been associated with seizures, including hyperthermia, acidosis, anoxic brain injury, and an eightfold increased risk of aspiration pneumonitis [3]. If intoxication is suspected, identification of the causative agent is imperative, as specific therapies aimed at toxin elimination may be required in parallel with antiepileptic treatment and supportive measures. Seizures may also occur as a result of withdrawal of recreational drugs while a patient is in the ICU for other reasons. Seizures then complicate the case and may interfere with treatment of the primary disease. Timely identification of the drug or the toxin involved is mandatory. Accompanying symptoms (e.g., delirium), the patient's history, and drug screens in blood and urine must be taken into consideration.

Toxin-induced seizures are typically generalized and self-limited and may not require antiepileptic treatment. However, SE has been reported to occur in 4–10% of cases [4], which has been associated with certain drugs/toxins more frequently (see Table 21.2). There are limited evidence-based approaches for treatment of drug- and toxin-induced seizures. For the majority of cases, antiepileptic treatment should be centered on GABA agonists. Benzodiazepines continue to be first-line therapy for drug- and toxin-related seizures. Propofol may be tried as a second-line treatment for refractory drug-induced seizures. Phenytoin is not considered first- or second-line therapy as it is ineffective for the majority of drug- and toxin-related seizures. In certain instances, phenytoin can exacerbate seizures associated with cocaine, lidocaine, theophylline, and organochlorine insecticides. Limited evidence exists for the efficacy of valproic acid or levetiracetam in treatment of drug- and toxin-related seizures, but could reasonably be considered as a third-line agent [4].

Epidemiology

The incidence of toxin-related seizures is unknown. A prospective study of patients presenting with their first convulsive seizure found that 8.5% of patients older than 25 years have a toxic/metabolic etiology; 11% of patients older than 60 years have a toxic/metabolic etiology; and 24% of patients between 40 and 65 years have a toxic/metabolic/vascular etiology [2].

M.L. McNulty (✉)
Department of Neurological Sciences, Rush Medical College, Rush University Medical Center,
600 S Paulina St, Chicago, IL 60612, USA
e-mail: maggie_mcnulty@rush.edu

A. Luft
Department of Vascular Neurology and Rehabilitation, University Hospital of Zurich, Rämistrasse 100, 8091 Zurich, Switzerland
e-mail: Andreas.luft@uzh.ch

T.P. Bleck
Department of Neurological Sciences, Neurosurgery, Anesthesiology, and Medicine, Rush Medical College, Chicago, IL, USA
e-mail: tbleck@rush.edu

Table 21.1 .Mechanisms associated with toxin-induced seizures

1.	Activity at NMDA and GABA receptors
2.	Disturbances of ion flux: typically involves sodium channels in which there is an alteration in the resting potential of nerve cells
3.	Adenosine antagonism
4.	Alterations in the concentration or activity of biogenic amines and catecholamines

Modified from Sharma AN, Hoffman RJ. Toxin-related seizures. Emerg Med Clin North Am. 2011 Feb;29(1):125–39, with permission from Elsevier

Table 21.2. Drugs/toxins that cause or precipitate status epilepticus

1.	Star fruit
2.	Endosulfan (pesticide)
3.	Domoic acid
4.	Soman (chemical weapon)
5.	Cocaine
6.	Tetramine (rodenticide)
7.	Camphor
8.	Aluminum-containing biomaterial
9.	Carbon monoxide
10.	Colloidal silver
11.	Ecstasy
12.	Lead
13.	Lysergic acid amide
14.	Maneb
15.	Neem oil
16.	Nitromethane
17.	Petrol sniffing

Modified from Tan RY, Neligan A, Shorvon SD. The uncommon causes of status epilepticus: a systematic review. Epilepsy Res. 2010 Oct;91(2–3):111–22, with permission from Elsevier

A retrospective review of the California Poison Control in 2003 evaluated the causes of all drug-related seizures [3]: of 386 cases, 7.5 and 6.9% were related to tramadol and amphetamine use, respectively, while 37% were related to antidepressants (tricyclics, bupropion, venlafaxine, of which 23% were related to bupropion), 8% to diphenhydramine, and 6% to isoniazid. The majority of these cases resulted in a single seizure, but 3.6% resulted in SE. Similarly, in a retrospective study of 142 pediatric drug-induced seizures, the antidepressant class of medications was the most common etiologic agent, representing 42% of the cases. Of those cases involving antidepressants, bupropion was the identified antidepressant in approximately 50% of cases [5].

Illicit or Abused Drugs

Chronic use, overdose (intoxication), and withdrawal are potential causes of seizures in illicit drugs users. A retrospective analysis identified 49 cases of recreational drug-induced seizures admitted to the San Francisco General Hospital between 1975 and 1987. Whereas the great majority had one single focal or generalized seizure, seven patients had multiple convulsions and two developed SE requiring ICU admission [6]. Identified drugs were cocaine (32 cases), amphetamine (11 cases), heroin (7 cases), and phencyclidine (4 cases). All except one patient had complete recovery.

This analysis demonstrates that hospital admissions for recreational drug-induced seizures are infrequent. Routine screening for recreational drugs in patients admitted to the hospital because of a seizure has a low yield and should only be considered if the patient's history raises suspicion for drug abuse, but, oftentimes, drug screens do not include the majority of drugs that can cause seizures [7]. However, if illicit drugs are suspected and seizure activity is prolonged, ICU care is necessary because management of drug-related seizures may be extremely difficult.

Opiates

Opiates include natural (endogenous, e.g., endorphin; exogenous, e.g., morphine, a constituent of the milky extract of opium poppy, *Papaver somniferum*) or synthetic compounds (e.g., fentanyl) acting on central opiate receptors and producing psychological and physical dependence. Heroin (diacetylmorphine, a lipophilic morphine analogue with faster blood-brain barrier passage) is the most commonly used recreational opiate leading to abuse and addiction. Intoxication usually caused by intravenous administration of an overdose presents with coma, respiratory depression, pinpoint but reactive pupils, and vomiting. Seizures are uncommon, which seems expected given the inhibitory actions of opiates on the brain: opiate receptors (μ, δ, κ) inhibit the adenylate cyclase and close Ca^{2+} channels via G-protein-mediated pathways and thereby reduce neuronal excitability. Pro-convulsant effects of morphine have been reported in an in vitro murine hippocampal preparation precipitated by selective stimulation of mu and kappa opiate receptors [8]. In humans, seizures have been reported in 2% of heroin overdose patients [9], which may be attributed to heroin itself [10] or to adulterants. Inadvertent intrathecal application of morphine has led to seizure in one reported case [11].

Because seizures related to opiates themselves are uncommon, other causes should be explored. These can be direct toxic effects of adulterant drugs, or the result of other diseases frequently observed in the addicted population (stroke, infection, neoplasms, and metabolic derangement). Adulterant drugs should be sought in laboratory analysis [12]. Acute opiate intoxication can be treated with the antagonist naloxone (0.8 mg iv, repeated as needed up to 20 mg). No specific recommendations exist for the use of antiepileptic drugs. Certain opioids are more commonly associated with seizures and those include tramadol, propoxyphene, and meperidine (see more details in the drug-induced seizures chapter of this book).

In contrast to acute overdose, chronic heroin abuse is an independent risk factor for seizures with an adjusted odds ratio of 2.8 that increased to 3.6 when concomitant brain pathology was present [13]. Seizures sometimes accompany opiate withdrawal which in adults typically presents with flu-like symptoms. A study by Wijdicks and Sharbrough evaluating patients with new onset seizures admitted to the medical or surgical ICU at the Mayo Clinic identified sudden withdrawal of narcotics as a cause of tonic-clonic seizures [14]. Among all admissions with first-ever seizure of identifiable cause, patients in opioid withdrawal constituted the largest group. However, they represented only a small fraction of all ICU admissions during the 10-year study period (0.066%). Therefore, opioid withdrawal seizure remains a rare cause of ICU admission. General withdrawal symptoms are usually well handled with methadone (20 mg once or twice daily). Withdrawal in the neonate (neonatal abstinence syndrome, NAS) who was exposed to opiates taken by the mother is more severe and more frequently associated with seizures. Its treatment should be based on substitution of opiates. If sedatives are required, phenobarbital should be preferred to diazepam [15].

The opiate oxycodone has been reported to lower seizure threshold in patients with a history of seizures or acute renal failure. One epileptic patient seized several times after ingestion of oxycodone. Seizures were controlled with carbamazepine and the opiate could be continued [16].

Sedatives and Hypnotics

Sedative agents used for recreational purposes include benzodiazepines, barbiturates, and others (e.g., glutethimide, methaqualone). Barbiturates especially have an addictive potential of psychological and physical dependence which is between stimulants (see below) and opiates. Benzodiazepines, with a lower abusive potential, may also lead to withdrawal symptoms. Seizures, however, are not as common as with withdrawal from barbiturates. In a study in which patients were withdrawn from therapeutic doses of benzodiazepines taken for several months, withdrawal seizures were not reported [17]. As benzodiazepines and barbiturates are powerful antiepileptic drugs, seizures have not been observed with overdose—mostly administered on suicidal purpose. However, flumazenil used as a benzodiazepine antidote has led to partial seizures [18] and fatal SE [19].

Withdrawal from benzodiazepines and barbiturates may be complicated by seizures along with delirium tremens (in many aspects similar to alcohol withdrawal) and often requires ICU care. Seizure susceptibility is explained in part by the downregulation of $GABA_A$ receptors by long-term use of these sedatives [20, 21]. Additionally, a role of the glutamatergic system is suspected because reduced susceptibility was observed after treating benzodiazepine-dependent mice with an NMDA antagonist [22].

Seizures are observed in 3% of patients going through benzodiazepine or barbiturate withdrawal [23]. They typically occur within 1–10 days after stopping the drug, depending on the specific agent's half-life and the previously ingested dose [24]. For example, with short-acting barbiturates, such as secobarbital, pentobarbital, or amobarbital, seizures are expected within the first 2–3 days after abrupt withdrawal of the drug and, as with alcohol, are followed occasionally by delirium tremens. Withdrawal from long-term use of pentobarbital is associated with seizures in 10% of subjects taking 600 mg per day and in 75% taking 900 mg. With lower daily doses of 400 mg, electroencephalographic changes consistent with epileptiform discharges can be found in up to one third of patients [25]. Sedative withdrawal seizures should be treated with titrated doses of benzodiazepine or barbiturate (determination of a "stabilization dose," usually 200 mg pentobarbital every 6 h, followed by gradual tapering over 2–3 weeks). Most other antiepileptic drugs are ineffective.

Other sedatives, such as chloral hydrate and meprobamate, can also cause seizures during withdrawal. In contrast, glutethimide [26] and pentazocine/tripelennamine (T's and blues) can produce seizures on ingestion [27].

Stimulants

Psychostimulants include amphetamines, ephedrine, and methylphenidate; these agents release monoamines at the synaptic nerve terminals. Clinical use of amphetamines is established for treatment of narcolepsy, hyperactivity in children, and the control of obesity. Due to their widespread use, amphetamines are easy to procure; after cannabis, amphetamines are the most common drugs of abuse. Use of methylenedioxymethamphetamine (MDMA, "ecstasy" or "molly"), an amphetamine with stimulant and hallucinogenic properties, has quadrupled over the past decade [28]. Another psychostimulant with properties similar to MDMA is cocaine. In contrast to amphetamines, cocaine blocks the reuptake of monoamines such as norepinephrine, dopamine, and serotonin at synaptic nerve endings.

The incidence of amphetamine-associated seizures is unknown; 4% (44/1019) of patients presenting to an Australian hospital with first-ever seizure were noted as having an amphetamine-associated seizure [29]. Reported frequencies of cocaine-induced seizures vary between 1 and 40% [30]. Seizures can occur with psychostimulant overdose but also after intentional administration of high doses. In one study, women were more likely to present with seizures than men (18% vs. 6%) [31]. Seizures occur with amphetamines, especially MDMA, even at intentional doses [32], but are less frequent than with cocaine [6] . MDMA causes euphoria and mental stimulation; however, it can also lead to more serious adverse effects such as hyperthermia, seizures, hyponatremia, rhabdomyolysis, and multi-organ failure [33]. An association exists between MDMA or cocaine use and acute catastrophic neurovascular events, such as subarachnoid hemorrhage, intraparenchymal hemorrhage, and ischemic stroke. These events can on their own produce seizures [34, 35]. These seizures are commonly focal, whereas the typical cocaine-induced seizure is generalized. Brain imaging studies should therefore be considered in stimulant users with focal seizures. Convulsions induced by cocaine are usually of short duration and occur immediately or within a few hours. MDMA produces a secondary clonic phase after the initial ictal event [36]. Rarely, SE develops, requiring ICU care. Complex partial SE has been reported with alkaloid "crack" cocaine abuse (smoked) in a patient who presented with bizarre behavior thought to be "cocaine psychosis" [14]. Seizures during stimulant withdrawal have not been reported. Newer, designer amphetamines, which oftentimes have little cross-reactivity with commercial urine toxicology screening, such as 2,5-dimethoxy-4-chloroamphetamine (DOC), have been reported to be associated with SE [37]. Benzodiazepines remain the first-line treatment for cocaine-induced seizures followed by barbiturates. If seizures are refractory still, then propofol may be useful. Current reports have not shown effectiveness or reduction in lethality with the use of phenytoin in the setting of cocaine intoxication [38]. In a mouse model, cannabidiol (CBD) pretreatment inhibited cocaine-induced acute seizure as well as associated liver injury [39]. However, SE after cocaine but also after MDMA is notoriously refractory to conventional treatment and requires ICU management [31, 40–42]. 4-Methylaminorex-related seizures can be treated with the calcium channel blocker flunarizine [34].

Solvents

Solvents include hydrocarbons, ketones, esters, and ethers and are commonly consumed by inhalation of glues, cleaning fluids, paint thinners, or anesthetics. Addictive effects resemble those of ethanol. Chronic abuse can lead to focal neurological deficits (e.g., cranial nerve palsies, internuclear ophthalmoplegia, and peripheral neuropathy) [43] and CNS demyelination [44]. Severe intoxication or oral administration can be accompanied by seizures [45, 46]. Seizures may be partial or generalized [47, 48]. Chronic solvent exposure may also lead to temporal lobe epilepsy as demonstrated by a case of occupational intoxication [49]. Seizures were fully controlled after stopping the exposure to cyclohexanone and isopropanol.

1,4-Butanediol is a solvent that is metabolized to gamma-hydroxybutyric acid (GHB), a metabolite that acts through GABA receptors. GHB and its derivative gamma-butyrolactone (GBL) have gained popularity as an illicit drug due to its sedative, anxiolytic, and euphoria-inducing effects. Poisoning leads to states of confusion, aggression, and combative behavior and later coma, respiratory depression, and death. Withdrawal is characterized by tremor, hallucinations, tachycardia, insomnia, and, in a few reported cases, epileptic seizures [50]. In Sweden, high dissemination of GHB and mortality rates comparable to those of heroin have been reported [51].

Hallucinogens

Marijuana is the illicit drug most frequently used for recreational purposes and is now approved in several states and countries legally for medical purposes. It is derived from the hemp plant *Cannabis sativa*. Its major hallucinogenic ingredient is Δ9-tetrahydrocannabinol (THC). THC acts via specific receptors which are called CB_1 and CB_2. These receptors are expressed in the brain and immune cells, respectively; certain brain lipids (anandamide and 2-arachidonoylglycerol) are endogenous ligands of CB_1 and operate as retrograde synaptic transmitters [52]. Cannabinoids have antiepileptic properties [13, 53], which are described as being similar to those of phenytoin [54] despite different mechanisms of action [55]. Pro-convulsant activity was also reported for THC in a rat model [56]; this discrepancy is likely related to species and seizure model. Cannabis withdrawal can produce a mild withdrawal syndrome consisting of anxiety, nausea, increased body temperature, and tremors. Seizures are not part of this syndrome.

Several case reports of seizures after ingestion of synthetic cannabinoids have been published [57, 58]. Since 2004, these herbal blends have been sold in specialty shops, convenient stores, and on the internet and claim to produce cannabis-like effects after smoking the blend. They are sold under various names such as Spice, K2, K3, and Mr. Nice Guy. In comparison to naturally occurring THC, certain formulations of synthetic cannabinoids have exhibited four times the potency for binding to the CB_1 receptor [58]. The binding to the CB_1 receptor is felt to be primarily responsible for the psychotropic effects, which can lead to psychosis, agitation, and unresponsiveness. It is important to note that a typical urine toxicology screen will be negative for THC after consumption of synthetic cannabinoids.

Other natural (mescaline, psilocybin) and synthetic hallucinogens (lysergic acid diethylamide, LSD) are not considered epileptogenic. However, one case of grand mal seizure after LSD overdose has been reported [59].

Phencyclidine ("angel dust"), a hallucinogenic anesthetic similar to ketamine, has antiepileptic properties [60]. Intoxication, however, can lead to a severe clinical syndrome characterized by agitation, violence, psychosis, and catatonia, which can be complicated by rhabdomyolysis, hyperthermia, and seizures [61]. Fatal SE has been reported in this setting [62].

Epileptogenic Environmental Toxins

Marine Toxins

Among various toxins produced by marine animals or plants, domoic acid and ciguatera toxins are most relevant in view of epileptogenicity. Domoic acid (DA) is a potent excitotoxin that is produced by algae (*Nitzschia pungens*). Humans are intoxicated via the food chain by eating mussels containing the poison. Domoic acid is an analog of kainic acid and binds to NMDA receptors and causes an influx of excessive calcium [63]. Administered to rats, DA produces seizures resulting from unspecific neuronal activation throughout many brain areas. Excitotoxic brain damage ensues within certain brain regions, hippocampus and cerebellum, being more vulnerable than others [64].

An epidemic DA intoxication was first identified in Canada in late 1987 [65]. After eating poisoned mussels, 107 patients developed acute gastrointestinal symptoms (76%), incapacitating headache (43%), and loss of short-term memory (25%). Twelve patients (11%) required intensive care because of seizures, coma, and respiratory or circulatory problems. One fourth of those patients died. Damage in hippocampus and amygdala was the leading neuropathological finding [66]. Hippocampal damage, also demonstrated in survivors by reduced glucose uptake in PET imaging [66], is likely responsible for persisting seizure activity until 4 months after intoxication and for delayed onset temporal lobe epilepsy after 1 year [67]. Acute DA-induced seizure activity was resistant to phenytoin but controlled by diazepam and phenobarbital [66].

Although less epileptogenic, ciguatera fish intoxication is the most common nonbacterial marine food poisoning syndrome in humans. Ciguatoxins are heat-stable polyether toxins which act by increasing the permeability of excitable membranes to sodium ions [68]. Produced by the benthic (bottom dwelling) dinoflagellate *Gambierdiscus toxicus*, they enter the food chain via carnivore fish (mackerel, barracuda, rabbitfish) to human. Ciguatera is endemic in tropical countries but has been observed in North America and Europe, where the diagnosis is often missed or the condition is misdiagnosed for multiple sclerosis [69]. This confusion stems from the typical ciguatera symptomatology being paresthesias, especially of thermo- and nociception with hot-cold inversion, occurring several hours after ingestion. Parasthesias usually begin periorally and then spread centrifugally. Complete restitution is common [70] but can take as long as several months and in some cases symptoms persist. Severe intoxication can lead to coma, flaccid paralysis, respiratory paralysis, and generalized tonic-clonic seizures [68, 71, 72]. Deaths have been reported [73]. Confirmation of diagnosis can be achieved by detecting the toxin in human blood using available bioassays [74, 70]. Treatment with intravenous mannitol (10 ml/kg of 20% solution infused slowly over 30–45 min) after initial fluid replacement reduces Schwann cell edema and completely reverses symptoms in up to 60% of patients [75, 68]. However, in a double-blind randomized study of mannitol versus normal saline treatment over 24 h, mannitol was not found superior and had more side effects [17]. Additional supportive therapy may be necessary.

Mushroom and Plant Toxins

The most poisonous mushrooms are of the *Amanita* species. These produce a variety of toxins (amatoxins) [76]. *A. phalloides* produces the cytotoxic amanitin, which can lead to acute hepatic and renal failure within days of ingestion [77]. Seizures can occur as part of fulminant hepatic failure (FHF) and are likely related to ammonia toxicity, which increases synaptic glutamate release [78]. Besides antiepileptic drugs and supportive therapy, specific treatments for *A. phalloides* poisoning include gastric decontamination, oral activated charcoal and lactulose, high doses of penicillin, ceftazidime, thioctic acid, or silibinin, and combined hemodialysis and hemoperfusion [79, 80]. Positive effects of acetylcysteine were also reported [81]. Benzodiazepines, as the first line drug for agitation and seizures, have been used in the past.

Inocybe; *Clitocybe*; other *Amanita* species, especially *A. pantherina* and *A. muscaria*; and *Psilocybe* produce neurotoxins [82]. Examples of these toxins are ibotenic acid, stizolobic acid, and muscimol. Intoxication occurs most commonly in children (unintentional ingestion) and produces a distinctive syndrome consisting of alternating phases of drowsiness, agitation plus hallucinations, and seizures occurring within 2–3 h after ingestion [83]. In a study of nine cases of *A. pantherina* or *A. muscaria* poisoning, seizures were observed in four [84]. All seizures were controlled by standard antiepileptic drugs. In contrast to *A. phalloides* poisoning, intoxication from neurotoxic *Amanita* species is usually time-limited and followed by complete recovery. However, mushroom identification should be sought, because syndromes differ in their course and treatment. Identification may be achieved from the remains of a meal [85]. Another species of mushrooms, *Gyromitra esculenta*, contains hydrazine that disrupts normal production of GABA by various mechanisms including blocking pyridoxal 5′-phosphate, which enhances the elimination of pyridoxine and ultimately may result in seizures due to inadequate GABA supply [2]. In this instance, use of benzodiazepines or barbiturates may be ineffective as they both require GABA to exert their clinical effect.

Besides mushrooms, ingestion of certain plants can induce seizures. Water hemlock or other members of the *Cicuta* genus and their toxin, cicutoxin, are mostly involved. Water hemlock grows along rivers in North America. Intoxication conveys an overall mortality rate of 70% [86]. Typical symptomatology includes nausea followed by loss of consciousness and generalized seizures. In one report a patient was successfully treated with hemodialysis and hemoperfusion, forced diuresis, and artificial ventilation [87]. Star fruit (*Averrhoa carambola*) is a tropical fruit that originates from Southeast Asia and has been shown to cause neurotoxicity among patients with chronic renal insufficiency [88]. In a series of 32 patients with star fruit toxicity, seven developed seizures and all but one died, which was felt related to SE [88]. The mechanism for toxicity is uncertain; however, animal studies have shown that star fruit inhibits GABA binding on synaptic membranes.

Another source of potential ingestions Toxins is herbal medications, which use has increased significantly in the past few decades. Some of these herbal medicines contain potential neurotoxic compounds. Borage seed oil is derived from the seeds of the borage plant (*Borago officinalis*) and is used medicinally as an anti-inflammatory, for menopause-related symptoms, and for diabetic neuropathy. A previously healthy 41-year-old woman presented with confusion with episodes of inappropriate staring and laughing that evolved into generalized tonic-clonic seizures and SE after taking borage oil daily for the week prior to presentation. Other toxic plants that can sometimes induce seizures (with severe intoxication) include members of the belladonna alkaloid family (jimsonweed, nightshade), azalea, and Christmas rose [89].

Besides direct toxicity, plant ingestion Toxins can lead to intoxication by insecticides or herbicides. Amitraz is a widely used insecticide that often leads to intoxication in children. Symptoms include loss of consciousness, vomiting, hypotension, hypothermia, and generalized seizures and evolve within 2 h after ingestion [90, 91]. Benzodiazepine treatment is effective against convulsions [90]. The outcome is usually good.

Carbon Monoxide (CO)

CO is a colorless and odorless gas that is contained in exhaust fumes of motor vehicles, smoke from fires, tobacco smoke, and fumes of faulty heating systems. Intoxication results from acute inhalation or from chronic exposure to low concentrations. Seizures can occur with either acute or chronic poisoning. CO has a higher affinity for hemoglobin (forming carboxyhemoglobin) than oxygen. It therefore competitively removes oxygen from hemoglobin, thereby producing tissue hypoxia. The brain is the organ most vulnerable to hypoxia which leads to neurological symptoms ranging from dizziness and headache to coma and death. CO intoxication is more common during the winter when heating systems are being used. Because initial symptoms are nonspecific, the diagnosis is often missed unless direct spectroscopic measurement of the whole blood COHb level is performed. In a prospective study, COHb levels were measured in 753 unselected patients admitted to the Emergency Department. Those with suspected diagnosis of CO intoxication were excluded. Two patients from the entire cohort (0.3%) and one of twenty (5%) admitted with seizures had COHb levels of greater than 10% [92]. In several case reports, mild to moderate CO poisoning (mild, 10–20% COHb; moderate, 20–40% COHb) presented as an isolated focal or generalized seizure [93–95]. Other symptoms of mild to moderate poisoning included headache (84%), dizziness (92%), visual disturbances, and fatigue [96]. The classic cherry-red discoloration of the skin (color of carboxyhemoglobin) is mostly seen with severe intoxication (40–60% COHb), which also leads to coma, generalized convulsions, and respiratory impairment. Global brain edema and signs of hypoxia (hypodensities in white matter or basal ganglia) are seen on computed tomography. In one report, the EEG was characterized by lateralized sharp waves and a focal electrographic seizure discharge within hours of the CO exposure associated with coma and focal motor seizures [97]. One case of CO-related nonconvulsive SE in a 70-year-old female patient has also been reported [98]. Long-term sequelae of severe intoxication range from memory deficits or extrapyramidal disorders to persistent vegetative state [99].

The therapy of choice for acute CO intoxication is hyperbaric oxygen therapy [100], which significantly reduces late sequelae [101]. Oxygen itself has neurotoxic properties: especially, when applied under high pressure, oxygen can induce seizures. In one study, seizures occurred in 0.3% of cases at 2.45 atm abs and in 2% at 2.80 atm abs [102]. Mortality remains at the 30% level if the patient is not treated with hyperbaric oxygen, but drops to less than 10% if this treatment is offered early [89, 100].

Heavy Metals

Introduction
Heavy metal poisoning stems from environmental pollution (e.g., herbicides, pesticides), occupational exposure (e.g., mining), iatrogenic (e.g., antimicrobials), or intentional ingestion of recreational drugs (e.g., gasoline sniffing).

Heavy metals can bind to various reactive groups (ligands) to inhibit their physiological function. Drugs designed to limit the toxic effects of heavy metals (chelators) compete with these endogenous ligands for heavy metal binding. Chelators have a greater affinity for heavy metals and form complexes which are easily eliminated from the body. Most heavy metal poisoning is secondary to chronic exposure.

Lead

Lead intoxication is common since Ancient Roman ages, when lead was ingested via water delivered through lead pipe systems. Today, most cases of lead poisoning are the result of occupational exposure. Large-scale prevention programs have been introduced to eliminate this health hazard [103]. Other cases of lead intoxication occur in children who accidentally ingest lead-containing paint or soil. Chronic lead poisoning is therefore more common in adults, whereas acute intoxication more often occurs in children. The symptoms differ: chronic exposure leads to gastrointestinal, hematological, and renal symptoms. CNS and neuromuscular symptoms predominate with acute intoxication. The neurological syndrome of lead poisoning includes vertigo, clumsiness, ataxia, headache, insomnia, restlessness, and convulsions [104, 105]. Seizures are often repetitive and tonic-clonic and are followed by somnolence with visual disturbances or coma [106, 107]. Lead binding to GABA thereby reducing inhibition in cortical circuits has been suggested as a possible pathophysiological mechanism for lead-induced seizures [108]. Antiepileptic drugs that increase GABA-mediated inhibition (sodium valproate, barbiturates, and benzodiazepines) are therefore preferred in lead-induced seizures [108]. Chronic lead exposure can also produce thiamine deficiency, which lowers seizure threshold [109]. In these cases thiamine should be substituted. Other treatments for lead intoxication include chelating agents—edetate calcium disodium, dimercaprol, D-penicillamine, or succimer (2,3-dimercaptosuccinic acid). Anemia with basophilic stippling of red cells and lead lines at the metaphyses of long bones are other diagnostic findings. Blood zinc protoporphyrin (ZPP) levels can be used to assess lead exposure over the prior 3 months [110]. Excretion of lead in the urine should be assessed before and after initiation of therapy with chelating agents. Asymptomatic patients with blood lead levels greater than 80 μg/dl or symptomatic patients with blood lead concentration greater than 50 μg/dl should be treated with edetate calcium disodium i.v., followed by oral administration of succimer for 19 days. Asymptomatic patients with blood lead concentration greater than 50 μg/dl can be treated with succimer alone. Edetate calcium disodium should be combined with dimercaprol in cases with CNS symptoms [110]. Dexamethasone and mannitol should be considered in cases of cerebral edema.

Mercury

Mercury poisoning used to be a common side effect of various drugs such as antimicrobials, laxatives, and antiseptics. Whereas these drugs have been replaced with nontoxic and more effective agents, chronic mercury exposure from cosmetics distributed in developing countries (e.g., skin whitening cream [111]) still occurs. Other sources of mercury are occupational exposure [112] and environmental pollution, especially fish containing organic mercury compounds. The FDA therefore recommends avoiding consumption of shark, swordfish, mackerel, and tilefish in pregnant or women of childbearing age and young children [113]. Mercury intoxication causes a variety of symptoms, including gastrointestinal, renal, pulmonary, hepatic, and neurological. Neurotoxicity may result from excitotoxic neuronal damage due to defective glutamate reuptake by astrocytes [114].

The symptomatology of mercury intoxication depends upon the route of ingestion and on whether the exposure was acute or chronic. Acute inhalation of vapors containing high doses of elementary mercury is the most hazardous form of intoxication. Clinical signs occur within hours, consisting of gastrointestinal, respiratory symptoms, visual impairment, and generalized tonic-clonic seizures [115, 116]. Intensive care is mandatory as respiratory, renal, and hepatic failure may be fatal. In contrast, intravenous injection of doses of metallic mercury as high as 8 g is not life-threatening: in a case of suicidal injection, gastroenteritis, stomatitis mercurialis, neuropsychological symptoms, and tremor mercurialis occurred without respiratory, hepatic, or renal abnormalities [117]. In one report, the patient was successfully treated with 2,3-dimercaptopropane-1-sulfonate (DMPS), a chelating agent, and surgical removal of mercury deposits. Chronic exposure to mercury, in metallic or organic form (methylmercury) causes a neuropsychological syndrome (erethism) characterized by irritability, personality change, depression, delirium, insomnia, apathy, memory disturbances, headaches, general pain, and tremors. Hypertension, renal disturbances, allergies, and immunological conditions occur [112]. Recurrent seizures and EEG abnormalities may also be present [118]. Standard antiepileptic drug therapy can be used for mercury-related seizures and epilepsy. The chelating agent DMPS should be given repetitively to remove approximately 1 mg of mercury per day of treatment [117].

Tin

Tin has neurotoxic properties as an organic compound (triethyltin, trimethyltin). These organotins are used as preservatives for textiles or wood and in the production of silicone rubber. Intoxication often occurs during occupational exposure. Symptoms include hearing loss, confusion, memory deficits, ataxia, sensory neuropathy, aggressiveness, and disturbed sexual behavior, complex partial and tonic-clonic seizures. Long-term effects include epilepsy, likely because trimethyltin intoxication produces damage in amygdala, piriform cortex, and hippocampus, requiring antiepileptic treatment.

Pesticides and Other Chemical Toxins

Introduction

Exposure to toxic chemicals that lead to excessive hyperactivity in the nervous system can originate from industrial accidents, misuse in agriculture, or occupational hazards [115, 119]. There is both short- and long-term neuropathology that is caused by excitotoxicity. The acute phase of excitotoxicity can be followed by long-term regional neurodegeneration that leads to functional consequences such as cognitive decline and/or sensorimotor deficits.

Cholinesterase Inhibitors

Pesticides and chemical warfare agents, which inhibit the enzyme acetylcholinesterase (AChE), are toxic to humans and can lead to severe neurological dysfunction, causing seizures, miosis, and alterations of consciousness. Compounds such as toxic VX and sarin ("nerve gases") are considered organophosphorus (OP) nerve agents that were developed for chemical warfare during World War II and are some of the most well-known epileptogenic compounds [119]. These nerve agents can rapidly cross the blood-brain barrier and initially induce seizures through overstimulation of cholinergic pathways [120]. OP pesticides are also one of the biggest classes of insecticides used both in the home and in agriculture. Another class of pesticides that have an anticholinesterase mode of action is the class of carbamate pesticides.

OP and carbamate cholinesterase inhibitors are epileptogenic due to the deactivation of AChE, which leads to overstimulation of cholinergic synapses in the brain. Seizures can begin in different brain regions and spread throughout causing multifocal lesions in areas such as the cortex, hippocampus, thalamus, and amygdala [119]. Epileptiform activity and the activation of glutamate receptors are triggered by the overstimulation of postsynaptic muscarinic acetylcholine (ACh) receptors.

Those affected from acute poisoning from OPs are treated with atropine in order to inhibit muscarinic effects and, typically, pralidoxime (2-PAM), which reactivates phosphorylated AChE. Benzodiazepines are the drugs of choice for stopping seizures and SE caused by nerve agents. Studies have recently favored the use of midazolam over diazepam as the benzodiazepine of choice due to its superior pharmacokinetic characteristics [121]. Midazolam is most effective when given early after seizure onset, but it loses its protective efficacy over time or when delayed in administration. Seizure activity-induced internalization or downregulation of synaptic $GABA_A$ receptors is theorized to lead to refractory SE that is observed later after OP exposure or seizure onset. If this occurs, newer antiepileptic drugs are required to effectively terminate nerve agent-induced seizures and SE [121]

Cyanide

Cyanide is toxic in its ionic form (CN-) and can be released as hydrogen cyanide or cyanogen chloride gases. Typical neurological symptoms after acute exposure include headache, vertigo, and seizures which are followed by coma, respiratory failure, cardiac arrest, and death [119]. Currently, there are two cyanide-specific antidotes available which are Cyanokit® and Nithiodote®. These agents work by binding free cyanide in the bloodstream and detoxifying cyanide, respectively.

Other Pesticides

Organochlorines such as dichlorodiphenyltrichloroethane (DDT) interfere with the function of sodium channels, which ultimately leads to repetitive nerve firing, clinically apparent as tremors and seizures. There are no specific antidotes for organochlorine pesticides. Another class of commercial and domestic insecticides that have similar effects on voltage-gated sodium channels are the pyrethroids. A case of SE has been reported after inhalational exposure to a type II pyrethroid, bifenthrin [122]. Type II pyrethroids additionally cause chloride channel inhibition, which lowers the threshold for action potential generation and increases neuronal hyperexcitability.

Conclusion

In summary, toxins and illicit drugs exert their effects and cause seizures via various pathophysiological mechanisms by altering the brain's excitatory and inhibitory pathways. Certain toxins and drugs are more commonly associated with SE. Unfortunately, most commercially available drug screens do not screen for the substances most commonly associated with provoking seizures and are therefore of uncertain utility. Treatment of toxin-related seizures typically focuses on supportive care with airway management to ensure proper oxygenation and ventilation in conjunction with blood pressure, heart rate, and temperature stabilization, followed by assessment of serum glucose and the administration of a benzodiazepine, if clinically indicated. Occasionally, a more specific treatment is necessary in cases of certain intoxications.

References

1. Judge BS, Rentmeester LL. Antidepressant overdose-induced seizures. Psychiatr Clin North Am. 2013;36(2):245–60.
2. Sharma AN, Hoffman RJ. Toxin-related seizures. Emerg Med Clin North Am. 2011;29(1):125–39.
3. Thundiyil JG, Kearney TE, Olson KR. Evolving epidemiology of drug-induced seizures reported to a poison control center system. J Med Toxicol. 2007;3(1):15–9.

4. Barry JD, Wills BK. Neurotoxic emergencies. Neurol Clin. 2011;29(3):539–63.

5. Finkelstein Y, Hutson JR, Freedman SB, Wax P, Brent J, Toxicology Investigators Consortium (ToxIC) Case Registry. Drug-induced seizures in children and adolescents presenting for emergency care: current and emerging trends. Clin Toxicol (Phila). 2013;51(8):761–6.

6. Alldredge BK, Lowenstein DH, Simon RP. Seizures associated with recreational drug abuse. Neurology. 1989;39(8):1037–9.

7. Steele MT, Westdorp EJ, Garza AG, Ma OJ, Roberts DK, Watson WA. Screening for stimulant use in adult emergency department seizure patients. J Toxicol Clin Toxicol. 2000;38(6):609–13.

8. Saboory E, Derchansky M, Ismaili M, Jahromi SS, Brull R, Carlen PL, et al. Mechanisms of morphine enhancement of spontaneous seizure activity. Anesth Analg. 2007;105(6):1729–35. table of contents

9. Warner-Smith M, Darke S, Day C. Morbidity associated with non-fatal heroin overdose. Addiction. 2002;97(8):963–7.

10. Volavka J, Zaks A, Roubicek J, Fink M. Electrographic effects of diacetylmorphine (heroin) and naloxone in man. Neuropharmacology. 1970;9(6):587–93.

11. Landow L. An apparent seizure following inadvertent intrathecal morphine. Anesthesiology. 1985;62(4):545–6.

12. Chiarotti M, Fucci N. Comparative analysis of heroin and cocaine seizures. J Chromatogr B Biomed Sci Appl. 1999;733(1–2):127–36.

13. Ng SK, Brust JC, Hauser WA, Susser M. Illicit drug use and the risk of new-onset seizures. Am J Epidemiol. 1990;132(1):47–57.

14. Ogunyemi AO, Locke GE, Kramer LD, Nelson L. Complex partial status epilepticus provoked by "crack" cocaine. Ann Neurol. 1989;26(6):785–6.

15. Osborn DA, Jeffery HE, Cole MJ. Sedatives for opiate withdrawal in newborn infants. Cochrane Database Syst Rev. 2002;3(3):CD002053.

16. Klein M, Rudich Z, Gurevich B, Lifshitz M, Brill S, Lottan M, et al. Controlled-release oxycodone-induced seizures. Clin Ther. 2005;27(11):1815–8.

17. Schnorf H, Taurarii M, Cundy T. Ciguatera fish poisoning: a double-blind randomized trial of mannitol therapy. Neurology. 2002;58(6):873–80.

18. Schulze-Bonhage A, Elger CE. Induction of partial epileptic seizures by flumazenil. Epilepsia. 2000;41(2):186–92.

19. Haverkos GP, DiSalvo RP, Imhoff TE. Fatal seizures after flumazenil administration in a patient with mixed overdose. Ann Pharmacother. 1994;28(12):1347–9.

20. Sandoval MR, Palermo-Neto J. GABAergic influences on barbital withdrawal induced convulsions. Gen Pharmacol. 1986;17(4):431–5.

21. Tseng YT, Wellman SE, Ho IK. In situ hybridization evidence of differential modulation by pentobarbital of GABAA receptor alpha 1- and beta 3-subunit mRNAs. J Neurochem. 1994;63(1):301–9.

22. Koff JM, Pritchard GA, Greenblatt DJ, Miller LG. The NMDA receptor competitive antagonist CPP modulates benzodiazepine tolerance and discontinuation. Pharmacology. 1997;55(5):217–27.

23. Martinez-Cano H, Vela-Bueno A, de Iceta M, Pomalima R, Martinez-Gras I. Benzodiazepine withdrawal syndrome seizures. Pharmacopsychiatry. 1995;28(6):257–62.

24. Systematic review of the benzodiazepines. Guidelines for data sheets on diazepam, chlordiazepoxide, medazepam, clorazepate, lorazepam, oxazepam, temazepam, triazolam, nitrazepam, and flurazepam. Committee on the Review of Medicines. Br Med J. 1980;280(6218):910–2.

25. Fraser HF, Wikler A, Essig CF, Isbell H. Degree of physical dependence induced by secobarbital or pentobarbital. J Am Med Assoc. 1958;166(2):126–9.

26. Bauer MS, Fus AF, Hanich RF, Ross RJ. Glutethimide intoxication and withdrawal. Am J Psychiatry. 1988;145(4):530–1.

27. Caplan LR, Thomas C, Banks G. Central nervous system complications of addiction to "T's and Blues". Neurology. 1982;32(6):623–8.

28. Landry MJ. MDMA: a review of epidemiologic data. J Psychoactive Drugs. 2002;34(2):163–9.

29. Brown JW, Dunne JW, Fatovich DM, Lee J, Lawn ND. Amphetamine-associated seizures: clinical features and prognosis. Epilepsia. 2011;52(2):401–4.

30. Zagnoni PG, Albano C. Psychostimulants and epilepsy. Epilepsia. 2002;43(2):28–31.

31. Dhuna A, Pascual-Leone A, Langendorf F, Anderson DC. Epileptogenic properties of cocaine in humans. Neurotoxicology. 1991 Fall;12(3):621–6.

32. Burgess C, O'Donohoe A, Gill M. Agony and ecstasy: a review of MDMA effects and toxicity. Eur Psychiatry. 2000;15(5):287–94.

33. Ridpath A, Driver CR, Nolan ML, Karpati A, Kass D, Paone D, et al. Illnesses and deaths among persons attending an electronic dance-music festival—New York City, 2013. MMWR Morb Mortal Wkly Rep. 2014;63(50):1195–8.

34. Auer J, Berent R, Weber T, Lassnig E, Eber B. Subarachnoid haemorrhage with "Ecstasy" abuse in a young adult. Neurol Sci. 2002;23(4):199–201.

35. Klausner HA, Lewandowski C. Infrequent causes of stroke. Emerg Med Clin North Am. 2002;20(3):657–70.

36. Hanson GR, Jensen M, Johnson M, White HS. Distinct features of seizures induced by cocaine and amphetamine analogs. Eur J Pharmacol. 1999;377(2–3):167–73.

37. Burish MJ, Thoren KL, Madou M, Toossi S, Shah M. Hallucinogens causing seizures? A case report of the synthetic amphetamine 2,5-dimethoxy-4-chloroamphetamine. Neurohospitalist. 2015;5(1):32–4.

38. Wiegand T. Phenytoin is not successful in preventing cocaine-induced seizures: a response to the article, "Cocaine body packing in pregnancy". Ann Emerg Med. 2007;49(4):543–4.

39. Vilela LR, Gomides LF, David BA, Antunes MM, Diniz AB, Moreira F d A, et al. Cannabidiol rescues acute hepatic toxicity and seizure induced by cocaine. Mediators Inflamm. 2015;2015:523418.

40. Schwartz RH, Estroff T, Hoffmann NG. Seizures and syncope in adolescent cocaine abusers. Am J Med. 1988;85(3):462.

41. Holmes SB, Banerjee AK, Alexander WD. Hyponatraemia and seizures after ecstasy use. Postgrad Med J. 1999;75(879):32–3.

42. Sue YM, Lee YL, Huang JJ. Acute hyponatremia, seizure, and rhabdomyolysis after ecstasy use. J Toxicol Clin Toxicol. 2002;40(7):931–2.

43. Szlatenyi CS, Wang RY. Encephalopathy and cranial nerve palsies caused by intentional trichloroethylene inhalation. Am J Emerg Med. 1996;14(5):464–6.

44. Aydin K, Sencer S, Demir T, Ogel K, Tunaci A, Minareci O. Cranial MR findings in chronic toluene abuse by inhalation. AJNR Am J Neuroradiol. 2002;23(7):1173–9.

45. Meredith TJ, Ruprah M, Liddle A, Flanagan RJ. Diagnosis and treatment of acute poisoning with volatile substances. Hum Toxicol. 1989;8(4):277–86.

46. Wells JC. Abuse of trichloroethylene by oral self-administration. Anaesthesia. 1982;37(4):440–1.

47. Littorin ME, Fehling C, Attewell RG, Skerfving S. Focal epilepsy and exposure to organic solvents: a case-referent study. J Occup Med. 1988;30(10):805–8.

48. Silva-Filho AR, Pires ML, Shiotsuki N. Anticonvulsant and convulsant effects of organic solvents. Pharmacol Biochem Behav. 1992;41(1):79–82.

49. Jacobsen M, Baelum J, Bonde JP. Temporal epileptic seizures and occupational exposure to solvents. Occup Environ Med. 1994;51(6):429–30.

50. Wojtowicz JM, Yarema MC, Wax PM. Withdrawal from gamma-hydroxybutyrate, 1,4-butanediol and gamma-butyrolactone: a case report and systematic review. CJEM. 2008;10(1):69–74.

51. Knudsen K, Greter J, Verdicchio M. High mortality rates among GHB abusers in Western Sweden. Clin Toxicol (Phila). 2008;46(3):187–92.

52. Wilson RI, Nicoll RA. Endocannabinoid signaling in the brain. Science. 2002;296(5568):678–82.

53. Mechoulam R, Parker LA, Gallily R. Cannabidiol: an overview of some pharmacological aspects. J Clin Pharmacol. 2002;42(11 Suppl):11S–9S.

54. Sofia RD, Solomon TA, Barry H. Anticonvulsant activity of delta9-tetrahydrocannabinol compared with three other drugs. Eur J Pharmacol. 1976;35(1):7–16.

55. Karler R, Turkanis SA. The cannabinoids as potential antiepileptics. J Clin Pharmacol. 1981;21(8–9 Suppl):437S–48S.

56. Turkanis SA, Karler R. Central excitatory properties of delta 9-tetrahydrocannabinol and its metabolites in iron-induced epileptic rats. Neuropharmacology. 1982;21(1):7–13.

57. Tofighi B, Lee JD. Internet highs—seizures after consumption of synthetic cannabinoids purchased online. J Addict Med. 2012;6(3):240–1.

58. Pant S, Deshmukh A, Dholaria B, Kaur V, Ramavaram S, Ukor M, et al. Spicy seizure. Am J Med Sci. 2012;344(1):67–8.

59. Fisher DD, Ungerleider JT. Grand mal seizures following ingestion of LSD. Calif Med. 1967;106(3):210–1.

60. Leander JD, Rathbun RC, Zimmerman DM. Anticonvulsant effects of phencyclidine-like drugs: relation to N-methyl-D-aspartic acid antagonism. Brain Res. 1988;454(1–2):368–72.

61. Baldridge EB, Bessen HA. Phencyclidine. Emerg Med Clin North Am. 1990;8(3):541–50.

62. Kessler Jr GF, Demers LM, Berlin C, Brennan RW. Letter: phencyclidine and fatal status epilepticus. N Engl J Med. 1974;291(18):979.

63. Stewart GR, Zorumski CF, Price MT, Olney JW. Domoic acid: a dementia-inducing excitotoxic food poison with kainic acid receptor specificity. Exp Neurol. 1990;110(1):127–38.

64. Cervos-Navarro J, Diemer NH. Selective vulnerability in brain hypoxia. Crit Rev Neurobiol. 1991;6(3):149–82.

65. Perl TM, Bedard L, Kosatsky T, Hockin JC, Todd EC, Remis RS. An outbreak of toxic encephalopathy caused by eating mussels contaminated with domoic acid. N Engl J Med. 1990;322(25):1775–80.

66. Teitelbaum JS, Zatorre RJ, Carpenter S, Gendron D, Evans AC, Gjedde A, et al. Neurologic sequelae of domoic acid intoxication due to the ingestion of contaminated mussels. N Engl J Med. 1990;322(25):1781–7.

67. Cendes F, Andermann F, Carpenter S, Zatorre RJ, Cashman NR. Temporal lobe epilepsy caused by domoic acid intoxication: evidence for glutamate receptor-mediated excitotoxicity in humans. Ann Neurol. 1995;37(1):123–6.

68. Pearn J. Neurology of ciguatera. J Neurol Neurosurg Psychiatry. 2001;70(1):4–8.

69. Ting JY, Brown AF. Ciguatera poisoning: a global issue with common management problems. Eur J Emerg Med. 2001;8(4):295–300.

70. Hashmi MA, Sorokin JJ, Levine SM. Ciguatera fish poisoning. N J Med. 1989;86(6):469–71.

71. Lange WR. Ciguatera toxicity. Am Fam Physician. 1987;35(4):177–82.

72. Bagnis R, Kuberski T, Laugier S. Clinical observations on 3,009 cases of ciguatera (fish poisoning) in the South Pacific. Am J Trop Med Hyg. 1979;28(6):1067–73.

73. Alcala AC, Alcala LC, Garth JS, Yasumura D, Yasumoto T. Human fatality due to ingestion of the crab Demania reynaudii that contained a palytoxin-like toxin. Toxicon. 1988;26(1):105–7.

74. Matta J, Navas J, Milad M, Manger R, Hupka A, Frazer T. A pilot study for the detection of acute ciguatera intoxication in human blood. J Toxicol Clin Toxicol. 2002;40(1):49–57.

75. Palafox NA, Jain LG, Pinano AZ, Gulick TM, Williams RK, Schatz IJ. Successful treatment of ciguatera fish poisoning with intravenous mannitol. JAMA. 1988;259(18):2740–2.

76. Chilton WS, Ott J. Toxic metabolites of Amanita pantherina, A. cothurnata, A. muscaria and other Amanita species. Lloydia. 1976;39(2–3):150–7.

77. McPartland JM, Vilgalys RJ, Cubeta MA. Mushroom poisoning. Am Fam Physician. 1997;55(5):1797–800. 1805–9, 1811–2

78. Albrecht J, Jones EA. Hepatic encephalopathy: molecular mechanisms underlying the clinical syndrome. J Neurol Sci. 1999;170(2):138–46.

79. Sabeel AI, Kurkus J, Lindholm T. Intensive hemodialysis and hemoperfusion treatment of Amanita mushroom poisoning. Mycopathologia. 1995;131(2):107–14.

80. Beer JH. The wrong mushroom. Diagnosis and therapy of mushroom poisoning, especially of Amanita phalloides poisoning. Schweiz Med Wochenschr. 1993;123(17):892–905.

81. Montanini S, Sinardi D, Pratico C, Sinardi AU, Trimarchi G. Use of acetylcysteine as the life-saving antidote in Amanita phalloides (death cap) poisoning. Case report on 11 patients. Arzneimittelforschung. 1999;49(12):1044–7.

82. Kohn R, Mot'ovska Z. Mushroom poisoning—classification, symptoms and therapy. Vnitr Lek. 1997;43(4):230–3.

83. Tupalska-Wilczynska K, Ignatowicz R, Poziemski A, Wojcik H, Wilczynski G. Amanita pantherina and Amanita muscaria poisonings—pathogenesis, symptoms and treatment. Pol Merkur Lekarski. 1997;3(13):30–2.

84. Benjamin DR. Mushroom poisoning in infants and children: the Amanita pantherina/muscaria group. J Toxicol Clin Toxicol. 1992;30(1):13–22.

85. Elonen E, Tarssanen L, Harkonen M. Poisoning with brown fly agaric. Amanita regalis. Acta Med Scand. 1979;205(1–2):121–3.

86. From the Centers for Disease Control and Prevention. Water hemlock poisoning—Maine, 1992. JAMA. 1994;271(19):1475.

87. Knutsen OH, Paszkowski P. New aspects in the treatment of water hemlock poisoning. J Toxicol Clin Toxicol. 1984;22(2):157–66.

88. Tan RY, Neligan A, Shorvon SD. The uncommon causes of status epilepticus: a systematic review. Epilepsy Res. 2010;91(2–3):111–22.

89. Kunisaki TA, Augenstein WL. Drug- and toxin-induced seizures. Emerg Med Clin North Am. 1994;12(4):1027–56.

90. Ertekin V, Alp H, Selimoglu MA, Karacan M. Amitraz poisoning in children: retrospective analysis of 21 cases. J Int Med Res. 2002;30(2):203–5.

91. Yilmaz HL, Yildizdas DR. Amitraz poisoning, an emerging problem: epidemiology, clinical features, management, and preventive strategies. Arch Dis Child. 2003;88(2):130–4.

92. Heckerling PS, Leikin JB, Maturen A, Terzian CG, Segarra DP. Screening hospital admissions from the emergency department for occult carbon monoxide poisoning. Am J Emerg Med. 1990;8(4):301–4.

93. Herman LY. Carbon monoxide poisoning presenting as an isolated seizure. J Emerg Med. 1998;16(3):429–32.

94. Mori T, Nagai K. Carbon-monoxide poisoning presenting as an afebrile seizure. Pediatr Neurol. 2000;22(4):330–1.

95. Durnin C. Carbon monoxide poisoning presenting with focal epileptiform seizures. Lancet. 1987;1(8545):1319.

96. Guzman JA. Carbon monoxide poisoning. Crit Care Clin. 2012;28(4):537–48.

97. Neufeld MY, Swanson JW, Klass DW. Localized EEG abnormalities in acute carbon monoxide poisoning. Arch Neurol. 1981;38(8):524–7.

98. Brown KL, Wilson RF, White MT. Carbon monoxide-induced status epilepticus in an adult. J Burn Care Res. 2007;28(3):533–6.

99. Mathieu D, Nolf M, Durocher A, Saulnier F, Frimat P, Furon D, et al. Acute carbon monoxide poisoning. Risk of late sequelae and treatment by hyperbaric oxygen. J Toxicol Clin Toxicol. 1985;23(4–6):315–24.

100. Hawkins M, Harrison J, Charters P. Severe carbon monoxide poisoning: outcome after hyperbaric oxygen therapy. Br J Anaesth. 2000;84(5):584–6.

101. Weaver LK, Hopkins RO, Chan KJ, Churchill S, Elliott CG, Clemmer TP, et al. Hyperbaric oxygen for acute carbon monoxide poisoning. N Engl J Med. 2002;347(14):1057–67.

102. Hampson NB, Simonson SG, Kramer CC, Piantadosi CA. Central nervous system oxygen toxicity during hyperbaric treatment of patients with carbon monoxide poisoning. Undersea Hyperb Med. 1996;23(4):215–9.

103. Roscoe RJ, Ball W, Curran JJ, DeLaurier C, Falken MC, Fitchett R, et al. Adult blood lead epidemiology and surveillance—United States, 1998–2001. MMWR Surveill Summ. 2002;51(11):1–10.

104. Shannon M. Severe lead poisoning in pregnancy. Ambul Pediatr. 2003;3(1):37–9.

105. Wedeen RP, Mallik DK, Batuman V, Bogden JD. Geophagic lead nephropathy: case report. Environ Res. 1978;17(3):409–15.

106. Kumar A, Dey PK, Singla PN, Ambasht RS, Upadhyay SK. Blood lead levels in children with neurological disorders. J Trop Pediatr. 1998;44(6):320–2.

107. Yu EC, Yeung CY. Lead encephalopathy due to herbal medicine. Chin Med J (Engl). 1987;100(11):915–7.

108. Healy MA, Aslam M, Harrison PG, Fernando NP. Lead-induced convulsions in young infants—a case history and the role of GABA and sodium valproate in the pathogenesis and treatment. J Clin Hosp Pharm. 1984;9(3):199–207.

109. Cheong JH, Seo DO, Ryu JR, Shin CY, Kim YT, Kim HC, et al. Lead induced thiamine deficiency in the brain decreased the threshold of electroshock seizure in rat. Toxicology. 1999;133(2–3):105–13.

110. Gordon JN, Taylor A, Bennett PN. Lead poisoning: case studies. Br J Clin Pharmacol. 2002;53(5):451–8.

111. Pelclova D, Lukas E, Urban P, Preiss J, Rysava R, Lebenhart P, et al. Mercury intoxication from skin ointment containing mercuric ammonium chloride. Int Arch Occup Environ Health. 2002;75(Suppl):S54–9.

112. Faria MA. Chronic occupational metallic mercurialism. Rev Saude Publica. 2003;37(1):116–27.

113. Evans EC. The FDA recommendations on fish intake during pregnancy. J Obstet Gynecol Neonatal Nurs. 2002;31(6):715–20.

114. Juarez BI, Martinez ML, Montante M, Dufour L, Garcia E, Jimenez-Capdeville ME. Methylmercury increases glutamate extracellular levels in frontal cortex of awake rats. Neurotoxicol Teratol. 2002;24(6):767–71.

115. Jaffe KM, Shurtleff DB, Robertson WO. Survival after acute mercury vapor poisoning. Am J Dis Child. 1983;137(8):749–51.

116. Abbaslou P, Zaman T. A Child with elemental mercury poisoning and unusual brain MRI findings. Clin Toxicol (Phila). 2006;44(1):85–8.

117. Winker R, Schaffer AW, Konnaris C, Barth A, Giovanoli P, Osterode W, et al. Health consequences of an intravenous injection of metallic mercury. Int Arch Occup Environ Health. 2002;75(8):581–6.

118. Brenner RP, Snyder RD. Late EEG findings and clinical status after organic mercury poisoning. Arch Neurol. 1980;37(5):282–4.

119. Jett DA. Chemical toxins that cause seizures. Neurotoxicology. 2012;33(6):1473–5.

120. de Araujo FM, Rossetti F, Chanda S, Yourick D. Exposure to nerve agents: from status epilepticus to neuroinflammation, brain damage, neurogenesis and epilepsy. Neurotoxicology. 2012;33(6):1476–90.

121. Reddy SD, Reddy DS. Midazolam as an anticonvulsant antidote for organophosphate intoxication—A pharmacotherapeutic appraisal. Epilepsia. 2015;56(6):813–21.

122. Rangaraju S, Webb A. Status epilepticus following inhalational exposure to bifenthrin, a Type II pyrethroid. Clin Toxicol (Phila). 2013;51(9):906.

Seizures and Status Epilepticus in Pediatric Critical Care

Nicholas S. Abend

Introduction

Status epilepticus (SE) and seizures are the most common neurologic conditions managed in pediatric intensive care units [1, 2]. However, while often encountered, management is highly variable and treatment delays have been reported [3–6]. Further, there is increasing evidence that many seizures in critically ill children are electrographic-only, so identification requires continuous electroencephalographic (EEG) monitoring. This chapter reviews the identification and management of seizures and status epilepticus in children in the pediatric intensive care unit (PICU).

Electrographic Seizure Incidence and Risk Factors

Few data are available regarding the incidence of clinically evident seizures in children receiving care in the PICU. However, observational studies by interdisciplinary neurological critical care teams describe seizures and SE as the most commonly managed conditions in the PICU [1, 2]. A study in a quaternary care children's hospital described 373 pediatric neurocritical care consultations over 1 year (2006–2007). SE was the admission diagnosis for 18% of patients receiving consults, and evaluation of seizures or possible seizures was the reason for neurologic consultation in 35% of patients. EEG was one of the most commonly used resources by the service. Forty-one percent of patients had EEGs performed, and 19% of patients had continuous EEG monitoring performed [1]. A second study from a quaternary care children's hospital describes 615 pediatric neurocritical care consultations over a 32-month period (2005–2008). The most common diagnoses are related to epilepsy, seizures, or SE, and these occurred in 48% of patients. The 615 patients underwent a total of 849 EEG studies of which 72% were standard 20–30 min EEG studies and 28% were continuous EEG monitoring studies [2].

Studies of critically ill children undergoing continuous EEG monitoring in PICUs have reported that 10–50% experience electrographic seizures. Further, about one-third of children with electrographic seizures have a sufficiently high seizure burden to be categorized as electrographic SE [7–26]. Although there is variability in the definition of electrographic SE across studies, a common criterion has been 50% of any 1 h epoch containing seizure activity. For example, this could constitute a single 30-minute seizure or ten 3-minute seizures. The indications for EEG monitoring varied across these studies. Some studies included only patients with known acute neurologic disorders, such as hypoxic-ischemic brain injury, encephalitis, or traumatic brain injury. Other studies had broader inclusion criteria and included patients with encephalopathy due to more heterogeneous diagnoses, including both primary neurologic and primary medical conditions. Inclusion criteria variability may explain the broad reported electrographic seizure incidences since lower electrographic seizure incidence is reported by studies with broader inclusion criteria.

The largest epidemiologic study of continuous EEG monitoring in the PICU was a retrospective study in which 11 tertiary care pediatric institutions each enrolled 50 consecutive subjects who underwent clinically indicated continuous EEG monitoring, thereby yielding 550 subjects. Electrographic seizures occurred in 30% of monitored subjects. Among subjects with electrographic seizures, electrographic SE occurred in 33% of subjects. Further, among subjects with electrographic seizures, 35% had exclusively EEG-only seizures [19]. These data are consistent with single-center studies [9, 12, 14–16, 18, 20–22, 24, 26].

N.S. Abend (✉)
Department of Neurology and Pediatrics, Children's Hospital of Philadelphia and Perelman School of Medicine, University of Pennsylvania, 3501 Civic Center Blvd, CTRB 10016, Philadelphia, PA 19104, USA
e-mail: abend@email.chop.edu

© Springer International Publishing AG 2017
P.N. Varelas, J. Claassen (eds.), *Seizures in Critical Care*, Current Clinical Neurology, DOI 10.1007/978-3-319-49557-6_22

Several studies have demonstrated that EEG-only seizures occur in children who have not received paralytics recently or ever during their PICU stay [21, 24]. This finding indicates the existence of electromechanical uncoupling, referring to a dissociation between the electrographic seizures and outwardly observable seizure manifestations. It indicates that clinically evident changes were not being simply masked by paralytic administration.

Continuous EEG monitoring is resource intense, and seemingly small changes in continuous EEG monitoring utilization and workflows may have substantial impacts on equipment and personnel needs [27, 28]. Thus, identifying children at higher risk of electrographic seizures may be very beneficial since limited continuous EEG monitoring resources could be directed optimally. Several risk factors have been reported consistently by multiple studies: (1) younger age (infants as compared to older children) [14, 17, 19, 22, 24], (2) the occurrence of convulsive seizures [15, 19, 20] or convulsive SE [14] prior to initiation of EEG monitoring, (3) the presence of acute structural brain injury [13–15, 17, 18, 20, 22, 26], and (4) the presence of interictal epileptiform discharges [14, 18–20] or periodic epileptiform discharges [9]. Although the reported risk factors are statistically significant, it is problematic that the absolute difference in the proportion of children with and without electrographic seizures based on the presence or absence of a risk factor is often only 10–20%. Thus, these risk factors may have limited clinical utility in selecting patients to undergo continuous EEG monitoring.

Seizure prediction models combining multiple known seizure risk factors could take into account multiple risk factors and allow targeting of continuous EEG monitoring to children at highest risk for experiencing electrographic seizures within the resource limitations of an individual medical center. A recent study derived a seizure prediction model from a retrospectively acquired multicenter dataset and validated it on a separate single-center dataset. The model had fair to good discrimination indicating that most, but not all, patients were appropriately classified as experiencing seizures or not.. The model could be applied clinically in three steps. First, the clinician would obtain two clinical variables (age and whether there were clinically evident seizures) and two EEG variables (background category and interictal epileptiform discharge presence) presence) from a routine 20-30 minute EEG. Second, the clinician could determine a model score based on those variables. Third, patients with model scores above an institutional cutoff score would be selected to undergo continuous EEG monitoring. Individual institutions could select different model cutoff scores based on center-specific resource criteria. A center with substantial continuous EEG monitoring resources might perform monitoring for any patient with a model score >0.10. At this cutoff, 14% of patients with electrographic seizures would not undergo continuous EEG monitoring, so their seizures would not be identified and managed. However, 58% of patients without electrographic seizures would be identified as not needing continuous EEG monitoring, so limited resources would be conserved. Given a seizure prevalence of 30%, this cutoff would have a positive predictive value of 47% and negative predictive value of 91% [29]. Further development of seizure prediction models in more homogeneous cohorts and with additional variables might yield improved performance characteristics.

Continuous EEG Monitoring Duration

Decisions regarding the duration of continuous EEG monitoring must balance the goal of identifying electrographic seizures with practical concerns regarding the substantial equipment and personnel resources required to perform continuous EEG monitoring. Observational studies of critically ill children undergoing clinically indicated continuous EEG monitoring have reported that about 50% of patients with electrographic seizures are identified with 1 h of EEG monitoring and 90% of patients with electrographic seizures are identified with 24–48 h of EEG monitoring [9, 12, 14, 15, 18, 20, 21, 24]. Monitoring for 48 h identifies about 5% more patients than monitoring for 24 h, but that duration requires substantial resource utilization [30]. Thus, using broad inclusion criteria for 24 h of EEG monitoring but then developing a seizure prediction model to determine which patients need additional monitoring may enable optimal resource utilization.

There are two important limitations regarding the electrographic seizure timing data described above. First, most of the studies calculated timing at the onset of continuous EEG monitoring and not the onset of the acute brain insult. This may be problematic since in clinical practice patients may present at varying durations after the onset of acute brain insult. Furthermore, patients may experience clinical changes potentially producing additional brain injury while in the intensive care unit, and it is unclear if the timing considerations should restart with each of these clinical occurrences. Second, patients in most of the studies underwent 1–3 days of clinically indicated continuous EEG monitoring, and none of the studies performed prolonged monitoring during the entire acute management course for all patients. Thus, some patients may have experienced electrographic seizures after EEG monitoring was discontinued.

Based on the data described above, the Neurocritical Care Society's Guideline for the Evaluation and Management of Status Epilepticus strongly recommends performing 48 h of continuous EEG monitoring to identify electrographic SE in comatose children following an acute brain insult [31]. The American Clinical Neurophysiology's Consensus Statement on Continuous EEG Monitoring in Critically Ill Children and Adults recommends performing continuous EEG monitoring for at least 24 h in children at risk for electrographic seizures [32].

Outcome

Several studies in critically ill children have reported associations between high electrographic seizure exposures and worse outcomes. However, the extent to which electrographic seizures are actually producing secondary brain injury versus serving as biomarkers of more severe acute brain injury remains unknown. Further, the extent to which seizures produce secondary brain injury is likely dependent on a complex interplay between acute brain injury etiology, seizure exposure (also referred to as seizure burden), seizure characteristics (possibly including anatomical extent, morphology, frequency, voltage), and seizure management strategies. As summarized below, a number of studies have reported an association between electrographic seizures, particularly with high electrographic seizure exposures, and worse outcomes even after adjustment for potential confounders related to acute encephalopathy etiology and critical illness severity [33].

Several studies have described an association between electrographic seizures and unfavorable short-term outcome. A prospective observational study of 1–3 channel EEGs in 204 critically ill neonates and children classified seizure exposure as present or absent. The study found that the occurrence of electrographic seizures was associated with a higher risk of unfavorable neurologic outcome (odds ratio 15.4) in a multivariate analysis that included age, etiology, pediatric index of mortality score, Adelaide coma score, and EEG background categories [16]. Several other studies aimed to evaluate the effect of seizure burden categorically classified children as no seizures, electrographic seizures, or electrographic SE (defined as more than 50% of any 1 h epoch containing seizure). A single-center study of 200 children in the PICU with outcome assessed at discharge identified an association between electrographic SE and higher mortality (odds ratio 5.1) and worsening pediatric cerebral performance category scores (odds ratio 17.3) in multivariate analyses including seizure category, age, acute neurologic disorder, prior neurodevelopmental status, and EEG background categories. Electrographic seizures not classified as electrographic SE were not associated with worse outcomes [34]. A larger multicenter study of 550 children in the pediatric intensive care unit reported an association between electrographic SE and mortality (odds ratio 2.4) in a multivariate analysis that included seizure category, acute encephalopathy etiology, and EEG background categories. Electrographic seizures not classified as electrographic SE were not associated with mortality [19]. A single-center prospective study evaluated 259 critically ill infants and children

who underwent continuous EEG monitoring. There were electrographic seizures in 36% of subjects, and 9% of those with seizures had electrographic SE. Seizure burden was calculated as the proportion of each hour containing seizures, and the maximum hourly seizure burden was identified for each subject. The mean maximum seizure burden per hour was 15.7% in subjects with neurological decline versus 1.8% in subjects without neurological decline. In a multivariate analysis that adjusted for diagnosis and illness severity, for every 1% increase in the maximum hourly seizure burden, the odds of neurological decline increased by 1.13. Maximum hourly seizure burdens of 10%, 20%, and 30% were associated with odds ratios for neurological decline of 3.3, 10.8, and 35.7, respectively. In contrast to some of the other studies described above, electrographic seizures were not associated with higher mortality [23].

A study addressing long-term outcome obtained follow-up data at a median of 2.7 years following admission to the PICU in 60 encephalopathic children who were neurodevelopmentally normal prior to admission and underwent clinically indicated continuous EEG monitoring. Multivariate analysis including acute neurologic diagnosis category, EEG background category, age, and several other clinical variables identified an association between electrographic SE and unfavorable Glasgow Outcome Scale (Extended Pediatric Version) category (odds ratio 6.36), lower Pediatric Quality of Life Inventory scores (median of 23.07 points lower), and an increased risk of subsequently diagnosed epilepsy (odds ratio 13.3). Children with electrographic seizures not classified as electrographic SE did not have worse outcomes [35].

Together, these studies suggest that there may be a dose-dependent or threshold effect of electrographic seizures upon outcomes, with high seizure exposures having clinically relevant adverse impacts. This threshold may vary based on age, brain injury etiology, and seizure characteristics such as the extent of brain involved and electroencephalographic morphology. While further study is needed, these data suggest that at least in some patients with high electrographic seizure exposures, electrographic seizures may be producing secondary brain injury. Thus, identifying and managing those seizures might mitigate such injury.

Clinical Practice and Guidelines Related to Continuous EEG Monitoring

A survey of continuous EEG monitoring use in the PICUs of 61 large pediatric hospitals in the United States and Canada reported about a 30% increase in the median number of patients who underwent continuous EEG monitoring per month from 2010 to 2011 [36]. Indications for continuous EEG monitoring included determining whether events of unclear etiology were seizures in 100% of centers and identifying electrographic seizures in patients considered "at risk" in about 90% of centers. Patients considered "at risk" included those with altered mental status following a convulsion, altered mental status in a patient with a known acute brain injury, and altered mental status of unknown etiology. About 30–50% of centers reported using continuous EEG monitoring as part of standard management for specific acute encephalopathy etiologies within a clinical pathway (i.e., following resuscitation from cardiac arrest or with severe traumatic brain injury). Further, although often referred to as "continuous EEG monitoring", at the vast majority of centers, EEG was recorded continuously but only intermittently reviewed. The EEG tracing was generally reviewed 2–3 times per day by a combination of physicians and technologists [36].

The Neurocritical Care Society's Guidelines for the Evaluation and Management of Status Epilepticus recommends the use of continuous EEG monitoring to identify electrographic seizures in at-risk patients including (1) patients with persisting altered mental status for more than 10 min after convulsive seizures or SE and (2) encephalopathic children after resuscitation from cardiac arrest, with traumatic brain injury, with intracranial hemorrhage, or with unexplained encephalopathy. The guideline strongly recommends 48 h of continuous EEG monitoring in comatose patients. If SE occurs (including electrographic SE), then the guideline recommends that management should continue until both clinical and electrographic seizures are halted [31].

The American Clinical Neurophysiology's Consensus Statement on Continuous EEG Monitoring in Critically Ill Children and Adults recommends continuous EEG monitoring for 24–48 h in children at risk for seizures. EEG monitoring indications include (1) recent convulsive seizures or convulsive SE with altered mental status, (2) cardiac arrest resuscitation or with other forms of hypoxic-ischemic encephalopathy, (3) stroke (intracerebral hemorrhage, ischemic, and subarachnoid hemorrhage), (4) encephalitis, and (5) altered mental status with related medical conditions. The consensus statement also provides detailed recommendations regarding personnel, technical specifications, and overall workflow [32].

Based on the available data, the Neurocritical Care Society's Guidelines for the Evaluation and Management of Status Epilepticus and the American Clinical Neurophysiology Society's Consensus Statement on Continuous EEG Monitoring in Critically Ill Children and Adults, an interdisciplinary workgroup at the Children's Hospital of Philadelphia composed of electroencephalographers, neurological critical care consultants, and intensivists developed an intensive care continuous EEG monitoring pathway which is available online (http://www.chop.edu/clinical-pathway/eeg-monitoring-clinical-pathway).

Quantitative EEG for Electrographic Seizure Identification

Increasing continuous EEG monitoring use among critically ill children [36, 37] is resource intense and would benefit from improved seizure identification efficiency. Quantitative EEG techniques separate the complex EEG signal into components (such as amplitude and frequency) and compress time, thereby permitting display of several hours of EEG data on a single image that may be interpreted more easily and/or more rapidly than conventional EEG. Quantitative EEG techniques may facilitate more efficient EEG monitoring review by encephalographers and perhaps even earlier identification of seizures by non-electroencephalographer clinicians providing bedside care. These quantitative EEG techniques are still being developed, and their test characteristics are still being established.

Several studies have examined the utility of quantitative EEG in critically ill children. In the first study, 27 color density spectral array and amplitude-integrated EEG tracings were reviewed by three encephalographers. The median sensitivity for seizure identification was 83% using color density spectral array and 82% using amplitude-integrated EEG. However, for individual tracings, the sensitivity varied from 0 to 100% indicating excellent performance for some patients and poor performance for other patients, likely related to individual patients' seizure characteristics. A false positive occurred about every 17–20 h [38]. In the second study, 84 color density spectral array images were reviewed by eight electroencephalographers. Sensitivity for seizure identification was 65%, indicating that some electrographic seizures were not identified. Further, only about half of seizures were identified by six or more of the raters indicating problems with inter-rater agreement. Specificity was 95%, indicating some non-ictal events were misdiagnosed as seizures [39]. A study of color density spectral array and envelope trend EEG found that seizure identification was impacted by both modifiable factors (interpreter experience, display size, and quantitative EEG method) and non-modifiable factors inherent to the EEG pattern (maximum spike amplitude, seizure duration, seizure frequency, and seizure duration) [40].

Critical care providers have expertise at screening multiple monitoring modalities and are generally continually available at bedside within the PICU. Thus, if critical care clinicians are able to use quantitative EEG techniques, then electrographic seizures might be identified more rapidly. A study provided 20 critical care physicians (attending and fellow physicians) and 19 critical care nurses with a brief training session regarding color density spectral array and then asked them to determine whether each of 200 color density spectral array images contained electrographic seizures.

The images were created from conventional EEG derived from critically ill children, and the true seizure incidence was 30% based on electroencephalographer review of the conventional EEG tracings. The sensitivity was 70%, indicating that some electrographic seizures were not identified. The specificity was 68%, indicating that some images categorized as containing EEG seizures did not contain seizures. These errors may be problematic since they could lead to exposure of non-seizing children to antiseizure medications with potential adverse effects. Given the 30% seizure incidence used in the study, the positive predictive value was 46% and the negative predictive value was 86% [41].

These data indicate that commercially available quantitative EEG techniques permit identification of many but not all seizures, and sometimes non-ictal events might be considered seizures based on isolated quantitative EEG review. Since seizures often occur early during EEG monitoring, recordings and EEG technologists may not be readily available when continuous EEG monitoring is needed [24]; rapid bedside implementation may be an important advantage of these quantitative EEG techniques. Seizure identification may improve with user training and experience, further development of quantitative EEG trends, and implementation of quantitative EEG panels with multiple trends. However, since quantitative EEG techniques lead to misclassification of some non-ictal events as seizures, potentially leading to unnecessary antiseizure medication administration, confirmation by conventional EEG review may be indicated when quantitative EEG techniques suggest seizures are present. With further development, these synergistic methods could make use of the efficiency and bedside availability of quantitative EEG methods and the accuracy of conventional EEG tracings.

Status Epilepticus Management Overview

SE describes a prolonged seizure or recurrent seizures without a return to baseline, and it is the most common pediatric neurological emergency with an incidence of 18–23 per 100,000 children per year [42]. The clinician's management aim is to rapidly institute care that simultaneously (1) stabilizes the patient medically, (2) identifies and manages any precipitant conditions, and (3) terminates clinically evident and electrographic-only seizures.

Historically, SE was defined as a seizure lasting longer than 30 min or a series of seizures without return to baseline level of alertness between seizures [43]. The *prodromal or incipient stage* occurred in the initial 5 min during which it is unknown whether the seizure will self-terminate or evolve into SE. The persisting SE period was divided into *early SE* (5–30 min), *established SE* (>30 min), and *refractory SE* (seizures persist despite treatment with adequate doses of two or three anticonvulsants). The temporal definition of SE has gradually shortened due to increasing recognition that most seizures are brief (3–4 min) [44] and delays in administration of antiseizure medication are associated with more refractory seizures. Additionally, the related terminology has been modified to convey a greater sense of urgency. The Neurocritical Care Society's Guideline for the Evaluation and Management of Status Epilepticus in Children and Adults defines SE as "5 minutes or more of (i) continuous clinical and/or electrographic seizure activity or (ii) recurrent seizure activity without recovery (returning to baseline) between seizures" and states that "definitive control of SE should be established within 60 minutes of onset" [31]. The antiseizure medication choices are referred to as "emergent," "urgent," and "refractory" to help convey that these medications should be administered sequentially and rapidly. Refractory SE is defined as clinical or electrographic seizures which persist after an adequate dose of an initial benzodiazepine and a second appropriate antiseizure medication. In contrast to prior definitions, there is no specific time that must elapse before initiation of refractory SE management if prior drugs have not terminated seizures.

Variability in SE management and treatment delays are common. Studies of SE management in children in emergency departments have described that laboratory parameters were often not checked, and some results were only available after long delays [6]. Additionally, benzodiazepine dosing was outside usual dosing guidelines in 23% of children with convulsive SE [6]. Excess benzodiazepine dosing, which often occurs when prehospital doses are administered, has been associated with respiratory insufficiency and need for intensive care unit admission [4–6], while inadequate dosing may reduce the likelihood of seizure termination.

Several studies have documented that antiseizure medication administration may be slower than optimal. In one study of children with convulsive SE, the median time to administer a second-line antiseizure medication was 24 min [45]. Additionally, a recent multicenter study of children who eventually experienced refractory SE found that the median time from seizure onset to medication administration was 28 min for the first medication, 40 min for the second medication, and 59 min for the third medication. Further, the first and second non-benzodiazepine antiseizure medications were administered at a median of 69 and 120 min [3]. These delays in antiseizure medication administration may be problematic since several studies have described associations between SE management delays and more prolonged seizures [46] and lower antiseizure medication responsiveness [47–50]. A study of children with convulsive SE found that for every minute delay between SE onset and emergency department arrival, there was a 5% increase in the risk of having SE that lasts more than 60 min [46]. A study of children with continued clinical seizures after the first- and second-line antiseizure medications reported that seizures were terminated in 100% of subjects when a third medication was administered within 1 h but were terminated in only 22% of subjects when the third medication was administered after 1 h [47]. Similarly, a study of children documented that the first-line and second-line medications terminated convulsive SE in 86% of children when administered in less than 15 min but only 15% of children when administered in more than 30 min [48]. A study of children with convulsive seizures lasting longer than 5 min found that treatment delays of more than 30 min were associated with seizure control delays [49]. Finally, midazolam efficacy has been found to be significantly lower when treatment was initiated more than 3 h after seizure onset, and there was a trend toward reduced efficacy even at 1 h [50]. Together, these data indicate that antiseizure medication administration delays are associated with reduced medication efficacy.

Based on this documented variability in care and management timing, a recent consensus document recommended that all units have a written SE management pathway [51]. However, a 2010–2011 survey of emergency departments in Illinois that received responses from 88% of 119 facilities reported that only 19% of facilities had an SE protocol and only 9% of facilities had a pediatric-specific SE protocol [52]. An example of SE management pathway is provided in Fig. 22.1 which is adapted from the Neurocritical Care Society's Status Epilepticus Evaluation and Management Guideline [31] and other recent publications [53–60]. An interdisciplinary workgroup at the Children's Hospital of Philadelphia composed of neurological critical care consultants, emergency medicine specialists, intensivists, and pharmacists developed a SE management pathway which is available online (http://www.chop.edu/clinical-pathway/status-epilepticus-clinical-pathway).

Status Epilepticus Management: Diagnostic Considerations

Medical stabilization is critical as part of the management of SE. The Neurocritical Care Society's Guideline for the Evaluation and Management of Status Epilepticus provides a timed treatment pathway [31]. Steps to be completed in the initial 2 min include (1) noninvasive airway protection with head positioning and (2) vital sign assessment. Steps to be included in the initial 5 min include (1) neurologic examination and (2) placement of peripheral intravenous access for administration of emergent antiseizure medications and fluid resuscitation. Steps to be completed in the initial 10 min include intubation if airway or gas exchange is compromised or intracranial pressure is elevated. Intubation may be necessary due to seizure-associated hypoventilation, medication-associated hypoventilation, inability to protect the airway, or other causes of oxygenation or ventilation failure. Steps to be completed in the initial 15 min include vasopressor support if needed [31].

Multiple studies have characterized the various potential etiologies for SE [42, 61–63]. Acute symptomatic conditions are identified in 15–20% of children with SE [42, 62, 64]. Rapidly reversible causes of seizures should be diagnosed and treated within minutes of hospital arrival, specifically evaluating for electrolyte disturbances such as hyponatremia, hypoglycemia, hypomagnesemia, and hypocalcemia. The American Academy of Neurology's practice parameter on the diagnostic assessment of the child with SE reported that abnormal results among children who underwent testing included low anticonvulsant levels (32%), neuroimaging abnormalities (8%), electrolytes (6%), inborn errors of metabolism (4%), ingestion (4%), central nervous system infections (3%), and positive blood cultures (3%) [65]. The Neurocritical Care Society's Guideline for the Evaluation and Management of SE provides suggestions regarding etiologic testing including bedside finger-stick blood glucose (0–2 min) and serum glucose, complete blood count, basic metabolic panel, calcium, magnesium, and antiseizure medication levels (5 min). In some patients, other diagnostic testing may include neuroimaging or lumbar puncture (0–60 min), additional laboratory testing (including liver function tests, coagulation studies, arterial blood gas, toxicology screen, and inborn errors of metabolism screening), and continuous EEG monitoring if the patient is not waking up after clinical seizures cease (15–60 min) [31]. These recommendations are similar to those of the prior American Academy of Neurology's practice parameter [65]. Rarer infectious, metabolic, autoimmune, and paraneoplastic etiologies may be considered in specific situations [66].

Among children with SE, neuroimaging abnormalities have been reported in 30% of children and are described to alter acute management in 24% of children [62]. If no etiology is identified by computerized tomography, magnetic resonance imaging may still identify lesions. For example, one study described that among 44 children who underwent head computerized tomography and magnetic resonance imaging, 14 had a normal head computerized tomography but an abnormal magnetic resonance imaging [62].

There are two main urgent EEG indications. First, if the diagnosis of psychogenic SE is suspected, then rapid diagnosis using EEG monitoring may avoid continued escalation of antiseizure medications with potential adverse effects. Second, if there is concern that EEG-only seizures (also referred to as subclinical seizures or nonconvulsive seizures) are ongoing despite cessation of clinically evident seizures, then EEG monitoring may be required for identification and to assess the impact of continued management [19, 24]. A multicenter study of children who underwent EEG monitoring while in the PICU reported that 33% of 98 children

Immediate Management

Non-invasive airway protection and gas exchange with head positioning. Intubation if needed.

Monitoring oxygen saturation, blood pressure, heart rate, temperature.

Finger stick blood glucose.

Establish peripheral IV access

Medical and Neurologic Examination.

Labs: basic metabolic panel, calcium, magnesium, complete blood count, liver function tests, coagulation tests, arterial blood gas, and anticonvulsant levels.

Emergent Initial Therapy

IV Access: Lorazepam 0.1mg/kg IV (max 4 mg) - may repeat if seizures persist in ~ 5 minutes.

No IV Access:

   Midazolam buccal or intranasal or intramuscular 0.3mg/kg (max 10mg) - may repeat if seizures persist in ~ 5 minutes.

   Diazepam rectal 0.5mg/kg (max 20mg) - may repeat if seizures persist in ~ 5 minutes.

Consider whether out-of-hospital benzodiazepines have been administered when considering how many doses to administer.

Urgent Management

Additional diagnostic testing as indicated:

   Lumbar puncture: opening pressure, cell count with differential, protein, glucose, gram stain and culture.

      Consider: oligoclonal band profile, IgG index, IgG synthesis rate, fungal culture, herpes simplex virus 1/2 PCR enterovirus PCR, parechovirus PCR.

   Imaging: computerized tomography, magnetic resonance imaging

   Consider: toxicology lab, inborn errors of metabolism, anti-thyroid peroxidase antibodies, anti-thyroglobulin antibodies, bacterial cultures.

Consider EEG monitoring if concern for psychogenic status epilepticus or persisting EEG-only seizures.

Neurology Consultation.

Urgent Control Therapy

Phenytoin   20mg/kg IV -may give another 10mg/kg if needed (max 1500mg)

OR Fosphenytoin 20 PE/kg IV -may give another 10 PE/kg if needed. (PE = phenytoin equivalents) (max 1500 PE)

OR Levetiracetam 50 mg/kg IV (max 2500mg)

OR Valproate Sodium 40 mg/kg IV (max 3000mg)

OR Phenobarbital 20mg/kg IV -may given another 20 mg/kg if needed.

If < 2 years, consider pyridoxine (100mg IV).

Refractory Status Epilepticus Management

If seizures continue after benzodiazepines and a second anti-seizure medication, then the patient is in refractory status epilepticus regardless of elapsed time. Continue management as plan for ICU admission/transfer and likely continuous EEG monitoring.

Administer another Urgent Control anticonvulsant or proceed to pharmacologic coma.

   Urgent Control Anticonvulsants (see above)

   Pharmacologic Coma Medications:

   Midazolam 0.2mg/kg bolus (max 10mg) and infusion at 0.1mg/kg/hr.

   Pentobarbital 5 mg/kg bolus and infusion at 0.5mg/kg/hour.

   For both medications, if dose escalation is needed, then re-bolus every 15-30 minutes and do not just increase the infusion rate.

Pharmacologic Coma Management

   Titrate medication to either seizure suppression or burst suppression based on continuous EEG monitoring.

   Continue pharmacologic coma for 24-48 hours.

   Continue diagnostic testing and implementation of etiology directed therapy.

   Modify anti-seizure medications so additional coverage is in place at the time of infusion wean.

Add-On Options

   Medications: phenytoin, phenobarbital, levetiracetam, valproate sodium, topiramate, lacosamide, ketamine, pyridoxine, pyridoxal-5-phosphate, folinic acid, biotin.

   Other: epilepsy surgery, ketogenic diet, vagus nerve stimulator, immunomodulatory therapy (methylprednisolone, IVIG, plasma exchange), hypothermia, electroconvulsive therapy.

Fig. 22.1 Example of management pathway for pediatric status epilepticus

who presented with convulsive SE had electrographic seizures identified. The seizure burden was often high with
electrographic SE in 47% of patients with seizures. Further,
34% of children with seizures had exclusively EEG-only seizures which would not have been identified without EEG
monitoring [67].

If no etiology is identified by the initial testing, then additional testing may be indicated. A targeted approach may be
useful for some patients, but in some patients sending a full
panel of tests initially may be optimal. Recent reviews have
summarized issues related to detailed etiologic testing [56,
66]. Central nervous system infections are a common cause of
acute symptomatic SE [62], accounting for 0.6–40% of all SE
[68, 69]. The clinical presentation of encephalitis and other
central nervous system infections is highly variable depending
on the pathogen involved and specific host factors. Additionally,
fever may be absent and clinical signs of infection may be
subtle or absent, particularly in young children, individuals
who are immunocompromised, or individuals who have
received recent antibiotics. Therefore, lumbar puncture should
be performed in all children with SE without an obvious non-
infectious etiology. A lumbar puncture should also be obtained
if an autoimmune etiology is suspected as neuro-inflammatory
processes will often yield cerebrospinal fluid pleocytosis, elevated cerebrospinal fluid protein, and intrathecal immunoglobulin synthesis (oligoclonal band profile, IgG index, and IgG
synthesis rate). Many causes of autoimmune encephalitis may
be associated with neoplasms, although the frequency of tumor
detection varies. Depending on the paraneoplastic autoantibody, distinct brain regions may be targeted, with seizures or
SE resulting from autoimmunity to either the limbic system or
cerebral cortex. Specific autoantibody testing for some of these
disorders is available, and, in general, testing of the cerebrospinal fluid has superior sensitivity and specificity as compared to
serum. Any patient with known or suspected paraneoplastic
disease should have appropriate tumor screening imaging performed. In addition to paraneoplastic processes, Rasmussen's
encephalitis (imaging showing progressive unihemispheric
cortical atrophy) and Hashimoto's encephalopathy (serum
antithyroid peroxidase antibodies or anti-thyroglobulin antibodies) may also cause autoimmune forms of SE. Some
genetic epilepsies may present with new-onset SE that do not
produce obvious metabolic or imaging changes. Thus, performing gene panel analysis or exome sequencing may be useful in some patients with unexplained SE.

Status Epilepticus Management: Emergent Benzodiazepine Management

The Neurocritical Care Society's Guideline for the Evaluation
and Management of SE states that "definitive control of SE
should be established within 60 minutes of onset" [31] with
termination of both clinical and electrographic seizures.
Benzodiazepines are the "emergent" medications of choice
with lorazepam for intravenous administration, diazepam for
rectal administration, and midazolam for intramuscular, buccal, or intranasal administration [31]. Repeat dosing may be
provided in 5–10 min if seizures persist. A double-blind randomized trial of 273 children with convulsive SE in the
emergency department compared intravenous lorazepam
(0.1 mg/kg) and diazepam (0.2 mg/kg). A half dose of either
medication could be administered if seizures persisted after
5 min. The primary outcome, SE cessation by 10 min without recurrence in 30 min, was not significantly different in
the two groups (72.1% with diazepam and 72.9% with lorazepam). Subjects receiving lorazepam were more likely to be
sedated (67% with lorazepam, 50% with diazepam), but
there was no difference in requirement for assisted ventilation (18% with lorazepam, 16% with diazepam) [70]. If
intravenous access cannot be obtained, then rectal, intramuscular, buccal, or intraosseous benzodiazepines can be administered. For buccal or nasal dosing of midazolam, the
intravenous version of the drug is generally used off-label in
the United States.

Status Epilepticus Management: Urgent Antiseizure Medication Management

About one-third to one-half of children will have persisting
SE after receiving benzodiazepines [45, 47, 70], yet there are
few comparative data evaluating the antiseizure medication
options available for this management stage. Options include
phenytoin, fosphenytoin, phenobarbital, valproate, and levetiracetam. Optimal decisions may depend on patient characteristics, seizure characteristics, and also practical
institutional factors such as which drugs are most rapidly
available since some need to be ordered and dispensed from
pharmacy as opposed to being immediately available in
medication carts.

Phenytoin is reported as the second-line agent by most
respondents in surveys of pediatric emergency medicine
physicians [71] and neurologists [72]. Phenytoin has demonstrated efficacy in pediatric SE management [73, 74].
Phenytoin is prepared with propylene glycol and alcohol at a
pH of 12 which may lead to cardiac arrhythmias, hypotension, and severe tissue injury if extravasation occurs (purple
glove syndrome). Fosphenytoin is a prodrug of phenytoin,
and it is dosed in phenytoin equivalents (PE). Cardiac
arrhythmias and hypotension are less common than with
phenytoin since it is not prepared with propylene glycol, but
they may still occur. Fosphenytoin is associated with less tissue injury (purple glove syndrome) if infiltration occurs.
Both phenytoin and fosphenytoin are considered focal anticonvulsants, and they may be ineffective in treating SE

related to epilepsy with a generalized mechanism of seizure onset. There are numerous drug interactions due to strong hepatic induction and high protein binding, so free phenytoin levels may need to be assessed [75]. There is little respiratory depression, particularly when compared to some of the other antiseizure medication options, such as phenobarbital, midazolam, or pentobarbital.

Phenobarbital is often considered a third-line or fourth-line drug in pediatric SE pathways. One study of 36 children with SE indicated that phenobarbital stopped seizures faster than a combination of diazepam and phenytoin and safety was similar, [76] and several reports have described the use of high-dose phenobarbital to control refractory SE and allow withdrawal of pharmacologic coma [77–79]. Phenobarbital may cause sedation, respiratory depression, and hypotension, so cardiovascular and respiratory monitoring is generally required. It is a hepatic enzyme inducer leading to drug interactions.

Valproate sodium is a broad-spectrum antiseizure medication reported to be safe and highly effective in terminating SE and refractory SE. Because it has mechanisms independent of GABA receptors, valproate may be effective later in refractory SE once GABA receptors have been targeted by other agents. Several studies and reports have reported that valproate sodium is effective in terminating SE [80] and refractory SE in children without adverse effects [80–84]. It may cause less sedation, respiratory depression, and hypotension than some other antiseizure medications, such as benzodiazepines, phenobarbital, or phenytoin. Black box warnings from the Federal Drug Administration include hepatotoxicity (highest risk in children younger than 2 years, receiving anticonvulsant poly-therapy, and with suspected or known metabolic/mitochondrial disorders), pancreatitis, and teratogenicity. Other adverse effects include pancytopenia, thrombocytopenia, platelet dysfunction, hypersensitivity reactions (including Stevens-Johnson syndrome and toxic epidermal necrolysis), and encephalopathy (with or without elevated ammonia). There are numerous drug interactions due to strong hepatic inhibition.

Levetiracetam is a broad-spectrum antiseizure medication. Several observational studies in children have reported that levetiracetam may be safe and effective for managing SE and acute symptomatic seizures [85–90]. Levetiracetam has no hepatic metabolism, which may be beneficial in complex patients with liver dysfunction, metabolic disorders, or in those at risk for major drug interactions. Additionally, in comparison to other intravenously available antiseizure medications, levetiracetam has a low risk of sedation, cardiorespiratory depression, or coagulopathy. Since levetiracetam clearance is dependent on renal function, maintenance dosage reduction is required in patients with renal impairment.

Refractory Status Epilepticus Management

Refractory SE is characterized by seizures that persist despite treatment with adequate doses of initial antiseizure medications. Definitions for refractory SE have varied in seizure durations (no time criteria, 30 min, 1 or 2 h) and/or lack of response to different numbers (two or three) of antiseizure medications. The Neurocritical Care Society's SE Evaluation and Management Guideline states that "patients who continue to experience either clinical or electrographic seizures after receiving adequate doses of an initial benzodiazepine followed by a second acceptable anticonvulsant will be considered refractory" [31]. In contrast to prior definitions of refractory SE, there is no specific time that must elapse to define refractory SE, thereby emphasizing the importance of rapid sequential treatment. Depending on refractory SE definitions and the cohorts described, refractory SE occurs in about 10–40% of children [48, 49, 73] with SE. Studies in children have indicated that SE lasted more than 1 h in 26–45% of patients [91, 92], longer than 2 h in 17–25% of patients [92, 93], and longer than 4 h in 10% of patients [92].

In a subgroup of patients, refractory SE may last for weeks to months, despite treatment with multiple antiseizure medications. This lengthy course has been referred to as malignant refractory SE [94] or super-refractory SE [95, 96]. Malignant refractory SE is associated with an infectious or inflammatory etiology, younger age, previous good health, and high morbidity and mortality [94, 97, 98]. It has also been referred to as de novo cryptogenic refractory multifocal SE [98], new-onset refractory SE (NORSE) [97, 99, 100], and febrile infection-related epilepsy syndrome (FIRES) [101–103]. Some of these entities in which refractory SE occurs in a previously healthy person with no identified cause except a recent infection may represent overlapping terms describing similar or identical entities [104].

The Neurocritical Care Society's SE Evaluation and Management Guideline states that "the main decision point at this step is to consider repeat bolus of the urgent control anticonvulsant or to immediately initiate additional agents" [31]. Additional urgent control antiseizure medications may be reasonable if they have not yet been tried or if the patient needs to be transferred or stabilized prior to administration of continuous infusions. However, if an initial urgent control medication fails to terminate seizures, then preparations should be initiated to achieve definitive seizure control with continuous infusions.

The management of refractory SE has been reviewed previously in children [56, 57, 105–107]. While there is variability in suggested pathways and reported management decisions [108], all pathways either administer additional antiseizure medications such as phenytoin/fosphenytoin, phenobarbital, valproate sodium, or levetiracetam or proceed to pharmacologic coma induction with intravenous or inhaled medications. The Neurocritical Care Society's SE Evaluation and Management Guideline recommends rapid advancement to pharmacologic coma induction rather than sequential trials of many urgent control antiseizure medications [31]. Few data are available regarding management of refractory SE with midazolam, pentobarbital, and other anesthetic therapies [59]. Midazolam dosing usually involves an initial loading dose of 0.2 mg/kg followed by an infusion at 0.05–2 mg/kg/h titrated as needed to achieve clinical or electrographic seizure suppression or EEG burst suppression. If seizures persist, escalating dosing through additional boluses is needed to rapidly increase levels and terminate seizures. Increasing the infusion rate without bolus dosing will lead to very slow increase in serum levels which is inconsistent with the goal of rapid seizure termination. Pentobarbital dosing usually involves an initial loading dose of 5–15 mg/kg (followed by another 5–10 mg/kg if needed) followed by an infusion at 0.5–5 mg/kg/h titrated as needed to achieve seizure suppression or EEG burst suppression. If seizures persist, escalating dosing through additional boluses is needed to rapidly increase levels and terminate seizures. Anesthetics such as isoflurane are effective in inducing a burst suppression pattern and terminating seizures. Propofol may also be used to terminate seizures, but is rarely used in children due to its Federal Drug Administration black box warning because of the risk of propofol infusion syndrome.

Patients treated with continuous infusions or inhaled anesthetics require intensive monitoring due to issues with:

1. Continuous mechanical ventilation both for airway protection and to maintain appropriate oxygenation and ventilation
2. Central venous access and arterial access due to frequent laboratory sampling and high likelihood of developing hypotension requiring vasopressor or inotropic support
3. Temperature management and regulation since high-dose sedatives and anesthetics can blunt the shivering response and endogenous thermoregulation
4. Assessment for development of lactic acidosis, anemia, thrombocytopenia, and end-organ dysfunction such as acute liver or renal injury
5. Risk of secondary infections due to indwelling catheters (central catheters, endotracheal tubes, Foley catheters), as well as some medications (pentobarbital)

The goals of pharmacologic coma induction are unclear. It remains unclear whether the EEG treatment goal should be termination of seizures, burst suppression, or complete suppression of EEG activity. The Neurocritical Care Society's SE Evaluation and Management Guideline states that "dosing of continuous infusions anticonvulsants for refractory SE should be titrated to cessation of electrographic seizures or burst suppression" [31]. Further, it remains unclear how long the patient should be maintained in pharmacologic coma. The guideline states that "a period of 24–48 h of electrographic control is recommended prior to slow withdrawal of continuous infusion anticonvulsants for refractory SE" [31], and a survey of experts in SE management across all age groups reported they would continue pharmacologic coma for 24 h [108].

Electrographic or electro-clinical seizures frequently recur during weaning of pharmacologic coma medications [109–112] indicating that pharmacologic coma should be considered as a temporizing measure, and during this period other antiseizure medications should be initiated which may provide seizure control as coma-inducing medications are weaned. Case reports and series have described several add-on medications, and other techniques have been reported useful in reducing seizure recurrence as pharmacologic coma is weaned, but there are no large studies. These options include topiramate, ketamine, pyridoxine, the ketogenic diet, epilepsy surgery, immunomodulation (steroids, intravenous immune globulin, plasmapheresis), hypothermia, and electroconvulsive therapy. These have been reviewed recently [56, 57].

Conclusions

Seizures and SE are common in critically ill children. Rapid management is needed to manage systemic complications, identify and manage precipitating conditions, and terminate seizures. While data are limited, a predetermined management plan that emphasizes rapid progression through appropriately dosed antiseizure medications may help streamline management. Children with or without prior convulsive seizures may experience electrographic seizures requiring EEG monitoring for identification.

References

1. Bell MJ, Carpenter J, Au AK, Keating RF, Myseros JS, Yaun A, et al. Development of a pediatric neurocritical care service. Neurocrit Care. 2008;10(1):4–10.
2. LaRovere KL, Graham RJ, Tasker RC. Pediatric neurocritical care: a neurology consultation model and implication for education and training. Pediatr Neurol. 2013;48(3):206–11.
3. Sanchez Fernandez I, Abend NS, Agadi S, An S, Arya R, Brenton JN, et al. Time from convulsive status epilepticus onset to anticonvulsant administration in children. Neurology. 2015;84(23):2304–11.
4. Chin RF, Verhulst L, Neville BG, Peters MJ, Scott RC. Inappropriate emergency management of status epilepticus in children contributes to need for intensive care. J Neurol Neurosurg Psychiatry. 2004;75(11):1584–8.
5. Tirupathi S, McMenamin JB, Webb DW. Analysis of factors influencing admission to intensive care following convulsive status epilepticus in children. Seizure. 2009;18(9):630–3.

6. Tobias JD, Berkenbosch JW. Management of status epilepticus in infants and children prior to pediatric ICU admission: deviations from the current guidelines. South Med J. 2008;101(3):268–72.

7. Abend NS, Wusthoff CJ, Goldberg EM, Dlugos DJ. Electrographic seizures and status epilepticus in critically ill children and neonates with encephalopathy. Lancet Neurol. 2013;12(12):1170–9.

8. Hosain SA, Solomon GE, Kobylarz EJ. Electroencephalographic patterns in unresponsive pediatric patients. Pediatr Neurol. 2005;32(3):162–5.

9. Jette N, Claassen J, Emerson RG, Hirsch LJ. Frequency and predictors of nonconvulsive seizures during continuous electroencephalographic monitoring in critically ill children. Arch Neurol. 2006;63(12):1750–5.

10. Abend NS, Dlugos DJ. Nonconvulsive status epilepticus in a pediatric intensive care unit. Pediatr Neurol. 2007;37(3):165–70.

11. Tay SK, Hirsch LJ, Leary L, Jette N, Wittman J, Akman CI. Nonconvulsive status epilepticus in children: clinical and EEG characteristics. Epilepsia. 2006;47(9):1504–9.

12. Shahwan A, Bailey C, Shekerdemian L, Harvey AS. The prevalence of seizures in comatose children in the pediatric intensive care unit: a prospective video-EEG study. Epilepsia. 2010;51(7): 1198–204.

13. Abend NS, Topjian A, Ichord R, Herman ST, Helfaer M, Donnelly M, et al. Electroencephalographic monitoring during hypothermia after pediatric cardiac arrest. Neurology. 2009;72(22):1931–40.

14. Williams K, Jarrar R, Buchhalter J. Continuous video-EEG monitoring in pediatric intensive care units. Epilepsia. 2011;52(6): 1130–6.

15. Greiner HM, Holland K, Leach JL, Horn PS, Hershey AD, Rose DF. Nonconvulsive status epilepticus: the encephalopathic pediatric patient. Pediatrics. 2012;129(3):e748–55.

16. Kirkham FJ, Wade AM, McElduff F, Boyd SG, Tasker RC, Edwards M, et al. Seizures in 204 comatose children: incidence and outcome. Intensive Care Med. 2012;38(5):853–62.

17. Arango JI, Deibert CP, Brown D, Bell M, Dvorchik I, Adelson PD. Posttraumatic seizures in children with severe traumatic brain injury. Childs Nerv Syst. 2012;28(11):1925–9.

18. Piantino JA, Wainwright MS, Grimason M, Smith CM, Hussain E, Byron D, et al. Nonconvulsive seizures are common in children treated with extracorporeal cardiac life support. Pediatr Crit Care Med. 2013;14(6):601–9.

19. Abend NS, Arndt DH, Carpenter JL, Chapman KE, Cornett KM, Gallentine WB, et al. Electrographic seizures in pediatric ICU patients: cohort study of risk factors and mortality. Neurology. 2013;81(4):383–91.

20. McCoy B, Sharma R, Ochi A, Go C, Otsubo H, Hutchison JS, et al. Predictors of nonconvulsive seizures among critically ill children. Epilepsia. 2011;52(11):1973–8.

21. Schreiber JM, Zelleke T, Gaillard WD, Kaulas H, Dean N, Carpenter JL. Continuous video EEG for patients with acute encephalopathy in a pediatric intensive care unit. Neurocrit Care. 2012;17(1):31–8.

22. Arndt DH, Lerner JT, Matsumoto JH, Madikians A, Yudovin S, Valino H, et al. Subclinical early posttraumatic seizures detected by continuous EEG monitoring in a consecutive pediatric cohort. Epilepsia. 2013;54(10):1780–8.

23. Payne ET, Zhao XY, Frndova H, McBain K, Sharma R, Hutchison JS, et al. Seizure burden is independently associated with short term outcome in critically ill children. Brain. 2014;137(Pt 5): 1429–38.

24. Abend NS, Gutierrez-Colina AM, Topjian AA, Zhao H, Guo R, Donnelly M, et al. Nonconvulsive seizures are common in critically ill children. Neurology. 2011;76(12):1071–7.

25. Gold JJ, Crawford JR, Glaser C, Sheriff H, Wang S, Nespeca M. The role of continuous electroencephalography in childhood encephalitis. Pediatr Neurol. 2014;50(4):318–23.

26. Greiner MV, Greiner HM, Care MM, Owens D, Shapiro R, Holland K. Adding insult to injury: nonconvulsive seizures in abusive head trauma. J Child Neurol. 2015;30(13):1778–84.

27. Gutierrez-Colina AM, Topjian AA, Dlugos DJ, Abend NS. EEG monitoring in critically ill children: indications and strategies. Pediatric Neurology. 2012;46:158–61.

28. Abend NS, Topjian AA, Williams S. How much does it cost to identify a critically ill child experiencing electrographic seizures? J Clin Neurophysiol. 2015;32:257–64.

29. Yang A, Arndt DH, Berg RA, Carpenter JL, Chapman KE, Dlugos DJ, et al. Development and validation of a seizure prediction model in critically ill children. Seizure. 2015;25:104–11.

30. Abend NS, Topjian AA, Williams S. How much does it cost to identify a critically ill child experiencing electrographic seizures? J Clin Neurophysiol. 2015;32(3):257–64.

31. Brophy GM, Bell R, Claassen J, Alldredge B, Bleck TP, Glauser T, et al. Guidelines for the evaluation and management of status epilepticus. Neurocrit Care. 2012;17(1):3–23.

32. Herman ST, Abend NS, Bleck TP, Chapman KE, Drislane FW, Emerson RG, et al. Consensus statement on continuous EEG in critically ill adults and children. Part I: Indications. J Clin Neurophysiol. 2015;32(2):87–95.

33. Abend NS. Electrographic status epilepticus in children with critical illness: epidemiology and outcome. Epilepsy Behav. 2015;49:223–7.

34. Topjian AA, Gutierrez-Colina AM, Sanchez SM, Berg RA, Friess SH, Dlugos DJ, et al. Electrographic status epilepticus is associated with mortality and worse short-term outcome in critically ill children. Crit Care Med. 2013;31:215–23.

35. Wagenman KL, Blake TP, Sanchez SM, Schultheis MT, Radcliffe J, Berg RA, et al. Electrographic status epilepticus and long-term outcome in critically ill children. Neurology. 2014;82(5):396–404.

36. Sanchez SM, Carpenter J, Chapman KE, Dlugos DJ, Gallentine W, Giza CC, et al. Pediatric ICU EEG monitoring: current resources and practice in the united states and canada. J Clin Neurophysiol. 2013;30(2):156–60.

37. Abend NS, Dlugos DJ, Hahn CD, Hirsch LJ, Herman ST. Use of EEG monitoring and management of non-convulsive seizures in critically ill patients: a survey of neurologists. Neurocrit Care. 2010;12(3):382–9.

38. Stewart CP, Otsubo H, Ochi A, Sharma R, Hutchison JS, Hahn CD. Seizure identification in the ICU using quantitative EEG displays. Neurology. 2010;75(17):1501–8.

39. Pensirikul AD, Beslow LA, Kessler SK, Sanchez SM, Topjian AA, Dlugos DJ, et al. Density Spectral Array for Seizure Identification in Critically Ill Children. J Clin Neurophysiol. 2013;30(4):371–5.

40. Akman CI, Micic V, Thompson A, Riviello Jr JJ. Seizure detection using digital trend analysis: factors affecting utility. Epilepsy Res. 2011;93(1):66–72.

41. Topjian AA, Fry M, Jawad AF, Herman ST, Nadkarni VM, Ichord R, et al. Detection of electrographic seizures by critical care providers using color density spectral array after cardiac arrest is feasible. Pediatr Crit Care Med. 2015;16(5):461–7.

42. Chin RF, Neville BG, Peckham C, Bedford H, Wade A, Scott RC. Incidence, cause, and short-term outcome of convulsive status epilepticus in childhood: prospective population-based study. Lancet. 2006;368(9531):222–9.

43. Commission on Epidemiology and Prognosis, International League Against Epilepsy. Guidelines for epidemiologic studies on epilepsy. Epilepsia. 1993;34(4):592–6.

44. Shinnar S, Berg AT, Moshe SL, Shinnar R. How long do new-onset seizures in children last? Ann Neurol. 2001;49(5):659–64.

45. Lewena S, Pennington V, Acworth J, Thornton S, Ngo P, McIntyre S, et al. Emergency management of pediatric convulsive status epilepticus: a multicenter study of 542 patients. Pediatr Emerg Care. 2009;25(2):83–7.

46. Chin RF, Neville BG, Peckham C, Wade A, Bedford H, Scott RC. Treatment of community-onset, childhood convulsive status epilepticus: a prospective, population-based study. Lancet Neurol. 2008;7(8):696–703.

47. Lambrechtsen FA, Buchhalter JR. Aborted and refractory status epilepticus in children: a comparative analysis. Epilepsia. 2008;49(4):615–25.

48. Lewena S, Young S. When benzodiazepines fail: how effective is second line therapy for status epilepticus in children? Emerg Med Australas. 2006;18(1):45–50.

49. Eriksson K, Metsaranta P, Huhtala H, Auvinen A, Kuusela AL, Koivikko M. Treatment delay and the risk of prolonged status epilepticus. Neurology. 2005;65(8):1316–8.

50. Hayashi K, Osawa M, Aihara M, Izumi T, Ohtsuka Y, Haginoya K, et al. Efficacy of intravenous midazolam for status epilepticus in childhood. Pediatr Neurol. 2007;36(6):366–72.

51. Shorvon S, Baulac M, Cross H, Trinka E, Walker M. The drug treatment of status epilepticus in Europe: consensus document from a workshop at the first London colloquium on status epilepticus. Epilepsia. 2008;49(7):1277–86.

52. Taylor C, Piantino J, Hageman J, Lyons E, Janies K, Leonard D, et al. Emergency department management of pediatric unprovoked seizures and status epilepticus in the state of illinois. J Child Neurol. 2015;30(11):1414–27.

53. Abend NS, Loddenkemper T. Pediatric status epilepticus management. Curr Opin Pediatr. 2014;26(6):668–74.

54. Abend NS, Loddenkemper T. Management of pediatric status epilepticus. Curr Treat Options Neurol. 2014;16(7):301.

55. Abend NS, Gutierrez-Colina AM, Dlugos DJ. Medical treatment of pediatric status epilepticus. Semin Pediatr Neurol. 2010;17(3):169–75.

56. Abend NS, Bearden D, Helbig I, McGuire J, Narula S, Panzer JA, et al. Status epilepticus and refractory status epilepticus management. Semin Pediatr Neurol. 2014;21(4):263–74.

57. Wilkes R, Tasker RC. Pediatric intensive care treatment of uncontrolled status epilepticus. Crit Care Clin. 2013;29(2):239–57.

58. Tasker R. Continuous infusions of anticonvulsants and anesthetics used in status epilepticus. Curr Opin Pediatr. 2014;26(6):682–9.

59. Wilkes R, Tasker RC. Intensive care treatment of uncontrolled status epilepticus in children: systematic literature search of midazolam and anesthetic therapies*. Pediatr Crit Care Med. 2014;15(7):632–9.

60. Shearer P, Riviello J. Generalized convulsive status epilepticus in adults and children: treatment guidelines and protocols. Emerg Med Clin North Am. 2011;29(1):51–64.

61. Hussain N, Appleton R, Thorburn K. Aetiology, course and outcome of children admitted to paediatric intensive care with convulsive status epilepticus: a retrospective 5-year review. Seizure. 2007;16(4):305–12.

62. Singh RK, Stephens S, Berl MM, Chang T, Brown K, Vezina LG, et al. Prospective study of new-onset seizures presenting as status epilepticus in childhood. Neurology. 2010;74(8):636–42.

63. Nishiyama I, Ohtsuka Y, Tsuda T, Inoue H, Kunitomi T, Shiraga H, et al. An epidemiological study of children with status epilepticus in Okayama, Japan. Epilepsia. 2007;48(6):1133–7.

64. Berg AT, Shinnar S, Levy SR, Testa FM. Status epilepticus in children with newly diagnosed epilepsy. Ann Neurol. 1999;45(5):618–23.

65. Riviello JJ, Ashwal S, Hirtz D, Glauser T, Ballaban-Gil K, Kelley K, et al. Practice parameter: diagnostic assessment of the child with status epilepticus (an evidence-based review). Neurology. 2006;67:1542–50.

66. Watemberg N, Segal G. A suggested approach to the etiologic evaluation of status epilepticus in children: what to seek after the usual causes have been ruled out. J Child Neurol. 2010;25(2):203–11.

67. Sanchez Fernandez I, Abend NS, Arndt DH, Carpenter JL, Chapman KE, Cornett KM, et al. Electrographic seizures after convulsive status epilepticus in children and young adults. A retrospective multicenter study. J Pediatr. 2014;164(2):339–46.

68. Neligan A, Shorvon SD. Frequency and prognosis of convulsive status epilepticus of different causes: a systematic review. Arch Neurol. 2010;67(8):931–40.

69. Saz EU, Karapinar B, Ozcetin M, Polat M, Tosun A, Serdaroglu G, et al. Convulsive status epilepticus in children: etiology, treatment protocol and outcome. Seizure. 2011;20(2):115–8.

70. Chamberlain JM, Okada P, Holsti M, Mahajan P, Brown KM, Vance C, et al. Lorazepam vs diazepam for pediatric status epilepticus: a randomized clinical trial. JAMA. 2014;311(16):1652–60.

71. Babl FE, Sheriff N, Borland M, Acworth J, Neutze J, Krieser D, et al. Emergency management of paediatric status epilepticus in Australia and New Zealand: practice patterns in the context of clinical practice guidelines. J Paediatr Child Health. 2009;45(9):541–6.

72. Claassen J, Hirsch LJ, Mayer SA. Treatment of status epilepticus: a survey of neurologists. J Neurol Sci. 2003;211(1–2):37–41.

73. Brevoord JC, Joosten KF, Arts WF, van Rooij RW, de Hoog M. Status epilepticus: clinical analysis of a treatment protocol based on midazolam and phenytoin. J Child Neurol. 2005;20(6):476–81.

74. Sreenath TG, Gupta P, Sharma KK, Krishnamurthy S. Lorazepam versus diazepam-phenytoin combination in the treatment of convulsive status epilepticus in children: a randomized controlled trial. Eur J Paediatr Neurol. 2010;14(2):162–8.

75. Wolf GK, McClain CD, Zurakowski D, Dodson B, McManus ML. Total phenytoin concentrations do not accurately predict free phenytoin concentrations in critically ill children. Pediatr Crit Care Med. 2006;7(5):434–9. quiz 40

76. Shaner DM, McCurdy SA, Herring MO, Gabor AJ. Treatment of status epilepticus: a prospective comparison of diazepam and phenytoin versus phenobarbital and optional phenytoin. Neurology. 1988;38:202–7.

77. Crawford TO, Mitchell WG, Fishman LS, Snodgrass SR. Very-high-dose phenobarbital for refractory status epilepticus in children. Neurology. 1988;38(7):1035–40.

78. Wilmshurst JM, van der Walt JS, Ackermann S, Karlsson MO, Blockman M. Rescue therapy with high-dose oral phenobarbitone loading for refractory status epilepticus. J Paediatr Child Health. 2010;46(1–2):17–22.

79. Lin JJ, Lin KL, Wang HS, Hsia SH, Wu CT. Effect of topiramate, in combination with lidocaine, and phenobarbital, in acute encephalitis with refractory repetitive partial seizures. Brain Dev. 2009;31(8):605–11.

80. Yu KT, Mills S, Thompson N, Cunanan C. Safety and efficacy of intravenous valproate in pediatric status epilepticus and acute repetitive seizures. Epilepsia. 2003;44(5):724–6.

81. Uberall MA, Trollmann R, Wunsiedler U, Wenzel D. Intravenous valproate in pediatric epilepsy patients with refractory status epilepticus. Neurology. 2000;54(11):2188–9.

82. Mehta V, Singhi P, Singhi S. Intravenous sodium valproate versus diazepam infusion for the control of refractory status epilepticus in children: a randomized controlled trial. J Child Neurol. 2007;22(10):1191–7.

83. Campistol J, Fernandez A, Ortega J. Status epilepticus in children. Experience with intravenous valproate. Update of treatment guidelines. Rev Neurol. 1999;29(4):359–65.

84. Hovinga CA, Chicella MF, Rose DF, Eades SK, Dalton JT, Phelps SJ. Use of intravenous valproate in three pediatric patients with nonconvulsive or convulsive status epilepticus. Ann Pharmacother. 1999;33(5):579–84.

85. Abend NS, Chapman KE, Gallentine WB, Goldstein J, Hyslop AE, Loddenkemper T, et al. Electroencephalographic monitoring in the pediatric intensive care unit. Curr Neurol Neurosci Rep. 2013;13(3):330.

86. Reiter PD, Huff AD, Knupp KG, Valuck RJ. Intravenous leveti-racetam in the management of acute seizures in children. Pediatric Neurology. 2010;43(2):117–21.

87. Abend NS, Monk HM, Licht DJ, Dlugos DJ. Intravenous leveti-racetam in critically ill children with status epilepticus or acute repetitive seizures. Pediatr Crit Care Med. 2009;10(4):505–10.

88. Goraya JS, Khurana DS, Valencia I, Melvin JJ, Cruz M, Legido A, et al. Intravenous levetiracetam in children with epilepsy. Pediatr Neurol. 2008;38(3):177–80.

89. Gallentine WB, Hunnicutt AS, Husain AM. Levetiracetam in children with refractory status epilepticus. Epilepsy Behav. 2009; 14(1):215–8.

90. McTague A, Kneen R, Kumar R, Spinty S, Appleton R. Intravenous levetiracetam in acute repetitive seizures and status epilepticus in children: experience from a children's hospital. Seizure. 2012; 21(7):529–34.

91. Maytal J, Shinnar S, Moshe SL, Alvarez LA. Low morbidity and mortality of status epilepticus in children. Pediatrics. 1989;83(3):323–31.

92. Dunn DW. Status epilepticus in children: etiology, clinical features, and outcome. J Child Neurol. 1988;3(3):167–73.

93. Eriksson KJ, Koivikko MJ. Status epilepticus in children: aetiology, treatment, and outcome. Dev Med Child Neurol. 1997;39(10): 652–8.

94. Holtkamp M, Othman J, Buchheim K, Masuhr F, Schielke E, Meierkord H. A "malignant" variant of status epilepticus. Arch Neurol. 2005;62(9):1428–31.

95. Shorvon S, Ferlisi M. The treatment of super-refractory status epilepticus: a critical review of available therapies and a clinical treatment protocol. Brain. 2011;134(Pt 10):2802–18.

96. Shorvon S. Super-refractory status epilepticus: an approach to therapy in this difficult clinical situation. Epilepsia. 2011;52(Suppl 8):53–6.

97. Wilder-Smith EP, Lim EC, Teoh HL, Sharma VK, Tan JJ, Chan BP, et al. The NORSE (new-onset refractory status epilepticus) syndrome: defining a disease entity. Ann Acad Med Singapore. 2005;34(7):417–20.

98. Van Lierde I, Van Paesschen W, Dupont P, Maes A, Sciot R. De novo cryptogenic refractory multifocal febrile status epilepticus in the young adult: a review of six cases. Acta Neurol Belg. 2003;103(2):88–94.

99. Rathakrishnan R, Wilder-Smith EP. New onset refractory status epilepticus (NORSE). J Neurol Sci. 2009;284(1–2):220. author reply -1

100. Costello DJ, Kilbride RD, Cole AJ. Cryptogenic new onset refractory status epilepticus (NORSE) in adults-Infectious or not? J Neurol Sci. 2009;277(1–2):26–31.

101. Kramer U, Chi CS, Lin KL, Specchio N, Sahin M, Olson H, et al. Febrile infection-related epilepsy syndrome (FIRES): pathogenesis, treatment, and outcome: a multicenter study on 77 children. Epilepsia. 2011;52(11):1956–65.

102. Kramer U, Shorer Z, Ben-Zeev B, Lerman-Sagie T, Goldberg-Stern H, Lahat E. Severe refractory status epilepticus owing to presumed encephalitis. J Child Neurol. 2005;20(3):184–7.

103. van Baalen A, Hausler M, Boor R, Rohr A, Sperner J, Kurlemann G, et al. Febrile infection-related epilepsy syndrome (FIRES): a nonencephalitic encephalopathy in childhood. Epilepsia. 2010;51(7):1323–8.

104. Ismail FY, Kossoff EH. AERRPS, DESC, NORSE, FIRES: multi-labeling or distinct epileptic entities? Epilepsia. 2011;52(11):e185–9.

105. Abend NS, Dlugos DJ. Treatment of refractory status epilepticus: literature review and a proposed protocol. Pediatr Neurol. 2008;38(6):377–90.

106. Owens J. Medical management of refractory status epilepticus. Semin Pediatr Neurol. 2010;17(3):176–81.

107. Wheless JW. Treatment of refractory convulsive status epilepticus in children: other therapies. Semin Pediatr Neurol. 2010;17(3):190–4.

108. Riviello Jr JJ, Claassen J, LaRoche SM, Sperling MR, Alldredge B, Bleck TP, et al. Treatment of status epilepticus: an international survey of experts. Neurocrit Care. 2013;18(2):193–200.

109. Kim SJ, Lee DY, Kim JS. Neurologic outcomes of pediatric epileptic patients with pentobarbital coma. Pediatr Neurol. 2001;25(3):217–20.

110. Morrison G, Gibbons E, Whitehouse WP. High-dose midazolam therapy for refractory status epilepticus in children. Intensive Care Med. 2006;32(12):2070–6.

111. Singhi S, Murthy A, Singhi P, Jayashree M. Continuous midazolam versus diazepam infusion for refractory convulsive status epilepticus. J Child Neurol. 2002;17(2):106–10.

112. Koul R, Chacko A, Javed H, Al Riyami K. Eight-year study of childhood status epilepticus: midazolam infusion in management and outcome. J Child Neurol. 2002;17(12):908–10.

Index

Printed in the United States
By Bookmasters